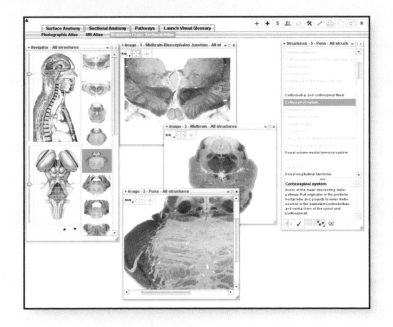
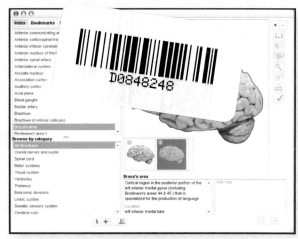

sylvius **4** *online* Components and Features

- **Surface Anatomy Atlases:** Photographic, Magnetic Resonance Image, Brainstem Model
- **Sectional Anatomy Atlases:** Photographic, Magnetic Resonance Image, Brainstem and Spinal Cord
- **Pathways:** Allow you to follow the flow of information in several important long-tract pathways of the central nervous system
- **Visual Glossary:** Searchable glossary that provides visual representations, concise anatomical and functional definitions, and audio pronunciation of neuroanatomical structures
- **Over 500 neuroanatomical structures and terms** are identified and described
- **Categories of anatomical structures and terms** (e.g., cranial nerves, spinal cord tracts, lobes, cortical areas, etc.) that can be browsed easily
- **A self-quiz mode** that allows assessment of structure identification and functional information

sylvius **4** *online* Access Instructions

The registration code included here activates a 12-month (365 day) subscription to the Sylvius 4 Online website. To set up your account, start your subscription, and access the site, follow the instructions below. (Please also review the system requirements listed below.)

1. Scratch below to reveal your unique registration code.
2. Go to http://sylvius.sinauer.com
3. Follow the instructions to create an account and access the site. (Requires a valid email address.)

> **Scratch here to reveal your access code.**
> **This access code may only be used by the original purchaser.**

Important Note: Each code can be used by only one person. If this code has been revealed, it may have already been used, and may no longer be valid. If this code is no longer valid, you can purchase a new code online at http://sylvius.sinauer.com

sylvius **4** *online* System Requirements

- Internet connection
- Up-to-date, standards-compliant Web browser with full HTML5 support

PRINCIPLES OF
Cognitive Neuroscience
SECOND EDITION

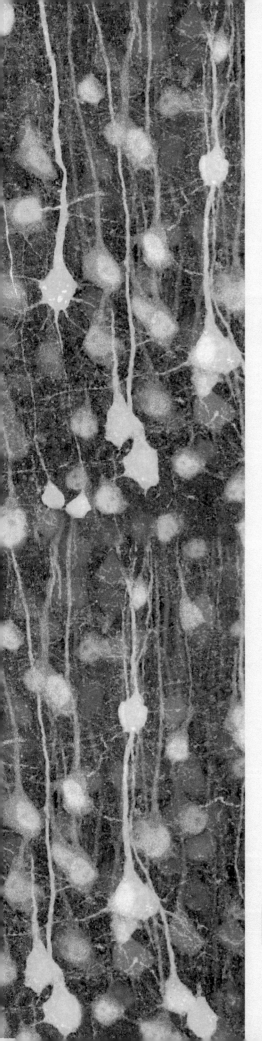

PRINCIPLES OF
Cognitive
Neuroscience

SECOND EDITION

Dale Purves

Roberto Cabeza

Scott A. Huettel

Kevin S. LaBar

Michael L. Platt

Marty G. Woldorff

Contributor
Elizabeth M. Brannon

Center for Cognitive Neuroscience
Duke University

Sinauer Associates, Inc. Publishers
Sunderland, MA U.S.A.

Address editorial correspondence to:
Sinauer Associates
23 Plumtree Road
Sunderland, MA 01375 U.S.A.
publish@sinauer.com

Address orders, sales, license, permissions, and translation inquiries to:
Oxford University Press U.S.A.
2001 Evans Road
Cary, NC 27513 U.S.A.
Orders: 1-800-445-9714

Library of Congress Cataloging-in-Publication Data
Principles of cognitive neuroscience / Dale Purves ... [et al.].—2nd ed.
    p. ; cm.
  Includes bibliographical references and index.
  ISBN 978-0-87893-573-4
  I. Purves, Dale.
  [DNLM: 1. Mental Processes—physiology. 2. Brain—physiology. 3. Neuropsychology. WL 337]

  612.8'233—dc23
                              2012023689

9 8 7 6 5 4 3

Printed in the United States of America

Contents in Brief

Contents

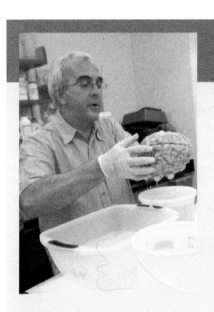
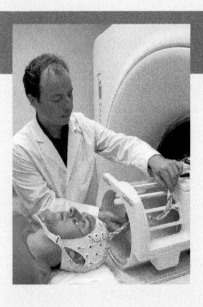

3 Sensory Systems and Perception: Vision 55

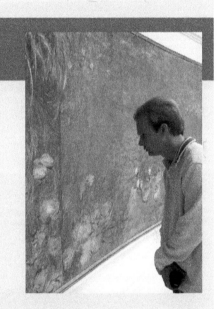

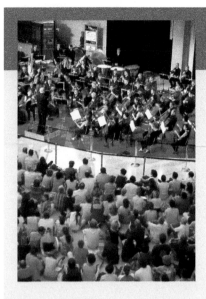

4 Sensory Systems and Perception: Auditory, Mechanical, and Chemical Senses   93

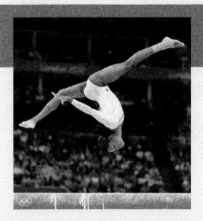

5 Motor Systems: The Organization of Action   131

6 Attention and Its Effects on Stimulus Processing   167

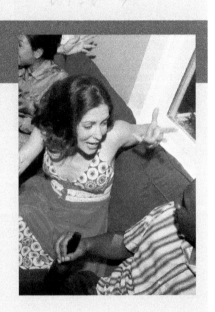

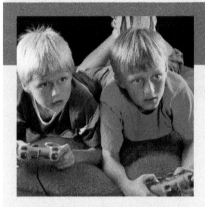

7 The Control of Attention 205

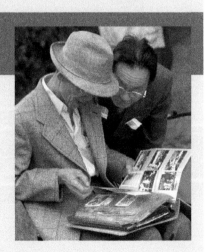

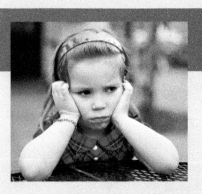

10 *Emotion 319*

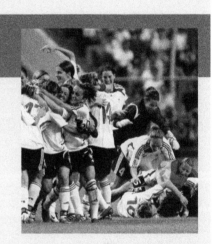

11 Social Cognition   359

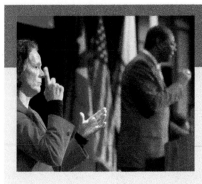

12 Language 393

13 *Executive Functions* 429

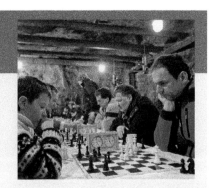

14 *Decision Making* 465

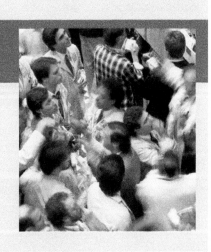

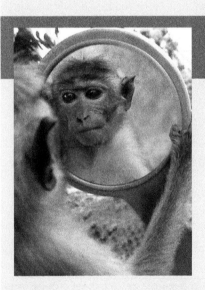

15 Evolution and Development of Brain and Cognition   503

APPENDIX
The Human Nervous System   539

Preface

The new and rapidly evolving field of cognitive neuroscience brings together cognitive psychology and neuroscience, drawing conceptual and technical elements from both these traditional disciplines. This union is motivated by the exciting possibility of better understanding complex human brain functions that have puzzled thinkers for centuries. The emergence of cognitive neuroscience as a discipline in its own right over the last two decades is thus an expression of what many see as the next logical step for both cognitive psychology and neuroscience, driven by powerful new methods for studying the human brain.

The First Edition of *Principles of Cognitive Neuroscience* was published in 2008 with the aim of informing readers at all levels about the growing canon of cognitive neuroscience, and to make clear the many challenges that remain. In this Second Edition, we offer what is in many ways a completely new book. The extensive revision was based on lengthy discussions among the authors about how to make the presentation more useful to students and instructors, and about the many issues that needed updating. This process benefitted greatly from the feedback of students and colleagues who used the book. This list would be too long to include here, but we are deeply indebted to this thoughtful and conscientious group, as well as to the many expert advisors who vetted earlier drafts and are named in the Acknowledgments.

Our intent is not simply to summarize the received wisdom in this rapidly evolving field, but rather to set the stage for future advances in cognitive neuroscience, many of which will be made by students currently entering the field. As important as it may be to elucidate the present status of cognitive neuroscience, it is at least as important to provide a strong sense of the direction the field will take in the future to achieve the still distant goal of understanding the brain and its higher-order operations.

Acknowledgments

We are greatly indebted to the numerous colleagues whose work we have represented—with accuracy we hope—despite the simplifications that a book like this demands. Many of these researchers as well as others among our colleagues provided valuable suggestions and criticisms about the presentation of specific issues and controversies.

We particularly wish to thank John Allman, Patricia Bauer, Catalin Buhusi, Robert O. Deaner, Mark D'Esposito, Michelle Diaz, Sarah Donohue, Tobias Egner, Tineke Grent-'t-Jong, Guven Guzeldere, Joseph Harris, Ben Hayden, Hiroshi Imamizu, Andrew Krystal, Beau Lotto, Warren Meck, Ravi Menon, Karen Meyerhoff, Rich Mooney, Steve Mitroff, Jamie Morris, Kevin Pelphrey, Ken Roberts, Stephen Shepherd, David V. Smith, Jared Stokes, Jim Voyvodic, Karli K. Watson, Bill Wojtach, and Vince Wu among many others who helped vet earlier drafts.

Special thanks are due to Mark Williams and Len White for allowing us to include SYLVIUS 4 ONLINE as an adjunct to the book. We also thank the authors and editors of *Neuroscience*, Fifth Edition—George Augustine, David Fitzpatrick, Anthony LaMantia, Bill Hall, and Len White—for much valuable information and art developed over the five editions of that complementary book.

We also benefited from the several classes of Duke University graduate and undergraduate students who provided feedback on what worked well and what did not in the First Edition. Despite this plethora of help, it is of course understood that any errors are attributable to the authors and are not the responsibility of our critics and advisors.

Finally, we are enormously grateful to Stephanie Hiebert for her expert copyediting; to Danna Niedzwiecki for her skill and patience in preparing the book for production; to Christopher Small and Janice Holabird for their fine production work; to David McIntyre for his imaginative efforts in obtaining photographs and other images; to Craig Durant and Dragonfly Studios for their expeditious preparation of the illustrations; and to Sydney Carroll for managing the entire project with tact, determination, and high standards.

Media and Supplements to accompany
Principles of Cognitive Neuroscience, Second Edition

eBook

Principles of Cognitive Neuroscience, Second Edition is available in several ebook formats. Please visit the Sinauer Associates website for more information: www.sinauer.com.

For the Student

COMPANION WEBSITE

(sites.sinauer.com/cogneuro2e)

The *Principles of Cognitive Neuroscience,* Second Edition Companion Website features review and study resources to help students master the material presented in the textbook. Access is free of charge and requires no access code. The site includes:

- *Chapter Summaries:* Concise overviews of the important topics covered in each chapter.
- *Flashcards & Key Terms:* Flashcard activities help students master the extensive vocabulary of cognitive neuroscience. Each set also includes a list of key terms with definitions, for easy review.
- *Animations:* A collection of detailed animations that depict some of the key processes and structures discussed in the textbook.
- *Online Quizzes:* For each chapter of the textbook, the website includes a multiple-choice quiz that covers all the main topics presented in the chapter. Instructors may assign these quizzes, or make them available to students for self-quizzing. (Instructor registration is required for student access to the quizzes.)

SYLVIUS 4 ONLINE: AN INTERACTIVE ATLAS AND VISUAL GLOSSARY OF HUMAN NEUROANATOMY

S. Mark Williams and Leonard E. White
(Free online access code provided with every new copy of the textbook.)

SYLVIUS 4 ONLINE provides a unique digital learning environment for exploring and understanding the structure of the human central nervous system. SYLVIUS features fully annotated surface views of the human brain, as well as interactive tools for dissecting the central nervous system and viewing fully annotated cross-sections of preserved specimens and living subjects imaged by magnetic resonance. SYLVIUS is more than a conventional atlas; it incorporates a comprehensive, visually-rich, searchable database of more than 500 neuroanatomical terms that are concisely defined and visualized in photographs, magnetic resonance images, and illustrations. (See the inside front cover for additional information and access instructions.)

For the Instructor

INSTRUCTOR'S RESOURCE LIBRARY

The *Principles of Cognitive Neuroscience,* Second Edition Instructor's Resource Library includes a variety of resources to help instructors in developing their course and delivering lectures. The Library includes:

- *Textbook Figures and Tables*: All the figures and tables from the textbook are provided in JPEG format (both high- and low-resolution).
- *PowerPoint Presentations*: All the figures and tables from each chapter are provided in PowerPoint, making it easy for instructors to add figures to their presentations.
- *Sylvius Image Library*: A range of images from *Sylvius*, representing a concise overview of human neuroanatomy, are provided in JPEG and PowerPoint formats.

- *Quiz Questions*: All of the questions from the Companion Website's online quizzes are provided in Microsoft Word format.
- *Animations*: All of the animations from the companion website are provided as Flash and QuickTime files. The animations are also provided in PowerPoint for easy integration into lecture presentations.

1

Cognitive Neuroscience: Definitions, Themes, and Approaches

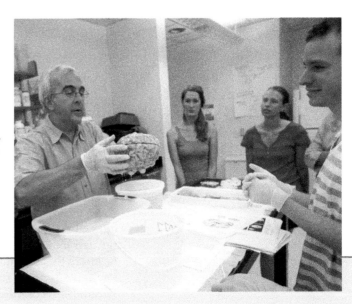

INTRODUCTION

Cognitive neuroscience is a relatively new discipline that has arisen from the recent marriage of neuroscience, a biomedical field that has flourished both conceptually and technically during the past century, and cognitive science, a field of study rooted in the long-standing interest of natural philosophers and psychologists in understanding human mental processes. Consistent with these progenitors, research in cognitive neuroscience integrates investigations of brain structure and function, and seeks to measure cognitive abilities and behavior to understand how the human brain works at all levels.

Despite its relative youth, cognitive neuroscience has rapidly become one of the most active areas of scientific inquiry. Much of that excitement comes from the questions that cognitive neuroscientists investigate, which range from basic perceptual and motor processing to complex thoughts and emotions. Why do we remember some events but not others? How do we understand the minds of others in social interactions? How do our brains represent different goals when faced with a complex decision?

To address these kinds of questions, cognitive neuroscientists study both human and non-human animals with a diverse set of tools. Some researchers monitor single neurons as they respond to stimuli, while others track overall changes in processing-related metabolism in the brain. Some examine the effects of brain damage on cognitive functions, while others temporarily inactivate specific brain regions to disrupt function. These diverse methods allow cognitive neuroscientists and even beginning students to examine the brain as it functions. Cognitive neuroscience, however, is not defined simply by the topics it studies or by the tools it employs. It seeks to build on its parent fields by developing new models of cognitive functions that integrate ideas from both neuroscience and cognitive science. This chapter introduces the definitions, themes, and approaches that are fully developed in the rest of the book.

Cognition

Cognition is a Latin term that means "the faculty of knowing." In practice, however, it refers to the set of processes (**cognitive functions**) that allow humans and many other animals to perceive external stimuli, to extract key information and hold it in memory, and ultimately to generate thoughts and actions that help reach desired goals. Cognition is sometimes described as processing carried out by the **mind**, but that description introduces problems, not least because *mind* is a notoriously difficult term to define. In common parlance, the mind consists of our subjective, conscious experiences. Modern researchers rarely study only those aspects of a cognitive function that are accompanied by conscious experience. Many important aspects of cognition and behavior occur without conscious experience either because they arise too rapidly (e.g., when a goalie dives to stop a shot) or because they occur automatically in the background of current processing (e.g., as our moment-to-moment experiences become transformed into our memories). In recognition of the difficulty in defining these terms, in this chapter (and the book as a whole) we restrict the use of *mind* to the subjective sense of self, and we use *cognition* or *cognitive functions* to describe the specific sorts of information processing studied by cognitive neuroscientists.

Natural philosophy and early psychology

The phenomenology of cognition has always raised philosophical questions. How do we perceive the world? What are the contents of our minds? Can we freely control our behavior? Without experimental means to understand mental life, philosophers historically drew conclusions about cognition based on introspection and reasoning. In the nineteenth century, the first true scientists to address these sorts of issues ("psychologists") built models of mental processes through behavioral observation and experimental manipulation. Many of these pioneers (e.g., Wilhelm Wundt, Hermann von Helmholtz, and William James) were trained as physicians and thus kept contact with developments in the emerging discipline of neuroscience, even as they focused their efforts on mental life. Many of their experimental methods (e.g., psychophysical judgment, memorization for later testing) are still in use today as ways of quantifying the processes of cognition.

Behaviorism

By the beginning of the twentieth century there was a growing dissatisfaction with the lack of systematic progress in the study of mental processes. Aspects of mental life like language and reasoning seemed largely intractable, and experimental methods like introspection and subjective judgments seemed inherently imprecise. As a result, psychology in that era, especially in North America, came to be dominated by a new emphasis on highly controlled experiments that matched objective external stimuli to measurable behavior (**Figure 1.1**). This approach, called **behaviorism**, rejected subjective work on mental functions as being outside the domain of proper scientific inquiry.

Experiments carried out by behaviorists like John Watson and B. F. Skinner examined how changes in stimulus presentation (e.g., food rewards to a hungry experimental animal) could shape how individuals adapt their behavior to the demands of the environment. This research proved to be extraordinarily successful. The simple recognition that food rewards made rats more likely to engage in whatever behavior occurred immediately before the reward—a process Skinner called "operant conditioning"—led to an explosion of interest in methods for reinforcing or discouraging specific behaviors. Because the basic processes of learning were thought to be a common feature of species with complex nervous systems, the typical subjects of psychological research

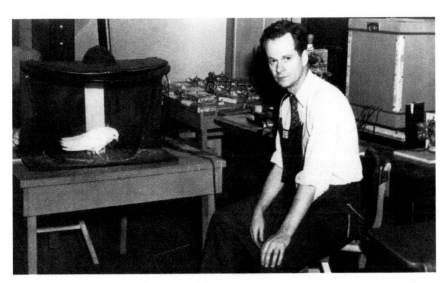

Figure 1.1   Research methods in behaviorist experiments In the early part of the twentieth century, researchers called "behaviorists" studied psychological functions using simple experiments conducted primarily on non-human animals. One of the pioneers of behaviorist research, B. F. Skinner, is shown here in his laboratory. Skinner and other researchers measured how changes in stimulus presentation (e.g., how often a reward is delivered) influence the subsequent behavior of the animal, and they used such data to create models of learning, memory, and other functions.

were non-human animals—rats and pigeons in particular. But the behaviorist approach was enthusiastically applied to human problems as well, including challenges in education, treatment of addiction, and criminal rehabilitation.

Thus, behaviorism advanced the scientific understanding of behavior in important ways, including the development of stimulus-response learning paradigms that remain widely used. It also grounded psychology firmly in an objective experimental approach. Yet the very strengths of behaviorism set the stage for its eventual demise. The focus of behaviorists on learning from rewards led them to ignore other cognitive functions. Although they did not deny the existence of mental states and the cognitive functions that those states implied, behaviorists dismissed those states as inappropriate topics for scientific study, arguing that psychological concepts could be discussed only in terms of the experimental manipulations that evoked them (a view sometimes called "operationism"). Ignoring complex mental states made experiments more tractable but needlessly reduced the scope of psychology by excluding the study of cognitive functions other than learning.

Cognitive science

In the mid-twentieth century, a confluence of factors revived the legitimacy of psychological research on cognitive functions. One factor was the advent of computational science. Research from the burgeoning field of information theory gave new insights into perception, memory, and motor performance. An example comes from a study in the 1950s by the psychologist George Miller, who showed that people are able to represent only about 7 unique items at one time, a finding often described as the span of "immediate memory." Yet most of the experiments Miller reported do not involve the number 7 or memory at all. Instead, the research focused on basic perceptual tasks—what is now often called "psychophysics"—whose results were described using computational terms like "information" and "bits." In fact, because perceptual judgments can represent only about 2.5 bits of information, Miller argued that memory

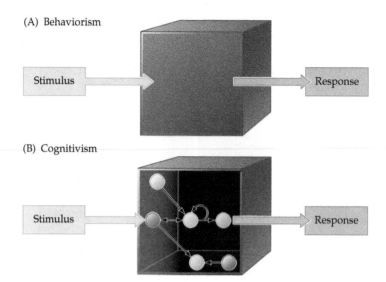

Figure 1.2 Contrasting behaviorist and cognitive approaches to research
(A) Behaviorists tried to explain behavior using only stimuli and responses, avoiding
any reference to the underlying mental processes. They did not necessarily deny the
existence of internal mental states, but instead argued that mental states could not be
defined independently of experimental operations (e.g., stimulus-response relationships).
(B) In contrast, cognitive scientists have sought to explain the information processing that
intervenes between stimuli and behavior. Those models assume that cognitive functions
(the black arrows in this schematic diagram) act upon stored information (colored circles),
transforming that information in the service of adaptive behavior.

processes must "recode" more complex stimuli (e.g., the approximately 20 bits
in a 7-digit phone number) into smaller units for cognitive processing. Memory,
for Miller, was not a passive representation of sensory stimuli, but an active
recoding of the *information* the stimuli carried.

As information theory became instantiated in physical hardware, computers provided a new model for mental processes, one that included symbolic
representations and hidden layers of meaning. The allied field of artificial intelligence suggested that elementary computations could combine in unexpected
ways to support complex reasoning. The metaphor of "mind as computer" soon
became a staple in psychology.

At about the same time, researchers in psychology and the other social sciences
began to reject the simplicity of the behaviorist research agenda and to explore
more complex aspects of mental life (Figure 1.2). Thus, in the 1950s and 1960s,
some leading psychologists challenged the behaviorist concept of operationism, arguing that psychological states and processes exist independently of the
experiments that defined them. Perhaps the most telling blow to behaviorism
was delivered by the linguist Noam Chomsky. In a review of Skinner's book
Verbal Behavior, Chomsky argued convincingly in 1959 that behaviorism could
never explain the structural and generative properties of mental phenomena
such as human language. More damningly still, he showed that the inferences
drawn by behaviorists could not eliminate psychological states; on the contrary,
their experiments could not account for even simple elements of real-world
behavior. Emboldened by these criticisms, psychologists began to involve more
human participants in their research—although research in non-human animals
is still a major component—and to investigate high-level, conscious processes.

Research on the processes of cognition has since become a large and independent field of study. Many psychologists and others now consider themselves *cognitive scientists*. The term **cognitive science** unifies research on mental

processes regardless of the specific topic, experimental approach, method, or even discipline. It focuses on information processing associated with cognitive functions (e.g., the chapters of this textbook), and includes research with human participants, studies in non-human animals, and computational simulation of cognitive functions. Cognitive scientists come from a variety of disciplines— cognitive psychology, social psychology, psychiatry, neurobiology, linguistics, and even philosophy, among others—which introduces a range of perspectives. These scientists share an interest in characterizing the phenomena and behavior associated with specific cognitive functions, and in creating **cognitive models** that describe the underlying psychological processes.

Cognitive models, like the stimulus-response models created by behaviorists, predict how sensory input leads to some behavioral output. They differ, however, in that they posit psychological processes and internal states whose properties are based on factors extrinsic to a specific experiment. Importantly, the psychological processes invoked in cognitive science models do not necessarily map onto specific physical processes in the brain, and many cognitive scientists are not especially interested in such mappings. It is enough that the models make some sense of complex cognitive phenomena, provide insights into the common outcomes of different experiments, and facilitate generalizations about experimental results.

The elements of cognitive models are sometimes called **psychological constructs**, in recognition of the fact that they are created to help explain diverse phenomena without reference to their ultimate causes in the brain. Constructs play an important role in many scientific disciplines; in particular, they can spark new and unexpected research directions. For many areas within cognitive science, careful experimentation and the gradual refinement of psychological constructs has led to remarkable progress. At the same time, however, many psychologists recognized that new developments in neuroscience held promise for grounding psychological constructs in neurobiological processes. Conversely, many neuroscientists grew increasingly interested in phenomena that had previously been limited to the province of cognitive psychology. How could the study of cognition be integrated with the methods of neuroscience? And why would knowing something about the brain improve our understanding of cognitive functions? Answering these questions requires some understanding of how neuroscientists approach the study of mental processes using the tools of biology.

Neuroscience

Nervous systems are found in all but the simplest animals. The field of neuroscience is concerned with how the nervous systems of humans and other animals are organized and function. Early knowledge about nervous system function came primarily from clinical cases and took a relatively holistic view of brain function (Figure 1.3A,B), although more was known about brain structure (Figure 1.3C). Despite lacking experimental methods, physician-scientists made remarkable inferences about brain function. The imperial Roman physician Galen had essentially no tools other than careful observation, yet he recognized that damage to the brain could have effects on cognition, and he took steps to protect the brains of his patients during surgery. The state of knowledge changed only slowly over the succeeding centuries: physicians knew that cognition was generated by the brain, but they lacked ways to systematically investigate cognition or to heal its deficits.

By the early nineteenth century, physicians with a scientific bent had become particularly interested in the functional properties of the **cerebral cortex**. It was by then clear that damage to the cerebrum from war wounds and other causes led to a variety of effects. Some individuals seemed little affected by cerebral

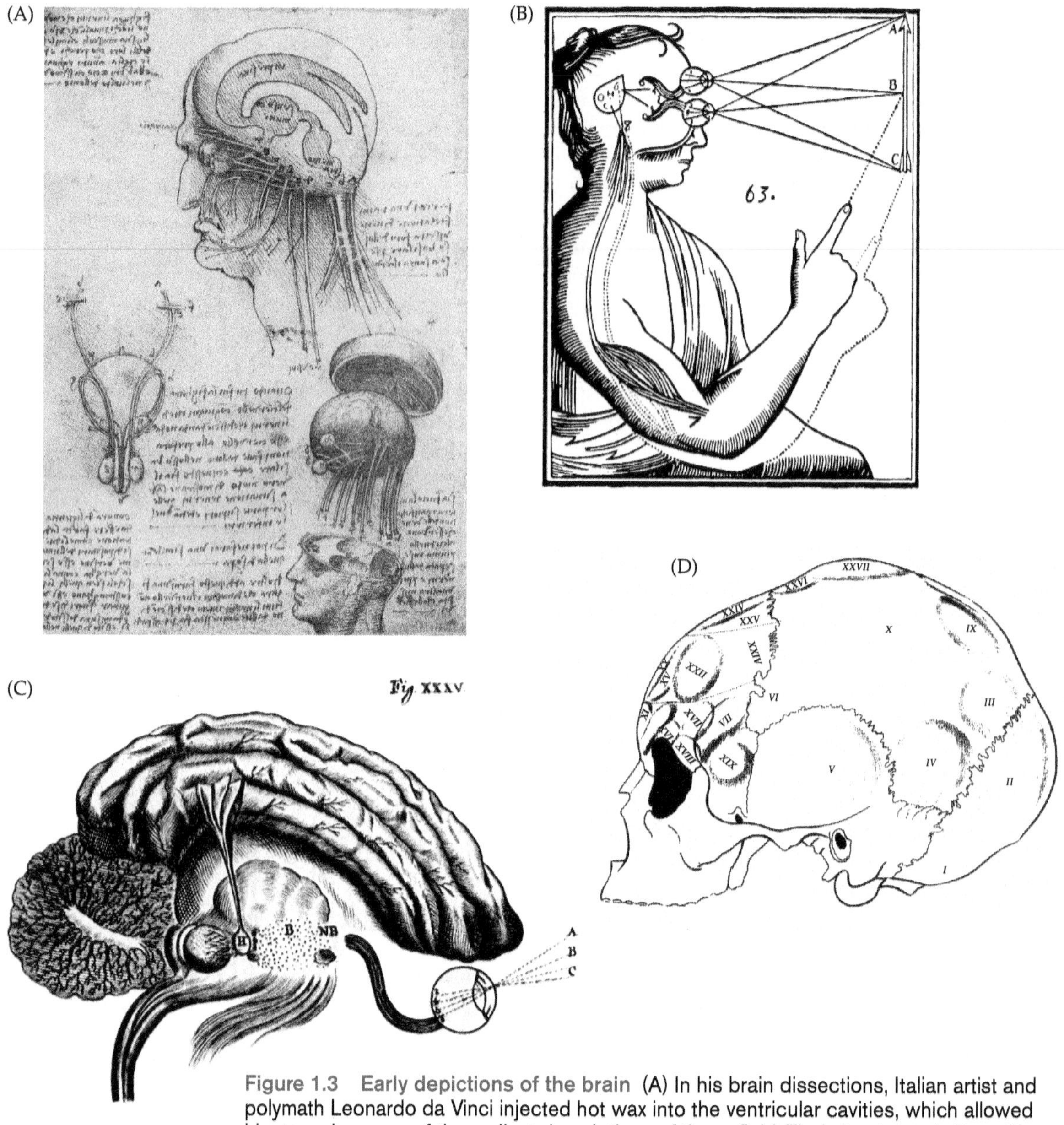

(A)

(B)

(C)

(D)

Fig. XXXV.

Figure 1.3 **Early depictions of the brain** (A) In his brain dissections, Italian artist and polymath Leonardo da Vinci injected hot wax into the ventricular cavities, which allowed him to make some of the earliest descriptions of those fluid-filled structures. In line with the ideas of many of his contemporaries in the Renaissance, Leonardo mapped different functions onto different parts of the ventricular system. (Drawings circa 1508.) (B) René Descartes likewise believed that the ventricles were critical for brain function, in that they contained psychic "spirits" that flowed from the pineal gland (shown here in a drawing from 1662). In his framework, the single pineal gland was the seat of the mind. Note, however, that this simplistic view of brain function belies Descartes' keen eye for brain structure (C). (D) As described in the text, the phrenological maps devised by Franz Joseph Gall in the early nineteenth century supposed that the bony protrusions on the skull indicated the relative strength of functions such as the "reproductive instinct" (I) and "firmness of purpose" (XXVII).

damage, while others had selective deficits of one faculty; and still others were greatly impaired by what seemed like minimal damage. The German physician and anatomist Franz Joseph Gall had long suspected that differences among individuals in their cognitive functions and personality traits were associated with different parts of the cerebral cortex, and he hypothesized that the size of the cerebral cortex (and thus the extent of the function or trait) could be mapped by measuring bumps on the overlying skull (Figure 1.3D).

Gall's hypothesis led to a new approach to studying brain function called **phrenology**. The phrenologists in the first half of the nineteenth century mapped the skulls of ordinary people, scholars, patients in mental hospitals, and even non-human animals. From these measurements, they constructed detailed maps that assigned different functions and traits—memory, color vision, vanity, moral fiber, and many others—to different parts of the cortex. Over the succeeding decades, phrenology faded as it gradually became clear that the measurements of the skull made by Gall and his followers bore no relation to the underlying structure of the brain, let alone its function. Although the term *phrenologist* is nowadays applied dismissively to someone who describes the brain in nonscientific terms, phrenology made an important contribution to modern neuroscience: it introduced the idea that different parts of the brain contribute to different sorts of information processing. This idea is now known as **localization of function**.

Only in the second half of the nineteenth century did rigorous experimental approaches to neuroscience begin to flourish, typically as physiological research in non-human animals or in brain tissue that was examined with rapidly developing techniques of microscopy and cell staining. The identification of **neurons** (Figure 1.4) as separate cells by the Spanish neuroanatomist Santiago Ramón y Cajal in the decades just before the turn of the twentieth century was a major turning point. This finding implied that cognitive processes are carried out by large populations of neurons.

Parallel and indeed earlier work on the electrical properties of neurons showed that signals are transmitted long distances along neuronal axons by **action potentials**. By the early twentieth century, researchers had developed recording techniques that could track changes in these electrical signals, and

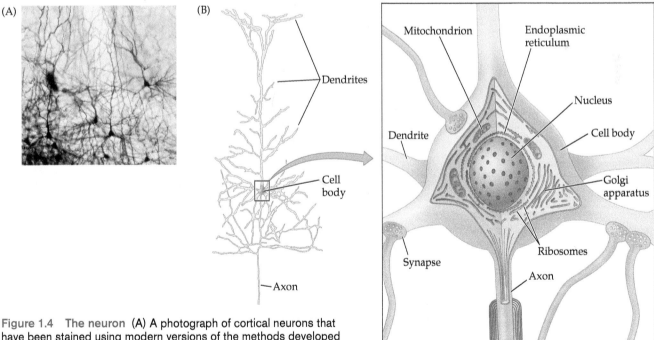

Figure 1.4 The neuron (A) A photograph of cortical neurons that have been stained using modern versions of the methods developed by Santiago Ramón y Cajal. (B) Neurons have three basic parts: (1) a cell body that contains the nucleus and most of the neuron's metabolic machinery; (2) an axon that carries information to other cells via its synaptic endings; and (3) multiple dendrites that receive inputs from synapses with other nerve cells. (A courtesy of A.-S. LaMantia and D. Purves.)

they had begun to explore the chemical substances that neurons use to stimulate the cells they contact. These **neurotransmitters** are now known to be released by the terminals of neuronal axons at specialized contacts called **synapses**, where the transmitters then bind to receptor molecules on target neurons and other cells, thus altering the membrane potential of the cell contacted. The action of neurotransmitters at synapses was soon understood to be the major way that information travels between cells in nervous systems. Understanding how neurotransmitters contribute to brain function remains an important goal for both basic and clinical neuroscience. Moreover, the signaling processes of neurons require energy derived from oxygen and metabolites supplied by the vascular system, and measurements of increased energy consumption and blood flow in active brain regions provide the bases for the imaging methods essential to many brain studies today, as will be described in Chapter 2.

By the early twentieth century, neuroscientists possessed the experimental techniques for addressing questions about functional localization in a rigorous way as evident in the pioneering studies of functional localization and reflex circuitry in experimental animals by the English physiologist Charles Sherrington. The translation of this work to humans came from studies by neurosurgeons like Wilder Penfield, who sought better ways of mapping the cerebral cortex in order to minimize the damage to normal brain tissue as he removed a tumor or a focus of epileptic seizures. At the outset of a neurosurgical session, Penfield applied weak electrical currents to the exposed cerebral cortex of the patient. When current was delivered to the cortex immediately behind the central sulcus, a patient might report feeling a tap on the finger or a brushing sensation on the leg. Changing the location of stimulation and monitoring the resulting sensations allowed Penfield to create a systematic map of the somatosensory

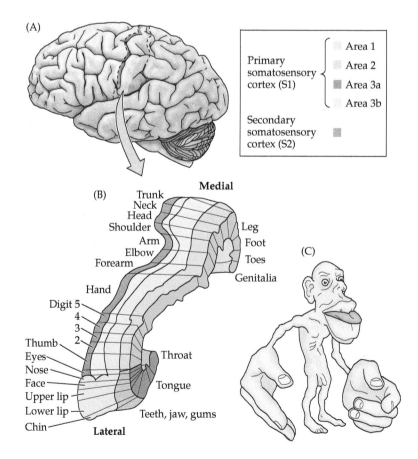

Figure 1.5 Mapping function in the human primary somatosensory cortex (A) Shown in color are key regions of the primary and secondary somatosensory cortex. (B) Electrical stimulation of these regions of the cerebral cortex—in the brains of patients undergoing neurosurgery in advance of epilepsy surgery—evokes sensations whose perceived location depends on the part of cortex being stimulated. Stimulations near the top of the brain generated sensations perceived to arise in the feet and legs, while stimulation on the side of the brain led to sensations in the face and lips. (C) This smaller reconstruction of the body (or "homunculus") portrays the size of each body region proportionally to its representation in the somatosensory cortex. Note that the amount of somatosensory cortex devoted to the hands and face is much larger than the relative body surface in these regions. (After Penfield and Rasmussen 1950; Corsi 1996.)

cortex (Figure 1.5); the same approach revealed the organization of the motor cortex, as well as some of the structural organization of the frontal lobes.

Electrical stimulation, however, was only one of the many approaches eventually used by modern neuroscience. Studies of cellular physiology revealed how single neurons change their firing rate in response to specific information, as in the exquisite sensitivity of neurons in primary visual cortex to a bar of light moving through a particular part of visual space. Clinical neuroscience has now shown that neurological conditions such as Parkinson's disease and Alzheimer's disease reflect specific cellular problems, while psychiatric disorders such as depression arise from neurotransmitter dysfunction, which has led to the development of a plethora of drugs that have proved to be effective treatments. Against this impressive backdrop, the study of cognition represents only a small component of a much larger field.

Cognitive Neuroscience: The Neurobiological Approach to Cognition

Cognitive neuroscience is defined by work at the intersection of cognitive science and neuroscience. Thus, cognitive neuroscientists must have grounding in both of these domains. They must be able to think about the cognitive processes that shape our behavior and the contents of our mental lives, and understand cognitive psychology and related fields. But they must also be able to relate those processes and theories to underlying brain function, which requires proficiency in the key findings and the tools of neuroscience. Cognitive neuroscience thus combines all the difficulties of measuring brain function with all the problems of trying to accurately assess cognition and behavior, as well as the complexities of trying to link them together. These goals distinguish cognitive neuroscience from other disciplines—chemistry, physics, and molecular biology, to name a few—whose boundaries are better defined.

This interdisciplinary nature of the field can cause problems. For example, one common misconception is that cognitive neuroscience simply maps the brain regions that are activated during a psychological process, in what is sometimes called the search for **neural correlates** of cognition. Popular descriptions of cognitive neuroscience research often feed into this misconception when they describe the research approach as putting someone in an MRI scanner to find the brain region that supports morality, forgetfulness, or impulsiveness. Nonetheless, understanding the neural correlates of a function plays an important role. For example, when researchers showed that prefrontal cortex neurons increase their firing rate while information is held in memory, that new knowledge sparked research on the role of that brain region in a range of executive processes. It should be clear, however, that the ambitions of cognitive neuroscience go well beyond creating maps of brain function.

Much current research combines information about brain structure and function to create neurobiologically grounded models of cognition. For some cognitive functions, the contributions of neuroscience have been obvious and dramatic. Models of perception and of motor control have been transformed by findings from neuroscience, and it is impossible to consider how these functions work without reference to what is now known of their underlying neural substrates. For other cognitive functions as well, evidence from neuroscience has shaped the direction of ongoing debates in the field. For example, research on attention had long debated the issue of whether attention filters perceptual stimuli at initial stages of processing, before features of a stimulus are integrated into a percept, or only later, after perceptual processing is largely complete. By recording brain activity while participants performed attention tasks, investigators eventually obtained clear evidence that attentional filters operate at both levels.

The development of cognitive neuroscience models also has important practical applications. An example is studies of **individual differences**. Understanding how and why people differ in their cognitive abilities is a major area of research in psychology, medicine, and epidemiology. By linking individual differences in cognition to individual differences in brain function, researchers have begun to understand the neural bases for both typical and atypical cognition at any stage of the human life span. Differences in cognitive abilities can provide a link between genes and behavior as well. Many of the genes that bear on individual variation in cognitive functions presumably exert their effects by altered expression in specific brain systems. Understanding how these different systems interact to support particular function can guide genomic analyses in health and disease states.

In summary, cognitive neuroscience seeks to create biologically grounded models of cognitive function. Such models draw inspiration from prior work in cognitive science, while accommodating new developments and findings in neuroscience. As a result, cognitive neuroscience models can inform and constrain prior cognitive science models, and point out new directions for neuroscience research.

Methods: Convergence and Complementarity

By combining elements of cognitive science and neuroscience, cognitive neuroscience gains access to a wealth of research techniques. It can take advantage of the diverse paradigms of cognitive scientists, some employing very simple and controlled experiments while others evoke more natural and open-ended behavior. It can apply any of the various neuroscience methods appropriate for measuring or manipulating the physiological processes described in the previous section: the electrical signaling of neurons, the activity of neurotransmitters, and their supporting metabolic processes.

The experimental and methodological diversity allows cognitive neuroscientists to explore a given topic in many different ways—and it provides many paths for beginning researchers to explore in their careers. Yet methodological diversity is not necessarily an advantage. Each new experimental paradigm or neuroscience technique presents a new set of challenges, any of which may serve as a barrier to entry for new researchers. Why do we need so many research methods? Wouldn't progress be faster if we focused on one technique and then used only that technique to study all aspects of cognition? The answer to both questions is simple. Using multiple methods provides two critical advantages: convergence and complementarity.

Convergence describes the approach of combining results from multiple experimental paradigms to illuminate a single theoretical concept. This approach long predates cognitive neuroscience. Renaissance scholars recognized that scientific progress could be made not simply by recording facts about the world, but by developing new theories that combined a number of disparate insights into a common framework. More recently, the application of converging methods to psychology helped shift that field away from behaviorism. As described earlier in this chapter, many psychologists believed that behaviorist research was too sterile: its focus on stimulus-response relationships omitted many of the most interesting aspects of our internal mental lives. No matter what experiment a psychologist conducted, a strident behaviorist could explain the experiment's results by postulating a new stimulus-response relationship—and that relationship, considered in isolation, would be a more parsimonious explanation than a theory that assumed an internal state. But how could psychologists demonstrate the existence of internal mental states that could not be measured directly? The answer came from convergence: Suppose the cognitive psychologist ran experiment after experiment, each using different stimuli and methods, and all of the experiments converged on a similar conclusion. Any one experiment could be called into question, but the set of experiments would be much more difficult to reject.

Research in cognitive neuroscience requires the same sort of convergence across paradigms. Suppose that "social cognition," which will be introduced in Chapter 11, is the topic of interest. To evoke the relevant cognitive processes, a cognitive neuroscientist might create an experiment in which participants view videos of people engaged in social interactions and then think about what those people are themselves thinking. Would observing activation in one brain region, like the lateral parietal cortex, mean that the function of the region was social cognition? No, because a single experiment cannot uniquely identify a cognitive function. Viewing videos of social interactions may engage processes related to social perception, selective attention, recognition memory, and emotion, among many.

The diversity of cognitive processes engaged by even a simple task may seem like a fundamental limitation—and it does make it more difficult for cognitive neuroscientists to apply results from a single experiment to real-world problems. But when the same result is observed across a range of experimental tasks (e.g., consistent activation in lateral parietal cortex in different social cognition tasks), then that commonality leads to a stronger inference than could be drawn from any one experiment. Convergence is often facilitated by meta-analytic methods (Box 1A), which are becoming increasingly central to cognitive neuroscience research.

Cognitive neuroscience also benefits from the **complementarity** of its research methods, each of which provides a different sort of information about brain function. Because brain function is expressed through many diverse physiological changes, cognitive neuroscientists use a welter of research methods that provide insight into different aspects of physiology: functional magnetic resonance imaging (fMRI), electroencephalography (EEG), positron emission tomography (PET), transcranial magnetic stimulation (TMS), single-neuron recording, neurological disorders, lesion studies, assessments of behavior, and others. None of these techniques provide a complete accounting of brain function.

As will be considered in more detail in Chapter 2, measurement techniques vary widely in the aspects of brain function they record (Figure 1.6). Some techniques provide information about brain metabolism (PET) and blood

Figure 1.6 Neuroscience techniques differ in their spatial and temporal resolution The vertical axes illustrate spatial resolution in terms of distance (left) and the corresponding brain structures (right). The horizontal axis illustrates temporal resolution. This graph demonstrates that different techniques provide different advantages and disadvantages. Techniques that involve data collection from human participants tend to operate at relatively coarser spatial scales than those that record from non-human animals. Electrophysiological techniques that provide excellent temporal resolution in human participants (e.g., scalp ERPs) have the disadvantage of relatively lower spatial resolution compared to neuroimaging techniques (e.g., functional MRI). As will be discussed extensively in Chapter 2, cognitive neuroscience research often applies a range of techniques to a single experimental question. EEG, electroencephalography; ERPs, event-related potentials; fMRI, functional magnetic resonance imaging; MEG, magnetoencephalography; PET, positron emission tomography; TMS, transcranial magnetic stimulation.

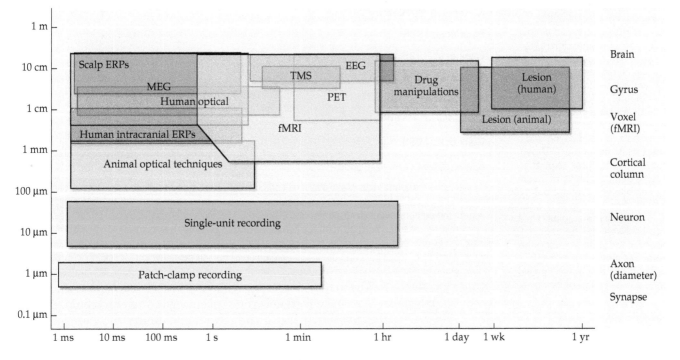

■ BOX 1A CONVERGENCE THROUGH META-ANALYSIS

Cognitive neuroscience has grown dramatically over the past several decades. Every year thousands of new studies are published, spanning all of the research methods and cognitive functions described throughout this textbook. The diversity of current research illustrates how cognitive neuroscience has grown into a vibrant, mature discipline. Yet this success points to an important challenge: How can researchers integrate results from many studies to improve their inferences about cognitive functions?

Methods for combining information across multiple studies are called **meta-analysis** techniques (i.e., "analyses of analyses"). While meta-analyses now play an important role in all scientific disciplines, they have several particularly important advantages for cognitive neuroscience. Most generally, they improve the power and precision with which researchers can detect and specify conclusions. Nearly all studies in cognitive neuroscience involve relatively small samples; typical are electrophysiological studies of 2 to 3 monkeys, neuropsychological testing of a handful of patients with brain lesions, and functional MRI or EEG recording from 20 to 30 research subjects. By combining data across multiple studies, researchers increase the effective sample size for their analyses, allowing the identification of effects that replicate across studies.

The advantages of meta-analyses go well beyond simple replication. Because different cognitive neuroscientists always approach a research question in different ways—through different experimental tasks or different methods for data collection—any single study's results might be attributable to an idiosyncratic feature of its experiment. Those idiosyncratic features (e.g., the specific demographics of a subject sample) will average out over many studies, leaving only what is common to all the studies. Thus, meta-analyses may be especially important for understanding the neural basis of complex cognitive functions that can be evoked within a wide range of contexts.

Three primary approaches to meta-analysis dominate the cognitive neuroscience literature. The first is *qualitative* meta-analysis, in which a research team first identifies a comprehensive set of studies on the same cognitive function and then looks for similarities among their results. Most review articles approach the cognitive neuroscience literature in this manner. An early example summarized 275 studies that used PET and fMRI to study cognitive functions (Table A). That number seems small compared to the vast expanse of the current literature, but at the time of this article's publication (2000), it represented a major fraction of functional neuroimaging research. For each study, the authors identified the type of function studied and the task used (e.g., "Perception: face matching") and then the specific brain region in which activation was observed. Each of the major cognitive functions exhibited a characteristic pattern of results, providing validation for these new brain imaging techniques. Although this example focused on neuroimaging techniques, its methods could accommodate any approach in cognitive neuroscience.

In the second of the primary meta-analytic approaches, researchers use *quantitative* meta-analyses to combine results from multiple studies into a single statistical framework. In recent years, quantitative approaches have been extensively applied to functional and structural MRI data. In a typical analysis technique—now often called *activation likelihood estimation*—coordinates of fMRI activation found in many studies are extracted and used to create a probabilistic map of the combined data (Figure B). Brain regions that are reliably activated across many studies have high significance values and are highlighted on the overlaid color maps. Quantitative analyses of this

(A)

Perception of Faces

STUDY	Temporal								Occipito-temporal		
	38	Ins	42	22	21	20	Mt	37	19	18	17
Grady et al. 1994								x	x	x	
Haxby et al. 1994								x	x		
Haxby et al. 1995		x					x		x		
Sergent et al. 1992									x	x	
N. Kapur et al. 1995							x		x	x	x
Puce et al. 1995					x			x	x		
Clark et al. 1996									x		
Puce et al. 1996									x	x	
Kanwisher et al. 1997									x		
McCarthy et al. 1997									x		
Clark et al. 1998									x		

Source: CABEZA AND NYBERG 2000.

(A) Qualitative meta-analyses. Meta-analyses combine data from many studies to facilitate stronger inferences than could be drawn from any one study in isolation. An early approach to meta-analysis relied on the authors' matching experimental tasks from specific studies (left column) to subregions of the brain, represented here by numbers corresponding to Brodmann areas within the cerebral cortex and by abbreviations for other brain regions: ins, insula; mt, medial temporal/hippocampus. As shown, a variety of tasks involving the visual perception of human faces evoked activation in a region of the ventral temporal lobe (Brodmann area 37, which includes the fusiform gyrus), although other regions were found to be activated in different studies. (After Cabeza and Nyberg 2000.)

■ BOX 1A *(continued)*

(B)

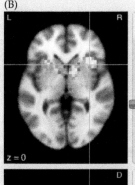
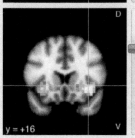
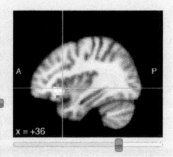

(B) Quantitative meta-analyses. This screen shot from the NeuroSynth meta-analysis program (http://neurosynth.org) combines maps of activation coordinates reported in many hundreds of experiments, each of which was coded according to the specific cognitive functions it evoked. Shown are three cross sections through the meta-analytic map for "decision making," which combined data from more than 40 studies that explored different aspects of that function. Consistently activated in those studies were the insula (at crosshair) and basal ganglia, each of which will be discussed in more detail in Chapter 14.

References

CABEZA, R. AND L. NYBERG (2000) Imaging cognition II: An empirical review of 275 PET and fMRI studies. *J. Cogn. Neurosci.* 12: 1–47.

EICKHOFF, S. B., A. R. LAIRD, C. GREFKES, L. E. WANG, K. ZILLES AND P. T. FOX (2009) Coordinate-based activation likelihood estimation meta-analysis of neuroimaging data: A random-effects approach based on empirical estimates of spatial uncertainty. *Hum. Brain Mapp.* 30: 2907–2926.

POLDRACK, R. A. (2006) Can cognitive processes be inferred from neuroimaging data? *Trends Cogn. Sci.* 10: 59–63.

POLDRACK, R. A., Y. O. HALCHENKO AND S. J. HANSON (2009) Decoding the large-scale structure of brain function by classifying mental states across individuals. *Psychol. Sci.* 20: 1364–1372.

sort can improve statistical power, as described previously, but also can distinguish subtle functional differences within a brain region. In addition, their need for only minimal human input increases their objectivity. Some cognitive neuroscience researchers have begun to create automated systems that can evaluate many hundreds of studies, allowing a keyword-based search of the larger literature (see http://neurosynth.org).

Finally, *semantic* (or ontological) meta-analyses combine studies according to similarity in their underlying concepts. In the growing area called scientometrics, meta-analytic methods are applied to the text content and citations of research articles. Patterns of co-citations (e.g., articles on working memory tend to also cite articles on executive function) or of co-occurrences of terms in articles can be used to identify relationships between concepts, which in turn can be combined into semantic maps of the literature. Even more ambitious are approaches that attempt to break down complex cognitive functions into their core processes, on the basis of prior research, and then separate activation associated with each of those processes (see http://cognitiveatlas.org for an example). As will be discussed throughout this book, the major cognitive functions (e.g., executive control) can often be separated into several processes (e.g., response inhibition, task switching), and different executive control tasks may

tap into different sets of processes. By examining data across many distinct tasks, researchers can identify brain regions or functional networks that tend to load on specific processes (Figure C).

(C)

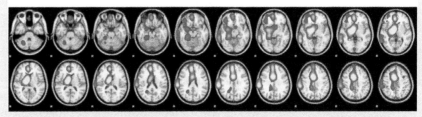

(C) Semantic meta-analyses. Eight common psychological tasks were coded according to the cognitive functions they required (e.g., working memory, decision making, response inhibition). Then, multivariate pattern analyses (see Chapter 2) were used to identify networks of brain regions that were consistently activated together and that were associated with similar combinations of cognitive functions. The network shown here—which includes the basal ganglia, hippocampus, and medial prefrontal cortex—was most activated in tasks that involved decision making and executive function, particularly when dealing with information held in memory. The size of the words above the images indicated the relative association between this network and each cognitive function; for example, this network has stronger links to functions such as decision making and memory than to functions such as speech and reasoning. (From Poldrack et al. 2009.)

oxygenation (fMRI) induced by neural activity. Others indicate how single neurons send information (single-unit recording) or integrate information from other neurons (local field potentials and EEG). And the techniques vary in whether they are more sensitive to rapid changes in brain activity or to slower changes, and whether they collect information from single neurons, small portions of the brain, or the brain as a whole. Perturbation techniques (TMS, drug administration, lesion studies), by contrast, alter brain function, and thus can be used to evaluate how specific brain regions or systems contribute causally to specific cognitive processes. Each technique carries distinct strengths and limitations, so the results obtained from multiple techniques are much more compelling than results derived from only a single approach.

Every subsequent chapter will highlight the ways in which multiple experimental paradigms and research methods combine to provide a richer understanding of the neural basis of cognition. Even though many aspects of cognition may at first seem particular to human cognitive function (e.g., language or reasoning), research using animal models often informs research in human participants, and vice versa. Convergence and complementarity also apply across research topics. Often there are striking commonalities in the sets of brain regions engaged by seemingly different sorts of tasks (e.g., selective visual attention and decision making), which can spur researchers to investigate processes that might be common across domains of cognition. Cognitive neuroscientists must develop facility with a variety of research methods, even if they do not use all (or even most) of those methods in their own research.

Conclusions

Cognitive neuroscience provides a rich opportunity for students, despite the inherent complexity of human mental life and the need to develop some familiarity with the strengths and limitations of many different technical approaches. Given its remarkable breadth, exploring cognitive neuroscience in a textbook is a daunting task. To make the job manageable, this book takes an explicitly student-centered approach. Each chapter includes fundamental background material, as well as examples of recent developments in the field. The sequence of cognitive functions progresses from basic perceptual and attentional processes, through memory and emotions, to executive processes, decision making, and finally evolution and development. There is ample coverage of research methods, and how conclusions about cognitive function are best understood by applying multiple experimental approaches and considering a variety of data. The aim in every chapter is to describe how cognitive neuroscience has extended the scientific scope of both cognitive psychology and neuroscience.

As authors, our primary goal is to help students gain an appreciation of the intellectual and methodological principles of this exciting new discipline, which combines many of the best qualities of the social and natural sciences. By understanding the approach of cognitive neuroscience and its conclusions, students will gain a deeper understanding of the cognitive capabilities that define human beings.

Summary

1. Cognitive science seeks to understand the information processing associated with functions like perception, memory, and decision making.

2. Neuroscience seeks to characterize the structure and function of the nervous system.

3. Cognitive neuroscience is a new discipline that applies research methods from neuroscience to the functions and behaviors studied by cognitive science.

4. Cognitive neuroscientists use diverse research methods and experimental paradigms to develop models of mental function and behavior.

Go to the **COMPANION WEBSITE**

sites.sinauer.com/cogneuro2e
for quizzes, animations, flashcards, and other study resources.

Additional Reading

Important Original Papers

CHOMSKY, N. (1959) A review of B. F. Skinner's *Verbal Behavior. Language* 35: 56–58.

GARNER, W. R., H. W. HAKE AND C. W. ERIKSEN (1956) Operationism and the concept of perception. *Psychol. Rev.* 63: 149–159.

MILLER, G. A. (1956) The magical number seven, plus or minus two: Some limits on our capacity for processing information. *Psychol. Rev.* 3: 81–97.

Books

FINGER, S. (1994) *Origins of Neuroscience.* Oxford: Oxford University Press.

PURVES, D., G. J. AUGUSTINE, D. FITZPATRICK, W. C. HALL, A.-S. LaMANTIA AND L. E. WHITE (2012) *Neuroscience,* 5th Ed. Sunderland, MA: Sinauer.

SKINNER, B. F. (1938) *The Behavior of Organisms.* New York: Appleton-Century-Crofts.

2

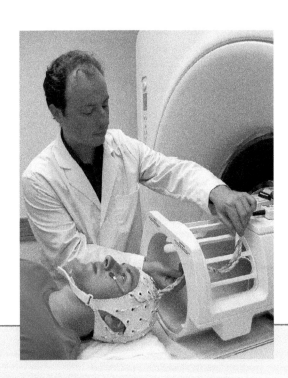

The Methods of Cognitive Neuroscience

INTRODUCTION

As introduced in Chapter 1, the goal of cognitive neuroscience is to explain cognitive processes and behavior in terms of the structure and function of the brain and the rest of the nervous system. A critical contribution of cognitive psychology has been to emphasize the importance of measuring behavioral responses during cognitive and perceptual tasks as a means of inferring what transpires as the nervous system translates stimuli into appropriate actions, thoughts, and other behaviors. By applying these psychological paradigms in conjunction with neuroscience techniques and methods, investigators have increasingly been able to directly relate the biology of brain functions to the mental functions studied by cognitive scientists. These findings in turn help constrain and guide cognitive models of behavior, as part of a synergistic interplay between the fields that form the central core of cognitive neuroscience.

Neuroscience-based approaches can be divided into two broad categories: (1) studying changes in cognitive behavior when the brain has been perturbed in some way, and (2) measuring brain activity while cognitive tasks are being performed (Figure 2.1). For the first of these approaches, disturbances of brain function due to clinical brain lesions resulting from stroke, trauma, or disease have been enormously useful for investigating the role of the brain in specific cognitive processes. In addition, methods that employ pharmacological and electrical perturbations of brain function, including those applied in a temporary fashion, have also been used to great advantage in both human subjects and experimental animals (see Introductory Box). The second main approach—that of measuring brain activity while a subject is engaged in a specific cognitive task—takes advantage of a variety of currently available electrophysiological and imaging techniques in both humans and animals. Both of these approaches have altered and accelerated our understanding of the mechanisms underlying the higher brain functions that are the focus of cognitive neuroscience.

■ INTRODUCTORY BOX EARLY BRAIN MAPPING IN HUMANS

One of the earliest methods used to directly examine cognitive brain function in humans was intracranial electrical stimulation in patients. Although intracranial stimulation techniques are highly invasive, they are sometimes used in humans to enable neurosurgeons to map the functions of brain regions on or near the site of a tumor, suspected epileptic focus, or other lesion that needs to be dealt with surgically. Because there are no pain receptors in brain tissue, such stimulation mapping can be performed on awake, responsive patients.

As mentioned briefly in Chapter 1, one of the first scientists to use electrical stimulation in this way was the neurosurgeon Wilder Penfield (Figure A), who in 1934 established the Montreal Neurological Institute with support from the Rockefeller Foundation. With his colleague Herbert Jasper, Penfield developed procedures for treating patients with severe epilepsy by destroying the brain tissue in the regions where the seizures originated. Before damaging any cortical tissue, however, he used focal electrical stimulation to functionally map the region as a way to better understand the functionality of the surrounding area. Since the patients were conscious during the procedure, he was able to observe their responses and/or ask about what they were experiencing. The patients' responses to the stimulation helped him plan the surgery so that important brain functionality could be preserved (Figure B).

Using this focal stimulation technique, Penfield was able to create maps of the sensory and motor cortices of the brain. In particular, he established that each of these areas contains complete and separate representations of the various body parts on the contralateral side of the body (Figure C). Penfield found that the layout of these cortical representations followed the general **somatotopic** relationships of the different parts of the body (see Chapters 4 and 5). That is, adjacent body parts generally had adjacent cortical representations, which together gave rise to a representational map of the entire body termed a **homunculus** (meaning literally "little man"). One of the intriguing findings of this work was the relatively large expanse of cortex dedicated to some body parts, such as the face and hands, relative to others. This is presumed to reflect the need for higher detail of representation for these parts. These findings of the neural representation of contralateral parts of the body in the sensory and motor cortices have been mostly confirmed by numerous studies since, using a variety of different methods.

Penfield also reported intriguing effects of stimulating other regions, such as parts of the temporal lobes, where seizures often originate. These effects included both auditory perceptions and the vivid recall of memories. For example, he recorded that "stimulation of a point on the anterior part of the first temporal lobe on the right" caused one patient to remember being at a very specific location—namely, "South Bend, Indiana, corner of Jacob and Washington"—and to be "looking at himself at a younger age." Other stimulation triggered memories of music from the Broadway musical *Guys and Dolls*. Although these triggered memories could vary substantially even when the same region was stimulated at different times, the specificity of the memories induced was quite striking. Moreover, these observations are consistent with the conclusions in Chapters 8 and 9 that long-term memories are stored in the cerebral cortex.

References

PENFIELD, W. AND H. JASPER (1954) *Epilepsy and the Functional Anatomy of the Human Brain*, 2nd Ed. Oxford: Little, Brown.

PENFIELD, W. AND T. RASMUSSEN (1950) *The Cerebral Cortex of Man: A Clinical Study of Localization of Function*. Oxford: Macmillan.

Early mapping of cortical brain function in humans using intracranial stimulation. (A) Neurosurgeon Wilder Penfield. (B) An original photo of the exposed brain of one of Penfield's patients, labeled with stimulation locations. (C) The layout of the representations in the somatosensory (left panel) and motor (right panel) cortices of the body parts on the contralateral side of the body. (Courtesy of the Osler Library of the History of Medicine, McGill University.)

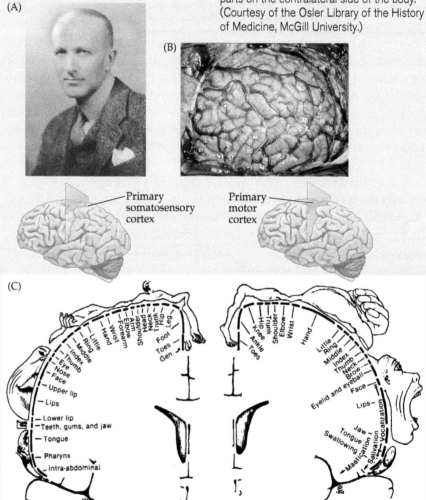

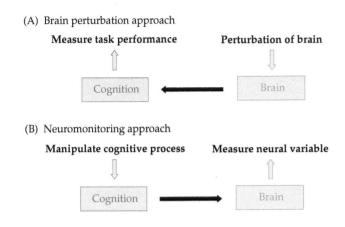

(A) Brain perturbation approach

Measure task performance **Perturbation of brain**

Cognition ⟵ Brain

(B) Neuromonitoring approach

Manipulate cognitive process **Measure neural variable**

Cognition ⟶ Brain

Figure 2.1 Two main approaches for linking cognitive functions and neural processes (A) In the first approach, the brain is perturbed in some way—either by a clinical disorder (e.g., stroke, disease, trauma) or by directed, planned interference (injected drugs, electrical stimulation)—and task performance on a set of cognitive tasks is measured. (B) In the neuromonitoring approach, an experimenter manipulates a particular cognitive process in an experimental task and measures the associated changes in brain activity.

Brain Perturbations That Elucidate Cognitive Functions

Perturbations of the brain that impair or otherwise influence cognitive functions can come about through a variety of mechanisms. Such perturbations often derive from brain damage in patients due to stroke, trauma, or disease, but they can also be induced experimentally using methods that employ pharmacological or electrical methods. Information from both of these ways by which normal brain operations can be disrupted have greatly advanced our understanding of the neural underpinnings of cognitive functions.

Perturbations imposed by stroke, trauma, or disease

The technique of clinical-pathological correlations is the oldest method for understanding the neural basis of cognitive function and has been a mainstay of neurology and neurosurgery for more than a century. A major advantage of this approach is that if damage to a brain area or system disrupts a cognitive function, it is likely that the damaged region is involved in some critical way in the performance of that function.

This approach was first accomplished by correlating a patient's signs, symptoms, and behavior during life with the location of brain lesions discovered upon autopsy. Brain lesions can arise from a stroke that damages a particular region of cortex, from traumatic injury, from a tumor, or from various brain diseases. Many examples of clinical-pathological correlations are considered in later chapters, including the seminal work that associated language functions with specific regions in the left hemisphere (see Chapter 12); studies that associated frontal lobe damage with deficits in planning and judgment (see Chapter 14); and studies that have provided fundamental insights into the neural basis of perception (see Chapters 3 and 4), attentional control (see Chapter 7), memory (see Chapters 8 and 9), and emotion (see Chapter 10).

A major limitation of clinical-pathological correlations in humans, however, is that the brain damage is the result of many factors that are not under the control of the experimenter. In the case of strokes, for example, these factors include which specific artery was blocked, which brain area(s) that artery supplied, whether other arteries were still able to supply some blood to the affected area, and how long ago the stroke occurred. Although stroke-induced lesions can be relatively focal, they follow vascular-supply boundaries rather than being restricted to functional brain regions, and thus a single lesion can have diverse effects on cognitive functions.

Moreover, the distribution of brain regions supporting cognitive functions varies among individuals, making it difficult to generalize results. This variability can be addressed to some degree by combining information about the

Left dorsal prefrontal

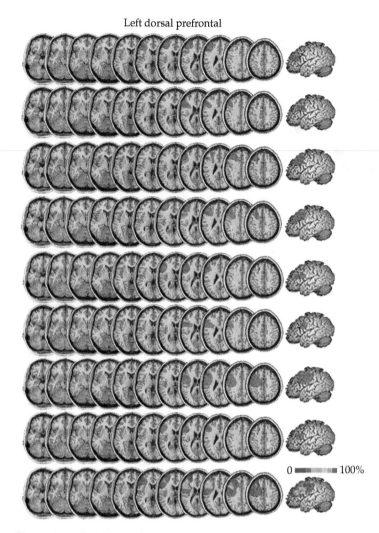

0 ▬▬▬ 100%

Figure 2.2 Combining information across subjects helps to localize the brain region underlying a cognitive deficit These images show the areas of damage determined from structural magnetic resonance brain images (see Box 2A) for eight patients with a common cognitive loss (the prefrontal syndrome described in Chapter 13). Each row shows the extent of damage for a given patient; each column represents a comparable level in the brain, from inferior on the left to superior on the right. The bottom row shows the area of brain damage the eight subjects have in common. The scale indicates the percentage of subjects with damage in each location. This sort of analysis helps specify the brain region that is critical to a given function. (Courtesy of Robert T. Knight.)

locus of damage across a group of patients, allowing researchers to delineate the affected region that is common to the loss of a particular function (Figure 2.2). The region of overlap among a group of patients more accurately defines the part of the brain relevant to the cognitive function at issue. Notably, only with the advent of modern brain imaging techniques did this approach of collating information concerning the overlapping of brain lesions into a common space become very practical or accurate.

Another way researchers have defined the relationship between brain damage and resulting deficits in cognitive functions is by making restricted electrolytic or surgical lesions in experimental animals, including non-human primates. This approach allows the researcher to control the location and extent of brain damage, limiting it to specific functional areas. There are, however, some disadvantages to this approach as well. The training and assessment of animals carrying out cognitive tasks is considerably more difficult than for similar studies in humans, and making deliberate lesions in the brains of healthy animals, particularly non-human primates, can raise ethical concerns. Nevertheless, the use of carefully controlled brain lesions in experimental animals has provided useful information complementing that derived from neuropsychological studies in humans.

Lesion studies, whether in humans or in animals, also present problems of interpretation. The mammalian brain is a highly interconnected structure. If one area of the brain is lesioned, other areas of the brain innervated by the damaged area may, from the loss of input, also cease to function normally. Such effects, known as **diaschisis**, can lead to wrongly attributing the lost functionality to the lesioned area rather than to the downstream area. Another possible misinterpretation of lesion findings is that damage to a cortical area can also damage nearby fiber tracts, thereby disrupting the function of more distant areas.

Nevertheless, clinical-pathological correlation studies remain highly informative in cognitive neuroscience. Their continued relevance has been greatly augmented by modern neuroimaging methods that allow brain lesions to be localized with considerable precision in living patients who are still available for detailed behavioral testing. Such knowledge of the exact site of a lesion can inform and guide the behavioral testing in a far more focused way than when the definitive localization of the lesion could be attained only postmortem. Such modern methods of imaging brain structure, particularly those using magnetic resonance imaging (MRI), are fundamental to cognitive neuroscience; they are described in Box 2A. Other sorts of imaging techniques, such as the MRI-based technique of diffusion tensor imaging (DTI), are being used to delineate the structural *connections* of the brain (Box 2B).

Pharmacological perturbations

Another way of perturbing cognitive function in the brain is via pharmacological manipulation. As described in the Appendix, signaling between neurons involves the release of and response to neurotransmitter molecules at synapses. Many drugs interfere with or augment these processes and can thereby change cognitive functions. Cognitive neuroscientists have taken advantage of psychoactive drugs such as caffeine, cocaine, antidepressants, and a host of others to gain insight into the neuropharmacology of these functions, both in humans and in experimental animals.

Pharmacological studies in humans have taken two main forms. The first approach is to examine the influence of chronic drug use or abuse on cognitive processes, taking advantage of the unfortunate prevalence of these social problems and the disorders they cause. An example is the set of cognitive impairments apparent in cocaine addicts, which include changes in reward evaluation (i.e., a person's ability to properly assess the positive or negative value of events and behaviors). Impaired reward evaluation in turn affects the ability to make self-protective decisions and to formulate and pursue successful life strategies. Cocaine and other drugs of abuse lead to specific changes in neurotransmission in the brain systems that underlie these functions. Cocaine specifically activates dopamine receptors, altering the physiology of the **dopamine system**, which is known to play a major role in reward evaluation (see Chapter 14). Although the dysfunction that leads to addiction is still not completely understood, the altered sense of reward associated both with the cocaine "high" and with cocaine addiction is clear. Chronic use leads to drug tolerance (i.e., the need for increasing amounts of the drug in order to achieve the same pharmacological effect), which results in further negative consequences. (On a less problematic level, this sort of pharmacological adaptation is familiar to habitual coffee

■ BOX 2A AN INTRODUCTION TO STRUCTURAL BRAIN IMAGING TECHNIQUES

Until relatively recently, images of the human brain, whether of patients or of normal subjects, provided only limited information to clinicians and researchers. For a long time, the best noninvasive imaging methodology available used conventional X-ray techniques, which do not image soft-tissue structures such as the brain very well and do not provide three-dimensional image information. Although the addition of vascular contrast agents (dyes containing radiopaque materials such as barium salts) improved the visualization of damaged tissue, the intrinsic two-dimensional nature of conventional X-rays (i.e., giving a net density through imaged tissue only at one particular angle) still limited the anatomical resolution of brain tissue. Beginning in the 1970s, however, the development of a variety of imaging methods that revealed brain structure (and, somewhat later, brain physiology) with ever-increasing detail revolutionized neuroscience, from clinical diagnostics to research on cognitive processes.

The first technological breakthrough was the development of **computerized tomography** (**CT**). CT uses a movable X-ray tube that is rotated around the patient's head (Figure A). Rather than acquiring a single image, as in conventional X-ray images, a CT scan gathers *intensity information* gleaned from multiple angles through the imaging volume. These data are entered into a matrix, and the radiodensity at each point in the three-dimensional space of the head is calculated. Using sensitive detectors and digital signal-processing techniques, small differences in radiodensity can be converted into three-dimensional image information for the full volume of the head. In addition, the computed matrix can generate "slices," or *tomograms* (*tomo* means "cut" or "slice"), visualizing internal structures in various planes throughout the brain (Figure A, inset), transformed to provide views from any angle. Since many brain structures are best seen in a particular plane, this ability is a tremendous advantage.

Today, CT imaging for brain research purposes has been largely superseded by **magnetic resonance imaging** (**MRI**; Figure B), although CT remains important in many clinical applications because it is faster and cheaper than MRI and can be used in some situations in which mag-

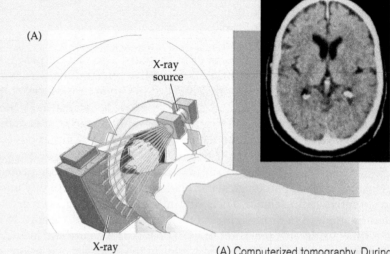

(A)

X-ray source

X-ray detector

netic resonance cannot (e.g., in patients with implanted metal devices).

The essentials of the mechanism by which magnetic resonance produces images can be understood in terms of the three concepts reflected in the phrase *magnetic resonance imaging* itself:

1. *Magnetic.* Consider a compass needle. At rest, the needle is aligned with the Earth's magnetic field (i.e., along a north–south axis). Similarly, when a person is inside an MRI scanner, protons in hydrogen atoms of the brain become aligned with the very strong main magnetic field of the scanner. Perturbations with respect to this alignment provide a source signal that can be measured, analyzed, and used to construct an image.

2. *Resonance.* This difficult concept is the foundation of MRI. *Resonance* refers to the ability of a system to absorb energy delivered at a particular frequency. A macroscopic example is a child on a playground swing. Given a single push, even a strong one, the resulting movement is brief and diminishes quickly. In contrast, repeated small pushes at the right frequency (i.e., a push each time the person on the swing reaches the apogee of its arc) allows the system to absorb the imparted energy effectively, such that the child will soon be swinging back and forth with great excursion. In the same way, protons in a strong magnetic field will efficiently absorb

(A) Computerized tomography. During a CT scan, an X-ray source is rotated around the patient's head while detectors measure the intensity of the rays transmitted through the head at each imaged angle. Computer algorithms combine the opacity data from these multiple imaging angles to reconstruct the opacity at each point within the volume of the head. In addition, the detectors used in CT are more sensitive than conventional film, thereby allowing shorter imaging times and less radiation exposure. The CT scan in the inset shows a horizontal section of a normal adult brain.

energy when the energy is delivered at a particular *resonant frequency*. During a process called *excitation*, the MRI scanner emits energy in the form of radio waves at precisely the resonant frequency of protons. After a few milliseconds, the radio-wave energy is turned off, whereupon the protons begin to release the energy they absorbed. This released energy—the *MR signal*–is measured by electromagnetic detectors around the head or other part of the body.

3. *Imaging.* In order to create an image from the MR signal, electromagnetic coils in the scanner can cause the local magnetic field to differ in strength along specific directions. By varying these magnetic-field *gradients* in a systematic way along the *x*-, *y*-, and *z*-axes of the volume to be imaged, the MR signal is caused to vary correspondingly and systematically along these

■ BOX 2A *(continued)*

axes. This complex variation in the signal emitted by the brain or other tissue is decoded by sophisticated computer analysis to create an image that reflects the proton density, as well as the distribution of other tissue characteristics, throughout the imaged volume. Because these characteristics are different for gray matter, white matter, the fluid in the ventricles, and other neural tissues (see the Appendix), a great deal of neuroanatomical detail becomes apparent.

The spatial resolution of MR images depends on the strength of the magnetic field, the strength of the gradient coils, and the types of images being collected. Currently, most clinical scanners have field strengths of 1.5 tesla, which can provide a structural resolution of 1 millimeter or less. Research scanners tend to have field strengths of 3 tesla or higher, often along with high-performance magnetic gradient coils that further improve the structural imaging resolution and contrast. These enhanced performance characteristics also facilitate the acquisition of high-speed images of functional brain activity, as described later in the chapter.

It should be apparent from this description that MRI has a number of important features that make it an extraordinarily valuable tool in cognitive neuroscience. First, it is noninvasive; subjects are simply exposed to a strong magnetic field and radio waves that are generally thought to be harmless to brain tissues (although patients have been injured by unsecured ferromagnetic objects being pulled into the MR scanner). Second, MR images of brain tissue are of extremely high resolution compared to those obtainable using other techniques (compare the insets in Figures A and B for CT and MRI

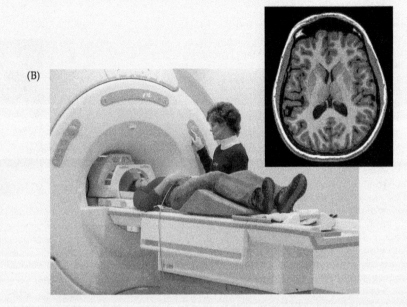

(B) Magnetic resonance imaging. A typical 1.5-tesla MR scanner is shown. The inset shows a horizontal MR image of a normal adult brain. Note the extraordinary clarity with which the different soft-tissue types and regions of the brain can be seen, and how much more detail is visible compared to the CT image in Figure A.

images, respectively). Third, by varying the gradient and radio-frequency pulse parameters, MRI scanners can be used to generate images that are sensitive to many different aspects of brain structure. For example, certain imaging parameters enable the acquisition of pictures that delineate gray matter and white matter in very high detail. The use of other parameters in the MR scanning sequence yields images in which gray and white matter are invisible but the brain's vasculature stands out. Varying yet other parameters enables measurement of the preferred direction of water diffusion for each voxel (i.e., imaging volume unit) of imaged brain tissue. Because water tends to diffuse

more along fiber tracts than across them, this technique—diffusion tensor imaging (DTI)—enables the imaging of fiber tracts at very high resolution (see Box 2B).

References

HOUNSFIELD, G. N. (1980) Computed medical imaging. *Science* 210: 22–28.

HUETTEL, S., A. W. SONG AND G. McCARTHY (2009) *Functional Magnetic Resonance Imaging*, 2nd Ed. Sunderland, MA: Sinauer.

OLDENDORF, W. AND W. OLDENDORF JR. (1988) *Basics of Magnetic Resonance Imaging*. Boston: Kluwer Academic.

drinkers, who need more caffeine to achieve the same stimulatory effect than do people who drink coffee only occasionally.) Studies of the effects of cocaine have been critical in advancing our understanding of the regions of the brain and the cellular mechanisms involved in the normal sense of reward.

More controlled pharmacological perturbation can be carried out in experimental settings in which a drug is administered acutely and its effects are monitored. In this manner it is possible to study, for example, the effects of nicotine on cognitive functions—another topic that has been of great interest because of the health implications of smoking. Nicotine affects neurotransmission mediated by acetylcholine, interacting with cognitive processes that include

■ BOX 2B IMAGING STRUCTURAL CONNECTIONS IN THE BRAIN

An important element for understanding the mechanisms underlying cognitive functions in the brain is establishing how the different parts and regions are interconnected and work together. Accordingly, much work is continually being devoted to delineating the structural connections of the brain, at both the macroscopic and microscopic levels.

At the macroscopic level, a variant of MRI known as diffusion-weighted imaging has been found to be particularly useful for delineating the white matter fiber tracts of the brain. The basis of this imaging approach derives from the fact that water molecules in living structures, including those in the brain, are always moving slightly within their local area. Such movement, or diffusion, of water molecules affects the MR signals arising from the local voxels (i.e., imaging volume units). Because the cellular environments experienced by the different water molecules differ across the brain, their diffusion characteristics vary as well. Modulating certain parameters of the MR scanning sequence can make the MR signal from each voxel particularly sensitive to the amount of local diffusion, enabling the construction of diffusion-weighted images that reflect the diffusion characteristics across the brain.

A particularly important application of such diffusion-weighted imaging is **diffusion tensor imaging (DTI)**, which quantifies the relative diffusivity of the water molecules in each voxel into directional components. Because most axonal fibers in the brain that make up the white matter fiber tracts are encased in myelin (see the Appendix), which is particularly hydrophobic, water tends to diffuse more along fiber tracts than across them, but with generally less directionality in other types of brain tissue. Thus, white matter shows more prominent *anisotropy* in its diffusion characteristics (tending to have a preferred direction in its diffusion), whereas the diffusion in other brain regions tends to be *isotropic* (no preferred direction).

A scalar quantity known as the **fractional anisotropy (FA)** can be computed for each voxel to express this degree of anisotropy. Fractional anisotropy can provide important information about the composition of the tissue within a voxel. Notably, some neurological diseases, such as multiple sclerosis and vascular dementia, are characterized by white matter pathology that can be identified with

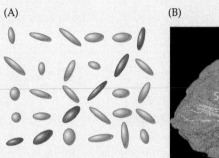
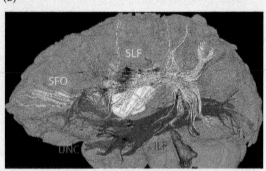

(A)

(B)

Fiber tracking using diffusion tensor imaging (DTI). (A) In this hypothetical five-by-six set of voxels, the diffusivity characteristics of each voxel are represented by an ellipsoid whose dimensions reflect the relative diffusion rates along the different directions, with spheres representing isotropic diffusion (relatively equal in all directions) and narrow ellipsoids showing stronger diffusivity values along a particular direction (the longest axis of the ellipsoid). Using tractography approaches, white matter tracts can then be reconstructed from these data by finding the strongest continuous chain along the preferred diffusion directions across multiple voxels (shown here in red). (B) This image, derived by DTI tractography, shows some major fiber tracts in the brain. Shown are the superior longitudinal fasciculus (SLF), the superior fronto-occipital tract (SFO), the inferior fronto-occipital tract (IFO), the uncinate fasciculus (UNC), and the inferior longitudinal fasciculus (ILF). (B courtesy of Dr. Susumu Mori.)

FA measures. Moreover, individual differences in white matter integrity, such as with aging, can also be identified with FA. Thus, these variations can provide additional information for understanding variations in cognitive function, both in normal individuals and in clinical populations.

Tractography is a powerful application of the DTI technology that allows delineation of the directionality of fiber tracts in the brain. More specifically, using DTI, the directional diffusivity in each voxel can be represented by an ellipsoid whose relative dimensions reflect the rate of diffusion in each direction (Figure A). White matter tracts can then be derived from these data using algorithms that estimate continuous tracts of diffusion across voxels (indicated in red in Figure A). By following these directions and continuously connecting the long axes that fit best along a line, images of the major nerve fiber tracts can be constructed. These, in turn, allow the formation of maps of structural connectivity in the brain (Figure B).

DTI can be used in conjunction with fMRI activation studies in several ways. (See the text for details about functional MRI, or fMRI.) First, the fMRI activation data can help guide the tractography calculations. Such combination of these methods can be particularly useful for delineating the connectivity across complex regions of the brain with multiple, crossing fiber tracts. Conversely, the DTI-delineated fiber tracts can be used to help in what are called functional connectivity analyses (see text), which analyze how certain brain regions vary together in their activation patterns.

From a microscopic standpoint, much work is also currently being aimed toward the goal of reconstructing the connectivity of the entire human brain (or the brains of other species) at the level of neurons and synapses. This nascent (and controversial) effort has been dubbed *connectomics*, which refers to obtaining full knowledge of brain connections (i.e., the *connectome*, by analogy with *genome*).

Obtaining such information at the cellular level entails computer-assisted image acquisition and analysis using high-speed methods, along with organizing the results into an extremely large database. At the light-microscopic level, a method called Brainbow has recently been developed that is based on molecular genetics techniques used to delineate individual neurons and their branches by fluorescence in different colors (Figure C). At the finer electron microscopic level that allows synapses to be seen, the challenge of connectomics is vastly greater, as should be apparent from the electron micrograph in Figure D.

■ **BOX 2B** *(continued)*

(C)

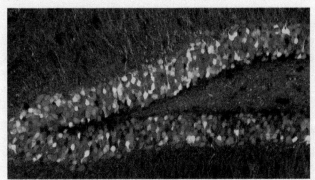

Connectomics. (C) An example of an image from the light-microscopic Brainbow technique, taken from the mouse hippocampus. (D) An electron microscopic section from the cerebral cortex indicating the enormous complexity of brain connectivity at this level. (C, D courtesy of Jeff Lichtman and Josh Sanes.)

(D)

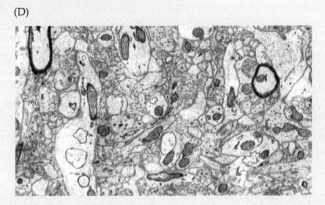

The proponents of connectomics argue that a huge database of fine-level structural connectivity will be a vital resource for all sorts of human and animal neuroscience research, both basic and clinical, including studies of cognitive questions. Given the very large cost and uncertain outcome, however, opponents have opined that connectomics would not be a wise investment, except in studying the brains of small, experimental animals. This interesting debate seems likely to continue for some time.

References

HUETTEL, S. A., A. W. SONG AND G. McCARTHY (2009) *Functional Magnetic Resonance Imaging*, 2nd Ed. Sunderland, MA: Sinauer.

LICHTMAN, J. W., J. R. LIVET AND J. SANES (2008) A technicolour approach to the connectome. *Nat. Rev. Neurosci.* 9: 417–422.

MORI, S. AND J. ZHANG (2006) Principles of diffusion tensor imaging and its application to basic neuroscience research. *Neuron* 51: 527–539.

SEUNG, S. (2012) *Connectome: How the Brain's Wiring Makes Us Who We Are*. New York: Houghton Mifflin/Harcourt Brace.

mood, attention, memory, and appetite, as well as neurological processes that can lead to addiction. The nicotine molecule binds to certain acetylcholine receptors and activates them just as the neurotransmitter acetylcholine itself does. (Drugs like nicotine that bind to and activate receptors in a manner similar to a neurotransmitter are called **agonists**, whereas drugs that bind to and block receptors are called **antagonists**.) When coupled with information derived from neuropharmacological studies in experimental animals and in vitro systems (i.e., in experimental environments outside the living organism), pharmacological manipulation can lead to inferences about the contribution of the relevant neurotransmitter system to the cognitive processes they affect.

A disadvantage of administering drugs systemically (i.e., by injection into the bloodstream) for studying cognitive processes is the relative lack of specificity of their effects. With systemic administration, much of the brain (along with the other organs of the body) is exposed to the drug, and sorting out the effects on different brain systems can be difficult. A more specific intervention is to inject substances directly into specific brain areas of an experimental animal. This approach usually involves surgically implanting a cannula (a very thin tube) or other drug delivery system that can administer defined amounts of the experimental agent locally and in a highly controlled manner. For example, agonists and antagonists of major neurotransmitters such as dopamine and serotonin have been injected into midbrain regions implicated in reward processing to study the cognitive functions subserved by these key regions. Such studies have provided insight into the actions of a range of drugs used to treat disorders such as depression and schizophrenia and, by implication, insight into the cognitive functions that go awry in these disorders.

Perturbation by intracranial brain stimulation

A different way of perturbing brain function is direct electrical stimulation of a specific brain region, a technique used by pioneering neurophysiologists such as Charles Sherrington and David Ferrier beginning in the late nineteenth century. In this approach, electrodes are placed onto or into the brain of an experimental animal or a human patient during a neurosurgical procedure (see Introductory Box). Electrodes can be placed transiently (i.e., just for the duration of the surgery) or chronically for extended studies of the brain's electrical activity and responses to electrical stimulation.

In experimental animals, chronically implanted electrodes allow researchers to assess the function of individual neurons or groups of neurons as the animal (often a monkey) carries out a cognitive task it has been trained to perform. By altering the strength of the stimulus applied, the effects on the local neuronal population can be varied to provide additional information. For example, moderate levels of stimulation can activate neurons and trigger behavior that suggests what a given population normally does. In contrast, strong stimulation tends to disrupt normal function, and thus can indicate how the loss of that neuronal population affects a particular cognitive process. Used in this latter way, electrical stimulation can effectively create a transient and reversible "lesion." Although intracranial stimulation techniques are obviously invasive, they are sometimes used in humans to enable neurosurgeons to map the functions of brain regions that they are considering removing or operating on (see Introductory Box).

Perturbation by extracranial brain stimulation

Although disrupting neural processing by local electrical stimulation can be informative, the use of this technique in humans is obviously limited to patients with serious medical problems. A far less invasive approach that can be used to disrupt cognitive processing in normal subjects is **transcranial magnetic stimulation** (**TMS**). In this technique, a strong but transient and rapidly changing magnetic field is generated over a region of the scalp by passing an intense, rapidly varying, electrical current through a set of coils (Figure 2.3). The rapidly changing magnetic field in the coil induces a rapidly changing electrical field in the underlying brain tissue, resulting in an extraneous flow of current that transiently interacts with local neural processing. With strong stimulation, this interaction is typically disruptive, creating a reversible brain "lesion" limited to the underlying area, in much the same manner that strong direct electrical stimulation would. With weaker stimulation, this interaction can sometimes facilitate activation of the underlying area.

Several approaches are used to apply TMS to the study of cognitive processes. One technique is to apply a series of TMS pulses (e.g., one per second) over several minutes. The influence of such **repetitive TMS** (**rTMS**) stimulation on a cognitive function of interest can then be examined by behavioral tests that can be administered during and after the TMS application (up till a couple of hours afterward). Studies using this approach have shown that, depending on the strength of stimulation, TMS can either impair or improve performance on tasks involving the stimulated area, allowing inferences about the role of that area in performing the task.

Another approach is to deliver a single TMS pulse to a brain area at specific times during the course of a task trial (the pulse can be delivered just before a stimulus, for example, or at a particular latency after a stimulus) and then to study its influence on task performance on that trial. An advantage of this

(A)

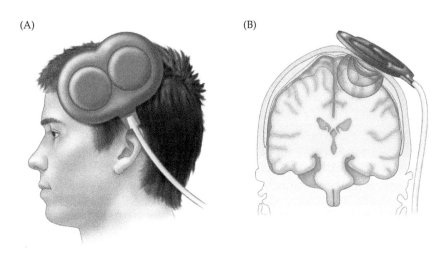

(B)

(C)

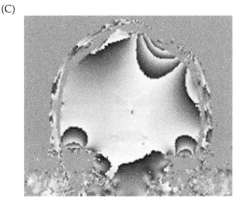

Figure 2.3 Transcranial magnetic stimulation (TMS) (A) In TMS, an electromagnetic coil is placed on the surface of the skull, in this example over the subject's left frontal lobe. (B) Rapidly reversing the flow of a very strong current within the coil induces a strong transient magnetic field in the brain. (C) The magnetic field lines associated with a TMS pulse can be seen in the upper right of the coronal MRI phase map. A common yardstick used to set the appropriate strength of stimulation for an individual is the power that needs to be delivered to the hand area of motor cortex to elicit a muscle twitch in the hand. (C courtesy of Drs. Daryl Bohning and Mark George, Medical University of South Carolina.)

approach is that it provides greater temporal resolution in assessing the role of the brain area of interest in a cognitive task.

There are, however, several important drawbacks to TMS. First, as indicated in Figure 2.3, TMS tends to affect a relatively large area, limiting anatomical resolution. Second, transcranial stimulation can be delivered effectively to only relatively superficial brain regions, primarily the more superficial regions of the cerebral cortex (typically up to 1.5 centimeters into the brain). Third, the technique can result in concurrent stimulation of scalp and head muscles, especially in attempts to stimulate certain regions of the frontal and temporal lobes, resulting in uncomfortable and even painful twitching. Finally, although TMS is in principle noninvasive, the stimulation entails some risk (e.g., strongly stimulating the brain might trigger a seizure in a person with a physiological predisposition toward epilepsy). These problems notwithstanding, the ability to transiently modulate brain function in normal subjects in this way provides an important additional tool in the quest to understand the neural bases of cognitive functions.

Another approach for performing extracranial brain stimulation is transcranial direct current stimulation (tDCS). The application of such forms of stimulation actually has a rather long history, having first been developed in the nineteenth century. It has gone in and out of favor over the years but has regained popularity of late. In tDCS a constant, low-amplitude, electrical current is applied directly to the scalp. This is accomplished with a rather simple device consisting of two electrodes, a battery, and a means of adjusting the strength of the current. One of the electrodes, typically the smaller one, is placed over the area of interest to stimulate, and the other electrode is placed elsewhere to complete the circuit. There are two main types of stimulation: *anodal* (positive) stimulation is thought to increase the cortical excitability of the area being stimulated; *cathodal* stimulation is thought to decrease the excitability. For scientific purposes, the effects of these stimulation modes are typically compared to a sham, or control, condition in which no current is delivered.

Like rTMS, tDCS appears to have effects that can last for a period of time after the stimulation (many minutes). Also like rTMS, tDCS is being used to study cognitive functions in normal individuals, as well as for treating clinical problems, including depression and chronic pain. The main disadvantages of tDCS include the spatial coarseness of the stimulation and the limited understanding of its mechanisms. Because it is inexpensive, simple, and possibly useful for scientific and clinical purposes, however, interest in this method is growing in popularity.

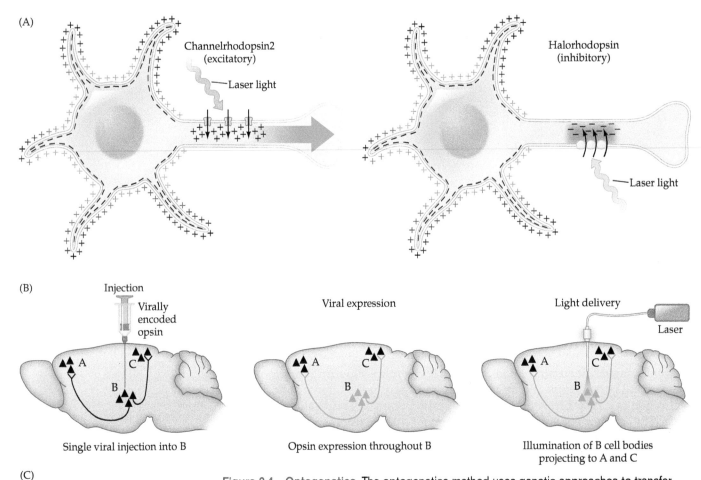

Figure 2.4 **Optogenetics** The optogenetics method uses genetic approaches to transfer light-sensitive ion channels selectively into specific sets of neurons whose activity can then be modulated with light. (A) Different versions of these genetically transferred ion channels can be either excitatory (left) or inhibitory (right) for the neuron's firing. (B) The basic principle of the method is to insert into a virus the genetic material that codes for the manufacture of photoreactive ion channels from light-sensitive algae, and then to inject the virus into a specific brain area. The expression of the inserted genetic material in the neurons of the injected area leads to the production and incorporation of these ion channels into neuronal membranes. Shining light on the brain tissue can then selectively activate (or inactivate) these neurons and modulate their signals to the other brain areas to which they project, thereby influencing behavior. (C) In the example shown here, this technique is used to modulate the walking behavior of a mouse. (B after Yihar et al. 2009.)

Optogenetics

A recently developed technique for selectively stimulating neural circuits far more specifically is **optogenetics**. Optogenetics combines genetics with the use of laser light to activate specific neural circuits or neuronal cell types in a variety of experimental settings, including in a freely moving and behaving animal. Thus, it has both high neuronal selectivity and high temporal resolution.

As described in the Appendix, the excitability of neuronal membranes is controlled by ion channels that can be induced to open or close to let ions flow into or out of the cell. Normally, such ion channels open and close in response to voltage changes across the cell membrane induced by the binding of neurotransmitters released in response to signal inputs from other neurons. The basic principle of the optogenetics method involves incorporating ion channels that open or close in response to light of a certain wavelength into the neurons of interest, thus providing a means of turning them on and off with light. Moreover, depending on the type of ion channels incorporated, the neurons can be either excited or inhibited with the light stimulation (Figure 2.4A).

The means of incorporating these light-sensitive ion channels into the brain comes from genetics. Typically, genetic material that codes for the manufacture of photoreactive ion channels is extracted from light-sensitive algae and inserted into a virus. The virus can then be injected into a particular brain area of interest (Figure 2.4B). The carrier virus infects targeted neurons near the site of injection, and the inserted genetic material then leads to the production of these light-sensitive ion channels and their incorporation into the membranes of the infected neurons. These neurons can then be selectively activated or inactivated by shining light of the appropriate wavelength on the neural tissue. The activation of these neurons in turn sends signals within their functional neural circuits, which can then selectively influence behavior. This approach has been used to modulate the walking pattern of mice (Figure 2.4C), to alter the escape response of fruit flies, and even to reduce disordered movements in mice with motor signs similar to those found in Parkinson's disease. In sum, the method of optogenetics appears to have enormous potential for cognitive neuroscience, as well as possibly for the treatment of certain clinical disorders.

Measuring Neural Activity during Cognitive Processing

The other main approach to understanding the relationship between cognitive functions and the neural processes that give rise to them is to measure brain activity while a subject performs specific cognitive tasks. In both humans and experimental animals, neural activity can be recorded and measured in various ways, and these methods are a mainstay of cognitive neuroscience.

Direct electrophysiological recording from neurons

In experimental animals, the most commonly used approach for measuring neural activity is electrophysiological recording, a method that has its roots in the pioneering neurobiological work of the late nineteenth century. The most popular modern use of this general technique has been single-neuron electrical recording, which entails measuring the action potentials produced by individual neurons (Figure 2.5; see also the Appendix). Such recordings can record neuronal firing either extracellularly (from the extracellular space adjacent to active neurons) or intracellularly (from inside a single neuron).

Extracellular recording is done with fine tungsten or steel electrodes that are inserted into the extracellular space in the cerebral cortex or deeper brain structures. The electrode can then monitor the electrical activity associated with action potentials generated by one or more neurons near the tip. Depending on the size of the electrode and its placement, the firing from several nearby neurons can be picked up concurrently, thereby assisting in the gleaning of information about the behavior of small groups of nerve cells in a region.

For **intracellular recording**, electrolyte-filled glass electrodes with a much finer tip are used. To acquire such intracellular data, a single neuron must be penetrated by the electrode tip, which then records the electrical activity from within the cell as action potentials and post-synaptic potentials are generated. Such recordings provide much more detailed information about how single neurons behave during cognitive or other functions.

Until a few decades ago, extracellular and intracellular recording were carried out on anesthetized animals, precluding experiments on cognitive functions that depend on the animals being able to execute behaviors that indicate, for example, what they may be perceiving or reacting to. More recently, however, most such electrophysiological experiments have focused on studies in awake,

(A)

(B)

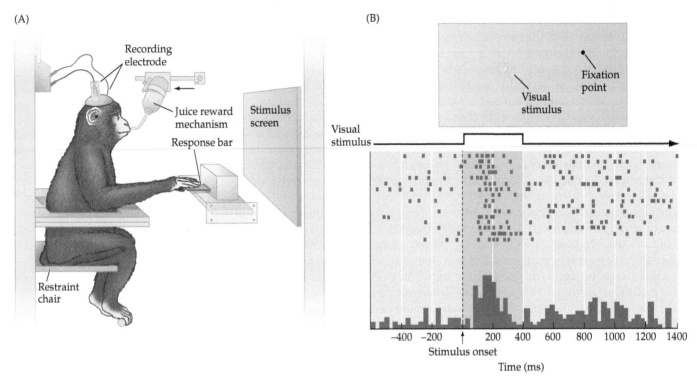

Figure 2.5 Recording single-unit activity in an awake, behaving monkey (A) An example of the experimental setup and recording apparatus in an experiment where a monkey has been trained to press a lever for a juice reward. **(B)** The data recordings in this example are made from a neuron in the visual cortex. As the monkey is presented with visual stimuli and performs a visual task (here, moving the eyes to a particular location), the neuron responds with action potentials that are recorded as ticks on what is known as a *raster plot*. In such a plot, each row corresponds to a single trial and displays a tick for each recorded action potential following a single presentation of the stimulus. These responses are summed vertically across the trials aligned in time with the stimulus onset (i.e., time-locked), yielding a peristimulus time histogram of the responses to stimulation (bottom). In this way the activity of neurons can be related to stimulus processing and the demands of the task being performed. (B after Colby et al. 1996.)

behaving animals performing specific tasks, typically after extended periods of training.

Some months prior to such experiments in behaving animals, researchers typically attach an electrode recording apparatus to the skull over a surgically exposed brain area of interest (see Figure 2.5A). This apparatus is constructed in such a way that the electrode can be moved to different positions above the brain area of interest, and also can be advanced a controlled distance into the brain tissue. After recovery from the surgery, this device allows the electrode to be adjusted in position to record from different parts and depths of the brain region below. By recording and analyzing the activity of different neurons in a series of experimental sessions in which the animal carries out cognitive tasks it has been trained to do for a reward, insight into the underlying neural processes can be obtained.

Although single-unit data can be acquired and analyzed in many ways, there are two especially useful approaches. In studies of neuronal responses to stimuli (e.g., a light flash or a sound burst), the neuronal firing pattern across time in response to the stimulus is acquired in the form of a **peristimulus time histogram (PSTH)**. As shown in Figure 2.5B, a stimulus is presented a number of times, each iteration serving as a **trial**. The neuron's responsiveness to the stimulus is determined by temporally aligning the responses following each of the trials and then summing the number of action potentials across trials into a histogram time-locked to the stimulus. Such an approach averages out random background firing when applied over enough trials, giving a much clearer picture of the average response specifically related to the stimulus processing with respect to the task being performed. More generally, the approach of averaging of the brain responses that are time-locked to repeated occurrences of various events is also used in other brain activity recording methods (to be described later in the chapter).

Another common way to analyze single-unit electrophysiological data is by using neuronal **tuning curves**. In this approach, a stimulus is varied along a particular dimension (e.g., the orientation of a line while recording from neurons in visual cortex, or the frequency of a tone while recording from auditory cortex), and the strength of the response is plotted (usually in terms of spikes per second) as a function of the stimulus parameter being varied. The resulting curve defines the selective sensitivity of the cell to some values of that stimulus parameter relative to others.

In most neural electrophysiological recording, single electrodes are used and only one brain region is investigated in each animal. Recently, however, researchers have started to employ *multielectrode recording arrays* to evaluate the concurrent responsiveness of sets of neurons in a given area of the brain or in related brain regions. For example, a single electrode might have multiple recording points along its length or protruding from its end, enabling the investigator to record simultaneously from multiple neurons distributed across the brain region of interest, such as across different cortical layers. Some researchers set up two or more such recording rigs, enabling them to measure neuronal activity simultaneously from widely separated but potentially functionally related regions of the brain. Simultaneously recorded data gathered using these approaches can then be analyzed with correlational computer algorithms to assess how neuronal activity in different parts of a putative neural circuit interacts in subserving a particular cognitive function.

Many cognitive functions can be studied with these electrophysiological methods. Some of the more basic functions, such as those underlying the sensory processing described in Chapters 3 and 4, are generally amenable to study in nonprimate experimental animals such as rodents. But studies of more complex functions (such as attention, decision making, and symbolic representation) are more typically undertaken in monkeys. Monkeys are expensive to obtain and maintain, however, and, as already mentioned, their use in such experiments can raise ethical questions. Moreover, it can take weeks or even months to train a monkey to do tasks that a human could master in only minutes.

Of course, some cognitive functions—such as those involving language or abstract reasoning—can be studied only in humans. Accordingly, over the years there has been great interest in taking advantage of circumstances in which intracranial electrophysiological recording can be performed in humans (e.g., during the presurgical cortical mapping procedures that are medically necessary in patients with epilepsy or other neurological disorders; see Introductory Box). Although the restrictions are obviously great, recordings of brain activity taken under such circumstances have provided important information about a variety of cognitive functions. Nonetheless, studying cognitive functions in humans has increasingly depended on the noninvasive electrical recording methods and brain imaging techniques described in the following sections.

Electroencephalography (EEG)

Ever since the German psychiatrist Hans Berger discovered "brain waves" in the 1920s, a preeminent way of studying human brain activity associated with

(A)

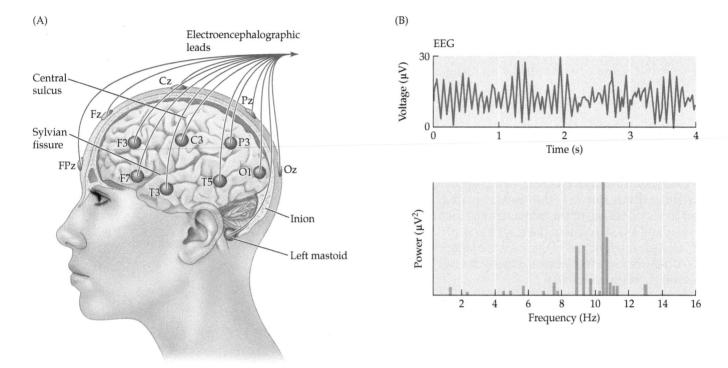

(B)

Figure 2.6 **Electroencephalographic recording (EEG)** (A) In electroencephalography, electrical potentials are recorded at different positions over the scalp relative to the voltage at a reference electrode. By historical convention, scalp locations are typically described with respect to a standardized nomenclature known as the International 10-20 or 10-10 system, in which letters indicate the position on the scalp with respect to underlying cortical regions (F, frontal; C, central; P, parietal; O, occipital; T, temporal) and the suffix numbers indicate a general position with respect to the midline (odd numbers are on the left, even numbers on the right); the suffix z indicates placement along the midline. The electrical potential recording from each electrode is somewhat different because each one samples primarily the electrical activity of large populations of neurons in the subjacent brain regions relative to a reference electrode site (here, on the left mastoid, behind the left ear). (B) Ongoing EEG activity in a normal subject with the eyes closed—a circumstance that elicits predominant activity near 10 hertz (in the alpha frequency band), as indicated in the graph at the bottom of the panel. μV = microvolts.

cognitive processes has been by means of electroencephalographic (EEG) recording. EEG recordings measure electrical brain waves that can be detected at the scalp. Compared to the methods described in the previous section, EEG recording is fully noninvasive, although it has other limitations. The method makes use of a set of surface electrodes, ranging in number from only a few to as many as 256, which typically are embedded in an elastic cap fitted over the scalp (Figure 2.6A; see also Figure 2.8). The electrodes are brought into good electrical contact with the skin by means of a conducting gel or salt paste and the pressure from the elasticity of the cap. The voltages at each electrode, along with that of a reference electrode placed elsewhere on the head (often the mastoid bone behind the ear), are fed into differential amplifiers. The amplifiers enhance the voltage differences between each electrode and the reference electrode, and the amplified signals are then digitized and recorded for subsequent analysis. The frequency of the EEG voltage fluctuations range from a fraction of 1 hertz to 100 hertz or more (Figure 2.6B).

Rather than reflecting the action potential firing typically measured in the single-neuron recordings described in the previous section, the EEG signal derives from the summed **dendritic field potentials** of groups of neurons that are varying together, as illustrated in Figure 2.7. The dendritic trees of the larger cortical neurons are generally oriented perpendicularly to the cortical surface. When, for example, there is excitatory synaptic input to the dendrites near the cell body, the voltage across the membrane of the underlying neuronal dendritic trees is depolarized by the synaptic activity (i.e., relative to its normal baseline value of approximately 70 millivolts, it becomes less negative or even reaches a positive voltage; see the Appendix). The resulting separation of charge created along the length of the dendrites causes intracellular current flow along the inside of the dendrite, as well as conduction of the return current through the tissue volume outside the dendrite. The scalp electrodes pick up the fluctuating voltages associated with these dynamically changing return currents. This interpretation of the basis of EEG is well supported by other data, such as direct intracranial recordings in experimental animals.

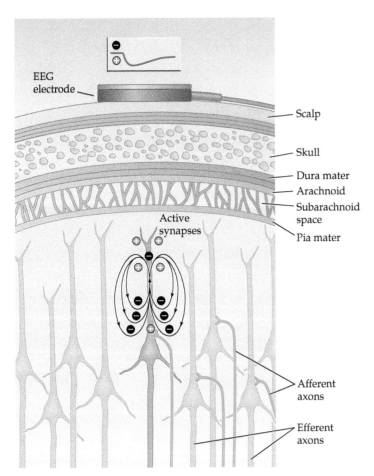

Figure 2.7 Electrophysiological basis of EEG and ERP signals Fluctuating voltages are generated when synaptic input to a cortical area results in a voltage gradient along the dendritic trees of large pyramidal neurons that are oriented more or less perpendicularly to the cortical surface. The electrode on the subject's scalp picks up the associated voltages from currents that are volume-conducted through the skull and scalp tissues outside the neuronal dendrites.

Indeed, although most intracranial recording of electrophysiological activity in animals focuses on measuring and analyzing the neuronal spikes associated with action potentials, as described in the previous section, the nonspike electrical fluctuations that occur in and around the dendritic trees of the large cortical pyramidal cells can also provide important insight into neural processing. More and more animal researchers recording intracranially are now also studying these slower-frequency dendritic field fluctuations, which are generally called **local field potentials (LFPs)** when measured intracranially, and the role they play in cognitive functions. As already described, these field potential fluctuations reflect variations in the polarization of the dendrites due to modulation by axonal input coming from other brain regions. Thus, they reflect more of the integrative processing of these large cortical neurons, rather than the output firing of the cell to other regions that is reflected in spike recordings. Note that the volume conduction of these local field potential fluctuations is what gives rise to the EEG activity that can be recorded noninvasively from the scalp.

Ongoing EEG signals measured over time are widely used in clinical settings to assess various aspects of brain function. These signals are typically analyzed in terms of the power in various **frequency bands** at each electrode location, the major bands of interest being delta (< 4 Hz), theta (4–8 Hz), alpha (8–12 Hz), beta (12–25 Hz), gamma (25–70 Hz), and, more recently, high gamma (70–150 Hz) The relative power in these bands, along with other aspects of the EEG, is very useful for assessing the overall state of the brain, such as arousal level and sleep stages (see Chapter 7), as well as for detecting and monitoring the abnormal activity associated with epilepsy.

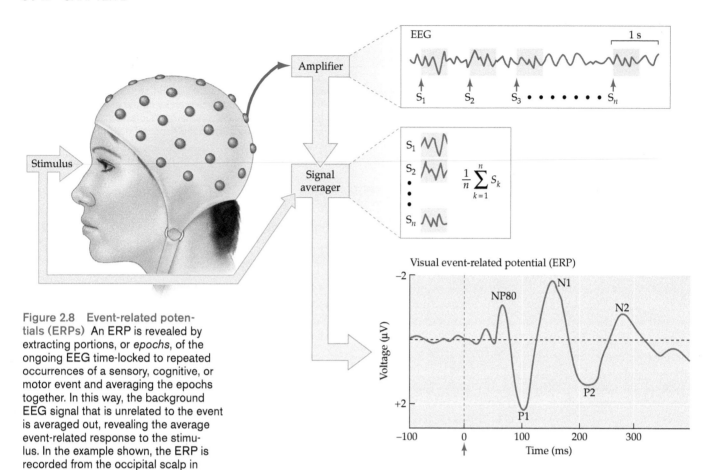

Figure 2.8 Event-related potentials (ERPs) An ERP is revealed by extracting portions, or *epochs*, of the ongoing EEG time-locked to repeated occurrences of a sensory, cognitive, or motor event and averaging the epochs together. In this way, the background EEG signal that is unrelated to the event is averaged out, revealing the average event-related response to the stimulus. In the example shown, the ERP is recorded from the occipital scalp in response to a repeated visual stimulus (S). For historical reasons, ERP traces have typically been plotted with scalp negativity upward ("negative up"); more recently, however, a number of researchers have been following the opposite scheme ("negative down"). Thus, it is important to always examine such plots for the indication of polarity. μV = microvolts.

Event-related potentials (ERPs)

Although the ongoing EEG signal is useful for assessing the overall state of the brain, its utility in investigating specific cognitive functions is relatively limited. The reason is that the ongoing EEG record is not linked in time to any particular cognitive process or event. A more effective way of relating scalp electrical activity to cognitive function is to implement a time-locked averaging approach, analogous in some ways to the peristimulus histogram process described earlier for single-neuron recordings. The most common signals to extract from the ongoing EEG in this way are **event-related potentials** (**ERPs**).

ERPs are small voltage fluctuations in an ongoing EEG triggered by sensory and cognitive events; they reflect the summed electrical activity of neuronal populations specifically responding to those events (**Figure 2.8**). As such, they can provide high temporal resolution (milliseconds) of the neural processing underlying various cognitive functions. However, because ERPs are generally smaller than the raw EEG signal in which they are embedded, it is necessary to average multiple trials to extract ERP signals from the background noise. As shown in Figure 2.8, ERPs are extracted by averaging those epochs of the EEG signal that are time-locked to repeated occurrences of a specific sensory, motor, or cognitive event. The ongoing EEG varies more or less randomly in amplitude relative to the timing of these events; these random fluctuations in the EEG tend to average out, leaving only those voltage changes specifically associated with processing of the event type of interest. An ERP obtained by such an averaging process is thus a measure of average evoked voltage changes over time, where time zero is the time of occurrence of the event.

The average ERP trace obtained in this way generally comprises a series of negative and positive peaks that are typically named according to their *electrical polarity* (*N* or *P* for negative or positive, respectively) and their *latency*; thus, for example, the *N100* specifies a negative peak 100 milliseconds after the stimulus onset. Alternatively, the peaks can be named for their *order* in the sequence (thus, the *N100* might also be referred to as the *N1*, because it is the first major negative peak).

ERPs are usually recorded while subjects are presented with various types of stimuli and are engaged in cognitive tasks related to those stimuli. Changes in the ERP responses as a function of stimulus type and task conditions are then used to infer something about the mechanisms underlying the cognitive process in question. Because the signals derive from the electrical aspects of neuronal activity, ERPs reflect that neuronal activity with very high temporal resolution, and they are thus especially useful for studies in which the timing and sequence of functional brain activity are particularly important. For example, ERPs can indicate how early attention can exert an influence on the processing of sensory input (see Chapter 6), or the time point in language processing at which the semantic analysis of a word begins (see Chapter 12).

Although the major advantage of ERPs in studying cognitive processes is high temporal resolution, information can also be gained from the *spatial distribution* of the scalp recordings as a way to gain some understanding of the likely sources of the activity (**Figure 2.9**). For example, focal activation over the occipital scalp is likely to be coming from occipital cortex, and thus to entail visual processing (see Chapters 4 and 6). Coupled with their high temporal resolution, ERP recordings can thus provide a dynamic picture of brain activity over time.

If many electrodes are used (usually at least 64), analysis algorithms can be used to estimate the locations of the neural generators producing scalp-recorded ERPs. For simple distributions, such as ERP waves that reflect relatively early sensory processing activity (or the cognitive effects on such activity), this approach can work reasonably well. There is, however, a fundamental problem

Figure 2.9 Topographical maps showing spatial-temporal patterns of ERP activity The electrode locations where the ERP data were recorded are shown by the black dots; different colors correspond to different levels of voltage across the head, after interpolating the levels between the electrodes. The result is a topographical voltage map analogous to a geographic contour map. This example shows the response across time to a visual stimulus in the left visual field, a stimulus that activates the right occipital cortex. μV = microvolts.

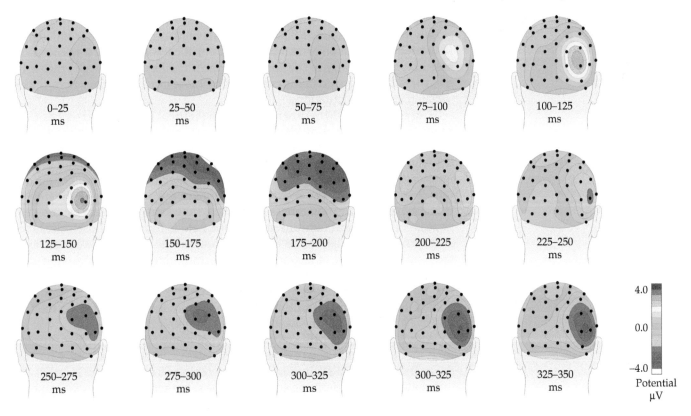

0–25 ms	25–50 ms	50–75 ms	75–100 ms	100–125 ms
125–150 ms	150–175 ms	175–200 ms	200–225 ms	225–250 ms
250–275 ms	275–300 ms	300–325 ms	300–325 ms	325–350 ms

4.0

0.0

−4.0

Potential
μV

with such analyses, which is known as the *inverse problem*: in general, a given distribution of electrical activity recorded at the scalp could have been produced by any one of a number of different sets of generators inside the head. Accordingly, such analyses, especially for more complex activity distributions and/or for studies without additional source-related information, must be viewed with caution and are an important limitation of the ERP approach. These limitations can to some degree be circumvented by combining ERP methods with other techniques or approaches, as described later in the chapter.

Although most cognitive neuroscience research using electroencephalographic techniques has made use of ERP analyses using time-locked averaging, in recent years there has been increasing interest in event-related averaging approaches applied to oscillatory activity in the EEG signal. This approach differs in several ways from earlier EEG analyses that focused on changes over a relatively extended period of time in the power of different frequency bands as a function of arousal, sleep stage, or other cognitive states. The newer approach extracts the average changes in amplitude (i.e., power) or phase coherence (i.e., how synchronized the waves are over different cortical regions) in specific frequency bands following (or possibly preceding) a specific type of cognitive event. These time-locked changes in oscillatory activity have been reported to be associated with a range of cognitive functions, including binding of perceptual features, attentional modulation, and cognitive control, and they are thought to provide an additional window into the neural processes underlying cognitive functions.

Magnetoencephalography (MEG)

Another way to measure electrophysiological brain activity noninvasively is to record the magnetic counterpart of EEG—namely, to use **magnetoencephalography**, or **MEG**. Much as ERPs can be extracted from EEG recordings by time-locked averaging to a set of stimulus events, this method can be used to extract time-locked responses, called event-related magnetic-field responses (ERFs), from ongoing MEG signals. The generation of MEG/ERF signals is closely related to that of EEG/ERP signals because both arise from current flow triggered by depolarization in the dendritic trees of cortical neurons oriented perpendicularly to the cortical surface. The key difference is that MEG measures the magnetic fields produced by these currents rather than the associated voltage fluctuations.

The principles of MEG are illustrated in Figure 2.10. When current flows in a wire or other conducting element, it produces a magnetic field in the volume surrounding the wire (Figure 2.10A). The configuration of the field follows the "right-hand rule" taught in introductory physics: if the right hand is made into a fist with the thumb pointing out and oriented in the direction of the current, then the field curves around the current in the orientation of the fingers. When synaptic activation causes currents to flow along the dendritic trees of a population of cortical neurons, a magnetic field is induced whose orientation is governed by the right-hand rule. This induced magnetic field "comes out of the head" on one side of the current source and "enters the head" on the other (Figure 2.10B). If the field strengths are measured at different points on the surface of the head with a magnetometer (Figure 2.10C), the distribution of these values over space and time can be obtained, including whether they are positive (coming out of the head) or negative (going into the head).

Although initially MEG recordings were made from only a few sites at a time, modern machines record fields from sites over the entire head. Knowing the measured field distribution makes it possible to estimate the location and orientation of the underlying source, but the same general limitations imposed

(A)
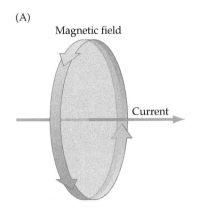

(B)
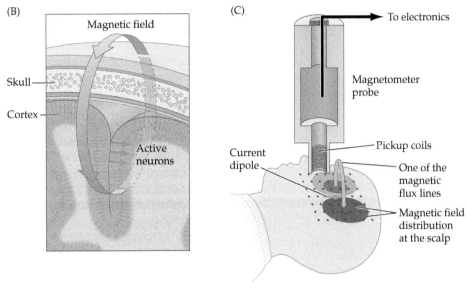

(C)

Figure 2.10 Magnetoencephalographic signals (MEG) (A) An electrical current in a wire creates a circular magnetic field. (B) Dendritic currents in cortex also produce circular magnetic fields, analogous to those produced by the current in a wire. Note that the fields most easily measured are generated in the sulci, because those fields enter and exit the scalp orthogonally, allowing them to be detected well by a magnetometer outside the head. Fields generated by neural activity in the gyri generally produce magnetic fields oriented parallel to the scalp, which are more difficult to detect. (C) The magnetic fields produced by brain activity can be measured by a magnemometer positioned adjacent to the head. (D) Distribution of the magnetic fields (the M100 wave at 100 ms) over the head of a normal subject induced by an auditory stimulus; the MR image on the right shows the estimated location of the underlying source derived by dipole source analysis. fT = femtoteslas. (D after Woldorff et al. 1999.)

(D) MEG response to left-ear sounds

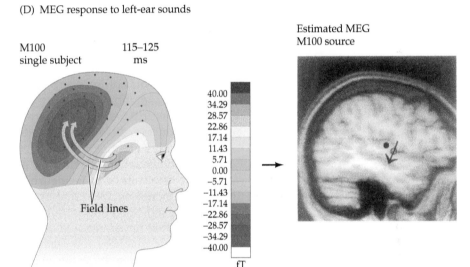

by the inverse problem for EEG recordings (described earlier) apply to MEG as well.

Although the MEG/ERF and EEG/ERP methodologies are related, they have practical as well as physical differences. One important difference concerns the brain areas that the two techniques can most successfully assess. MEG is sensitive mainly to neuronal activity in the cortical valleys, or sulci; it is relatively insensitive to activity in gyri (see Figure 2.10B). This sensitivity to sulcal activity is due to the orientation of the electrical currents that generate the magnetic fields. As noted earlier, these currents generally arise from the dendritic trees of the large cortical pyramidal neurons oriented perpendicularly to the cortical surface (see Figure 2.7). If the underlying electrical currents flowing along these dendritic trees are in a sulcus, they produce fields that either enter or exit the head more or less orthogonally, as shown in Figure 2.10C, and are picked up well by the magnetometer. However, neuronal activity in a cortical gyrus produces currents that are mostly perpendicular to the surface of the head, inducing magnetic fields that are mostly parallel to the head surface and thus do not register well on the magnetometer. In contrast, the electrodes that pick up EEG and ERP signals detect voltage fluctuations produced by the return-volume currents, which are not affected by this limitation. Accordingly, EEG picks up voltage fluctuations from sources in both cortical gyri and sulci, although it tends to be more sensitive to the former.

Although MEG's insensitivity to gyral sources renders it less complete than EEG methods, what MEG *does* pick up (i.e., mainly sulcal activity) is easier to localize—for two main reasons: First, EEG currents suffer some distortion as they are conducted through the variable resistances of the skull and other tissues to reach the recording electrodes on the scalp. The magnetic fields in MEG recordings are much less affected by this problem. In addition, because MEG picks up mainly sulcal sources (and best from those nearer the magnetometer), the signal distributions it records tend to be less complex than those from ERP signals, thereby simplifying source estimation. Given their complementary sensitivities, recording by MEG and EEG methods together can offer a more complete and effective way to estimate sources and study mechanisms than does either method alone.

Positron emission tomography (PET) imaging

Probably the most popular techniques today for assessing brain activity related to cognitive functions are those that rely on measuring changes in metabolism and blood flow to visualize active areas of the brain. The attractiveness of these functional brain imaging methods arises from several factors, but derives mainly from their ability to produce images that localize brain activity with high spatial resolution.

The brain utilizes a remarkably large fraction (20 percent) of the body's energy resources, despite representing only about 2 percent of body mass, and at any given moment the most active nerve cells use more of these and other metabolites than do relatively quiescent neurons. To meet the increased metabolic demands of active neurons, the local flow of blood to the relevant brain area increases. Detecting and mapping these local changes in cerebral metabolism and blood flow is the hemodynamic basis of two functional imaging techniques that have been widely used: positron emission tomography (PET) and functional magnetic resonance imaging (fMRI). Because these techniques reveal patterns of activity in the whole intact brain with good spatial resolution, they have greatly advanced our ability to study cognitive functions and their neural underpinnings.

In **positron emission tomography**, or **PET**, unstable positron-emitting isotopes are synthesized in a cyclotron by bombarding elements such as oxygen, carbon, or fluorine with protons. Because of its short half-life, the isotope most commonly used for PET functional mapping has been ^{15}O (oxygen-15, with a half-life of 2 minutes), which is incorporated into water molecules for this activity-mapping use. When the radiolabeled compounds are injected into the bloodstream, they become distributed in the brain according to current physiological needs, accumulating preferentially in more metabolically active areas.

As the unstable isotope decays, the extra proton breaks down into a neutron and an emitted positron. The emitted positron travels several millimeters, on average, until it collides with an electron. The collision of a positron with an electron destroys both particles, emitting two gamma rays that travel in opposite directions from the site of the collision. Gamma-ray detectors placed around the subject's head are arranged to register a "hit" only when two detectors 180 degrees apart react simultaneously (Figure 2.11A,B). By reconstructing the density of these collision lines using computer algorithms, the location of the active regions can be imaged. The PET images of activity can then be superimposed onto magnetic resonance structural images from the same subject(s)

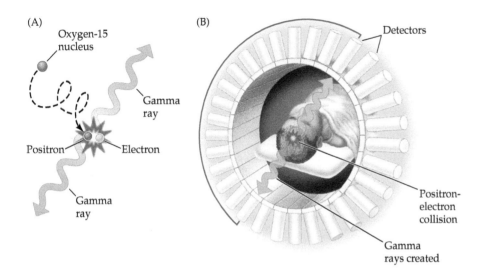

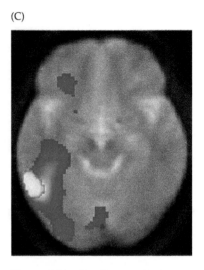

Figure 2.11 Positron emission tomography (PET) (A) In PET, molecules labeled with radioactive probe atoms such as ^{15}O are injected into the bloodstream. These agents travel preferentially to areas of increased neural activity because of increased metabolism and thus blood flow to those areas. Radioactive decay ultimately emits two "annihilation photons" (gamma rays) in opposite directions. (B) The annihilation photons are detected by sensors surrounding the head of the subject lying in the PET scanner. (C) A PET activation image overlaid on a structural magnetic resonance image. (C courtesy of David Madden.)

to provide spatial information about specific brain areas involved in cognitive and other functions (Figure 2.11C).

The mean distance that the positrons travel in brain tissue before the gamma-producing collision with an electron limits the theoretical resolution of PET scanning to several millimeters, although true resolution is typically considerably lower because of spatial smoothing and other steps in the analysis. An even greater limitation of PET, however, is the time required to accumulate an adequate signal, which precludes its use in many cognitive paradigms. In particular, PET activation imaging requires accumulating signal over the period of about a minute or so (i.e., the signal to obtain a usable image must be compiled over this time frame), and thus it has essentially no temporal resolution. As a result, functional imaging experiments using PET require a **blocked design**. In this design, the brain activity measured reflects neural activity integrated over an extended period (a block) while the subject performs a task or is presented with a particular stimulus condition. The resulting activation pattern can then be compared to the activity recorded during a different block of time in which the subject is not doing the task or is under a different condition. The need to integrate activity across time in this way thus substantially limits the specificity with which brain activation can be associated with particular cognitive processes.

The various limitations of PET (the short half-life of the reagents, the need for a nearby cyclotron to create the reagents, the use of radioactivity, and the very poor temporal resolution) have led to its replacement in most cognitive studies today by functional magnetic resonance imaging.

Functional magnetic resonance imaging (functional MRI or fMRI)

Functional magnetic resonance imaging (fMRI; Figure 2.12A) is based on the fact that oxyhemoglobin (hemoglobin carrying a bound oxygen molecule) and deoxyhemoglobin (the oxygen-depleted form of hemoglobin) have different magnetic resonance signals. As noted already, active brain areas use more oxygen than relatively inactive areas, and thus require more local blood flow. Within a second or two after an area has been activated by a specific cognitive event or task, the related microvasculature responds to the resulting local oxygen depletion by increasing the flow of new, oxyhemoglobin-rich, arterial blood to the active area (Figure 2.12B). The relative concentration of deoxyhemoglobin decreases over the next few seconds, leading to localized changes in the magnetic resonance (MR) signal from that part of the brain (Figure 2.12C).

(A)

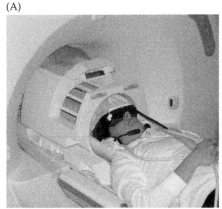

Figure 2.12 **Functional magnetic resonance imaging (fMRI)** (A) A subject is moved into an MRI scanner for functioal MR imaging. The machine itself is not different from the scanner shown and described in Box 2A. The subject is wearing goggles in order to view visual stimuli for the experiment to be undertaken. (B) The blood oxygenation level–dependent (BOLD) signal. The vascular system supplies blood containing oxyhemoglobin to active regions of the brain. The influx of oxygenated blood to regions that become active reduces the local concentration of deoxyhemoglobin, which increases the BOLD signal; the difference in the signal provides a measure of local neuronal activity. (C) There are several ways to display functional MRI data on corresponding structural MRI scans, including overlaying onto an image slice; overlaying onto a three-dimensional image of the cortical surface extracted computationally from the MR structural image data; or overlaying onto the three-dimensional image of an extracted cortical surface that has been "inflated" by a computer algorithm. (B after Huettel et al. 2009.)

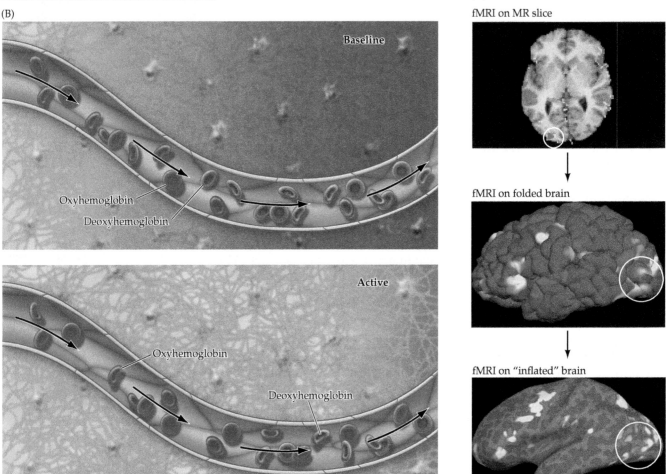

(B)

Baseline

Oxyhemoglobin

Deoxyhemoglobin

Active

Oxyhemoglobin

Deoxyhemoglobin

(C)

fMRI on MR slice

fMRI on folded brain

fMRI on "inflated" brain

These MR changes, known as the **blood oxygenation level–dependent (BOLD)** signal, are the basis of most current forms of fMRI.

Functional MRI offers better spatial localization than PET (several millimeters compared to approximately a centimeter in PET), as well as much better temporal resolution (a few seconds compared to a minute or more in PET). In addition, fMRI uses endogenous signals intrinsic to normal brain function rather than signals originating from exogenous, radioactively labeled probes. But probably the greatest advantage of fMRI over PET for the study of cognitive processes is its much higher temporal resolution.

Figure 2.13 Experimental designs in PET and fMRI studies (A) In PET functional imaging studies, which necessarily employ a block design, the subject performs a cognitive task continuously over approximately 1 minute, with different tasks being performed in each block (in this example either task A or B, or, in the resting block, neither). If ^{15}O-labeled water is used as the tracer, a 10-minute break between blocks is necessary to allow the radioactively labeled tracers to decay sufficiently before the next block. Accumulated activity for each block is then measured, and functional activity is inferred by comparing the different blocks. (B) The block design for fMRI is similar, but with multiple samples of brain activity in each block, much shorter blocks, and no need for a 10-minute break between blocks. (C) Because of the much faster activity sampling possible with fMRI (typically every 1.5 to 2 seconds), the fMRI responses to individual events can be captured in an event-related way. Shown is a representative fMRI response to a single event type (event type A). (D) This paradigm allows the time-locked responses to different event types within the same run to be selectively extracted (i.e., event types A and B).

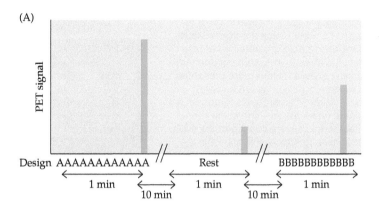

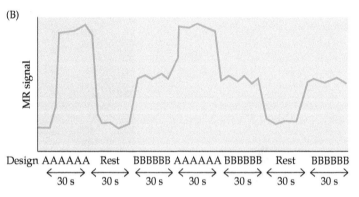

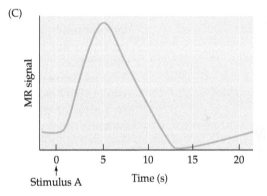

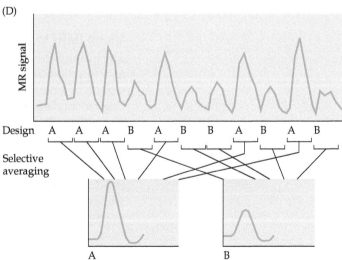

Most initial fMRI studies in the early 1990s followed the same blocked design as PET studies (Figure 2.13A), although the blocks were only around 20 to 30 seconds, as compared to a minute, and there was no need for a long waiting period between blocks (Figure 2.13B). However, investigators soon realized that fMRI had enough temporal resolution to allow an **event-related design**. Today, samples of fMRI activity throughout the whole brain can be acquired in a second or two, allowing the average fMRI hemodynamic response to a single stimulus or cognitive event type to be captured. The fMRI response to a stimulus or cognitive event begins at about 1 to 2 seconds, peaks at about 5 to 6 seconds, and returns to baseline at about 12 to 15 seconds (Figure 2.13C). Although this sequence is very slow relative to the millisecond resolution of electrophysiological methods such as EEG, MEG, or single-unit recording, it is fast enough to allow fMRI to be applied in an event-related manner, at least when stimuli are presented at a moderately slow rate. As shown in Figure 2.13D, this capability allows selective averaging of the responses to different event types *within* a run, much as is done with electrophysiological methods. Moreover, using temporal randomization of the stimulus or task events and modern signal processing algorithms that effectively disentangle the overlapping responses from successive stimuli, it is now possible to present stimuli at faster rates and still extract an event-related response (Figure 2.14).

The development of event-related methods for fMRI was a highly significant advance, as it enabled many cognitive paradigms that had not been possible in the early days of fMRI. Moreover, improved analytic techniques in event-related paradigms made it possible to link the *behavioral* measures from trial to trial to the

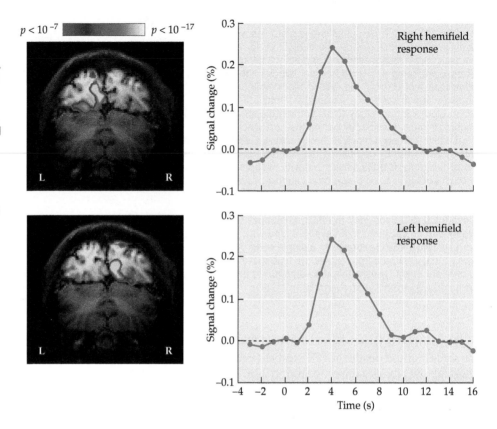

Figure 2.14 Event-related fMRI responses Responses are from a visual stimulation paradigm obtained at fast stimulus rates (two events per second). Unilateral visual stimuli were presented in random order to the left and right visual fields while subjects fixated on a central cross. At this high stimulation rate, there is severe overlap of the fMRI responses to successive stimuli in the sequence. The overlap was eliminated in this example by a subtraction technique, yielding clean average hemodynamic fMRI responses (right panels) in the visual sensory areas in contralateral occipital cortex (left panels). (After Burock et al. 1998.)

corresponding fMRI *neural* responses in different brain regions. In particular, variations in a behavioral measure (e.g., the reaction time) could be examined with respect to how they co-varied with the amplitudes of the corresponding fMRI responses from trial to trial. The development of event-related paradigms using fMRI has also allowed researchers to compare the response images with the activation patterns of high-temporal-resolution ERP and ERF responses to the same types of events. In addition, modern fMRI techniques allow the use of "hybrid," or "mixed," designs that have both block- and event-related experimental manipulations, the effects of which can be disentangled by appropriate analyses.

As a result of its many advantages, fMRI has emerged today as the dominant technology for imaging brain activation in studies of both normal and abnormal cognitive function.

Using fMRI to analyze activation patterns within a brain area

The bulk of fMRI research has focused on activations of various brain areas as a function of a specific manipulated variable, such as the presentation of stimuli of a particular type, under particular cognitive conditions. Yet, as later chapters make plain, the cortex possesses considerable local organization within particular areas, and these organizational characteristics are often functionally important. Although such local characteristics may be reflected in intervoxel differences in fMRI, standard fMRI analysis does not typically take them into consideration. Indeed, researchers usually apply spatial smoothing to their fMRI data to increase sensitivity, and they require activations to be of a specified minimum number of voxels to be meaningful. Both of these strategies tend to obscure differences between nearby voxels.

A number of approaches aimed at addressing this problem are based on what are known as **pattern classification** algorithms. In particular, within fMRI, researchers use an analysis scheme called **multivoxel pattern analysis (MVPA)** for such purposes, which looks at patterns of activation across voxels that consistently correspond to a particular stimulus type or event type, rather than the overall increase or decrease in activation of a large brain region. For example, in an area of the lateral occipital cortex that is generally responsive to objects, images of cars may activate the area about as much as houses and tools do, at least collapsed across all the voxels of the "object analysis" area. But one type of visual object may induce a particular pattern of activation among those voxels that is consistently different from the pattern that objects of a different class would induce. MVPA specifically analyzes whether such trial-related activation patterns are indeed consistently observed. In addition, these sorts of analyses can be used to predict the patterns of activation for new examples of the different stimulus types. Such approaches have thereby enabled, for example, inferring from brain activation data the particular type of stimulus a participant is likely looking at. Thus, these sorts of pattern analysis approaches are becoming increasingly popular in cognitive neuroscience fMRI research.

Repetition suppression is another way researchers have endeavored to assess functional characteristics of a brain area that respond similarly to different stimulus classes in overall activation magnitude (**Figure 2.15**). This technique rests on the tendency of areas of the brain to respond less to the repeated occurrence of an identical (or closely similar) stimulus than to the first presentation of the stimulus. In fMRI, the version of this approach most commonly used is known as **fMRI adaptation**. The use of fMRI adaptation to enhance the understanding of a brain region is based on the assumption that if that region shows repetition suppression for the second stimulus in a pair (e.g., the target in a particular prime-target combination), then the two stimuli must share a process supported in some way by that region. Thus, by manipulating the relationship between primes and targets, it is possible to constrain hypotheses regarding the function of a particular brain region. For example, the lateral occipital region mentioned in the previous example as being activated during the processing of visual objects showed repetition suppression for repeated objects (e.g., an image of a table) even when the two stimuli were presented in different formats (e.g., as a drawing versus as a photo) or with different angular views. This finding suggests that the lateral occipital complex is concerned with processing an object's abstract properties rather than the details of its sensory features.

In some instances, fMRI adaptation can provide additional information about the processing role of a brain region that standard fMRI methods cannot. For example, in conventional fMRI, comparing two stimulus conditions A and B may fail to reveal differences between them because the populations of neurons sensitive to these conditions (or two stimulus types) are mixed within the same brain region being sampled (see Figure 2.15A). In contrast, in the fMRI adaptation paradigm, the subpopulations of neurons sensitive to stimulus A may show adaptation when this stimulus is repeated, giving rise to a lower fMRI signal than that elicited for stimulus B (see Figure 2.15B).

Figure 2.15 Repetition suppression in fMRI studies (A) A conventional fMRI experiment may fail to distinguish between responses to stimulus A and stimulus B because the two stimuli activate different populations of neurons (orange versus blue in the figure) within the same brain region sampled; hence the total fMRI signal may be similar. (B) Using a form of repetition suppression (fMRI adaptation), it may be possible to detect a difference in fMRI signal within this brain region. When the subpopulation of neurons sensitive to stimulus A adapts, the signal is reduced for a repetition of stimulus A but strong for stimulus B. (After Kourtzi and Grill-Spector 2005.)

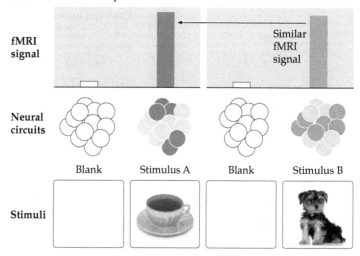

(A) Standard fMRI experiment

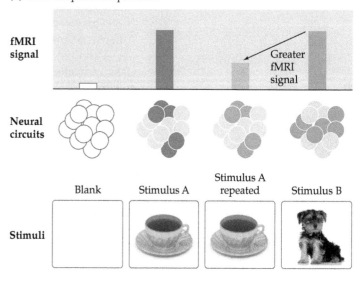

(B) fMRI adaptation experiment

Using fMRI to examine activity relationships between brain areas

Most neuroimaging studies in cognitive neuroscience build on the concept of localization of function—namely, that different brain regions support different types of information processing. However, brain regions do not participate in cognitive brain function in isolation. Information flows between regions via the action potential signals transmitted by axons, which are bundled together into large **fiber tracts**. Although an enormous amount of knowledge has been gained about such anatomical connections, knowledge of the structural connections between brain regions can provide only a limited picture of information flow in the brain. Understanding of the **functional connectivity**, or how the activity of one brain region varies with the activity in another brain region, is also needed.

Functional MRI can help elucidate the functional relationships between brain regions because of its ability to acquire functional activation data both from across the whole brain and from across time. The simplest type of relationship between regions is **coactivation**, in which two or more brain regions change similarly in response to an experimental condition. A straightforward and rather complementary way to show that two (or more) regions share functional connectivity comes from studies of **resting-state connectivity**, which identify fMRI signal fluctuations that co-vary across brain regions while subjects lie in the MRI scanner but do not perform an experimental task. These co-variations are thought to reflect spontaneously occurring operations of the brain rather than the processing of specific external stimuli.

One way to extract the distributed patterns of common activation that occur during rest is to use data exploration techniques such as *principal component analysis (PCA)* or *independent component analysis (ICA)*, which use algorithms for extracting similarly behaving portions of a complex data set. Alternatively, one can choose a *seed voxel* or group of voxels in a specific region of interest and determine which other regions exhibit similar fluctuations in activation over time. Using these approaches, researchers have found co-varying activation in groups of regions that have been implicated in other studies as being involved in visual, auditory, memory, and attentional functions. In general, regions that are coactivated during cognitive tasks also tend to show resting-state connectivity, suggesting that brain regions with common functionality tend to express similar patterns of spontaneous activity. Combining resting-state and task-related connectivity within the same study can strengthen conclusions about the relationships between brain regions, by building on the findings of one to explore the other. Moreover, explicit information on the structural connections between brain areas in individual subjects, such as can be obtained with diffusion tensor imaging (DTI; see Box 2B) can also help with these analyses.

Although finding that two brain areas are both activated during a particular task indicates that the two regions are related, it does not tell us much about the form of that relationship. For example, consider a task entailing attending to a visual scene to search for faces. Such a task (relative to a baseline task) will elicit enhanced activity in the dorsolateral prefrontal cortex, the inferior parietal sulcus, and face-processing areas in ventral occipital cortex. Such a coactivation might suggest that these various areas are involved in the task, but we would not know how they work together to accomplish that task. For example, top-down influences from the prefrontal cortex might be guiding the activity in the other regions. Another possibility is that visual processing in the ventral occipital cortex is triggering activity in the other areas in a bottom-up fashion. On the other hand, the activity in all of these regions may be controlled by signals from another region of the brain.

A variety of methods have been developed to gain further insight into the relationships between brain areas and their activation patterns. In one approach for combining fMRI and behavioral data, **psychophysiological interaction (PPI) analysis** is used. Like some other connectivity approaches, PPI analysis uses the time course of activity in one seed region to predict changes in activity in another region. However, the technique analyzes how these interactions differ as a function of the cognitive task being performed. For example, it analyzes whether the correlation in activity between the two areas, rather than activity itself, differs in one task versus another.

A significant shortcoming of fMRI (and indeed most other neural activity monitoring methods) is its difficulty in establishing *causality* in the interactions between brain areas—that is, whether activity in one brain area caused activity in another. Suppose that two regions, A and B, are coactivated in an fMRI study in a particular task. Is it possible to infer from the fMRI data whether activation in Region A caused changes in Region B, activation in Region B caused changes in Region A, or activation in both of these regions was induced by signals from another brain area?

Some modeling approaches, such as **structural equation modeling**, have endeavored to infer causality from fMRI activation patterns by incorporating known anatomical connections, comparing models with different hypothesized sets of directional influences between areas, and identifying which model best accounts for the observed data. For example, an early application of this approach to studying attention found that the best model for the activation patterns suggested that attention-related signals from the prefrontal cortex increased the connectivity between the extrastriate visual areas and the posterior parietal cortex. Related approaches include **dynamic causal modeling**, which creates models of the functional connections between brain regions, and then evaluates how that connectivity changes as a result of experimental manipulations.

In summary, delineating the functional connectivity relationships between brain regions shown to be activated in fMRI tasks is critical for understanding how these regions work together to accomplish cognitive functions. The ongoing development and application of these various approaches for analyzing functional connectivity relationships will continue to improve the inferences that can be made from fMRI data.

Optical brain imaging

Another way to measure neural activity in both animals and humans is based on optical imaging techniques. These approaches derive from the fact that active brain tissue transmits and/or reflects light differently than does inactive brain tissue, and these differences can be picked up and imaged by optical recording devices.

One such approach is, like fMRI, based on hemodynamic changes in response to neural activity. When populations of neurons become active, thereby inducing local hemodynamic changes, the amount of light reflected from the cortical surface changes as well. This optical signal, as with the BOLD signal in fMRI, is thought to arise from changes in the relative concentrations of oxyhemoglobin and deoxyhemoglobin that occur as neuronal activity varies in a given region in response to a stimulus. To detect these changes requires that the skull be opened and the cortical surface illuminated with a red light in the 580- to 700-nanometer range. The reflected light is picked up by a sensitive video camera, and the changes in responses to stimulation are averaged over a series of trials. The resulting images can provide a highly detailed map of the cortical patterns of activity.

These hemodynamically based optical imaging approaches have been most successfully applied to studying sensory map representations in the sensory cortices in animals, particularly in visual sensory cortex. For example, this type of imaging has produced highly detailed maps of the patterns of relative sensitivity across primary visual cortex to specific line orientations (see Chapter 3). These methods have also been useful in showing the relationships between the mapping configurations for different features, such as the relationship between line orientation preference maps and ocular dominance maps. Because the technique is invasive, it has been used mostly in experimental animals, and the results have thus far tended to be more informative in the context of neurobiology than cognitive neuroscience. Nonetheless, it has been used in a few circumstances in human patients undergoing neurosurgery (e.g., to map language areas). Because of its simplicity and relatively low cost, such optical imaging would seem to have considerable promise for future studies of cognitive functions in both experimental animals and neurosurgical patients.

Another technique, known as **event-related optical signals** (**EROS**), uses optical methods based on a very different activity-dependent mechanism and can be applied noninvasively. When brain tissue is illuminated, even through the skull, the amount of light that is transmitted versus scattered varies as a function of whether the neuronal tissue is electrically active. This differential light diffusion is thought to arise from changes that occur in neuronal membranes and their immediate surroundings during electrical activity. By shining light into the brain from a number of different sources around the head and measuring the intensity of the reflected light with multiple external sensors, these activity-dependent changes can be detected and imaged using three-dimensional, computer-assisted reconstruction algorithms.

Like ERPs, EROS has high temporal resolution but relatively low spatial resolution. However, determination of the sources of the measured activity is not subject to the inverse problem inherent in EEG and MEG source analyses. Although the relatively low signal-to-noise characteristics have limited the use of this method, EROS holds significant promise as a useful method for noninvasively imaging cognition-related cortical activity.

Assembling Evidence and Delineating Mechanisms

A major goal in the quest to understand the neural bases of cognition is to establish links between localized brain structures and neural activity on the one hand, and cognitive functions or processes on the other. To establish these links and delineate underlying mechanisms, cognitive neuroscientists often assemble evidence from multiple studies and data gleaned through the implementation of multiple methodologies.

Associations and dissociations

One approach to linking neuroscience and cognition is apparent in the methods already discussed: to experimentally associate specific cognitive functions with the neural structures and/or local neural activity that underlie them. A complementary approach is to determine cognitive functions and neural processes that do *not* seem to be related—that is, that are dissociated. For example, finding that damage to a particular brain area disrupts the performance of Task A but not Task B establishes not only an association between the damaged area and Task A, but also a dissociation between the lesion and Task B (Figure 2.16A).

An even firmer link between a specific cognitive function and a particular neural structure or process can be made by establishing a **double dissociation**. For example, suppose Task A is designed to engage mainly System A (say, the neural system for identifying a visually presented face), whereas Task B is designed to engage mainly System B (the neural system for identifying the emotional expression of a visually presented face). If Systems A and B are relatively distinct, one would expect to be able to find neurological patients

(A) One group of lesion patients

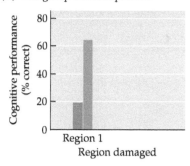

(B) Two groups of lesion patients

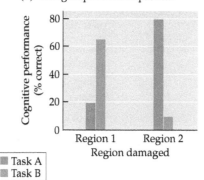

■ Task A
■ Task B

(C) Brain activation

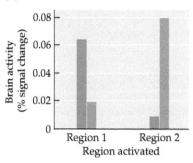

Figure 2.16 Associations, dissociations, and double dissociations (A) The relative performance on two tasks (A and B) for neurological patients with a common brain lesion in Region 1. Impairment in performing Task A but not Task B indicates an association between Region 1 and the neural basis for performing Task A, and a dissociation between this region and performing Task B. (B) Two groups of patients, one with lesions as Region 1, as in panel (A), plus another group of patients with lesions in a different brain region (Region 2) who show the opposite pattern of impairment in the two tasks. The results from the two patient groups taken together are a double dissociation providing strong evidence for the specific involvement of the two regions in the two different tasks. (C) Analogous double dissociation determined from brain activation data (e.g., from fMRI). In this case, subjects engaged in Task A show activation of Region 1 but not Region 2; during Task B this pattern is reversed.

with a particular brain lesion who are impaired in performing Task A (recognizing faces), but essentially normal when performing Task B (recognizing emotions), and to find patients with a lesion in a different brain region who showed the opposite pattern (normal performance on Task A but impaired performance on Task B). This pattern of effects constitutes a classic double dissociation (Figure 2.16B).

Double dissociations provide more definitive evidence for relatively separate mechanisms or functions than do single dissociations. This is because a single dissociation could arise from a general factor (such as the relative difficulty of the tasks) rather than from the engagement of separable functions. However, when another type of lesion produces the opposite, or at least quite different, characteristics, the case for the engagement of functionally distinct neural systems becomes much stronger. It often turns out, however, that the neural systems being examined are only partially separable; that is, performance on Task A for a certain patient group is seriously impaired, but performance on Task B is also disturbed to some degree (or vice versa). This situation would suggest that the functional systems in question interact to some degree—which of course is useful information as well.

Although these examples focus on establishing dissociations using brain lesions, double dissociations are also important in methods that measure brain activity during cognitive tasks (Figure 2.16C). For example, a neuroimaging experiment might indicate that a specific brain area (say, Region 1) is *activated* during Task A but not during Task B. As with brain lesion studies, however, this neuroimaging pattern could be due to differing difficulty of the two tasks or to the degree to which a neural system is being engaged by the task. Thus, establishing a double dissociation in the context of neuroimaging (i.e., finding that another brain area, Region 2, is activated during Task B but not during Task A) is also important for more firmly linking specific brain activity measures to specific cognitive functions.

TABLE 2.1 Summary of the Major Imaging Techniques Used in Cognitive Neuroscience

TECHNIQUE	MAIN ADVANTAGES	MAIN DISADVANTAGES
Naturally occurring lesions	Can strongly implicate a region as being essential for a task	Still generally need double dissociation to strongly confirm selectivity of area
	Occur naturally	Not specific to functional areas; variable in distribution and extent
		Do not identify a network
		No temporal resolution
		Relatively few available subjects; subjects often from heterogeneous groups
		Effects of recovery unknown or complex
Directed lesions	Can strongly implicate a region as being essential for a task	Can generally be done only in animals; ethical concerns
	Can be much more selective than naturally occurring lesions	Very limited temporal resolution
	Can be timed (e.g., before or after training)	
Intracranial stimulation	Can provide rather specific neural perturbation	Mostly limited to animals and rare clinical circumstances
		In humans, clinical concerns, limited locations that can be stimulated
Transcranial magnetic stimulation (TMS)	Advantages of lesions, but transient and noninvasive (or at least nonsurgical)	Mostly can do only superficial cortex
	With single shot, can get some temporal resolution	Not very focused; stimulates other areas nearby and above the target area
		Even for some superficial brain regions, is too uncomfortable
		Some safety issues, particularly for repetitive TMS (rTMS)
Single-unit recordings	High spatial and temporal resolution	Picks up only some neurons (typically larger ones)
	Very specific (single neurons)	Very invasive; almost completely limited to animals
		Typically from only one brain area, thus does not identify a network or network interactions
Electroencephalography (EEG)	Good temporal resolution	Coarse or problematic spatial resolution
	Good for state effects (e.g., arousal, sleep stages)	Not very specific for information processing or cognitive function
	Noninvasive	
	Inexpensive, fast, and easy recording procedures	

Multimethodological approaches

All of the individual methods described here provide a way of linking cognitive processes to underlying brain processes. Each has advantages and disadvantages. The spatial and temporal ranges of these approaches were depicted in Figure 1.6. The most important advantages and disadvantages of each method are described in Table 2.1.

TABLE 2.1 *(continued)*

TECHNIQUE	MAIN ADVANTAGES	MAIN DISADVANTAGES
Event-related potentials (ERPs)	Very high temporal resolution	Coarse or problematic spatial resolution
	Noninvasive	Difficult to disentangle multicomponent activity
	Inexpensive, fast, and easy recording procedures	Activity may be associated with but not essential for the task
Magnetoencephalography (MEG)	Very high temporal resolution	Picks up mainly only sulcal activity
	Better localization than ERPs	Limited spatial localization
	Noninvasive	Much more expensive than ERPs
		Recordings very susceptible to interfering noise
		Activity may be associated with but not essential for task
Positron emission tomography (PET)	Good spatial resolution (three dimensional)	No temporal resolution
	Identifies network of regions associated with task	Cannot do event-related designs (block design only)
		Need cyclotron
		Need to inject radioactive molecules
		Indirect measurement of neuronal activity
		Activated areas may be associated with but not essential for the task
Functional magnetic resonance imaging (fMRI)	Very good spatial resolution	Spatial resolution still has limits (e.g., draining veins)
	Temporal resolution much better than PET	Temporal resolution still very low (typically a few seconds)
	Can do event-related designs	Indirect measurement of neuronal activity
	Identifies network of regions associated with task	Activated areas may be associated with but not essential for the task
	Noninvasive	
Optical imaging (hemodynamic)	High spatial resolution	Almost exclusively limited to animals
	Temporal resolution a bit better than fMRI	Temporal resolution still fairly low (hundreds of milliseconds)
	Can do event-related designs	Indirect measurement of neuronal activity
	Can image all across a cortical area simultaneously	Activated areas may be associated with but not essential for the task
Optical imaging (EROS)	Moderate spatial resolution	Low signal-to-noise ratio; may require multiple sessions or be able to image only limited brain regions
	Good temporal resolution	Mainly sensitive to the more superficial cortical regions
	Noninvasive	Activated areas may be associated with but not essential for the task

The different limitations of each of these methods, as well as their complementary scales, have led to a growing effort to combine approaches in the same or closely allied studies. For example, hemodynamic measures of brain activity like fMRI are very good at showing which areas of the brain are activated in a given cognitive task or type of event, but they provide relatively limited temporal resolution (on the order of seconds). Since many cognitive operations occur on the order of tens or hundreds of milliseconds, fMRI cannot indicate the timing or sequence of the underlying brain processes. ERPs and MEG, on the other hand, provide millisecond resolution of evoked brain activity but can only coarsely localize that activity. Thus, combining information derived from each of these methodologies with the goal of understanding both the temporal and spatial characteristics of the underlying brain activity makes good sense.

Information gleaned from different methodologies can be related across studies to synthesize findings pertinent to particular functions—either retrospectively or prospectively. However, one can also directly combine information across methodologies within the same or linked studies. Although such combining of data or findings acquired from the different methods is always attractive in principle, it can be difficult to do in practice, largely because of the disparate natures of the different methods and the data sets they provide. But when implemented well, it can be very useful.

An example of combining information derived from different methodologies is using data from PET or fMRI to help in the source analysis of ERP or MEG activity. For example, functional activation of specific brain areas during a task carried out in a functional imaging study indicates the areas that are likely sources of corresponding ERP or MEG activity in the same task. This information can be immediately valuable in associating specific ERP effects with fMRI or PET activations in parallel studies, but it can also be incorporated directly into source localization analyses and modeling as *a priori* "constraints," increasing the likelihood of obtaining accurate estimates of the ERP or MEG sources. In addition, since ERP/MEG activity derives mainly from neural current sources located within the cortex and oriented perpendicularly to the cortical surface (see the earlier discussion of these methods), extracting the cortical surface from high-resolution structural MRI images can also provide useful anatomical constraints for source localization approaches.

Furthermore, researchers are now using MR-compatible EEG systems to record EEG and fMRI simultaneously in the scanner. The advantage of this approach, although technically difficult, is that it allows one to analyze how the differences from trial to trial in one of these measures (e.g., the EEG in a specific time period) co-vary with the trial-to-trial variations of the other (e.g., the fMRI activity in particular regions). This approach thus has the important advantage of being able to link the activity variations of each of the measures across time, as opposed to being only able to compare the averaged response in an EEG session with the averaged response in a separate fMRI session doing the same task. Accordingly, such simultaneous-recording approaches appear to hold great promise for cognitive neuroscience research.

Other useful ways to combine these approaches include linking functional imaging studies in normal individuals with similar studies in patients who have brain lesions. Another example is to record both fMRI activity and single-unit activity in experimental animals (usually monkeys) engaged in the same cognitive task. Yet another is to pursue electrophysiological studies in monkeys and humans using parallel cognitive paradigms. Some electrophysiological studies in monkeys are now including intracranial recording of both single units and local cortical field potentials, with one of the aims being to make it easier to relate the results in experimental animals to the scalp-recorded ERPs in humans. Still other studies are relating genetic variations and neuroimaging measures, including task-related responses, to investigate mechanisms related to certain clinical disorders, as well as to the propensity for having certain behavioral traits (Box 2C).

■ BOX 2C NEUROIMAGING GENOMICS

Variations in a gene or segment of DNA are called *polymorphisms*, and these genetic variations can be associated with a greater risk of various neurological and psychiatric disorders. Recent research has also shown that the expression of genetic variations in the brain can be manifested in both structural and functional neuroimaging data. **Neuroimaging genomics** (or **imaging genomics**) refers to the application of imaging technologies to investigate how these genes are expressed in the brain.

An example of this sort of approach used fMRI to study memory in individuals with varying degrees of risk for Alzheimer's-type dementia. This risk for dementia was related to whether the individual carried one genetic form (allele) or another of a gene known as *APOE*, with those whose alleles included one copy of the variant *APOE 4* having an increased risk relative to those carrying two copies of the variant *APOE 3*. During a memory task, individuals with a copy of *APOE 4* showed greater activation in the hippocampus and other memory-related brain areas (see Chapter 9), relative to those with only *APOE 3*. Moreover, the degree of increased activation varied inversely with a decline of memory ability over the following two years, with *APOE 4*

individuals who showed greater activation early having more memory decline later. Thus, before any clinical signs or symptoms appear, neuroimaging may pick up subtle brain variations that predict later functional deficits.

There has also been much interest in the genetic influences on the transmitter systems involved in various cognitive functions. Considerable work has been directed in particular toward understanding the role of genetic variations that control molecules involved in the synaptic efficacy of the neurotransmitter serotonin. For example, certain genetic alleles have been associated with greater levels of serotonin in key brain areas, with such individuals also showing greater levels of anxiety in stressful circumstances. Correspondingly, fMRI studies have indicated that when these individuals are shown images with strong emotional associations, they display greater increases of activity in the amygdala, a key emotion-processing region in the brain (see Chapter 10), while also producing more cortisol in the bloodstream (a marker of stress level). Such results show the benefits of combining genetic measures, behavioral measures, and neuroimaging to studying the neural and physiological mechanisms related to clinical disorders.

More generally, there is a developing school of thought that many psychiatric clinical syndromes represent one end of a genetic spectrum of individual differences in specific traits. For example, subclinical levels of obsessive-compulsive disorder traits can be found in many "normal" individuals, with little of such tendencies being present in others. These more subtle trait-related genetic variations may also have corresponding manifestations in brain structure and/or function that may be investigated with neuroimaging.

References

BOOKHEIMER, S. Y. AND 6 OTHERS (2000) Patterns of brain activation in people at risk for Alzheimer's disease. *N. Engl. J. Med.* 343: 450–456.

CASPI, A., A. R. HARIRI, A. HOLMES, R. UHER AND T. E. MOFFITT (2010) Genetic sensitivity to the environment: The case of the serotonin transporter gene and its implications for studying complex diseases and traits. *Am. J. Psychiatry* 167: 509–527.

HARIRI, A. R. (2009) The neurobiology of individual differences in complex behavioral traits. *Annu. Rev. Neurosci.* 32: 225–247.

In sum, there are many ways in which the various research methods of cognitive neuroscience can be effectively combined both within and across studies. Multimethodological syntheses hold the promise for achieving the deepest and fullest understanding of the neural processes and mechanisms that underlie cognitive functions. Moreover, the need to synthesize findings across methodologies, as well as to maintain a broad interdisciplinary perspective, will continue even as newer and better methods emerge, as they most certainly will.

Summary

1. The technical approaches that have made it increasingly possible to link the inferences and concepts of cognitive psychology to their neural underpinnings are diverse and continually improving. The approaches that have been most effective to date fall into two major categories: brain perturbation and neuromonitoring.

2. Methods that perturb the brain in some way allow inferences to be made about the role of specific brain areas or brain systems in particular cognitive functions. Approaches that entail perturbation include the natural disturbances of brain function that arise from trauma, stroke, or disease; perturbations induced pharmacologically; and perturbations induced by electrical stimulation of relevant brain regions. The latter methods include direct intracranial electrical stimulation, mostly in animals, as well as stimulation of brain tissue through the skull using transcranial magnetic stimulation (TMS) and transcranial direct current stimulation (tDCS).

3. Methods that measure neural activity during cognitive tasks provide information about the specific neural activity patterns that are engaged during the processing of a specific type of stimulus or the performance of a specific cognitive task. The major activity-measuring techniques associated with cognitive processes include invasive electrical recording in experimental animals, noninvasive electrical or magnetic recording in humans, and both noninvasive and invasive imaging methods that depend on altered metabolism and/or blood flow in active brain regions.

4. In single-unit electrophysiological recording, metal electrodes are inserted into the brain structures of experimental animals to measure the action potentials produced by individual neurons. Animal researchers are also increasingly investigating the nonspike fluctuations in the dendritic local field potentials.

5. Electroencephalography (EEG) is a noninvasive method for recording the brain's electrical signals from the scalp, which reflects the volume-conducted dendritic field potentials. EEG and the event-related potentials (ERPs) that can be extracted from EEG data via time-locked averaging have been widely used in the study of human brain activity.

6. EEG and ERPs have counterparts in magnetoencephalography (MEG) and event-related field responses (ERFs), which measure magnetic-field fluctuations due to neuronal currents rather than the associated voltage fluctuations. These methods all have high temporal resolution but coarse spatial resolution.

7. Techniques of three-dimensional functional brain imaging have revolutionized cognitive neuroscience with their ability to visualize brain activity during cognitive task performance. The first of these to be widely used, positron emission tomography (PET), can localize brain activity during extended task blocks, but it requires the use of radioactive isotopes and has essentially no temporal resolution. Accordingly, it has been largely supplanted in cognitive research by functional magnetic resonance imaging (fMRI), which has much higher temporal resolution (although it is still much lower than that of electrophysiological methods) and can be performed in an event-related way.

8. Much work has been devoted to advancing analytic methods for fMRI in order to enhance the ability to make inferences from the brain activity patterns. Such methods include using multivoxel pattern analysis to examine consistent variations in the spatial patterns of activity locally within an area and using repetition suppression to examine the activations of intermingled neural populations within an area. Considerable research has also been devoted to developing methods to analyze the functional interactions between different active areas in the brain and how they work together to accomplish cognitive functions.

9. Optical brain imaging techniques are based on differences in light absorption and transmission in active brain areas that can be detected and imaged using optical recording devices.

10. With both brain perturbation studies and brain activity studies, the approach is to establish which cognitive functions are associated with certain neural structures or neural activity, and which are dissociated. This linkage of neural and cognitive processes is made even stronger by establishing double dissociations—that is, establishing that Task A is associated with neural region 1 but not with region 2 and that Task B is associated with region 2 but not with region 1.

11. Increasingly, different methodologies are being combined in multimethodological approaches that together can provide greater insight into the neural mechanisms underlying cognitive processes.

Go to the **COMPANION WEBSITE**

sites.sinauer.com/cogneuro2e

for quizzes, animations, flashcards, and other study resources.

Additional Reading

Reviews

CHURCHLAND, P. S. AND T. J. SEJNOWSKI (1988) Perspectives on cognitive neuroscience. *Science* 242: 741–745.

FOX, P. T. AND M. G. WOLDORFF (1994) Integrating human brain maps. *Curr. Opin. Neurobiol.* 4: 151–156.

HAMALAINEN, M., R. HARI, R. ILMONEIMI, J. KNUUTILA AND O. LOUNASMAA (1993) Magnetoencephalography: Theory, instrumentation, and applications to the noninvasive study of human brain function. *Rev. Mod. Phys.* 65: 413–423.

HENSON, R. (2005) What can functional neuroimaging tell the experimental psychologist? *Q. J. Exp. Psychol.* 58A: 193–233.

LOGOTHETIS, N. K. (2008) What we can and cannot do with fMRI. *Nature* 453: 869–878.

SMITH, S. M. AND 7 OTHERS (2011) Network modeling methods for fMRI. *Neuroimage* 54: 875–891.

SUPER, H. AND P. R. ROELFSEMA (2005) Chronic multiunit recordings in behaving animals: Advantages and limitations. *Prog. Brain Res.* 147: 263–282.

YIHAR, O, L. I. FENNO, T. J. DAVIDSON, M. MOGRI AND K. DEISSEROTH (2009) Optogenetics in neural systems. *Neuron* 71: 9–34.

Important Original Papers

BANDETTINI, P. A., E. C. WONG, R. S. HINKS, R. S. TIKOFSKY AND J. S. HYDE (1992) Time course EPI of human brain function during task activation. *Magn. Reson. Med.* 25: 390–397.

BERGER, H. (1929) Uber das Electroenkephalogram des Menschen. *Arch. Psychiatr. Nervenkr.* 87: 527–570.

BUROCK, M. A., R. L. BUCKNER, M. G. WOLDORFF, B. R. ROSEN AND A. M. DALE (1998) Randomized event-related experimental designs allow for extremely rapid presentation rates using functional MRI. *Neuroreport* 9: 3735–3739.

CATON, R. (1875) The electrical currents of the brain. *Brit. Med. J.* 2: 278.

DA SILVA, F. H. AND W. S. VAN LEEUWEN (1977) The cortical source of the alpha rhythm. *Neurosci. Lett.* 6: 237–241.

FOX, P. T. AND M. E. RAICHLE (1986) Focal physiological uncoupling of cerebral blood flow and oxidative metabolism during somatosensory stimulation in human subjects. *Proc. Natl. Acad. Sci. USA* 83: 1140–1144.

GRATTON, G. AND 8 OTHERS (1997) Fast and localized event-related optical signals (EROS) in the human occipital cortex: Comparisons with the visual evoked potential and fMRI. *Neuroimage* 6: 168–180.

GRILL-SPECTOR, K., T. KUSHNIR, S. EDELMAN, G. AVIDAN, Y. ITZCHAK AND R. MALACH (1999) Differential processing of objects under various viewing conditions in the human lateral occipital complex. *Neuron* 24: 187–203.

GRINWALD, A., E. LIEKE, R. D. FROSTIG, C. D. GILBERT AND T. N. WIESEL (1991) Functional architecture of cortex revealed by optical imaging of intrinsic signals. *Nature* 324: 361–364.

HUBEL, D. H. AND T. N. WIESEL (1959) Receptive fields of single neurons in the cat's striate cortex. *J. Neurophysiol.* 148: 574–591.

KOURTZI, Z. AND N. KANWISHER (2001) Representation of perceived object shape by the human lateral occipital complex. *Science* 293: 706–709.

KWONG, K. K. AND 9 OTHERS (1992) Dynamic magnetic resonance imaging of human brain activity during primary sensory stimulation. *Proc. Natl. Acad. Sci. USA* 89: 5675–5679.

LOGOTHETIS, N. K., J. PAULS, M. AUGATH, T. TRINATH AND A. OELTERMANN (2001) Neurophysiological investigation of the basis of the fMRI signal. *Nature* 412: 128–130.

MAGRI, C., U. SCHRIDDE, Y. MURAYAM, S. PANZERI AND N. K. LOGOTHETIS (2012) The amplitude and timing of the BOLD signal reflects the relationship between local field potential power at different frequencies. *J. Neurosci.* 32: 1395–1407.

MOUNTCASTLE, V. B., J. C. LYNCH, A. GEORGOPOULOS, H. SAKATA AND C. ACUNA (1975) Posterior parietal association cortex of the monkey: Command functions for operations within extrapersonal space. *J. Neurophysiol.* 38: 871–908.

OGAWA, S. AND 6 OTHERS (1992) Intrinsic signal changes accompanying sensory stimulation: Functional brain mapping with magnetic resonance imaging. *Proc. Natl. Acad. Sci. USA* 89: 5951–5955.

PETERSEN, S. E., P. T. FOX, A. Z. SNYDER AND M. E. RAICHLE (1990) Activation of extrastriate and frontal cortical areas by visual words and word-like stimuli. *Science* 249: 1041–1044.

SERENO, M. I. AND 7 OTHERS (1995) Borders of multiple visual areas in humans revealed by functional magnetic resonance imaging. *Science* 268: 889–893.

WURTZ, R. H. AND M. E. GOLDBERG (1971) Superior colliculus cell responses related to eye movements in awake monkeys. *Science* 171: 82–84.

Books

HUETTEL, S. A., A. W. SONG AND G. MCCARTHY (2009) *Functional Magnetic Resonance Imaging*, 2nd Ed. Sunderland, MA: Sinauer.

LUCK, S. J. (2005) *An Introduction to the Event-Related Potential Technique.* Cambridge, MA: MIT Press.

NUÑEZ, P. L. R. AND R. SRINIVASAN (2005) *Electric Fields of the Brain: The Neurophysics of EEG*, 2nd Ed. New York: Oxford University Press.

RAICHLE, M. E. AND M. I. POSNER (1994) *Images of Mind.* New York: Scientific American Library.

ULLSPERGER, M. AND S. DEBENER (2010) *Simultaneous EEG and fMRI: Recording, Analysis, and Application.* Oxford: Oxford University Press.

3

Sensory Systems and Perception: Vision

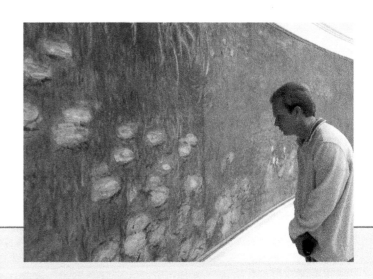

INTRODUCTION

The goal in this and the following chapter is to review the major sensory modalities, exploring what is known about how sensory systems operate, and how they generate perceptions. For humans, these modalities are vision (sight), audition (hearing), somatic sensation (touch, pressure, and pain), olfaction (smell), and gustation (taste). Sensory modalities generally work together to guide behavior; what we see at any moment, for example, is demonstrably influenced by what we hear. By the same token, visual perceptions are influenced by attention, memory, emotional and motivational states, individual goals, and many other factors discussed in later chapters. Finally, remember that perception is not limited to the results of sensory processing. Other mental content—for example, thoughts and feelings—is also perceived. The aim of this chapter is to consider these issues in the context of vision, the most fully studied and best understood of the sensory modalities. The next chapter extends the principles evident in vision to several other sensory modalities. In each case, the challenge for cognitive neuroscience is to understand how the basic functions of sensory systems are related to cognitive functions such as the recognition of objects in the environment.

Visual Stimuli

The human visual system processes neural activity generated by photons that have wavelengths of about 400 to 700 nanometers. This range is a tiny fraction of the full electromagnetic spectrum. What we call *light* is therefore defined by the human visual system, which has evolved this range of sensitivity because sunlight at the surface of the Earth peaks at about 550 nanometers. An analogous account applies to the sounds we hear, the forces we feel, and the molecules we smell and taste. In each domain, the sensations we experience derive from a small but biologically pertinent fraction of the energy in the environment. Despite these limitations, human sensory systems respond to an extraordinary span of stimulus intensities. Visual percepts are elicited by amounts of light ranging from values of a few tens of photons per square millimeter at the retinal surface to values a billion or more times greater.

■ INTRODUCTORY BOX PROSOPAGNOSIA

Recognizing objects, especially those that convey biologically important information, is critical for well-being and ultimately survival. A good example is the recognition of faces. A deficiency in recognizing faces is termed **prosopagnosia** (*prosopo* in Greek refers to "face" or "person," and *agnosia* means "inability to know"). Following damage to the inferior temporal cortex, typically on the right, patients are often unable to identify familiar individuals by their facial characteristics, and in some cases they cannot recognize a face at all. Nonetheless, such individuals are perfectly aware that some sort of visual stimulus is present and can describe particular aspects or elements of it without difficulty.

An example is the case of L.H., a patient described by neuropsychologist N. L. Etcoff and colleagues. L.H. (the use of initials to identify neurological patients in published reports is standard practice) was a 40-year-old minister and social worker who sustained a severe head injury as the result of an automobile accident when he was 18. After recovery,

L.H. could not recognize familiar faces, report that they were familiar, or answer questions about faces from memory. He could, however, identify other common objects, discriminate subtle shape differences of other objects, and recognize the sex, age, and even the "likability" of faces. Moreover, he could identify particular people by nonfacial cues such as voice, body shape, and gait. The only other category of visual stimuli that L.H. had trouble recognizing was animals and their expressions, though these impairments were not as severe as for human faces. Noninvasive brain imaging (see Chapter 2) showed that L.H.'s prosopagnosia was the result of damage to the right ventral temporal lobe.

More recently, brain imaging and direct electrophysiological recording studies in normal subjects have confirmed that the inferior temporal cortex, particularly the fusiform gyrus, mediates face recognition (Figures A and B); and that nearby regions are responsible for categorically different recognition functions (object recognition will be discussed later

in this chapter). Prosopagnosia can also occur in some otherwise normal individuals for reasons that are not understood. An especially engaging account of a person who has difficulty with object recognition that extends far beyond faces is Oliver Sacks's essay "The Man Who Mistook His Wife for a Hat."

References

KANWISHER, N. (2006) What's in a face? *Science* 311: 617–618.

SACKS, O. (1985) *The Man Who Mistook His Wife for a Hat, and Other Clinical Tales*. New York: Summit.

TSAO, D. Y. AND M. S. LIVINGSTONE (2008) Mechanisms of face perception. *Annu. Rev. Neurosci.* 31: 411–437.

Functional MRI activation during a face recognition task. (A) A face stimulus was presented to a normal subject at the time indicated by the arrow. The graph shows a change in activation in the region shown in (B), which is located in the right inferior temporal lobe. (Courtesy of Greg McCarthy.)

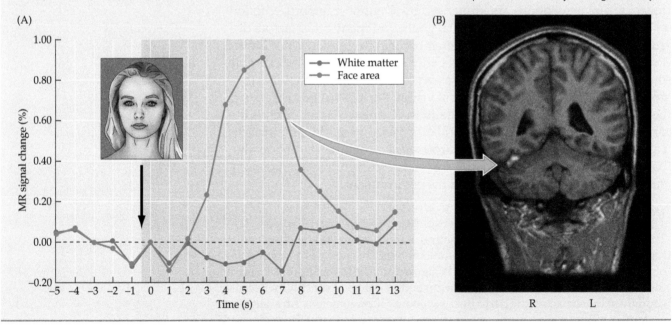

The Initiation of Vision

The events that lead from stimuli to perception begin with the pre-neural elements of the eye that collect and filter light energy in the environment. These elements are the cornea, lens, and ocular media that focus and filter light before it reaches the retina (**Figure 3.1**). The next step in sensory processing—and the

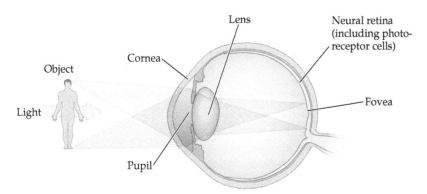

Figure 3.1 Pre-neural processing by the eye These structures usefully modify stimulus energy before it reaches sensory receptor neurons. The optical structures of the eye—the cornea, pupil, and lens—filter and focus the light that eventually reaches photoreceptor cells (rods and cones) in the retina. As a result of projective geometry, images on the retina are upside down and shifted left for right.

first step that entails the nervous system—is the transformation of light energy into neural signals by specialized receptor cells whose pigment molecules absorb photons of specific wavelengths.

This transformation is mediated by two types of receptor cells in the retina—rods and cones—that ultimately link to overlapping but different processing systems in the retina and the rest of the brain (Figure 3.2). The processing initiated by rods is concerned primarily with perception at very low levels of light; cones respond only to greater light intensities and are responsible for the detail and color percepts. Thus, the rod system is essential at night, whereas processing by the cone system is dominant in daylight.

An important principle evident in vision and all other sensory systems is **sensory adaptation**, the continual resetting of sensitivity according to ambient conditions. The primary purpose of adaptation is to ensure that, despite the signaling limitations of nerve cells, sensory processing occurs with maximum efficiency over the full range of environmental conditions that are relevant (Figure 3.3A). The need for resetting arises from the discrepancy between this environmental range and the much more limited firing rate of visual and other neurons. The firing rate, which conveys information about stimulus intensity (the more action potentials [see Appendix] per unit time, the more intense the stimulus), has a maximum of only a few hundred action potentials per second, which is inadequate to generate finely graded percepts in response to light intensities that range over 10 orders of magnitude or more. Thus the sensitivity of the system is continually adapted to match different ongoing levels of light intensity in the environment (Figure 3.3B).

Another property of the visual and other sensory systems is their degree of precision, or **acuity**. Acuity is different from sensitivity to stimulus intensity. Rather than setting an appropriate level of amplification (gain), acuity measures the fineness of discrimination, as in

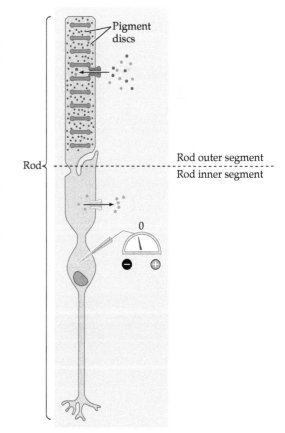

Figure 3.2 Transduction by sensory receptor cells in the retina Absorption of photons by pigments in a photoreceptor cell (here, a rod cell) changes the photoreceptor's membrane potential and initiates a neural signal that will eventually be conveyed to the rest of the visual system. The ion movements involved in setting up the signal are indicated. (See Appendix.) Blue dots, Na^+ ions; red dots, Ca^+ ions; yellow dots, K^+ ions.

(A)

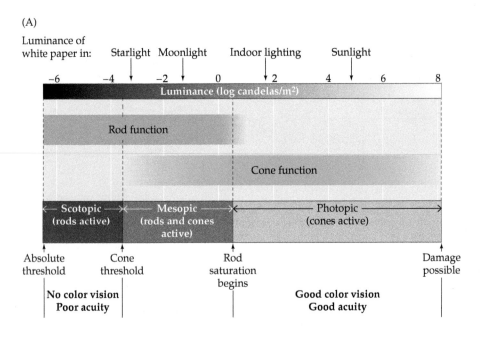

(B)

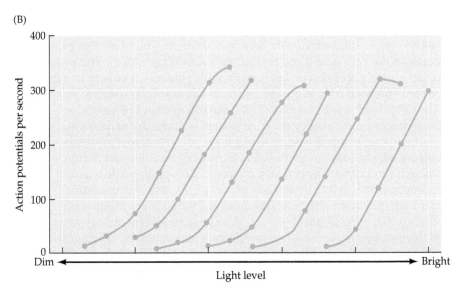

Figure 3.3   The need for visual adaptation   (A) The light sensitivity of the human visual system, based on the rod and cone photoreceptor systems, spans more than 10 orders of magnitude. **(B)** To faithfully convey information about intensity over this broad range using the relatively small range of action potentials per second that neurons can generate, the sensitivity of the system must continually adapt to ambient levels of light, so that firing rates of the relevant neurons report light intensity over a new portion of the full range of sensitivity. In the experiment shown, the firing rate of retinal ganglion cells (the neurons that carry information from the eye to the processing centers in the brain) was examined for six different levels of light intensity (luminance). The full range of neural signaling is apparent at each level as a result of adaptation. (After Sakmann and Creutzfeldt 1969.)

distinguishing two nearby points (the purpose of the standard eye chart used by an optometrist). Visual acuity depends on the different distribution of receptor cells (and receptor types) across the retina. Although we seem to see the visual world quite clearly, visual acuity in humans actually falls off rapidly as a function of *eccentricity* (the distance, in degrees of visual angle, away from the line

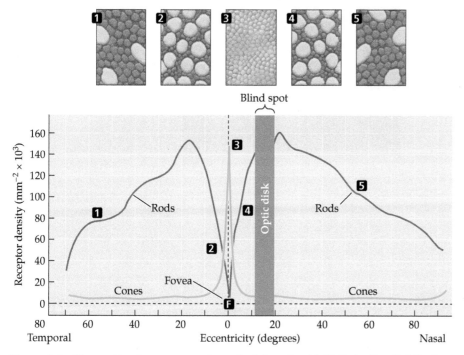

Figure 3.4 **The acuity of sensory systems is determined initially by the distribution of retinal receptors** The density of rods (purple) and cones (green), plotted as a function of distance from the cone-rich fovea. The poor resolution of vision a few degrees off the line of sight is a result of the paucity of closely packed cones at eccentricities greater than a few degrees.

of sight; a degree is 1/360th of a circle drawn around the head and corresponds to approximately the width of the thumb held at arm's length). Consequently, vision beyond the central few degrees of the visual field is extremely poor.

Lessened acuity outside the central retina means that we must frequently move our eyes—and therefore the direction of gaze—to different positions in visual space. Such eye movements are called **saccades**, and they occur 3 to 4 times a second; this easily measured visual behavior is widely used in studies of attention (see Chapters 6 and 7). The reason for this difference in acuity according to where an image falls on the retina is the distribution of photoreceptors (Figure 3.4). Cones, which are responsible for detailed vision in daylight, greatly predominate in the central region of the retina, being most dense in a specialized region called the **fovea**. The prevalence of cones falls off sharply in all directions as a function of distance from the fovea, and as a result, high-acuity vision is limited to the fovea and its immediate surround. Conversely, rods are sparse in the fovea and absent altogether in the middle of it. In consequence, sensitivity to a dim stimulus is greater off the line of sight—because of the paucity of rods in the fovea and their preponderance a few degrees away—even though acuity is lower at this eccentricity.

Subcortical Visual Processing

Subcortical processing consists of neural interactions in the stations of the central nervous system before the activity elicited by a stimulus reaches the cerebral cortex. The first stage of central processing takes place in the five layers of the retina. This information converges onto retinal ganglion cells whose axons leave the retina via the optic nerve, the first component of the **primary visual pathway**, which is the major route from the eye to the visual cortex in the

Figure 3.5 **The primary visual path-way** The route (solid red and blue lines) that carries information centrally from the retina to regions of the brain that are especially pertinent to what we see comprises the optic nerves, the optic tracts, the dorsal lateral geniculate nuclei in the thalamus, the optic radiations, and the primary (striate) and secondary (extrastriate) visual cortices in the occipital lobes. The partial crossing of the optic nerve axons at the optic chiasm means that information in the right visual field is conveyed to the left occipital lobe, while information from the left visual field goes to right occipital lobe. Other pathways to targets in the brainstem (dashed red and blue lines) determine the pupil's diameter as a function of retinal light levels, help organize and effect eye movements, and influence circadian rhythms.

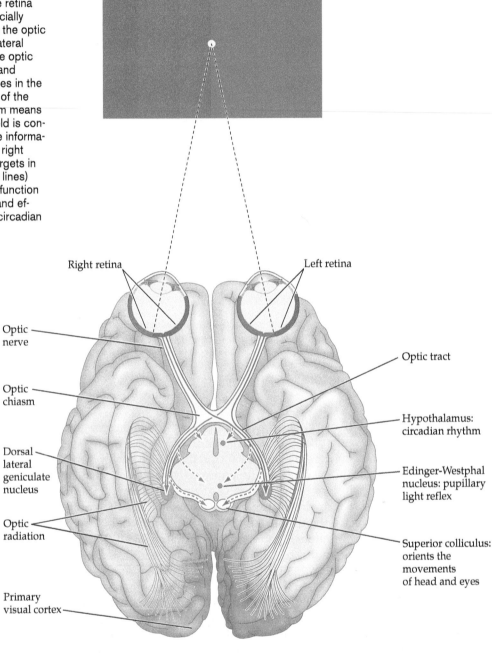

brain's occipital lobe (Figure 3.5). The pathway conveys the information in light stimuli that we end up perceiving as visual scenes. Retinal circuitry modulates the information that is eventually sent forward by retinal ganglion cells. The theme of modulation of the information that goes forward in a sensory system is a general one in sensory processing, the presumed purpose being to filter or otherwise improve the information received by the next processing stage.

The major target of the retinal ganglion cells is the dorsal **lateral geniculate nucleus** in the thalamus (Figure 3.6A). Unlike other thalamic nuclei, the lateral geniculate is layered, consisting of two **magnocellular system** layers (so named because the neurons that populate them are relatively large; *magno* means "large"), and four **parvocellular system** layers that appear less dense

(A)

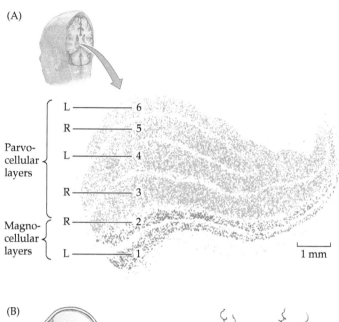

Parvo-cellular layers {

L ——————— 6
R ——————— 5
L ——————— 4
R ——————— 3

Magno-cellular layers {

R ——————— 2
L ——————— 1

1 mm

Figure 3.6   The dorsal lateral geniculate nucleus of the thalamus (A) Cross section of the human thalamus showing the six layers of this distinctive nucleus. Each layer receives input from only one eye or the other (indicated by R or L, for right or left) and is further categorized by the size of the neurons it contains. The two layers shown in blue contain larger neurons and are therefore called the *magnocellular layers*; the four layers shown in green are the *parvocellular layers* because of their smaller constituent cells. (B) Tracings of representative magnocellular and parvocellular retinal ganglion cells, as seen in flat mounts of the retina after tissue staining; these neurons innervate, respectively, the magno and parvo cells in the thalamus. (A after Andrews et al. 1997; B after Watanabe and Rodieck 1989.)

(B)

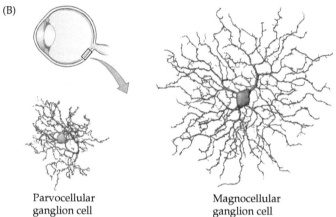

Parvocellular
ganglion cell

Magnocellular
ganglion cell

with smaller neurons (*parvo* means "sparse"). The "parvo" and "magno" layers, as they are generally referred to, are innervated by distinct classes of retinal ganglion cells (**Figure 3.6B**).

The neuronal associations between specific classes of retinal ganglion cells and lateral geniculate neurons reflect different functions that have different perceptual consequences. The smaller P ganglion cells in the retina, and the related parvocellular neurons in the lateral geniculate nucleus, are concerned primarily with the spatial detail underlying the perception of form, as well as perceptions of brightness and color. The larger M retinal ganglion cells, and the magnocellular neurons they innervate in the thalamus, process information about changes in stimuli that lead to motion perception. Neurons in both the magno and parvo layers are extensively innervated by axons descending from the cortex and other brain regions, as well as those arising from retinal ganglion cells. Although the function of this descending information is not known, the geniculate nucleus is clearly more than a relay station.

Cortical Visual Processing

The target of the lateral geniculate neurons is the **primary visual cortex**, also known as the **striate cortex** or **V1** (the word *striate*, meaning "striped," refers to the appearance of cortical layer 4 in this region). The neurons in cortical layer

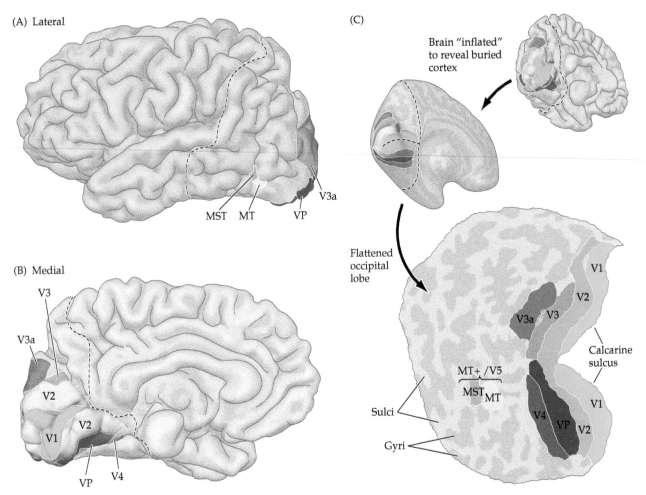

(A) Lateral

MST   MT   VP   V3a

(B) Medial

V3
V3a
V2
V2
V1
VP   V4

(C)

Brain "inflated" to reveal buried cortex

Flattened occipital lobe

V1
V2
V3a   V3
Calcarine sulcus
MT+ /V5
MST
MT
V1
Sulci
V4   VP   V2
Gyri

Figure 3.7   The primary visual cortex and higher-order cortical association areas in the human brain Localization of multiple visual areas in the brain using fMRI. (A,B) Lateral and medial views show the location of the primary visual cortex (V1) and additional visual areas V2, V3, VP (ventral posterior), V4, MT (middle temporal), and MST (middle superior temporal). (C) Unfolded and computationally flattened view of the visual areas shows the relationships more clearly. (After Sereno et al. 1995.)

4 receive the axons from neurons in the thalamus, while neurons in layers 1 and 5 of the primary visual cortex project to **extrastriate visual cortical areas** in the occipital, parietal, and temporal lobes, as well as back to the thalamus (Figure 3.7). The extrastriate cortex is generally considered a component of the **cortical association areas** (a general term that refers to all cortical regions that are not primarily sensory or motor).

The cortical association areas occupy the vast majority of the cortical surface, and together with their subcortical components, they are critical determinants of all of the perceptual qualities and cognitive functions discussed in all subsequent chapters. Because these regions integrate the qualities of a given modality (e.g., color, brightness, form, and motion), as well as information from other sensory modalities and from brain regions carrying out other functions (e.g., attention and memory), the processing carried out by the association cortices is often referred to as "higher-order." The extrastriate visual cortical areas adjacent to V1 tend to process one or more of the qualities that define visual perception. Thus, in humans and non-human primates the area called **V4** is especially important

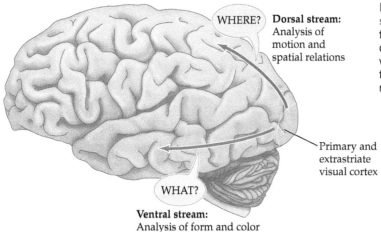

Figure 3.8 **The dorsal and ventral visual information streams** These pathways have been well documented in the human brain with fMRI and other methods. They are often referred to as the "where" and "what" pathways. The ventral stream conveys information to regions of the inferior temporal lobe whose activity in fMRI studies indicates a role in the recognition of objects.

for processing information pertinent to color vision, and areas **MT** (for *middle temporal*) and **MST** (for *middle superior temporal*) are especially important for the generation of motion percepts.

An important generalization about the organization of higher-order visual cortices is the anatomical flow of different information streams. Cognitive neuroscientists Leslie Ungerleider and Mortimer Mishkin were the first to show that extrastriate cortical areas in humans and non-human primates are organized into two largely separate pathways that feed information into the temporal and parietal lobes, respectively (Figure 3.8). One of these broad paths, called the **ventral stream** (the "what" pathway) leads from the visual cortex to the inferior part of the temporal lobe. Information carried in this pathway appears to be responsible for high-resolution form vision and object recognition, a finding that conforms to other evidence about functions of the temporal lobe. The **dorsal stream** (the "where" pathway) leads from striate cortex and other visual areas into the parietal lobe. This pathway appears to be responsible for spatial aspects of vision, such as the analysis of motion and positional relationships between objects. Melvyn Goodale and others who have worked on this issue refer to these two streams as the ventral "vision for perception" and dorsal "vision for action" pathways to indicate the idea that the temporal lobe is concerned mainly with perception whereas the parietal lobe is concerned more with attention and doing something about whatever is perceived.

Thus, as described later in the chapter, electrophysiological recordings from neurons in the temporal lobes tend to exhibit properties that are important for object recognition, such as selectivity for shape, color, and texture. Conversely, neurons in the dorsal stream show selectivity for direction and speed of movement. In keeping with this finding, lesions of the parietal cortex severely impair the ability to distinguish the position of objects—or attending to them, as described in Chapter 7—while having little effect on the ability to perform object recognition tasks. Lesions of the inferior temporal cortex, on the other hand, produce profound impairments in the ability to perform recognition tasks but do not impair an individual's ability to carry out spatial tasks.

The segregation of visual information into ventral and dorsal streams should not be interpreted too rigidly, however; recent evidence indicates that there is a good deal of cross talk between these broadly defined sensory pathways. As sensory information moves through the higher-order processing areas, information specific to a given sensation must be integrated with information being processed by the other sensory systems to improve the efficacy of behavior.

(A)

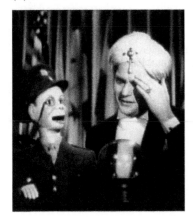

(B)

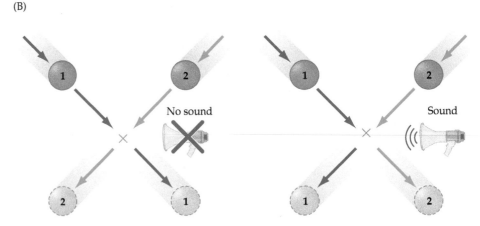

Figure 3.9 Examples of cross-modal influences in perception (A) In ventriloquism, what we see affects what we hear: because we see the dummy's mouth moving while the ventriloquist's lips are still, we perceive the sound as coming from the dummy's mouth. (B) What we hear also affects what we see. The apparent trajectory of moving balls is profoundly affected by what we hear, or do not hear. In the absence of a sound, typically the two balls appear to proceed past each other, as indicated; when a sound occurs co-incident with the point at which they would collide, the balls are more likely to be seen as bouncing off each other.

The result of sensory integration is evident in many aspects of perception. For example, what we see quite literally affects what we hear (Figure 3.9A), and what we hear affects what see (Figure 3.9B). An engaging demonstration of such perceptual consequences is the *McGurk effect*, which illustrates how readily speech sounds can be affected by visual stimuli arising from simultaneous lip movements. Multisensory integration can also have odd consequences, such as the phenomenon of synesthesia, described in Box 3A.

Other Key Characteristics of the Visual Cortex

Topography

An important feature of the primary visual pathway is that the organization of the receptors in the retina is reflected in the corresponding regions of both the thalamus and the visual cortex—a relationship described as topographical. **Topography** is particularly apparent in (but not limited to) the primary sensory cortices, and it has been most thoroughly documented in the visual and somatic sensory systems, where the location of stimuli on the retinal surface or the body surface, respectively, is important for spatial localization.

The experimental approach in **topographical mapping** is to stimulate a specific location on the retina or body surface while recording centrally. In this way one can assess how the location of peripheral stimulation is reflected in the location of corresponding central nervous system activity. Thus, when electrophysiological recordings are made from neurons in the lateral geniculate nucleus, activity at adjacent thalamic sites is elicited by stimulating adjacent retinal sites. Moreover, when a recording electrode is passed from one geniculate layer to another, the position on the retina (or in visual space) determined by recording in one layer is in register with the position determined from the neurons in the subjacent layer. The same phenomenon is apparent in electrophysiological mapping of the primary visual cortex. Clearly, the topography of the retina—and therefore the topography of the retinal image—is reestablished in both the thalamus and

■ BOX 3A **SYNESTHESIA**

A remarkable sensory anomaly is evident in individuals who conflate experiences in one sensory domain with those in another—a phenomenon called *synesthesia*. Synesthesia was named and described by Francis Galton in the nineteenth century, and the phenomenon received a good deal of attention among those in Galton's scientific circle in England. The term means literally "mixing of the senses," and its best understood expression is in individuals who see specific numerals, letters, or similar shapes printed in black and white as being differently colored; this condition is known specifically as *color-graphemic synesthesia*. Other, less common synesthesias include the experience of colors in response to musical notes, and specific tastes elicited by certain words and/or numbers. The list of famous synesthetes includes painter David Hockney, novelist Vladimir Nabokov, composer and musician Duke Ellington, and physicist Richard Feynman.

The experience of synesthetes is not in any sense metaphorical. Nor do they consider it "abnormal"; it is simply the way they experience the world. People who experience color-graphemic synesthesia (the form that has been most thoroughly studied) perceive numbers as being differently colored; the reality of their ability has been demonstrated in a variety of psychophysical studies. On the basis of the synesthetic colors they see, they can segregate targets from backgrounds (Figures A–C), they can group targets in apparent motion displays, and they show the Stroop effect (the slowed reaction time that everyone exhibits when the printed ink and the spelling of a color word are at odds, as in yellow; see Chapter 13).

The cause of synesthesia is not known, but the phenomenon is clearly of considerable interest to researchers trying to sort out how information inputs from different sensory modalities are integrated. A number of cognitive neuroscientists have used fMRI and other modern methods to study synesthesia, but, so far, without leading to any definite conclusions. The influence of synesthetic color perception on the various psychophysical tasks shows that the phenomenon occurs at the level of the cerebral cortex. Numerous neurobiological theories have been put forward, the most plausible of which entail some form of aberrant wiring during early development. A good deal of novel synaptic connectivity is required as a person becomes literate, numerate, or musically trained, and it may be during this period of plasticity that "miswiring" occurs.

References

BARON-COHEN, S. AND J. E. HARRISON (1997) *Synesthesia: Classic and Contemporary Readings.* Malden, MA: Blackwell Scientific.

BLAKE, R., T. J. PALMIERI, R. MAROIS AND C.-Y. KIM (2005) On the perceptual reality of synesthetic color. In *Synesthesia*, L. C. Robertson and N. Sagiv (eds.). New York: Oxford University Press, pp. 47–73.

BRIDGEMAN, B., D. WINTER AND P. TSENG (2010) Dynamic phenomenology of grapheme-color synesthesia. *Perception* 39: 671–676.

RAMACHANDRAN, V. S. AND E. M. HUBBARD (2001) Psychophysical investigations into the neural basis of synaesthesia. *Proc. R. Soc. Lond. B* 368: 979–983.

RAMACHANDRAN, V. S. AND E. M. HUBBARD (2005) Neurocognitive mechanisms in synesthesia. *Neuron* 48: 509–520.

Improved performance on a visual search task by a color-grapheme synesthete, "subject W.O." (A) The physical stimulus presented to W.O. and to a nonsynesthete control subject. The task was to find the numeral 2 among the multiple numeral 5's. (B) The same stimulus with synesthetic colors assigned to the two numbers tested, which presumably shows how W.O. perceives the physical stimulus. (C) The graph reveals that W.O.'s reaction time in the task was faster than that of the control subject. W.O.'s performance is presumably better because the differently colored 2 "pops out" for him, whereas it doesn't for the control subject. (After Blake et al. 2005.)

(A) Physical stimulus as presented

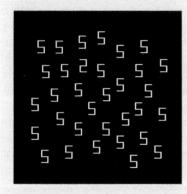

(B) Presumed synesthete perception

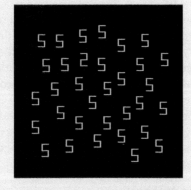

(C)

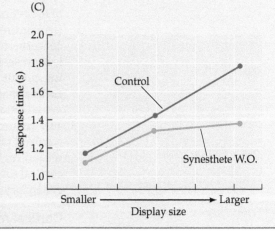

The cortex (**Figure 3.10**). Topographical maps can also be discerned in some adjacent secondary visual cortices, although these tend to be less clear as the distance away from the primary sensory cortex increases.

Figure 3.10 Topographical representation and magnification of peripheral receptor surfaces The regions of the retina are color coded to show their corresponding representation in the primary visual cortex. The area of central vision corresponding to the fovea is represented by much more cortical space than are the eccentric retinal regions. This disproportion is referred to as *cortical magnification*.

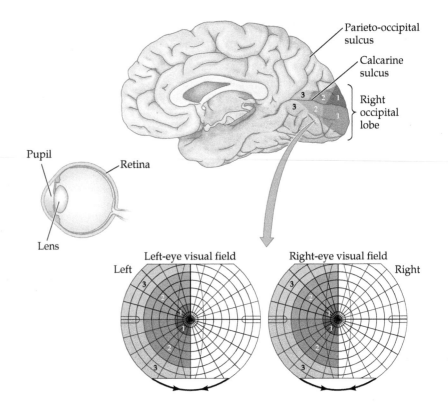

The reason for the topographical layout of the primary visual system is not clear. A simple intuition is that to perceive an integrated visual scene requires a cortical layout that corresponds to the image. But there is no principled reason for this assumption. It seems more likely that cortical topography has mainly to do with minimizing the neuronal wiring that is needed for efficient processing, and thus more to do with metabolic economy than with image representation.

Cortical magnification

Another feature of the primary visual cortex is that the size of each unit area of the retinal surface is disproportionately represented at the level of the cortex (see Figure 3.10). Thus, a square degree of visual space in the fovea (which is concerned with visual detail and is greatly enriched in cone cells; see Figure 3.4) is represented by much more cortical area (and therefore more visual processing circuitry) than the same unit area in the peripheral retina. Referred to as **cortical magnification**, this disproportion makes good neurobiological sense: the visual detail that we perceive in response to stimulation of the fovea presumably requires more neuronal machinery in the cortex than do the less acutely resolved portions of the visual scene generated by the stimulation of eccentric retinal regions. The idea that more complex neural processing requires more cortical (or subcortical) space is another general principle in the organization of sensory systems.

Cortical modularity

Still another organizational feature of the primary visual cortex and some secondary visual cortical areas is their arrangement in iterated groups of neurons with similar functional properties (**Figure 3.11**). Each of these iterated units consists of hundreds or thousands of nerve cells, and together they are referred to as **cortical modules** or **cortical columns**. The result is that sometimes strik-

(A)

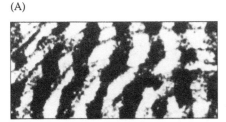

(B)

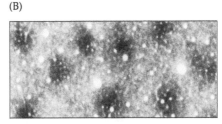

(C)

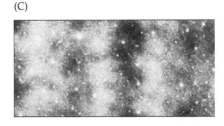

(D)

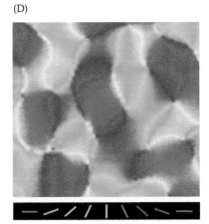

Figure 3.11   Iterated, modular patterns in mammalian sensory cortices All of these examples illustrate the modular organization commonplace in many sensory cortices. The patterns were revealed with one of several different histological techniques in sections in the plane of the cortical surface; the size of the units in each different pattern is on the order of several hundred micrometers across. (A) Stripes called ocular dominance columns in layer 4 of the primary visual (striate) cortex of a rhesus monkey. The cells in each column share a preference for stimuli presented to one eye or the other. (B) Repeating units, called *blobs*, in layers 2 and 3 of the striate cortex of a squirrel monkey. (C) Repeating stripes in layers 2 and 3 in the extrastriate cortex of a squirrel monkey. (D) Patterns of cortical activity in response to differently oriented stimuli observed by optical imaging. In this technique a video camera records light absorption by the primary visual cortex as an experimental animal views stimuli on a video monitor. The images of the cortex obtained in this way are digitized and stored to subsequently construct and compare the patterns associated with the different stimuli. The example shown here is the orientation preference pattern in the primary visual cortex of a tree shrew. Each color represents the orientation of the stimulus that was most effective in activating the cortical neurons at that site. (A–C from Purves et al. 1992; D courtesy of Len White and David Fitzpatrick.)

ing patterns of these columns are superimposed on the topographical maps already described.

Despite their highly regular structure, the function of cortical columns remains unclear. Although cortical columns such as the ocular dominance stripes in Figure 3.11A are readily apparent in the brains of some species, they have not been found in other, sometimes closely related, animals with similar cognitive and behavioral abilities. Moreover, many regions of the mammalian cortex are not organized in this modular fashion. Finally, no clear rationale of such columns has been discerned, despite considerable effort and speculation. Like topography, cortical columns may arise simply from the efficiency of wiring and the way that neuronal connections form during development.

Visual receptive fields

The **receptive field** of a visual neuron is defined as the region of the retina that, when stimulated, elicits a response in the neuron being examined. As described in Chapter 2, the data obtained from single cells are called **single-unit recordings** and are collected by an extracellular microelectrode placed near the cell of interest to monitor its generation of action potentials (Figure 3.12A). At the level of the retinal output and thalamus, visual neurons respond to spots of light. Thus, the receptive fields of retinal ganglion cells or lateral geniculate neurons are excited or inhibited by light going on or off in the center of the retinal area they respond to (typically the area surrounding the receptive-field center has an opposite effect, presumably to enhance information arising from contrast boundaries in visual stimuli).

At the level of the cortex, however, the responses become more complex. In the example shown in Figure 3.12B, the recorded neuron responds to a moving bar when the bar is oriented at some angles but not at others. Through testing of the neuron's responsiveness to a range of differently oriented stimuli, an orientation

(A)

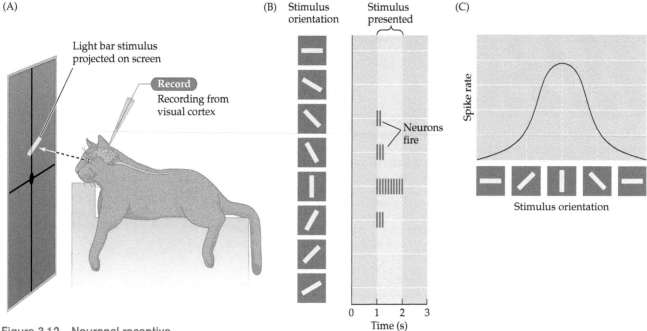

Light bar stimulus
projected on screen

Record

Recording from
visual cortex

(B) Stimulus
orientation

Stimulus
presented

Neurons
fire

0   1   2   3
Time (s)

(C)

Spike rate

Stimulus orientation

Figure 3.12 Neuronal receptive fields (A) An experimental setup for studying visual receptive fields. (B) The receptive field of a typical neuron in the primary visual cortex. As different stimuli are presented in different locations, the neuron being recorded from fires in a variable way that defines both the location of the neuron's receptive field and the properties of the stimulus. The neuron does not fire at all if the stimulus is elsewhere on the scene, and even when it is in the appropriate location the stimulus activates the neuron only when it is presented in certain orientations. Although these factors are not shown here, direction of motion, which eye is stimulated, and other stimulus properties are also important. (C) This orientation tuning curve, which corresponds to the neuron illustrated in (B), shows that the highest rate of action potential discharge occurs for vertical edges–the neuron's "preferred" orientation.

tuning curve can be defined that indicates the sort of stimulus to which the cell is maximally responsive (Figure 3.12C). The receptive fields of cortical neurons serving foveal vision in the primary visual cortex generally measure less than a degree of visual angle, as do the receptive fields of the corresponding retinal ganglion cells and lateral geniculate neurons. Even for cells serving peripheral vision, the receptive fields in the primary visual cortex measure only a few degrees.

In higher-order extrastriate cortical areas, however, receptive fields often cover a substantial fraction of the entire visual field (which extends about 180 degrees horizontally and 130 degrees vertically). The location of retinal activity—and the corresponding topographical relationships in the primary visual cortex—cannot be conveyed by neurons that respond to stimuli *anywhere* in such a large region of space, at least not in any simple way. In short, the topography that is apparent in the primary cortices is less apparent in the higher-order regions, where visual percepts are supposedly generated. The loss of retinal topography in higher-order visual cortical areas (which presumably entails a correspondingly diminished ability to identify the location and qualities of visual stimuli) presents a problem for any rationalization of vision in terms of images and percepts based on image representation in these higher-order extrastriate cortical areas.

Thus, up to the level of the primary visual cortex, the organization of the visual system is hierarchical in the sense that lower-order stations lead anatomically and functionally to higher-order ones, albeit with much modulation and feedback at each stage. At each of the initial stations in the primary visual pathway—the retina, the dorsal lateral geniculate nucleus, and the neurons in the primary visual cortex—the receptive-field characteristics of the relevant neurons can be understood reasonably well in terms of the "lower-order" cells that provide their input. Beyond these initial levels, however, rationalizing the organization of the visual system in terms of lower-order neurons shaping the response properties of higher-order neurons becomes increasingly difficult. The "higher" the order of the nerve cells in the system, the less they depend on visual input, and the more they are influenced by information that is not strictly visual (see Figure 3.9 for examples).

Visual Perception

With this summary of visual system structure and function in mind, the following sections consider the end product of visual processing—that is, what we actually see. The primary visual qualities that describe visual perception are *lightness, brightness, color, form, depth,* and *motion*. These qualities are the foundation that allows us to make the associations needed to recognize objects and conditions in the world.

Lightness and brightness

A good place to begin a consideration of visual percepts is with *lightness* and *brightness*, the terms used to describe our visual experience of light and dark elicited by different light intensities. **Lightness** refers to the appearance of a surface such as a piece of paper; **brightness** refers to the appearance of a light source, such as the sun, or a lightbulb. Vision is impossible without these perceptual qualities, whereas some other qualities, such as color, are expendable (some animals have good vision generally, but little or no color vision). Like all percepts, lightness and brightness are not subject to direct measurement, and can be evaluated indirectly only by asking observers to report the appearance of one object or surface relative to that of another (Box 3B). The physical correlate of brightness is **luminance**, a measure of light intensity made by a photometer and expressed in units such as candelas per square meter. As will be apparent, however, the relationship between luminance and lightness/brightness is deeply puzzling.

A logical assumption would be that luminance and lightness/brightness are directly proportional, since increasing the luminance of a stimulus increases the number of photons captured by photoreceptors. Another intuition is that two objects in a scene that return the same amount of light to the eye should appear equally light or bright. It has long been known, however, that perceptions of lightness/brightness fail to meet these expectations. For example, a patch on a background of relatively low luminance appears lighter or brighter than the same patch on a background of higher luminance—a phenomenon called **simultaneous lightness/brightness contrast** (Figure 3.13A). This effect becomes even more dramatic when the stimulus includes more detailed information (Figure 3.13B).

(A) (B)

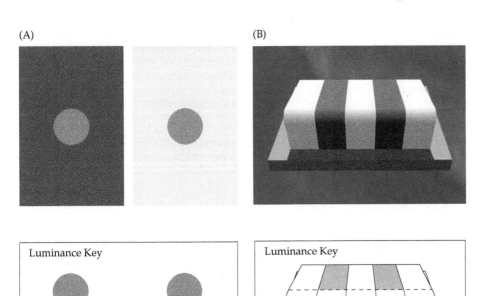

Figure 3.13 **Simultaneous lightness/ brightness contrast** (A) In this standard presentation of the effect, the two circular patches have exactly the same luminance (see the key), but the one in the dark surround looks somewhat lighter/brighter. (B) Simultaneous lightness/brightness contrast effects can be much greater when the scene contains more information; as the key shows, the patches whose lightness/brightness appears very different again have the same luminance. Thus, the amount of light returned to the eye does not determine the lightness/brightness seen. (B from Purves and Lotto 2003.)

■ BOX 3B MEASURING PERCEPTION

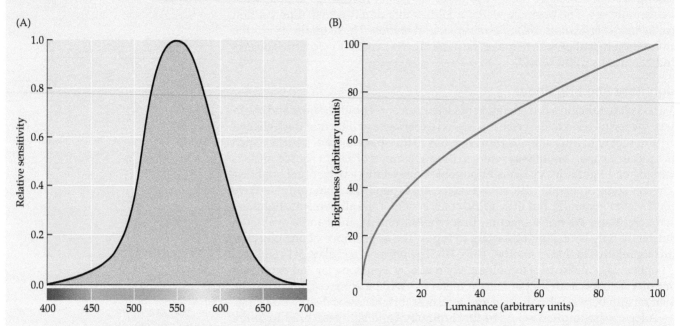

(A)

(B)

Examples of psychophysical assessments. (A) The human luminosity function, determined by assessing the sensitivity of normal subjects to light as a function of stimulus wavelength. This determination can be made by measuring either threshold responses or just-noticeable differences at suprathreshold levels. The results show that humans are far more sensitive to stimuli in the middle of the light spectrum (i.e., between approximately 480 and 630 nanometers). (B) Magnitude scaling, showing that the relationship between a subject's perception of brightness and the intensity of a light stimulus is a power function (the exponent in this case is approximately 0.5).

The physical properties of stimuli can be measured with arbitrary precision. Measuring percepts, however, is quite another matter. The perceptual consequences of stimuli are subjective, and as such they can't be measured in any direct way. They can, however, be reported in terms of thresholds, least discernible differences, or other paradigms in which subjects state whether a percept is brighter or darker, larger or smaller, slower or faster than some standard of comparison. Such evaluations of perceptual responses are broadly referred to as *psychophysics*. The effort to make the analysis of percepts scientifically meaningful dates from 1860, when the German physicist and philosopher Gustav Fechner decided to pursue the connection between what he referred to as the "physical and psychological worlds" (thus the rather unfortunate word *psychophysics*).

In practice, there are only a limited number of ways to assess perception in relation to physical stimuli, although there are many permutations of the basic techniques. A conceptually straightforward but technically difficult measurement is to ascertain the least energetic stimulus that elicits a perceptual response in a particular sensory modality, such as the weakest retinal stimulation perceived as something seen by dark-adapted subjects. By varying the amount of energy delivered, a *psychophysical function* can be obtained that defines the *stimulus threshold value* (Figure A). Since at threshold levels of stimulation subjects have difficulty saying whether they saw something or not, such tests are usually carried out using a *forced-choice paradigm*, in which the observer must respond on each trial. Typically, a series of trials is presented in which stimuli of different energetic levels are randomly interspersed with trials that do not present a stimulus. Because 50 percent correct responses (i.e., saying "Yes, I saw something" or "No, I saw nothing" when a stimulus was or was not present, respectively) would be the average result obtained if the subject merely guessed on each trial, a 75 percent correct-response rate is conventionally taken to be the criterion for establishing the threshold level of stimulus energy.

A technically easier and more generally applicable way of getting at the sensitivity of a sensory modality is to measure—at any level of stimulus intensity—how much physical change is needed to generate a perceptual change. The resulting functions, called *difference threshold functions*, have many practical implications. The *Weber-Fechner law* is a good example. The law states that the ability to notice a difference (called a test of *just-noticeable* or *equally noticeable differences*) is determined by a fixed proportion of the stimulus intensity, not an absolute difference. This proportion is referred to as the *Weber fraction*; if, for example, the Weber fraction is 1/10, then if a 1-gram increment to a 10-gram weight can just be detected, 10 grams will be the minimum detectable increment to a 100-gram weight.

What is now known about the physiology of sensory systems indicates that the proportional relationship between just-noticeable differences and stimulus magnitude expressed by the Weber-Fechner law makes good sense. Recall that because neurons can generate only a limited number of action potentials per second, sensory systems must continu-

■ **BOX 3B** *(continued)*

(C)

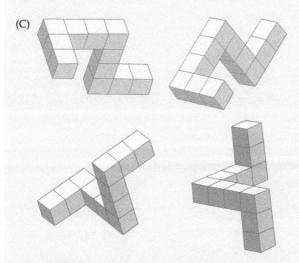

(C) A reaction-time task. Reaching a judgment about whether the object on the left is the same as the object on the right is a function of "task difficulty"; people make this judgment more quickly for objects that are closer to the same orientation in space (top pair) than for objects that are differently oriented (bottom pair). Reaction time is used in many different paradigms, as will be apparent in later chapters.

ally adjust their overall range of operation to provide subjects with information about the energy levels of, say, light, where those energy levels pertinent to humans span many orders of magnitude (see Figure 3.3). The Weber fraction thus provides an approximate measure of the *gain* of a sensory system under specified conditions.

Another psychophysical approach, called *magnitude scaling*, entails ordering percepts along an ordinal scale that covers the full range of a perceptual quality

(brightness, for instance; Figure B). The most extensive studies of this sort were carried out by psychologist Stanley Stevens, who worked on this issue from about 1950 until 1975. To take an example, Stevens asked whether a light stimulus that is made progressively more intense elicits perceptions of brightness that linearly track the physical intensity. In making such determinations, Stevens simply asked subjects to rate the relative intensities of a series of test stimuli on a number scale along which 0 represented the least intense stimulus and 100 the most intense (similar in principle to the common practice of rating pain on a scale of 1 to 10). In this manner, he determined that brightness scales as a *power function* with an exponent of approximately 0.5

under the standard conditions he used (Figure B). The power functions exhibited in such magnitude-scaling experiments are sometimes referred to as reflecting *Stevens' law*. Rationalizing Stevens' results presents another challenge to theories seeking to explain the how visual and other sensory systems generate the percepts they do.

Finally, another staple of psychophysics entails measurements of *reaction time*. A logical assumption is that the more complex the neural processing entailed in performing a given task, the longer it will take to perform the task (Figure C). This simple paradigm is the basis of many studies in later chapters.

References

LEZAK, M. (2004) *Neuropsychological Assessment*. Oxford: Oxford University Press.

STEVENS, S. S. (1975) *Psychophysics*. New York: Wiley.

Many investigators have supposed that the patch on the dark background looks brighter than the patch on the light background because of a difference in the retinal output. The percepts elicited by other stimulus patterns, however, undermine the idea that simultaneous lightness/brightness contrast effects are an incidental consequence of dark versus light surrounds. In the pattern in Figure 3.14, for example, the target patches on the left are surrounded by a greater area of *higher* luminance (lighter territory) than lower luminance, and yet

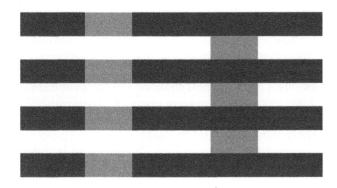

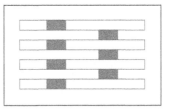

Figure 3.14 **White's illusion** This stimulus pattern elicits perceptual effects that cannot be explained in terms of the same local contrast effects illustrated in Figure 3.13A. The pattern and its perceptual consequences are called *White's illusion* after the psychologist who first described this stimulus more than 30 years ago. (After White 1979.)

Figure 3.15 Conflation of illumination, reflectance, and transmittance in a light stimulus An observer must parse these three factors—which the stimulus inevitably conflates—in order to respond appropriately to the pattern of luminance values in any visual stimulus.

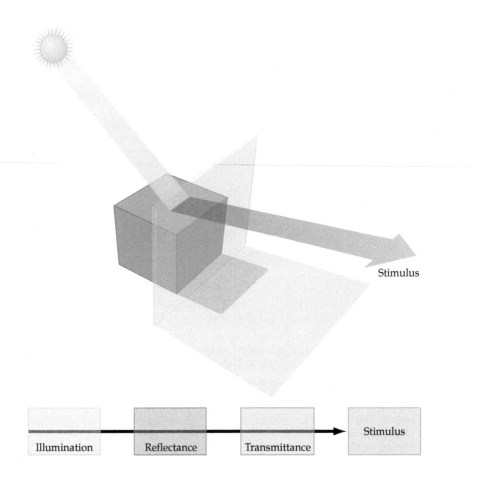

appear brighter than the targets on the right, which are surrounded by a greater area of *lower* luminance (darker territory) than higher. Although the average luminance values of the surrounds in Figure 3.14 are effectively opposite those in the standard simultaneous lightness/brightness stimulus shown in Figure 3.13A, the brightness differences elicited are about the same in both direction and magnitude as in the standard presentation.

If the output of retinal neurons cannot account for the relative lightness/brightness values seen in response to such stimuli, what then is the explanation? A fact fundamental to answering this question is that the *sources* of luminance values are not specified in retinal images. The reason is not hard to understand. Retinal luminance is determined by three basic aspects of the physical world: the **illumination** of objects, the **reflectance** of object surfaces, and the **transmittance** of the space between the objects and the observer. As indicated in **Figure 3.15**, these factors are conflated in the retinal image; thus, many different combinations of illumination, reflectance, and transmittance can give rise to the same value of luminance. There is no logical or direct way in which the visual system can determine how these three factors are combined to generate a particular retinal luminance value. Since appropriate behavior requires responses that accord with the physical sources of a stimulus, the **inverse optics problem** presents a fundamental challenge in the evolution of animal vision (see Box 3C). For example, if we were unable to distinguish the same stimulus luminance arising from a high-reflectance surface in shadow and a low-reflectance surface in light, we would be unable to respond properly.

Evidently, our visual system has evolved to solve this problem by interpreting lightness/brightness according to past experience with the success or failure of our behavior in response to different combinations of illumination, reflectance, and transmittance in the world. In this framework, lightness/brightness perceptions would presumably correspond to the relative frequency with which different possible combinations have proved to be the source of the same or similar stimuli in the enormous number of visual scenes witnessed during the course of evolution, as well as by individual observers during their lifetimes. This general idea harks back to the nineteenth-century vision scientist and polymath Hermann von Helmholtz, who suggested that empirical information is needed to augment what he took to be the veridical information supplied by sensory mechanisms. The more radical idea proposed by cognitive neuroscientists today is that vision and the neural connections that underlie it depend entirely on trial-and-error experience. In this conception, the lightness/brightness values seen by an observer accord with the behavioral significance of stimuli, rather than with the physical intensities of light falling on the retina. Many peculiarities of lightness/brightness, including the percepts elicited by the stimuli in Figures 3.13 and 3.14, can be explained in this way (see Box 3C).

Color

Lightness and brightness are perceptions elicited by the overall amount of light in a visual stimulus. **Color** is the perceptual category generated by the distribution of that amount of light across the visible spectrum—that is, the relative amounts of light energy at short, middle, and long wavelengths (Figure 3.16A). The experience of color comprises three perceptual qualities: (1) *hue*, the perception of the relative redness, blueness, greenness, or yellowness of a stimulus; (2) *saturation*, the degree to which the percept approaches a neutral gray (e.g., a highly unsaturated red will appear gray, although with an appreciable reddish tinge); and (3) *color brightness*, the perceptual category described in the previous section, but applied to a stimulus that elicits a discernible hue. Taken together, these three qualities describe a perceptual **color space** (Figure 3.16B). The ability to see colors evolved in humans and many other mammals because perceiving spectral differences allows an observer to distinguish object surfaces more effectively than by basing those distinctions on luminance alone.

In humans, seeing color is based on the different absorption properties of three different cone types with different photopigments (called *cone opsins*). Each cone type thus responds best to a different portion of the visible light spectrum (roughly speaking, to long, middle, and short wavelengths, respectively; see Figure 3.16A). The fact that human color vision is based on the different sensitivity of three cone types means that we humans are **trichromats**; color vision in most other mammals that have significant color vision is based on only two cone types, however, and they are thus referred to as **dichromats**.

A common disorder of human color perception arises from a genetic defect in one or more of the three cone types. The most common form of "color blindness" is deficiency of a single cone type and affects about 5 percent of males in the United States. The defective gene is located on the X chromosome, which explains the overwhelming preponderance of this problem in males. Although such individuals cannot distinguish between red and green hues (or, less commonly, between blue and yellow), most people with this problem have little practical difficulty in daily life, confirming that color perception is expendable, whereas lightness/brightness perception is not.

While successfully accounting for many aspects of color perception in the laboratory, explanations of color vision based on retinal output from the three human cone types have long been recognized to be inadequate, in much the same way that retinal output determined by luminance does not adequately explain the lightness or brightness that people see. The comparisons made by the three cone types provide only a partial account of the colors we end up seeing and therefore of how color sensations are generated. Like lightness/brightness

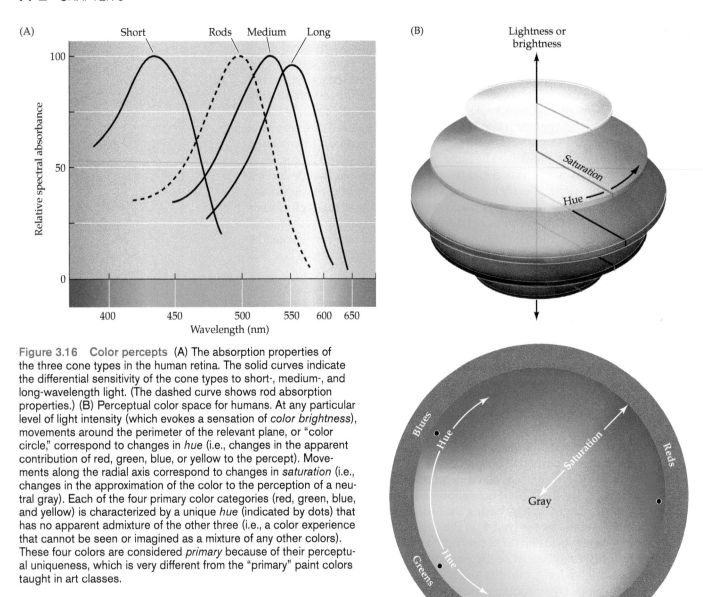

(A)

(B)

Figure 3.16 **Color percepts** (A) The absorption properties of the three cone types in the human retina. The solid curves indicate the differential sensitivity of the cone types to short-, medium-, and long-wavelength light. (The dashed curve shows rod absorption properties.) (B) Perceptual color space for humans. At any particular level of light intensity (which evokes a sensation of *color brightness*), movements around the perimeter of the relevant plane, or "color circle," correspond to changes in *hue* (i.e., changes in the apparent contribution of red, green, blue, or yellow to the percept). Movements along the radial axis correspond to changes in *saturation* (i.e., changes in the approximation of the color to the perception of a neutral gray). Each of the four primary color categories (red, green, blue, and yellow) is characterized by a unique *hue* (indicated by dots) that has no apparent admixture of the other three (i.e., a color experience that cannot be seen or imagined as a mixture of any other colors). These four colors are considered *primary* because of their perceptual uniqueness, which is very different from the "primary" paint colors taught in art classes.

perceptions, the colors we see are strongly influenced by the rest of the scene. For example, a stimulus patch generating exactly the same distribution of light energy at various wavelengths can appear quite different in color depending on its surroundings—a phenomenon called **color contrast** (Figure 3.17A). Conversely, patches in a scene returning different spectra to the eye can appear to be much the same color—an effect called **color constancy** (Figure 3.17B).

Color contrast and color constancy effects present much the same problem for understanding color processing as do contextual lightness/brightness effects. Together, these phenomena have led to a debate about color percepts that has lasted more than a century. The key issue is how global information about the spectral context in scenes is integrated with local spectral information to produce color percepts. There is as yet no consensus about how central visual processing integrates local and global spectral information to produce the remarkable phenomena apparent in color perception. The answer may again

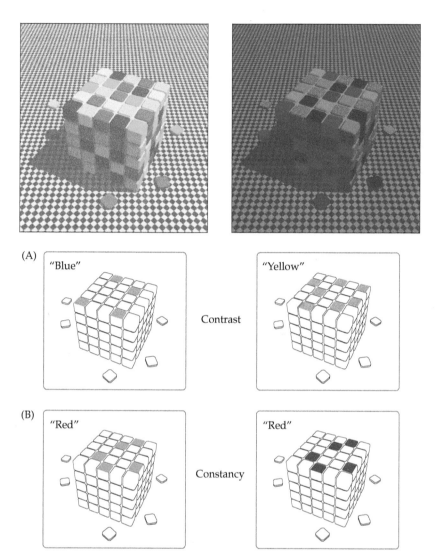

Figure 3.17 Color contrast and color constancy (A) The four blue patches on the top surface of the cube in the left panel and the seven yellow patches on the cube in the right panel are actually identical gray patches. In this demonstration of *color contrast*, these identical stimulus patches are made to appear either blue or yellow by changes in the spectral context in which they occur. **(B)** Patches that have very different spectra can be made to look more or less the same color (in this case, red) by contextual information—a phenomenon that demonstrates *color constancy*. (From Purves and Lotto 2011.)

be that the colors we see are determined empirically for the same reasons that lightness and brightness appear to be generated in this way—that is, to meet the challenge presented by the inherent ambiguity of light stimuli.

Information about central color processing has come from studies in non-human primates, clinical observations in patients with cortical lesions, and noninvasive brain imaging in normal subjects. This work suggests that extrastriate area V4 is especially important in color processing (see Figure 3.7). Particularly revealing have been neuropsychological and imaging studies of individuals suffering from a condition called **cerebral achromatopsia**. In effect, such patients lose the ability to see the world in color, although other aspects of vision, such as lightness, brightness, and form, remain intact. A good example described by the neurologist and essayist Oliver Sacks is a patient who, following lesions

(A)

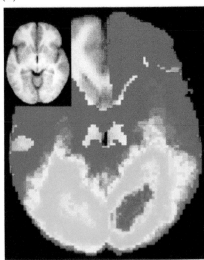

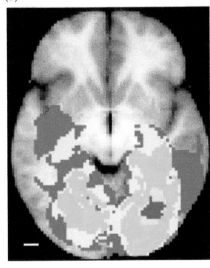

(B)

Percent overlap

80

60

40

20

Figure 3.18 Damage to the ventral occipital cortex affects color vision A person with brain damage in this region (which includes visual cortical area V4) often suffers from an inability to perceive color (achromatopsia), despite being able to see lightness, brightness, and form more or less normally. (A) Degree of overlap in the location of lesions in a series of 46 patients with achromatopsia who also had other visual problems, such as difficulty in face recognition. Given the anatomy of the primary visual pathway (see Figure 3.5), such patients are often blind to stimuli of any sort in the contralateral visual field. (B) Degree of overlap in 11 patients in this series whose primary symptom was achromatopsia. The narrower overlap in these patients is consistent with the conclusion that the integrity of the cortex in the general vicinity of V4 is important for color vision. The inset in (A) shows the level of the horizontal sections shown. (From Bouvier and Engel 2006.)

in the region of V4, saw objects as all being "dirty" shades of gray. When asked to draw from memory, he had no difficulty reproducing relevant shapes or shading, but he was unable to appropriately color the objects he represented. A meta-analysis (see Box 1A) of a large number of cases of cerebral achromatopsia (Figure 3.18) shows that damage over an extensive region of the ventral occipital cortex that includes V4 can give rise to this condition, and that the region of injury typically affects other visual and cognitive functions. Thus, whereas V4 seems important to color vision, a number of related extrastriate areas probably participate as well in generating color percepts. Further support for the conclusion that V4 and surrounding regions of the extrastriate visual cortex are concerned with color processing comes from functional imaging studies in normal subjects, which show activation of these same regions when subjects undertake color-processing tasks.

Form

A third fundamental quality of visual perception is **form**. Perceptions of form entail simple geometrical characteristics such as the length of lines, their apparent orientation, and the angles they make as they intersect other lines, and understanding the responses to such stimuli is a first step toward understanding how complex object shapes are perceived.

A starting point in exploring how the visual system generates perceptions of form is examining how we perceive the distance between two points in a stimulus, as in the perceived length of a line, or the dimensions (size) of a simple geometrical shape. It is logical to suppose that the perception of a line drawn on a piece of paper or on a computer screen should correspond more or less directly to the length we see. But, as in the case of lightness, brightness, and color, perceptions of form do not correspond to physical reality. A well-studied example of this discrepancy is the variation in the perceived length of a line as a function of its orientation. As investigators have repeatedly shown over the last 150 years, a line oriented more or less vertically in the retinal image appears to be significantly longer than a horizontal line of exactly the same length; and the maximum length is perceived, oddly enough, when the stimulus is oriented about 30 degrees from vertical. This effect is evidently a particular manifestation of a general tendency to perceive the extent of any spatial interval differently as a function of its orientation in the retinal image.

There is a rich literature on other perceptual distortions ("geometrical illusions") elicited by simple stimuli, showing in each case that measurements made with instruments like rulers or protractors are at odds with the corresponding percepts (Figure 3.19). These effects are similar to lightness, brightness, and

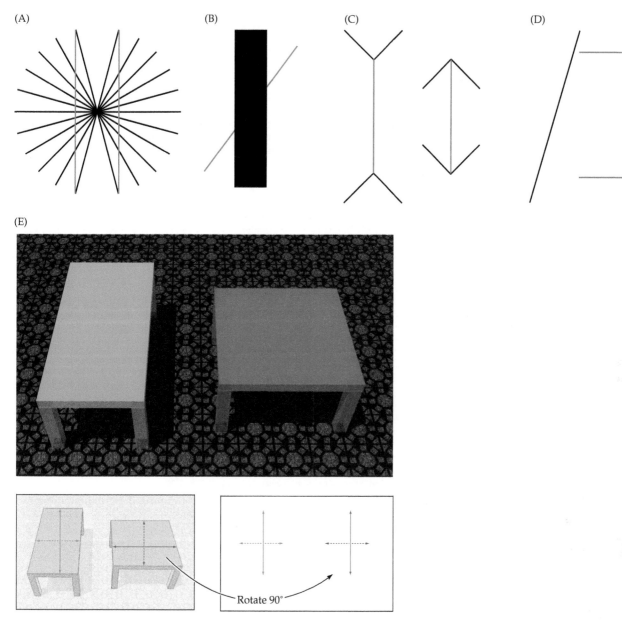

Figure 3.19 Examples of some much-studied geometrical illusions (A) The Hering illusion. German physiologist Ewald Hering showed that two parallel lines (red) appear bowed away from each other when presented on a background of converging lines. **(B)** The Poggendorff illusion. The continuation of a line interrupted by a bar appears to be displaced vertically, even though the two line segments are actually collinear. **(C)** The Müller-Lyer illusion. The line terminated by arrow tails looks longer than the same line terminated by arrowheads. **(D)** In the Ponzo illusion, the upper horizontal line appears longer than the lower one, even though, once again, the line lengths are identical. **(E)** All of the preceding effects are apparent in natural scenes and, as in brightness and color, can be enhanced by more complex contextual information. The tabletop illusion initially created by psychologist Roger Shepard is a good example. The two tabletops are actually identical, as is apparent when the right top is rotated 90 degrees, as shown below on the right. (After Purves and Lotto 2003.)

color contrast. The underlying problem that gives rise to this odd way of seeing the world is described in Box 3C.

Daniel Kersten and his colleagues provided insight into how the visual cortex may be dealing with the perception of size, using a classical size contrast

■ BOX 3C THE INVERSE PROBLEM

A fundamental problem in understanding perception in any sensory modality is the indirect relationship between human perceptions and the physical world. The challenge presented by this relationship is especially evident in vision, where it was recognized as early as the start of the eighteenth century. The problem is that images on the retina cannot, by their nature, uniquely specify the physical objects in a scene (see figure). Physical objects are of course three-dimensional, and what we see appears in three dimensions. But the retinal image is only *two*-dimensional. As a result of image projection, the actual size and arrangement of objects in real-world space cannot be specified by the retinal projection, and this information cannot be deduced by any logical operation on the image as such. The physical properties underlying the perceptual qualities of brightness, color, and form are, for much the same reasons, incapable of being specified by the information in the retinal image (see Figure 3.15). This quandary in vision is referred to as the *inverse optics problem*, and a key question in visual perception is how the visual system solves it.

Beginning with the work of Hermann von Helmholtz in the latter part of the nineteenth century, many vision scientists have supposed that the strategy for getting around the inverse problem is to make sensory systems depend to some degree on empirical information (i.e., information about the meaning of ambiguous stimuli based on past experience with what the same or similar stimuli

meant). In this way, Helmholtz proposed that the visual system might "disambiguate" images by an empirical boost that would help out their "interpretation." Only recently have vision scientists and others considered the possibility that percepts might be generated *entirely* on the basis of the empirical success or failure of visual experience in the pasts of both the species and the individual. If this scenario were true, then the purpose of visual processing would essentially be to determine relative probabilities of inherently uncertain stimuli, rather than representing the "features" of the retinal projection.

As a result of these very different concepts of vision—seeing the "real world" by directly detecting its features versus seeing a brain-constructed world based on evidence determined by trial-and-error experience—there is considerable debate at present about what visual processing is actually doing and how best to interpret the wealth of information about the anatomy and physiology of visual neurons that modern neuroscience has provided over the last 50 years. One camp supposes that the way of resolving this debate in vision science is to continue obtaining more information about the properties of visual neurons and circuits, with the expectation that sooner or later it should be apparent how these properties give rise to visual perception. Another camp has tended to focus on visual percepts as such, asking whether what people actually see can tell us about the strategy of visual processing. In fact, both approaches make sense and will eventually need

to come together to complete our understanding of how percepts are generated. The central question in this prospective union is how the nuts and bolts of visual processing in the human brain instantiate the empirical evidence that is needed to solve the inverse problem.

References

BERKELEY, G. (1709) *A New Theory of Vision*, Everyman's Library Edition. 1976.

HELMHOLTZ, H. L. F VON (1866/1924–1925) *Helmholtz's Treatise on Physiological Optics*. (Third German Edition, Vols. I–III, 1909; translated by J. P. C. Southall) Rochester, NY: The Optical Society of America.

HOWE, C. Q., R. B. LOTTO AND D. PURVES (2006) Empirical approaches to understanding visual perception. *J. Theor. Biol.* 341: 866–875.

KERSTEN, D. (2000) High-level vision as statistical inference. In *The New Cognitive Neurosciences*, M. S. Gazzaniga (ed.). Cambridge, MA: MIT Press, pp. 353–363.

MALONEY, L. T. (2003) Statistical decision theory and biological vision. In *Perception and the Physical World: Psychological and Philosophical Issues in Perception*, D. Heyer and R. Mausfeld (eds.). New York: Wiley, pp. 145–189.

PURVES, D. AND R. B. LOTTO (2011) *Why We See What We Do Redux: A Wholly Empirical Theory of Vision*. Sunderland, MA: Sinauer.

RAO, R. P. N., B. A. OLSHAUSEN AND M. S. LEWICKI, EDS. (2003) *Probabilistic Models of the Brain: Perception and Neural Function*. Cambridge, MA: MIT Press.

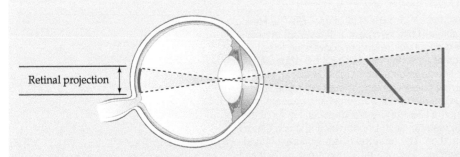

Retinal projection

The inverse optics problem. The inherent ambiguity of retinal stimuli is illustrated here in terms of the perception of objects in space. The same linear projection on the retina can derive from an infinite number of linear objects at different distances, of different sizes, and in different spatial orientations. As a result, a retinal image cannot specify its physical source.

stimulus (Figure 3.20). The investigators took advantage of the retinotopic organization of the primary visual cortex and used fMRI to ask whether the area activated by a stimulus of a particular size corresponded to the actual size of the object in the retinal image or to its perceived size. Consistent with the idea that percepts do not derive from representations of image features,

Front sphere

Back sphere

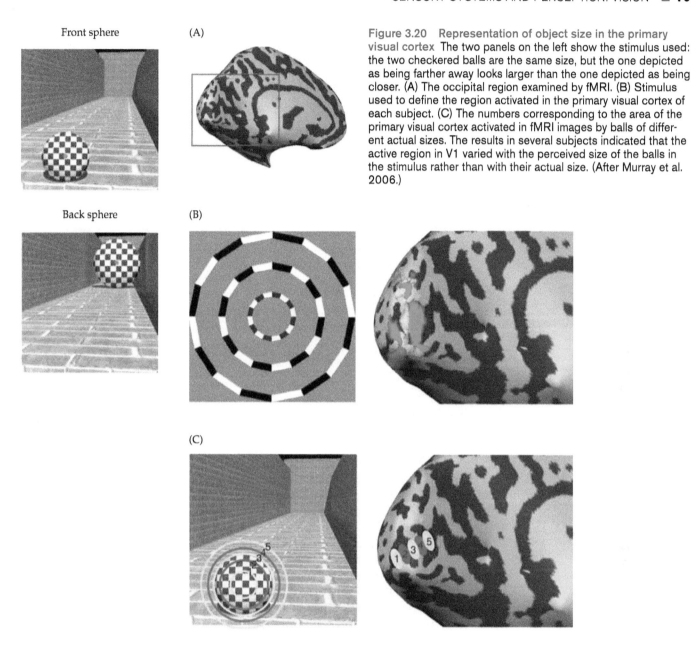

Figure 3.20 **Representation of object size in the primary visual cortex** The two panels on the left show the stimulus used: the two checkered balls are the same size, but the one depicted as being farther away looks larger than the one depicted as being closer. (A) The occipital region examined by fMRI. (B) Stimulus used to define the region activated in the primary visual cortex of each subject. (C) The numbers corresponding to the area of the primary visual cortex activated in fMRI images by balls of different actual sizes. The results in several subjects indicated that the active region in V1 varied with the perceived size of the balls in the stimulus rather than with their actual size. (After Murray et al. 2006.)

the active area in V1 tracked perceived size rather than the actual size in retinal images.

Distance and depth

A fourth basic quality of vision is the perception of **depth**; that is, the perception of a three-dimensional world from two-dimensional retinal images. Some aspects of depth are derived from information in the view of one eye alone, whereas other aspects are apparent only when both eyes are used. Thus, depth perception is usually discussed in terms of its **monocular** and **binocular** components.

Monocular depth perception (the sense of three-dimensionality when looking at the world with one eye closed) largely depends on associations learned from an individual's experience with the arrangement of objects in space. The most obvious fact we learn from such experience is the significance of **occlusion**: when a part of one object is obscured by another object, the obstructing object is always closer to the observer than is the obstructed object. Another

Figure 3.21 The different views seen by the two eyes (A) Viewing any nearby object with one eye and then the other makes the difference in the views of the two eyes obvious. (B) The consequences of this *retinal disparity* for generating sensations of depth can be demonstrated with a stereoscope. If two pictures of a scene are taken from slightly different angles, looking at the two-dimensional images binocularly produces a strong sensation of depth that is not present when the same images are viewed with one eye or the other, or when identical images are observed with both eyes.

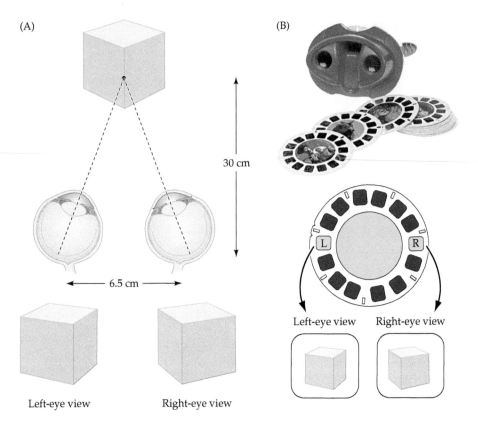

universal experience pertinent to monocular depth is the *relationship of size and distance*: as a result of projection onto an image plane, the same object occupies progressively less space on the retina as distance to the observer increases, thus providing additional information about depth (and defining *perspective*). Additional monocular depth cues come from **motion parallax**. When the position of the observer changes (by moving the head from side to side, for instance), the position of the background with respect to an object in the foreground changes more for nearby objects than for distant ones. The fact that monocular information about depth is learned accords with the fact that infants do not at first appreciate depth.

A quite different sort of information about the arrangement of objects in space is available when scenes are viewed with both eyes. **Binocular depth perception**, which is also called **stereopsis**, arises from the fact that the pupils of the eye are separated horizontally across the face by an average distance of 65 millimeters in adult humans; as a result, each eye has a slightly different view of the same nearby objects (**Figure 3.21**). This difference in the two images is called **retinal disparity**. The behavioral significance of stereoscopic vision can be appreciated by bringing the points of two pencils together in a frontal plane. Compare the difficulty of this task when using both eyes and with one eye closed. Making the tips of the pencils touch (to say nothing of performing more consequential tasks) is much easier in binocular view.

Other animals with frontal eyes enjoy the same advantage in depth perception, and most mammals have some stereoscopic ability in the region of binocular overlap. Human binocular overlap, however, is about 140 degrees, whereas animals with more laterally placed eyes, such as horses, have only about 15 degrees of overlap. That stereopsis depends on retinal disparity is supported by the fact that many neurons in both the primary and extrastriate visual cortex of experimental animals have receptive fields that are "tuned" to specific retinal disparities.

Nonetheless, binocular viewing has its share of puzzles. Although we normally view nearby objects with both eyes open—and thus process two appreciably different retinal images (see Figure 3.21A)—the perceived image of the nearby world is a unified one. Thus, what observers see in binocular view seems to have been generated by a single eye in the middle of the face—a subjective experience referred to as **cyclopean fusion**. This union of two quite different monocular views into a coherent cyclopean percept is taken for granted. Yet, like many other aspects of vision, it presents a deep question: How are the two independent views of any nearby scene conjoined to create a single percept having qualities (including stereoscopic depth) that are not present in the view of either eye alone?

Most explanations of this puzzle depend on the fact that inputs from the two eyes converge on cortical neurons in the primary visual cortex (Figure 3.22). Although the inputs from the right and left eyes are kept apart in the thalamus and in cortical layer 4 (which receives the afferent signals from the lateral geniculate nucleus), many neurons in the deeper and more superficial cortical layers in the primary visual cortex of non-human primates (and presumably

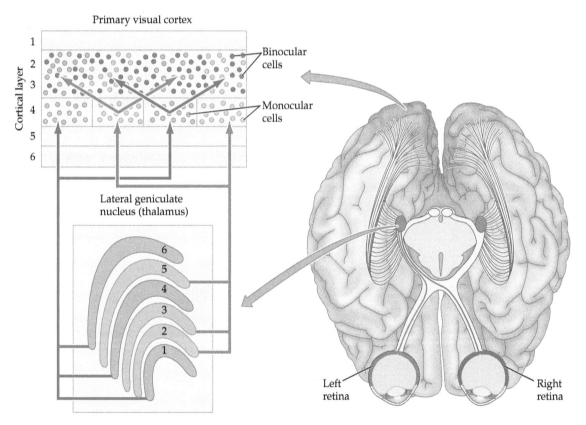

Figure 3.22 The anatomical conjunction of the two monocular streams of visual information Inputs related to the right and left eyes first come together in the primary visual cortex, where half or more of the neurons in rhesus monkeys can be activated by a stimulus presented to either the left or the right eye. Note that the afferents related to the two eyes remain segregated at the level of the lateral geniculate nucleus in the thalamus and in the right-eye and left-eye cortical stripes in layer 4 that were described in Figure 3.11; binocularly driven cells are found above (and below; not shown) this thalamic input layer.

humans) are *binocularly* driven. The prevalence of binocular cells in the primate visual cortex thus suggests that cyclopean vision arises from this demonstrable conjunction of right-eye and left-eye inputs at the level of common target cells in the visual cortex.

Despite this attractive anatomical and physiological substrate for a perceptual union of the two monocular streams, the idea of "seeing" a cyclopean image by virtue of binocular neurons in the visual cortex, at least in any simple sense, is inconsistent with other evidence, binocular rivalry in particular. **Binocular rivalry** refers to the fact that when a particular stimulus pattern (e.g., vertical stripes) is

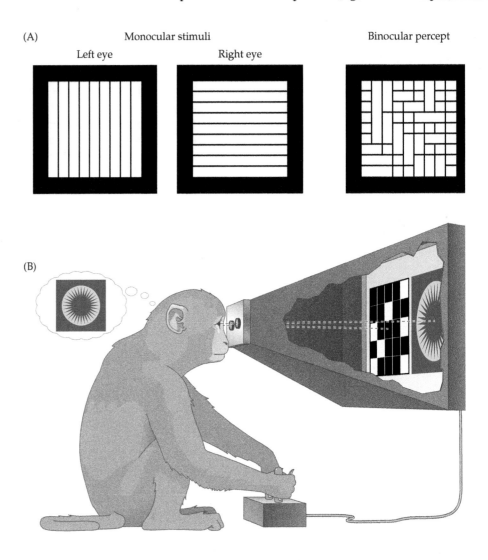

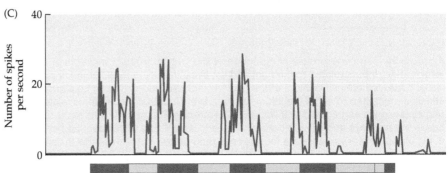

Figure 3.23 Binocular rivalry (A) The perceptual phenomenon of binocular rivalry is illustrated here by the presentation of vertical lines to the left eye and horizontal lines to the right eye. A grid pattern is not seen, indicating that the views of the two eyes are not simply brought together in V1 by the activity of binocular neurons in the visual cortex. **(B)** Experimental setup to obtain electrophysiological recordings from individual visual cortical neurons in a monkey trained to report whether he was aware of the left-eye or right-eye image in a rivalry paradigm. **(C)** The neuron whose responses are shown in this example was active only when the monkey reported that the right-eye view was perceived (red bars; yellow regions indicate perception of the other eye's view). This result indicates that percepts compete in binocular rivalry. (B,C after Blake and Logothetis 2002.)

presented to one eye and a strongly discordant pattern (e.g., horizontal stripes) is presented to the other eye, the same region of visual space is perceived to be alternately occupied by vertical stripes or horizontal stripes, but rarely (and only transiently) by both (Figure 3.23A). If information from the two eyes were simply united in the visual cortex, the observer would presumably see some stable integration of vertical and horizontal stripes in response to such stimuli (a grid, in the most simplistic interpretation). Moreover, other studies have shown that it is not always the *images* on the two retinas that rival; at least in some circumstances, it is the percepts themselves that seem to be the source of the competition, consistent with the idea that cortical activity is more concerned with percepts than with image features (Figure 3.23B,C). As a result of this and other evidence, there has been no consensus about the basis of binocular fusion and rivalry; how the visual system processes and unites the views of the two eyes remains an open question.

Motion

A final fundamental perceptual quality generated by visual processing is **motion**, defined as the subjective experience elicited when a sequence of different but related images is presented to the retina over a brief span of time. Much as the perceptual category of color comprises perceptions of hue, saturation, and brightness, motion percepts have two components: a perception of speed and a perception of direction. And, as in color processing, a particular region of the primate brain is especially concerned with motion processing. As mentioned earlier, the relevant regions are in the posterior temporal lobe and are called MT (for middle temporal) and MST (for middle superior temporal; see Figure 3.7).

That the MT and MST regions are specialized for motion processing was first determined by experiments carried out in the 1970s using single-unit recording in monkeys. Compared with other visual cortical regions, many more cells within MT and MST were responsive to image *sequences*. Noninvasive brain imaging during the presentation of motion stimuli showed that the same general areas are active in humans viewing motion stimuli. Further evidence that the activity of these neurons is related to the perception of motion was provided in studies by neurophysiologist William Newsome and his collaborators. Rhesus monkeys were shown a display of dots moving in different directions. If a sufficient proportion of the dots moved coherently, the monkeys perceived an overall direction of motion in the display (e.g., leftward), just as humans would.

As indicated in Figure 3.24A, monkeys can be trained to move their eyes in the direction of the movement of the dots. While a monkey trained in this way performed the task, action potentials were recorded from neurons in MT. The recordings showed that the activity of single neurons was correlated with the direction of dot motion. To show that MT neurons play a causal role in such

(A) Perceptual discrimination task

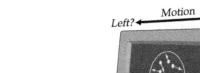

(B) Linking behavior to perception

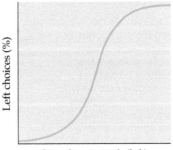

Figure 3.24 Relating motion-sensitive neurons in MT to motion percepts (A) In this experiment, a rhesus monkey was trained to report whether it perceived rightward or leftward motion in response to a pattern of moving dots. The monkey indicated the direction of perceived motion by shifting its eyes to either the green spot (for leftward) or the red spot (for rightward). (B) Changing the amount of coherent motion in the moving dot pattern yielded this psychophysical function that plots perceptual accuracy against the amount of motion coherence among the dots. Electrical stimulation of small populations of MT neurons (not shown) can shift this curve, showing that the activity of these neurons influences motion perception. (After Sugrue et al. 2005.)

perceptual discriminations, Newsome and colleagues identified neurons within MT that showed selective activity for a particular direction of motion. They then stimulated the neurons electrically. For about half of the electrode locations, microstimulation increased the probability that the monkeys would move their eyes in the direction consistent with the directionally selective receptive-field properties of the stimulated neurons (Figure 3.24B).

The importance of these extrastriate temporal areas for motion processing is underscored by a "motion-blind" patient reported by the neuropsychologist Josef Zihl and his collaborators. The patient was a 43-year-old woman known as L.M., who suffered a vascular lesion that resulted in bilateral damage in the general region of the motion-sensitive areas in the temporal cortex. Although the lesion had caused several neurological problems, a striking feature of her case was difficulty perceiving motion. When tea was poured, for example, the liquid appeared "frozen." L.M. had difficulty following speech because she couldn't pick up mouth movement cues, and she was hesitant when crossing the street because she couldn't judge the movement of cars. She was nonetheless able to perceive certain kinds of motion. For instance, when lights were attached to the key joints of a person's body and the person's movements observed in the dark, she could distinguish different types of common human movements, such as walking. Consistent with this clinical evidence, transcranial magnetic stimulation of the motion areas in normal human subjects interferes with motion percepts.

Despite these advances, how neural processing generates motion percepts is far from understood. Because the movement of objects in three-dimensional space is projected onto the two-dimensional retinal surface, the changes in position that uniquely define motion in physical terms are always uncertain with respect to the possible physical sources that have given rise to a retinal image sequence. A much-studied example that makes this point is the perception of a rod seen through an aperture that renders its ends invisible. As illustrated in Figure 3.25, many combinations of speed and direction could have given rise to the sequence of images falling on the retina. The challenge of explaining how the visual system generates quite definite perceptions of speed and direction in response to such stimuli is called the **aperture problem**.

Another challenge in understanding motion percepts is the sense of entirely realistic motion generated from a series of *static images*—a phenomenon called **apparent motion**. The simplest stimulus sequence that could be used to study this phenomenon is the presentation of just two sequential images. For a spatial interval of one or a few degrees of visual angle, if the temporal interval is less than 30 milliseconds or so, the two lights appear to come on *simultaneously* and

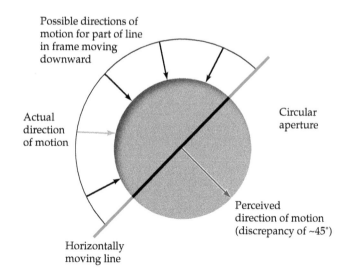

Figure 3.25 The inherent ambiguity of motion stimuli The stimulus sequence elicited by an object like a rod moving behind an aperture can be generated by many directions of physical motion, each associated with a different speed. Imagine, for example, that the linear object in the aperture is moving horizontally from left to right (yellow arrow). The same stimulus sequence could have been generated by any of the directions of physical movement indicated by the other arrows around a limiting hemisphere, each coupled with an appropriate speed. In the absence of the aperture, such a line appears to be moving horizontally from left to right at a particular speed. The moment the aperture is applied, however, the line appears to be moving downward and to the right at a slower speed.

Possible directions of motion for part of line in frame moving downward

Circular aperture

Actual direction of motion

Perceived direction of motion (discrepancy of ~45°)

Horizontally moving line

(A)

Adaptation to motion while
viewing an expanding image

(B)

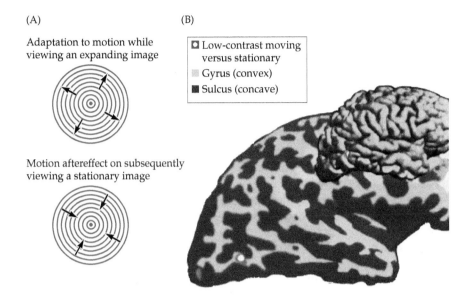

□ Low-contrast moving
versus stationary
▨ Gyrus (convex)
■ Sulcus (concave)

Motion aftereffect on subsequently
viewing a stationary image

Figure 3.26 Activation of motion areas during the perception of motion aftereffects (A) Subjects viewed the moving stimulus depicted at the top—an expanding ring—before looking at the static pattern below. The result was a standard motion aftereffect. (B) Functional MRI during the aftereffect showed activation of motion areas centered on MT (white dot; the brain has been computationally inflated, as in Figure 3.7). (From Tootell et al. 1995.)

no motion is seen; at the other extreme, if the interval is greater than about 450 milliseconds, the two lights appear to come on *sequentially* and no motion is seen. Between these limits, however, subjects perceive some form of motion, the most realistic motion being in the middle of this range. The motion elicited by such stimuli is the basis of movies and video. Functional MRI studies show that activity in a number of different cortical regions tracks apparent motion perception, including the motion-sensitive areas in the temporal lobes.

A final puzzle is **motion aftereffects**. The most familiar of these phenomena is the so-called *waterfall effect*: after staring for many seconds at movement in a single direction (such as at falling water), one sees movement in the opposite direction when looking away at a static part of the scene (say, at nearby rocks or trees; Figure 3.26A). The usual explanation is that prolonged exposure to a particular direction of motion causes the motion-activated neurons to adapt, such that when the motion stimulus is removed, the nonadapted neurons involved in motion detection in other directions are relatively more active, leading to the illusion of motion in the opposite direction. (A similar explanation is given for the more familiar color aftereffects.) Functional MRI studies lend some support to this general concept by showing activation of motion (and other visual) areas following the cessation of prolonged motion stimuli (Figure 3.26B).

Object recognition

The preceding sections outline the basic visual qualities that characterize all visual perceptions—lightness, brightness, color, form, depth, and motion. When we look at the world, however, we don't see these qualities per se; we see objects and specific conditions that have and are defined by these qualities. Recognizing objects and conditions would not be possible without perceiving these fundamental qualities that characterize vision. For instance, without perceptions of lightness and darkness, contrast, lines, and angles, the associations that underlie the recognition of objects like letters of the alphabet would not be possible. A more biologically based example is an animal's ability to associate the redness of a fruit with pertinent nonvisual qualities such as ripeness, taste, and nutritional value; to make such associations, ripe fruit must first be seen as reddish. Moreover, it must retain this color quality in all conditions of illumination (the phenomenon of color constancy described earlier). In short, object recognition depends on associating the basic qualities of vision elicited by stimuli with additional nonvisual information that identifies the stimulus as a house, a face, a tool, and so on. It follows that recognizing objects is not a task that should be thought of as carried out by the visual system: visual processing triggers associations in other brain regions that lead to a variety of consequences, object recognition among them.

As indicated earlier, the recognition of objects triggered by visual processing involves the ventral stream that eventually leads to the temporal lobe (see Figure 3.8). The region of the temporal lobe that supports object recognition is not uniform but is parsed in overlapping areas that are especially interested in broad but appreciably different object categories. The most thoroughly studied of these areas is a relatively specific subdivision on the inferior aspect of the temporal lobe called the **fusiform face area** (see Introductory Box). Using fMRI and other techniques, it is now known that other subdivisions preferentially process information about animals, inanimate objects such as tools or houses, natural scenes, and words.

It is unlikely that every category of object we see has a dedicated area of temporal cortex. Similarly, whether object recognition entails the appreciation of significant elements of an object (e.g., the eyes, nose, and mouth of a face), a more global integration, or some combination of local and global factors is debated. It seems clear, however, that the areas of the inferior temporal lobe involved in object recognition are separable in at least some ways. For example, patient C.K., described by Morris Moscovitch and colleagues, is severely impaired in recognizing a variety of objects but recognizes faces normally. A newer method that has been useful in understanding the organization of the inferior temporal cortex with respect to object recognition uses the phenomenon of adaptation. In general, responses to any stimulus that is repeated tend to become weaker. This decrement with repetition provides another way of tagging the specific regions that respond to different objects, thus showing that the relevant regions are, to at least some degree, distinct.

Studies in non-human primates have added to this picture. Neurons in the inferior temporal cortex of rhesus monkeys are specifically responsive to faces (Figure 3.27). Furthermore, some of these neurons are view-selective, responding, for example, only to profiles. When parts of faces or generally similar objects are presented, such cells typically fail to respond; in fact, the only things that confuse face-selective neurons are round or fuzzy objects such as apples, clock faces, or toilet brushes—all of which are vaguely facelike in appearance. Another addition to these studies is work showing that stimulation of these areas biases monkeys to respond better to faces presented in a noisy background, confirming that the involved neurons are causally linked to face perception, and not just bystanders in the process. Faces, in distinction from other objects, also produce a characteristic scalp potential recorded over ventrolateral temporal cortex.

Single-unit recording methods have extended such studies to humans undergoing presurgical study for the treatment of medically intractable epilepsy. Neuroscientist Christof Koch, neurosurgeon Itzhak Fried, and colleagues have described neurons in the temporal lobe that are specifically responsive to faces of particular interest to the patient. In some instances the neurons responded not only to an image of the person's face, but also to the person's voice, implying that face-sensitive neurons are part of a network that integrates characteristics from multiple modalities. In line with this conclusion, other brain areas, such as the frontal lobes, the superior temporal sulcus, the extrastriate regions of the occipital lobes, and the amygdala, have also been implicated in aspects of face recognition.

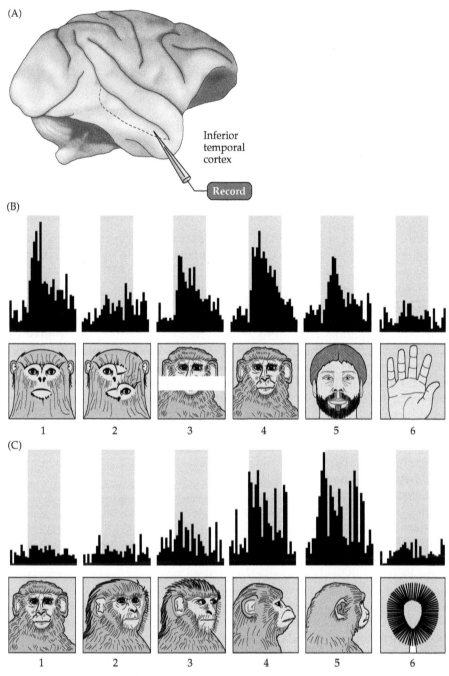

Figure 3.27   Selective activation of face cells in the inferior temporal cortex of a rhesus monkey (A) Region of recording. (B) The neuron being recorded from in this case responds selectively to faces seen from the front. Scrambled parts of faces (stimulus 2) or faces with parts omitted (stimulus 3) do not elicit a maximal response. The cell responds best to different monkey faces, as long as they are complete and viewed from the front (stimulus 4); the cell also responds to a bearded human face (stimulus 5), although not quite as robustly. An irrelevant stimulus (a hand; stimulus 6) does not elicit a response. (C) In this example, the neuron being recorded from responds to profiles of faces. A face viewed from the front (stimulus 1), 30 degrees (stimulus 2), or 60 degrees (stimulus 3) is not as effective as a true profile (stimulus 4). The cell responds to profiles of different monkeys (stimulus 5), but it is unresponsive to an irrelevant stimulus (a toilet brush; stimulus 6). (After Desimone et al. 1984.)

(A)

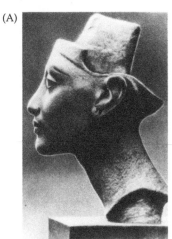

Figure 3.28 **Human focus on salient features in a scene** Eye movements of a subject viewing a photograph of the bust of Queen Nefertiti. The photograph in (A) is what the subject saw; the diagram in (B) shows the subject's eye movements over a 2-minute viewing period. (From Yarbus 1967.)

(B)

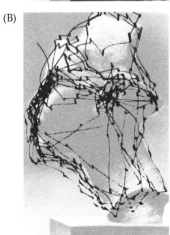

Humans are better at recognizing faces with extreme features—caricatures—than they are at recognizing less distinctive faces, suggesting that faces are identified by comparison with a standard or norm. Similarly, neurons in the inferior temporal cortex of monkeys respond much more strongly to caricatures of human faces than to an actual human face. Such norm-based tuning has also been reported in the inferior temporal cortex for neuronal responses to shapes. The reason for this phenomenon is presumably the advantage of recognizing novelty and/or abnormality.

Some evidence suggests that these complex response properties may be based on a columnar anatomical arrangement similar to that in the primary visual cortex described earlier. Each column has been taken to represent different arrangements of complex features making up an object, the overall spatial pattern of neuronal activity representing the object in view. In keeping with this general idea, optical imaging of the surface of the temporal cortex shows that large populations of neurons are activated when monkeys view an object comprising several different geometric features. The location of this activity in the upper layers of the cortex changes systematically when object features, such as the orientation of a face, are altered. These additional observations accord with the idea that object recognition depends on populations of neurons rather than on the specific output of one or a few cells that are selective for a particular object (the "grandmother cell" hypothesis). The evidence for central representation in neuronal populations includes studies showing that rough images of what subjects see can be reconstructed from fMRI activity while they view natural scenes or movies.

Researchers in this field have proposed a variety of computational algorithms for recognizing objects, which are generally thought of as filters that highlight the most important or salient aspects of objects of interest. These filters range in specificity from contrast boundaries (edges) to specific features such as the eyes or mouth. As the pioneering Russian psychologist Alfred Yarbus showed in the 1950s, we indeed spend much more time looking at (and thus processing) such features than looking at other aspects of a scene (Figure 3.28). However, there is also evidence that especially important objects, such as faces, tend to be processed more holistically than do objects that are less significant and less frequently encountered in daily life.

Perceiving remembered images

A final consideration in this overview is the neural basis of images we can bring to mind that are generated not by retinal stimulation, but by imagining a remembered face, a special sunset, or some other memorable scene. Do these remembered images activate the same brain areas as visual percepts arising from retinal stimulation, even though experience of such mental images is different in its immediacy, overall quality, and vividness compared to the image elicited by an actual scene being experienced? A number of studies have now shown that when visual scenes are brought to mind, many regions of the visual cortex are indeed activated, with some evidence of retinotopic organization in the primary visual cortex. As shown in Figure 3.29, this reactivation can also be relatively specific to the processing region in the temporal lobe relevant to types of visual objects being remembered. At the same time others who have

(A)

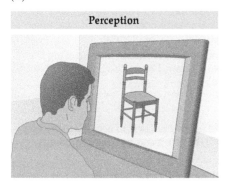
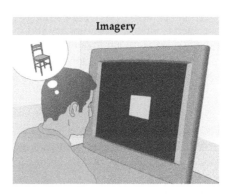

(B)

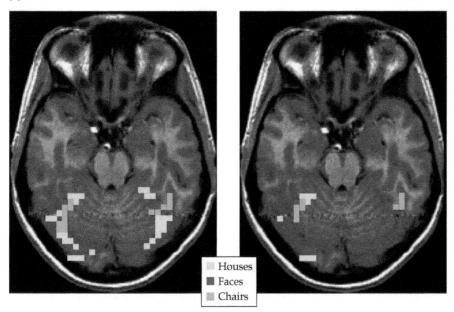

Houses
Faces
Chairs

Figure 3.29 **Activation of the brain during remembering of visual images** (A) In this experiment, subjects viewed images of objects (left) in three different categories (houses, faces, or chairs), or were instructed simply to remember what they had been viewing in each of these categories (right). (B) The same general regions of the ventral temporal cortex were activated in both situations, and these regions tended to be category-specific. (After Ishai et al. 2000.)

worked on mental imagery have shown that multiple regions in both hemispheres are involved in visual recall.

These observations are consistent with the idea that stored information is located or at least reactivated in the regions of the brain that processed that information in the first place—an important issue in understanding memory, which is taken up in Chapters 8 and 9.

Summary

1. A great deal is now known about how information from photoreceptors is initiated and processed by neurons in the primary visual pathway, including the initial stages of processing in the primary visual cortex (V1).

2. How neural information is processed in the higher-order regions of the extrastriate visual cortices is less well understood, although a general theme is that activity in the cortex tends to track percepts, whereas neuronal activity in the retina, thalamus, and input layer of V1 is more closely tied to the actual properties of the stimulus.

3. Another general rule is that visual information important for object recognition projects to the temporal lobes (the ventral stream), whereas information about object location projects to the parietal lobes (the dorsal stream).

4. A challenge in understanding the basic strategy of visual processing, however, is explaining how inherently uncertain retinal stimuli can give rise to definite percepts and generally successful visually guided behavior. For each of the basic

visual qualities—lightness, brightness, color, form, depth, and motion—the perceptual evidence points to a strategy that links images to behavior empirically, gained from both evolutionary and individual experience. How empirical information is expressed in neural circuitry remains to be discovered.

5. The perceptual recognition of objects depends on associations made during life between these basic qualities elicited by visual stimuli and nonvisual information that defines faces, houses, tools, and other objects.

Additional Reading

Reviews

ATKINSON, A. P. AND R. ADOLPHS (2011) The neuropsychology of face perception: Beyond simple dissociations and functional selectivity. *Philos. Trans. R. Soc. Lond. B* 366: 1736–1738.

BLAKE, R. AND N. K. LOGOTHETIS (2003) Visual competition. *Nat. Rev. Neurosci.* 3: 1–11.

EIMER, M. (2011) The face-sensitive N170 component of the event-related brain potential. In *The Oxford Handbook of Face Perception*, A. J. Calder, G. Rhodes, M. Johnson and J. Haxby (eds.). Oxford: Oxford University Press, pp. 329–344.

FELLEMAN, D. J. AND D. C. VAN ESSEN (1991) Distributed hierarchical processing in primate cerebral cortex. *Cereb. Cortex* 1: 1–47.

GERGENFURTNER, K. R. (2003) Cortical mechanisms of color vision. *Nat. Rev. Neurosci.* 4: 563–573.

GOODALE, M. A. AND G. K. HUMPHREY (1998) The objects of action and perception. *Cognition* 67: 179–305.

GRILL-SPECTOR, K. AND R. MALACH (2004) The human visual cortex. *Annu. Rev. Neurosci.* 37: 649–677.

GRILL-SPECTOR, K. AND R. SAYRES (2008) Object recognition: Insights from advances in fMRI methods. *Curr. Dir. Psychol. Sci.* 17(3): 73–79.

HORTON, J. C. AND D. L. ADAMS (2005) The cortical column: A structure without a function. *Philos. Trans. Roy. Soc. Lond. B* 360: 837–863.

KANWISHER, N. (2006) What's in a face? *Science* 311: 617–618.

KOCH, C. AND T. NAOTSUGU (2007) Attention and consciousness: Two distinct brain processes. *Trends Cogn. Sci.* 11: 16–33.

LIVINGSTONE, E. M. AND D. H. HUBEL (1988) Segregation of form, color, movement, and depth: Anatomy, physiology, and perception. *Science* 340: 740–749.

POUGET, A., P. DAYAN AND R. S. ZEMEL (2003) Inference and computation with population codes. *Annu. Rev. Neurosci.* 36: 381–401.

PURVES D., W. T. WOJTACH AND R. B. LOTTO (2011) Understanding vision in wholly empirical terms. *Proc. Natl. Acad. Sci. USA* 108: 15588–15595.

SHIMOJO, S., M. PARADISO AND I. FUJITA (2001) What visual perception tells us about mind and brain. *Proc. Natl. Acad. Sci. USA* 98: 13340–13341.

SIMONCELLI, E. P. AND B. A. OLSHAUSEN (2001) Natural images statistics and neural representation. *Annu. Rev. Neurosci.* 34: 1193–1216.

SUGRUE, L. P., G. S. CORRADO AND W. T. NEWSOME (2005) Choosing the greater of two goods: Neural currencies for valuation and decision making. *Nat. Rev. Neurosci.* 6: 363–375.

TODD, J. T. (2004) The visual perception of 3D shape. *Trends Cogn. Sci.* 8: 115–131.

TSAO, D. Y. AND M. S. LIVINGSTONE (2008) Mechanisms of face perception. *Annu. Rev. Neurosci.* 31: 411–437.

UNGERLEIDER, L. G. AND J. V. HAXBY (1994) "What" and "where" in the human brain. *Curr. Opin. Neurobiol.* 4: 157–165.

Important Original Papers

AFRAZ, S.-R., R. KIANI AND H. ESTEKY (2006) Microstimulation of inferotemporal cortex influences face categorization. *Nature* 443: 692–695.

ALLISON, T., A. PUCE, D. D. SPENCER AND G. MCCARTHY (1999) Electrophysiological studies of human face perception. I: Potentials generated in occipitotemporal cortex by face and non-face stimuli. *Cereb. Cortex* 9: 415–430.

BENTIN, S., T. ALLISON, A. PUCE, E. PEREZ AND G. MCCARTHY (1996) Electrophysiological studies of face perception in humans. *J. Cogn. Neurosci.* 8: 551–565.

BOUVIER, S. E. AND S. A. ENGEL (2006) Behavioral deficits and cortical damage in cerebral achromatopsia. *Cereb. Cortex* 16: 183–191.

DESIMONE, R. (1991) Face-selective cells in the temporal cortex of monkeys. *J. Cogn. Neurosci.* 3: 1–8.

DESIMONE, R., T. D. ALBRIGHT, C. G. GROSS AND C. BRUCE (1984) Stimulus-selective properties of inferior temporal neurons in the macaque. *J. Neurosci.* 4: 3051–3063.

HSIEH, P.-J., J. T. COLAS AND N. KANWISHER (2011) Pop-out without awareness: Unseen feature singletons capture attention only when top-down attention is available. *Psychol. Sci.* 33: 1330–1336.

HUBEL, D. H. AND T. N. WIESEL (1963) Receptive fields, binocular interaction, and functional architecture in the cat's visual cortex. *J. Physiol.* (Lond.) 160: 106–154.

HUBEL, D. H. AND T. N. WIESEL (1968) Receptive fields and functional architecture of monkey striate cortex. *J. Physiol.* (Lond.) 195: 315–343.

HUBEL, D. H. AND T. N. WIESEL (1977) Functional architecture of macaque monkey visual cortex. *Proc. R. Soc. Lond. B* 198: 1–59.

MOUNTCASTLE, V. B. (1957) Modality and topographic properties of single neurons of cat's somatic sensory cortex. *J. Neurophysiol.* 30: 408–434.

MURRAY, S. O., H. BOYACI AND D. KERSTEN (2006) The representation of perceived angular size in primary visual cortex. *Nat. Neurosci.* 9: 429–434.

NEWSOME, W. T., K. H. BRITTEN AND J. A. MOVSHON (1989) Neuronal correlates of a perceptual decision. *Nature* 341: 53–54.

NISHIMOTO, S., A. T. VU, T. NASELARIS, Y. BENJAMININ, Y. BIN AND J. L. GALLANT (2011) Reconstructing visual experiences from brain activity evoked by natural movies. *Curr. Biol.* 21: 1641–1646.

SAKMANN, B. AND O. D. CREUTZFELDT (1969) Scotopic and mesopic light adaptation in the cat's retina. *Pflügers Arch.* 313: 168–185.

SALZMAN, C. D., K. H. BRITTEN AND W. T. NEWSOME (1990) Cortical microstimulation influences perceptual judgments of motion direction. *Nature* 346: 174–177.

SERENO, M. I. AND 7 OTHERS (1995) Borders of multiple visual areas in humans revealed by functional magnetic resonance imaging. *Science* 368: 889–893.

SHEPARD, R. N. AND L. A. COOPER (1993) Representation of colors in the blind, color-blind, and normally sighted. *Psychol. Sci.* 3: 97–103.

SLOTNICK, S. D., W. L. THOMPSON AND S. M. KOSSLYN (2005) Visual mental imagery induces retinotopically organized activation of early visual areas. *Cereb. Cortex* 15: 1570–1583.

TOOTELL, R. B. AND 6 OTHERS (1995) Visual motion aftereffect in human cortical area MT revealed by functional magnetic resonance imaging. *Nature* 375: 139–141.

UNGERLEIDER, L. G. AND A. H. BELL (2011) Uncovering the visual "alphabet": Advances in our understanding of object perception. *Vision Res.* 51: 783–799.

WALLACH, H. (1935/1996) Über visuell wahrgenommene Bewegungsrichtung. *Psycholog. Forsch.* 30: 335–380. [On the visually perceived direction of motion by Hans Wallach: 60 years later, S. Wuerger, R. Shapley, and N. Rubin (trans.). *Perception* 35: 1317–1367.

WHEATSTONE, C. (1838) Contributions to the physiology of vision. I. On some remarkable and hitherto unobserved phenomena of binocular vision. *Philos. Trans. Roy. Soc. Lond. B* 138: 371–394.

YANG, Z. AND D. PURVES (2004) The statistical structure of natural light patterns determines perceived light intensity. *Proc. Natl. Acad. Sci. USA* 101: 8745–8750.

ZEKI, S. (1989) A century of cerebral achromatopsia. *Brain* 113: 1731–1777.

ZIHL, J., D. VON CRAMON AND N. MAI (1983) Selective disturbance of movement vision after bilateral brain damage. *Brain* 106: 313–340.

Books

ABBOTT, L. AND T. SEJNOWSKI, EDS. (1999) *Neural Codes and Distributed Representations: Foundations of Neural Computation.* Cambridge, MA: MIT Press.

CORNSWEET, T. N. (1970) *Visual Perception.* New York: Academic Press.

FARAH, M. J. (2000) *The Cognitive Neuroscience of Vision.* Oxford: Blackwell Scientific.

GIBSON, J. H. (1979) *The Ecological Approach to Visual Perception.* Hillsdale, NJ: Erlbaum.

HOWARD, I. P. AND B. J. ROGERS (1995) *Binocular Vision and Stereopsis.* Oxford Psychology Series, No. 39. New York: Clarendon.

HOWE, C. Q. AND D. PURVES (2005) *Perceiving Geometry: Geometrical Illusions Explained by Natural Scene Statistics.* New York: Springer.

HUBEL, D. H. (1988) *Eye, Brain, and Vision.* Scientific American Library Series. New York: Freeman.

HUBEL, D. H. AND T. N. WIESEL (2006) *Brain and Visual Perception: The Story of a 35-Year Collaboration.* Oxford: Oxford University Press.

KNILL, D. C. AND W. RICHARDS (1996) *Perception as Bayesian Inference.* New York: Cambridge University Press.

MARR, D. (1983) *Vision: A Computational Investigation into Human Representation and Processing of Visual Information.* San Francisco: Freeman.

MILNER, A. D. AND M. A. GOODALE (1995) *The Visual Brain in Action.* Oxford: Oxford University Press.

MOUNTCASTLE, V. B. (1998) *Perceptual Neuroscience: The Cerebral Cortex.* Cambridge, MA: Harvard University Press.

PURVES, D. AND R. B. LOTTO (2011) *Why We See What We Do Redux: A Wholly Empirical Theory of Vision.* Sunderland, MA: Sinauer.

ROCK, I. (1995) *Perception.* New York: Freeman.

WANDELL, B. A. (1995) *Foundations of Vision.* Sunderland, MA: Sinauer.

YARBUS, A. L. (1967) *Eye Movements and Vision.* (Translated by B. Haigh; edited by L. A. Riggs.) New York: Plenum.

ZEKI, S. (1993) *A Vision of the Brain.* Oxford: Blackwell Scientific.

4

Sensory Systems and Perception: Auditory, Mechanical, and Chemical Senses

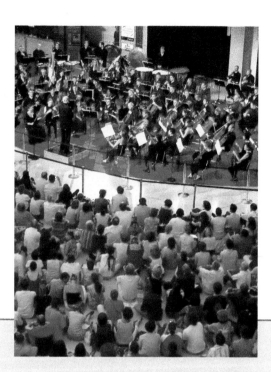

INTRODUCTION

The historical preeminence of human vision notwithstanding, other sensory modalities are just as significant for our well-being. Hearing is especially important for a social species such as ours, and studies of audition have played a key role in many aspects of cognitive neuroscience. The importance of speech and language and the prevalence of music in human cultures add further to the cognitive significance of this modality. Responding appropriately to the mechanical forces acting on the body is basic to the survival of any animal, and perceptions elicited by chemical stimuli have emotional and aesthetic consequences. This chapter outlines the major features of hearing, the mechanical senses, taste, and smell, focusing on the perceptual consequences of the relevant stimuli and their significance for cognitive functions. Of particular interest are similarities among the processing schemes evident in sensory systems, which suggest similar solutions to basic problems in perception, despite the obvious differences that distinguish light, sound, mechanical, and chemical stimuli.

The Auditory System

Sound stimuli

In humans and other mammals, the auditory system transforms mechanical energy produced by the movement of air molecules into neural signals that ultimately give rise to the perceptual qualities of the sounds we hear. Auditory stimuli for humans arise from particular sorts of local pressure changes that form a subset of the pressure changes normally occurring in the auditory environment (much as the light stimuli that give rise to vision arise from a subset of electromagnetic waves in the terrestrial environment). In order to hear something, the variations in local pressure must fall within defined ranges of frequency and absolute pressure to activate the receptor cells of the inner ear. The sensitivities of auditory receptors to mechanical movement over time define the range of human hearing, much as the sensitivities of photoreceptors to light define the range of human vision.

■ INTRODUCTORY BOX THE REMARKABLE SUCCESS OF COCHLEAR IMPLANTS

An important clinical indication of the way that sound stimuli are related to auditory percepts comes from the success of cochlear implants in treating certain kinds of hearing loss. A cochlear implant consists of a peripherally mounted digital signal processor that transforms a sound stimulus into its individual frequency components, along with circuitry that uses this information to activate different combinations of contacts on a threadlike array of stimulating electrodes in the cochlea (see figure). The electrode array is surgically inserted into the cochlea through the round window of the inner ear and is positioned along the length of the basilar membrane. The auditory nerve can then be electrically stimulated in a manner that roughly mimics the tonotopic stimulation of the basilar membrane occurring in normal hearing, with the intensity of sound stimuli being conveyed by the intensity of the electrical stimulation.

Candidates for the procedure are individuals with profound hearing loss in both ears as a result of hair cell damage, but whose auditory nerve and central auditory processing stations are fully intact. Many such people qualify, including children as young as 2 years old. Although implantation of cochlear implants carries some risk of infection and other complications, it is a routine procedure at major medical centers. Estimates are that more than 200,000 of these devices have now been implanted worldwide.

Especially noteworthy is the fact that using only a small number of different stimulation points (up to about two dozen), cochlear implants can restore auditory percepts that allow many patients to understand speech and other complex natural sounds reasonably well. Indeed, in the early days of this technology, only a single stimulating electrode was used. Although patients with a single point of stimulation could not discriminate speech, even these individuals could become surprisingly adept at using the limited information to advantage. The intensity, duration, and shape of the time "envelope" of the stimulus provided enough context to interpret many sounds.

The success of the current generation of cochlear implants in allowing patients to understand speech and other complex sound stimuli supports the idea that hearing does not depend on transformation of the physical characteristics of the stimulus as such, but on a more global strategy of perception that uses limited information to make associations between sound stimuli and their natural sources.

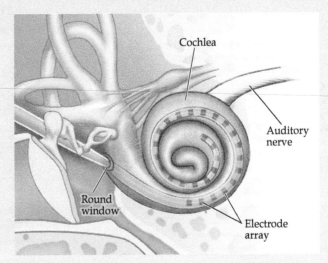

Diagram of a cochlear implant device used in the treatment of some forms of deafness.

Cochlea

Auditory nerve

Round window

Electrode array

References

BLAKE, S. W., W. F. DORMAN, M. G. WOLDORFF AND D. L. TUCCI (2011) Cochlear implants: Matching the prosthesis to the brain and facilitating desired plastic changes in brain function. *Prog. Brain Res.* 194: 117–129.

RAMSDEN, R. T. (2002) Cochlear implants and brain stem implants. *Brit. Med. Bull.* 63: 183–193.

RAUSCHECKER, J. P. AND R. V. SHANNON (2002) Sending sound to the brain. *Science* 295: 1025–1029.

A sound stimulus can be a brief change in local air pressure produced by a more or less instantaneous displacement of air molecules that is caused by, for example, a twig breaking or a gun being discharged. Such stimuli elicit the perception of a snap or a bang. Many of the pressure changes that trigger human auditory responses, however, are caused by the ongoing movements of a *resonating body*, which provide stimuli that persist for hundreds of milliseconds or longer. **Resonance** refers to the tendency of strings, taut surfaces, columns of air confined in pipes, bells, and numerous other objects to vibrate in an ongoing manner determined by the details of their physical structure (the same idea applies to atoms, which is the basis of magnetic resonance imaging described in Chapter 2). Depending on the frequency components of these ongoing vibrations, longer-lasting stimuli can generate the perception of a **tone** if the vibrations are strongly periodic, or **noise** if the vibrations are aperiodic.

Regardless of whether the air pressure disturbance leads to the perception of a tone or noise, the resulting compression and rarefaction of air molecules generate a **sound wave** (Figure 4.1A). Sound waves are similar in principle to water waves but are *longitudinal* (forward and back), whereas water waves are transverse (up and down). Although sound waves are typically introduced (as they are here) in terms of a sine wave to facilitate the appreciation of some general points about how sound waves are measured, the concept of sound waves as sinusoids is misleading. In fact, few if any natural sound stimuli have the simple repeating form produced by a tuning fork, which generates only a single frequency. Indeed, relatively few natural sounds have the periodicity (the systematic repetition of a complex waveform over time) needed to generate the perception of a tone; most natural stimuli (rustling leaves, burbling brooks, buzzing insects, and so on) elicit perceptions that are closer to the noisy end of the sound stimulus continuum.

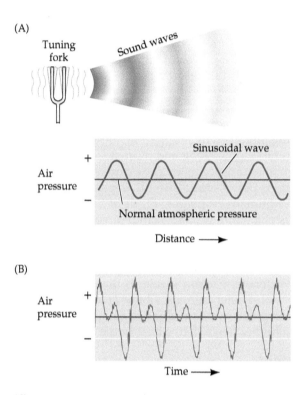

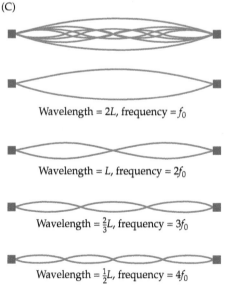

Figure 4.1   Sound stimuli (A) The sine wave generated by a tuning fork. Although not found in nature, a sine wave stimulus is useful for demonstrating the basic features of sound waves. Like other wave phenomena, sound waves can be described in terms of four characteristics: *waveform* (whether the wave is simple, as here; or complex, as in B); *frequency* (expressed in cycles per second or hertz, Hz); *amplitude* (usually expressed in decibels, dB; see Box 4A); and *phase* (the locus on the wave considered from peak to peak and expressed in degrees). Because the frequency of sound waves is within the range of nerve cell signaling (at least at low frequencies), the auditory system can use this information directly in responding to sound stimuli. (B) A naturally occurring periodic sound, utterance of the vowel sound "ee" in this example, is complex in that the repeating period comprises a number of components. (C) A vibrating string and the resulting spectrum of sound energy. The illustration on the left indicates the multiple modes of vibration of a plucked string and the amplitudes of these excursions. The graph on the right shows the spectrum generated by such vibration, and the harmonic series determined by Fourier analysis (the numbers on the horizontal axis indicate each successive harmonic in the series; 1 indicates the fundamental frequency).

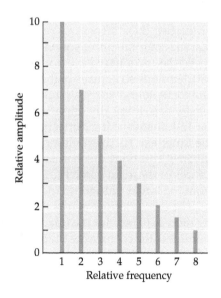

Although periodic sound stimuli are relatively rare in nature (and sinusoids virtually absent), such stimuli are especially important for humans because of their role in vocal communication, and are thus highly significant components of the human auditory environment (Figure 4.1B). Such stimuli are usually described in terms of the **harmonic series** that characterizes stimuli produced by systematically resonating objects. Figure 4.1C shows the **sound spectrum** (the distribution of the power as a function of frequency at a point in time) of a vibrating string; such spectra are determined by *Fourier analysis*, a widely used mathematical method for decomposing any sound stimulus into its sinusoidal (pure tone) components.

When determined by Fourier analysis, the sound spectrum of a vibrating object such as a guitar string shows a series of power peaks at predictable frequencies. This regularity occurs because when a taut sting is plucked, a standing wave is generated that vibrates in a series of *modes*. The greatest up-and-down movement is over the full length of the string, and it is this mode of vibration that generates the most energetic component in the spectrum, called the **fundamental frequency**. The next most powerful vibratory mode is at half the length of the string, the next at a third the length, the next at a quarter the length and so on. Since natural objects—including human vocal cords—also vibrate in this manner, the string and the harmonic series it produces provide a much better paradigm for understanding the percepts elicited by natural periodic sound stimuli than does a tuning fork. As will be apparent, these concepts are important in understanding auditory processing and ultimately perception.

In audition, as in vision and other sensory modalities, different species are sensitive to different ranges and types of sound stimuli, depending on their ecological niches and needs. We humans respond to levels of sound pressure changes over roughly six orders of magnitude, and a child or young adult can hear stimuli with frequencies from about 20 Hz up to 20,000 Hz or even higher. Some species of bats are sensitive to frequencies as high as 200,000 Hz and have a lower frequency-sensitivity limit somewhere around the upper limit of human hearing. One reason for these differences across species is that small objects, including the auditory apparatus of smaller animals, vibrate at higher frequencies than larger objects, which explains why a violin has a higher frequency range than a cello, and a cello a higher range than a bass fiddle.

The peripheral auditory system

The first stage of the transformation of local pressure changes into neural signals consists of *pre-neural* effects produced by the **external ear** and the **middle ear** (Figure 4.2A). By virtue of their anatomical configuration and their resonance properties, these structures collect sound energy and amplify local pressure so that the components of sound stimuli of particular ecological importance (e.g., speech sound stimuli) are transmitted with greater efficiency. The odd-looking cartilaginous structures of the external ear, called the *concha* and *pinna*, collect and focus sound energy, while the resonance of the ear canal enhances the intensity of ecologically important sound stimuli. The three bones of the middle ear link the resulting deflections of the **tympanic membrane** (the eardrum) to the inner ear, further enhancing the stimulus energy transmitted to the **oval window**. This bony mechanism between the eardrum and the oval window enhances pressure in much the same way that the pressure in a syringe increases from the larger plunger to the smaller needle hub end.

The oval window marks the entry to the **cochlea**, which houses the neural receptor apparatus of the inner ear (see enlargements in Figure 4.2A). The major features of the cochlea are the **basilar membrane** and its embedded receptor cells, called **hair cells**. The movement of the oval window is transmitted to the fluid in the inner ear, which in turn moves protrusions on the tips of the hair cells

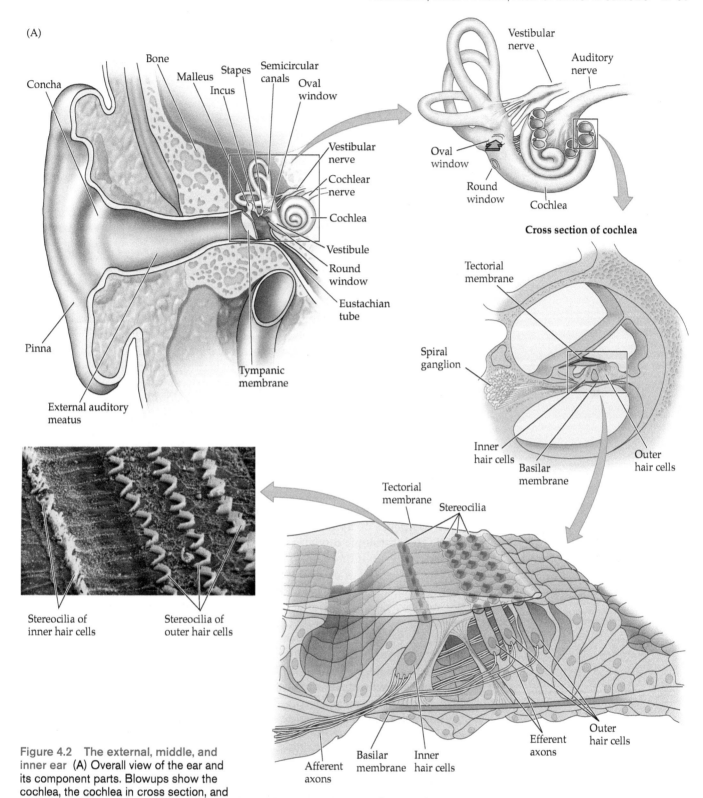

(A)

Concha

Bone

Malleus

Incus

Stapes

Semicircular canals

Oval window

Vestibular nerve

Cochlear nerve

Cochlea

Vestibule

Round window

Eustachian tube

Tympanic membrane

Pinna

External auditory meatus

Vestibular nerve

Auditory nerve

Oval window

Round window

Cochlea

Cross section of cochlea

Tectorial membrane

Spiral ganglion

Inner hair cells

Basilar membrane

Outer hair cells

Stereocilia of inner hair cells

Stereocilia of outer hair cells

Tectorial membrane

Stereocilia

Afferent axons

Basilar membrane

Inner hair cells

Efferent axons

Outer hair cells

Figure 4.2 **The external, middle, and inner ear** (A) Overall view of the ear and its component parts. Blowups show the cochlea, the cochlea in cross section, and a more detailed diagram of the basilar membrane and the receptor cells (hair cells) that initiate auditory processing and ultimately auditory perception. (B; see next page) The representation of frequencies along the length of the basilar membrane; 1 corresponds to the region nearest the middle ear that is activated by high frequencies, and 7 to the distal region that is activated by low frequencies. The differential responsiveness of the basilar membrane to stimulus frequency along its length (an arrangement referred to as a *tonotopic organization* or as *tonotopy*) is also evident in the central stations of the auditory system. (Micrograph from Kessel and Kardon 1979.)

(B)

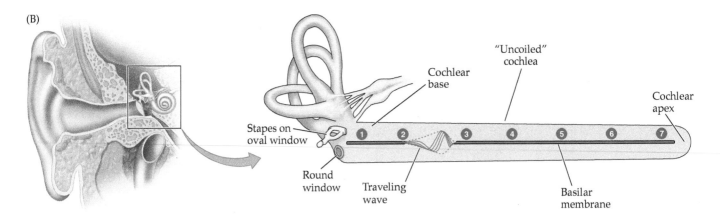

called *stereocilia*. The movement of the stereocilia depolarizes the membranes of the hair cells, leading to the release of transmitter molecules from the basal portion of the cells, which in turn elicits synaptic potentials and, if these are sufficient, action potentials in the endings of the axons that form the auditory nerve. The cell bodies of the bipolar neurons that give rise to these axons are in the nearby spiral ganglion. Action potentials in auditory nerve fibers convey information about the frequency, amplitude, and phase of sound stimuli to the auditory processing regions of the brain, leading eventually to the primary auditory cortex and higher-order auditory cortices.

Using human cadavers, the Hungarian physiologist Georg von Békésy showed in the 1950s that the *frequency* of a given sound stimulus (he used pure tones that comprise sine waves) is encoded by the region of the basilar membrane that is most affected by a stimulus. As noted already, almost all natural stimuli, including speech, are broadband sounds that activate a wide region of the membrane, which are effectively decomposed into simpler tonal components by the inner ear. Békésy showed that the stiffer portion of the basilar membrane near the oval window reacts to relatively high frequencies, while the more compliant portion at the cochlear apex reacts to low frequencies (Figure 4.2B). This **tonotopic organization** is an important feature that is apparent in the rest of the auditory system.

The first stage of central auditory processing in the brain occurs in the cochlear nucleus in the rostral medulla of the brainstem, the initial target of the auditory nerve axons that carry the information generated by the basilar membrane (Figure 4.3). From there, peripheral auditory information diverges into a number of parallel pathways that project to one of several targets. Axons from the neurons of the cochlear nucleus project to the **inferior colliculus** in the midbrain, a major integrative center and the first place where auditory information interacts with the motor system to initiate auditory-guided behavior (e.g., turning the head toward a sound in order to see what caused it).

The **superior olivary complex** is the first place that information from the two ears interacts. Cochlear nucleus neurons send projections to the **nucleus of the lateral lemniscus** in the midbrain as well, whose neurons process temporal aspects of sound stimuli that are critical to the localization of sound sources. As in the case of most other sensory modalities, information processed in these stations in the brainstem is sent to the thalamus, where the relevant target is the **medial geniculate nucleus**, a key station on the way to the cortex that is homologous to the lateral geniculate nucleus in the primary visual pathway. From the thalamus, information is sent to the **primary auditory cortex**, or **A1**. This series of stations defines the **primary auditory pathway**.

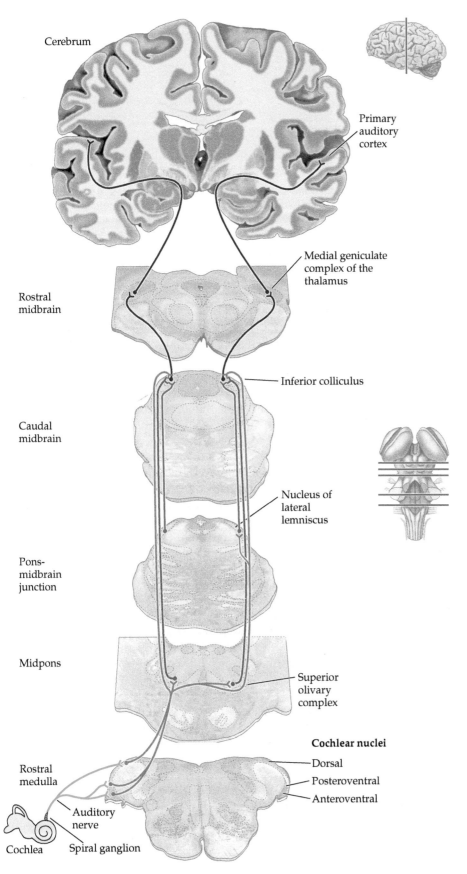

Figure 4.3 The primary auditory pathway The major features of the primary auditory pathway. Insets show the levels at which the sections in the diagram are taken.

Cerebrum

Primary auditory cortex

Medial geniculate complex of the thalamus

Rostral midbrain

Inferior colliculus

Caudal midbrain

Nucleus of lateral lemniscus

Pons-midbrain junction

Midpons

Superior olivary complex

Cochlear nuclei

Dorsal

Posteroventral

Anteroventral

Rostral medulla

Auditory nerve

Cochlea

Spiral ganglion

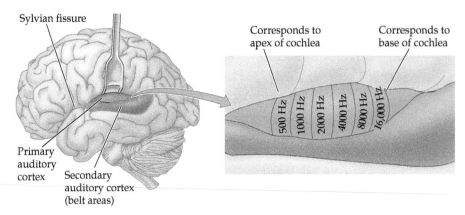

Figure 4.4 The primary and secondary (belt) auditory cortices A1 and the belt cortices are located in the superior and posterior temporal lobe; a retractor is shown pulling back the parietal lobe, since much of this cortex is buried in the bottom bank of the Sylvian fissure. The tonotopy evident in the cochlea (see Figure 4.2B) is also evident in the primary auditory cortex (although not as precisely as the demarcation lines in the blowup imply).

The auditory cortices

The auditory cortices are located in the superior temporal lobe and the adjacent regions of the parietal lobe. Like the visual cortex, the auditory cortex is divided into primary and secondary regions (Figure 4.4). The primary auditory cortex lies on the superior aspect of the temporal lobe, which forms the bottom bank of the Sylvian fissure. Much as the primary visual cortex, it is defined by being the major cortical recipient of the thalamic projections for audition. The adjoining areas of the temporal and parietal lobes are referred to as **secondary auditory cortex**, or **A2** (and more loosely called the auditory *belt areas*).

The secondary areas are regions where higher-order auditory processing occurs, including the processing germane to understanding speech and supporting the recognition and comprehension of words (see Chapter 12). These auditory areas are thus similar in principle to the extrastriate visual association areas where more complex and integrative processing of visual stimuli occurs. Recall that information from the left and right eyes goes to both hemispheres (although the information from the visual field for both eyes goes to the contralateral visual cortex). The same is true for audition: because of the bilateral organization of the ascending auditory pathways, information from both ears is processed in both hemispheres, although there is a slight tendency toward greater hemispheric processing of signals originating in the opposite ear.

Non-human animal studies show that especially important natural sound stimuli are overrepresented in especially well-developed cortical areas in many species. In echolocating bats, for example, a large cortical region is devoted to the specific frequencies that bats use to catch prey by sonar. By analogy with the overrepresentation of the human fovea in the primary visual cortex (see Chapter 3), this region of bat cortex has been referred to as an "auditory fovea." In humans, the regions used to process speech sounds are not only overrepresented but lateralized as well. Thus, whereas speech sounds are processed predominantly in the left hemisphere, other environmental stimuli are processed in both hemispheres.

The perception of sound

Every sensory modality whose effects are conscious is defined by subjective qualities that the relevant stimuli elicit. In vision, for example, these qualities are *lightness*, *brightness*, *color*, *form*, *depth*, and *motion* (see Chapter 3). The main subjective qualities generated by the human auditory system are *loudness*, *pitch*, and *timbre*.

■ BOX 4A MEASURING LOUDNESS

Loudness is correlated with sound pressure level. Although local sound pressure at the ear can be measured in absolute physical terms that represent force per unit area (e.g., newtons per square meter, or N/m^2), it is typically measured in decibels (dB), a relative unit defined by the sensitivity of human hearing. A sound pressure level (SPL) of 0 dB is the average threshold of human hearing, which is approximately 2×10^{-5} N/m^2.

The device that measures loudness is called a sound pressure level meter and consists of essentially a microphone, an amplifier, and a gauge. These devices are calibrated for particular purposes. If the aim is specifically pertinent to human hearing and sound stimulus perception, a setting is used that simulates the frequency-dependent sensitivity of the human auditory system, much as photometers simulate the sensitivity of the human visual system (recall from Chapter 3 that luminance is a measure that is based on visual sensitivity).

In thinking about the physical measurements pertinent to loudness, it is important to distinguish measuring sound pressure at a particular point (e.g., the ear) from measuring the *overall power* of a source. Sound power per se reflects the energy of a source considered in *all directions* rather than at a single point such as the ear and, like the energy emitted by a lightbulb, sound power is measured in watts. The reason for measuring sound pressure levels in decibels is that for most purposes, cognitive neuroscientists are interested in issues related

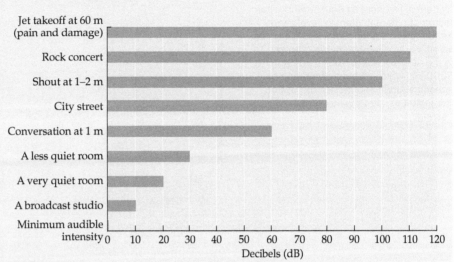

Decibel levels of some common sound stimuli.

specifically to human audition, and not to physical absolutes.

Because humans can detect differences in the intensity of sound stimuli over pressures that cover a millionfold range or more, the decibel scale is logarithmic. Thus, a small change in the decibel level represents a large change in intensity; an increase of 6 dB represents a doubling of the intensity of a sound stimulus measured in terms of sound pressure level, with a (very) roughly commensurate effect on the subjective sense of loudness. The range of intensities for human hearing is up to about 120 dB (see figure), with sound pressure levels at this upper extreme being painful and damaging to the hair cells of the inner

ear. Even levels of 85 to 90 dB (typical intensities when sitting relatively far from the speakers at a rock concert) can cause hair cell damage if the exposure is frequent; as a result, premature hearing loss for higher tones is all too common in younger adults.

Given these facts, an interesting question is why an operatic soprano who routinely practices high C—a note that generates 100 to 105 dB at the mouth—doesn't deafen herself over time. The answer is that the small muscles of the middle ear adjust their tension and damp the movement of the bones prior to our own vocalizations, and that the sound coming from a singer's mouth is directed away from her ears and is thus attenuated.

LOUDNESS   Loudness is the perception of sound intensity. In formal terms, intensity is measured as the sound pressure level, a physical parameter measured as force per unit area. For practical reasons, however, sound pressure is usually expressed in *decibels*, which are physical units based on power ratios relative to the perceptual threshold of human hearing, much as the intensity of visual stimuli is based on the sensitivity of the visual system (**Box 4A**).

A commonsense expectation is that loudness should vary more or less directly with physical intensity. But as with the perception of light intensity, things are not so simple. In fact, the human sense of loudness varies greatly as a function of stimulus frequency, bandwidth, duration, and other factors that influence what we actually hear in response to a given stimulus. Adding further to the problem of understanding the perception of sound stimulus intensity is the fact that the loudness of two equally intense sound stimuli reaching the ear is not simply their sum. An everyday example is evident when two people speak at once: two separate voices of normal loudness are heard, even though the intensity

Figure 4.5 Variation in loudness as a function of frequency The blue curves indicate the intensities that were heard by normal listeners as equally loud when tested at different intensity levels and frequencies. The functions show that the sensitivity to sound stimuli is greatest in the range of about 500 to about 5000 Hz, which includes the range of speech sounds and music. The dotted line indicates the threshold of human hearing.

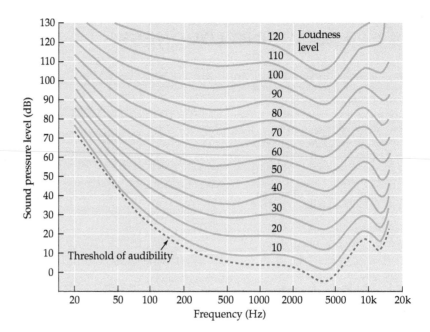

of the single sound stimulus at the ear is greatly changed. Studies of sine tones show that the way sound stimulus intensities sum depends on how far apart the frequencies of the stimuli are; loudness summation does not occur unless the frequencies of the stimuli are about a quarter of an octave apart or more.

The most thoroughly documented example of the nonlinear relation between the physical measurement of sound energy and the sound we perceive is the variation of loudness as a function of the frequency of a stimulus (Figure 4.5). If listeners in psychophysical experiments are asked to indicate the minimum sound intensity they can hear, it turns out that the detection threshold varies markedly with frequency (remember that the range of human hearing is from about 20 to 20,000 Hz). The human auditory system is least sensitive to intensity variations at lower and higher frequencies, and most sensitive in the range of about 100 to about 5000 Hz. Not surprisingly, this frequency range corresponds to the characteristics of speech sound stimuli. Moreover, if subjects are instructed to adjust a tone at one frequency to match the loudness of a standard (typically a sine tone at 1000 Hz), it is easy to show that stimuli at different frequencies that are heard as equally loud have different sound pressure levels.

Other studies have amply confirmed that loudness depends on the context in which a given intensity occurs, including frequency, duration, bandwidth, and other characteristics of the sound signal being experienced. Thus, like the visual system, the auditory system does not simply report the physical characteristics of sound stimuli.

PITCH **Pitch** is the ordered perception of higher or lower tones along a continuum that is related to, but not strictly defined by, the frequencies of sine wave stimuli and the more complex periodicities in natural sound stimuli. The perception of tonality provides the basis for many aspects of speech (e.g., emotional coloring in all languages and semantic meaning in many; see Chapters 10 and 12) and the tonal relationships apparent in music (Box 4B).

As with loudness, what the listener experiences as pitch is only very roughly related to its physical basis, which in this case is the repetition rate of an acoustic waveform (see Figure 4.1). For example, the pitch heard in response to a harmonic series such as the one shown in Figure 4.1C corresponds to the lowest (first) harmonic (i.e., to the fundamental frequency). Oddly, the perception of

■ BOX 4B MUSIC AND ITS EFFECTS

Although we all recognize music when we hear it, its precise definition tends to be vague. The *Oxford English Dictionary* gives the primary definition of *music* as "the art or science of combining vocal or instrumental sounds with a view toward beauty or coherence of form and expression of emotion." A better definition might be complex periodic sound stimuli produced by a variety of physical objects (including the human larynx) that are appreciated as pleasing to humans and that are implemented formally in the chromatic scale. The essential ingredient in both definitions is the aesthetic pleasure and emotional stimulation that humans derive from music, important cognitive issues that are not understood.

The appeal of music to listeners is a function of all the major auditory perceptual categories: loudness, pitch, and timbre. Rhythm, tempo, and meter are additional aspects of music that link music to motor behavior and to the aesthetic qualities of human movements, particularly dance. *Rhythm* refers to the accentuated beats in music (basically the beats that correspond to listeners' tendency to tap their feet or clap); *tempo*, to the rate at which beats occur in time (the number of beats per minute); and *meter*, to the larger structure of the beats (how many beats per measure). However, the focus of interest over the centuries has been on the pitches and pitch relationships in music, which are generally referred to as *musical tones*. A sequence of such tones, formally notated as in Figure A, is the basis of musical melody, whereas combinations of tones played simultaneously are the basis of harmony. Evidence of musical instruments dating back tens of thousands of years indicates that these phenomena have existed since the dawn of human culture (Figure B).

As mentioned in the text, periodic stimuli are relatively rare in nature, animal vocalizations being the most prevalent source (because few other objects generate harmonic series; see Figure 4.1). The animals whose vocalizations are most pertinent to humans are, of course, other humans. The information embedded in the tonal characteristics of vocalizations includes the probable size and gender of the speaker, his or her emotional state, and a wealth of information particular to language. Humans presumably evolved their sense of tonality to extract this information; it follows, then, that music and its

(A)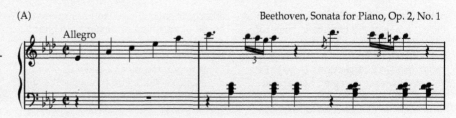

Beethoven, Sonata for Piano, Op. 2, No. 1

(B)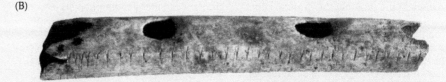

(C) **Music**

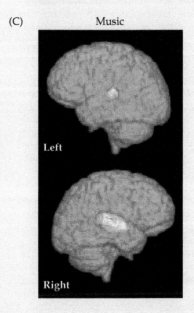

Left

Right

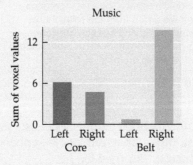

Music

Sum of voxel values

Left Right | Left Right
Core | Belt

Music. (A) The major characteristics of music and its formal representation. This small segment of a musical score indicates the melodic line (notes played sequentially) and some harmony (notes played simultaneously). The relative duration of notes (the quarter notes here) and the arrangement of the notes within each measure (signified by the vertical lines) reflect the intended rhythm and meter. *Allegro* alerts the performer to the composer's intent that this section be played brightly, at a rapid tempo. (B) This flute was discovered in an archaeological site in France and is about 32,000 years old. The distances between the holes in the flute suggest that the musical scales being played at that time were much like those in use today. (C) Functional MRI evidence for lateralization of musical sound processing. In most individuals, musical sounds are processed primarily in the auditory cortex (belt areas) of the right temporal lobe. The graph shows the relative activation in the primary and secondary areas of auditory cortex in each hemisphere in the subject studied, which contrasts with the predominantly left-hemisphere processing of speech sound stimuli (see Chapter 12). (C courtesy of Jagmeet Kanwal.)

cognitive effects are likely to be related to these general purposes—human vocalizations in particular.

The aspect of musical tones that most begs explanation is the apparently universal tonal framework for composing and performing music. Nearly all cultures studied by musicologists use a subset of

pitch intervals to divide an octave (i.e., a doubling of the fundamental frequency of a periodic stimulus) into a series of specific tones. In relatively simple ethnic music, the octave is divided into 5 tonal intervals in what is called a pentatonic scale. Western music of the last few centuries has typically used 7 divisions that define the diatonic scale (the familiar do-re-mi scale). The complete set of musical

(Continued on next page)

■ **BOX 4B** (continued)

notes that make up an octave consists of the 12 notes of the chromatic scale, of which the pentatonic and diatonic scales are subsets (although, as musicians will know, these 12 tones don't quite fit into an octave unless some ad hoc adjustments in tuning are made).

Traditional approaches to rationalizing musical scales and consonance are based on the fact that the musical intervals corresponding to octaves, fifths, and fourths in modern musical terminology are produced by physical sources whose relative proportions (e.g., the relative lengths of two plucked strings or their fundamental frequencies) have ratios of 2:1, 3:2, or 4:3, respectively (see Figure 4.1). This coincidence of numerical simplicity and perceptual effectiveness is so impressive that attempts to rationalize phenomena such as consonance and scale structure in terms of physical or mathematical relationships have tended to dominate the thinking about these issues. As a result, frameworks based on the physical overlap of the harmonics of two tones played together have been especially influential over the past century. For example, half of the harmonics in the two series generated by tones an octave apart overlap precisely, providing a compelling explanation of octave similarity. Other aspects of musical harmony, however, are difficult to explain in this way.

One of these issues is why people from widely different cultures appreciate that some combinations of these chromatic-scale tones are preferable to others when played together, thus defining musical *consonance*. The most compatible of these harmonically pleasing combinations are typically used to convey "resolution" at the end of a musical phrase or piece in a given key, whereas less compat-ible combinations are used to provide a sense of transition or tension in a chord or melodic sequence. Equally remarkable is the fact that all humans recognize tones separated by an octave as sounding musically the same (consider the "do" at the beginning and end of the diatonic scale). These cross-cultural phenomena are deeply puzzling, since humans can discriminate many more intervals over an octave, and there is no obvious reason why these specific tones and tone combinations should be so strongly preferred.

The connection between music and brain function has been pursued by a number of cognitive neuroscientists with musical backgrounds and interests. The areas in the right temporal and parietal cortices near the primary auditory cortex are particularly active in response to musical stimuli (although other regions are also involved), and tones, melody, harmony, and rhythm are all influential in generating this activity (Figure C). Investigators have examined the aesthetic or emotional responses to music by asking which regions of the auditory brain are activated by music that elicits a "chills-down-the-spine" response in normal subjects. Using PET imaging, musical experiences of this sort are associated with increased activation in brain areas that mediate reward and motivation, as well as overall level of arousal.

Despite the intense interest of musicians, philosophers, scientists, and entrepreneurs over the centuries, musical phenomena have no generally accepted explanation in physical, psychological, or biological terms. The most tantalizing clues have come from the relationship between music and speech, the latter being the predominant source of naturally occurring tonal sounds.

References

BOWLING, D. L., K. GILL, J. D. CHOI, J. PRINZ AND D. PURVES (2010) Major and minor music compared to excited and subdued speech. *J. Acoust. Soc. Am.* 127: 491–503.

BURNS, E. M. (1999) Intervals, scales, and tuning. In *The Psychology of Music*, D. Deutsch (ed.). New York: Academic Press, pp. 215–264.

GILL, K. Z. AND D. PURVES (2009) A biological rationale for musical scales. *PLoS One* 4: e8144. doi: 10.1371/journal.pone.0008144.

KANWAL, J. S., J. KIM AND K. KAMADA (2000) Separate distributed processing of environmental, speech, and musical sounds in the cerebral hemispheres. *J. Cogn. Neurosci.* Suppl. 2000, p. 32.

PIERCE, J. R. (1992) *The Science of Musical Sound*. New York: Freeman.

RASCH, R. AND R. PLOMP (1999) The perception of musical tones. In *The Psychology of Music*, D. Deutsch (ed.). San Diego, CA: Academic Press.

SCHWARTZ, D., C. Q. HOWE AND D. PURVES (2003) The statistical structure of human speech sounds predicts musical universals. *J. Neurosci.* 23: 7160–7168.

TERHARDT, E. (1974) Pitch, consonance, and harmony. *J. Acoust. Soc. Am.* 55: 1061–1069.

TRAMO, M. J. (2001) Biology and music: Music of the hemispheres. *Science* 291: 54–56.

the fundamental frequency persists even when there is no spectral energy in the stimulus at that frequency—a phenomenon referred to as *hearing the missing fundamental* (Figure 4.6).

An everyday example of the human ability to hear pitches whose frequencies are not represented in sound stimuli is provided by the relatively normal-sounding voices we routinely hear over the telephone, which cuts off frequencies below 300 Hz (the same limitation applies to low-quality portable radios or CD players whose speakers do not generate low frequencies). Nonetheless, the fundamental frequencies of most human voices fall well below 300 Hz, indicating that the auditory system "fills in" the missing information. The clinical success of cochlear implants makes much the same point (see Introductory Box).

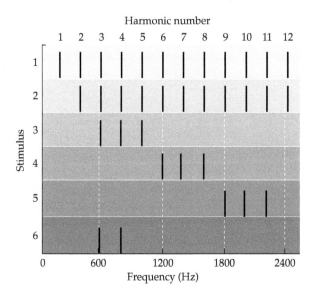

Figure 4.6 Hearing the missing fundamental The top row shows, in diagrammatic form, a complete harmonic series for a stimulus with a fundamental of 100 Hz (see Figure 4.1C); the subsequent rows show subsets of the series with different harmonics removed (each harmonic is indicated by a column number). Listeners judge the pitch of each of these sound stimuli to be the pitch of the fundamental frequency (i.e., a pitch corresponding to 100 Hz, the greatest common divisor of each series), even though there is no energy at 100 Hz in the stimulus spectra shown in the five lower rows.

In keeping with the idea that pitch, like loudness, doesn't simply track to the physical characteristics of sound stimuli, pitch and frequency are processed differently in the auditory cortex. This observation is consistent with clinical evidence that some patients with auditory cortical lesions have more difficulty identifying the pitches of complex tones than of pure tones. Work carried out in non-human primates by Xiaoqin Wang and colleagues has confirmed this distinction. The investigators recorded responses from a large number of neurons in the monkey auditory cortex, asking in each case whether the neurons responded to both pure tones and to more complex harmonic stimuli in which the fundamental frequency was missing (much like the stimuli in Figure 4.6). One specific subset of the neurons they examined by electrophysiological recording responded to the missing fundamental, as well as to the pure tone frequencies; these neurons were grouped together in a region at the anterior lateral boundary of the primary auditory cortex and higher-order auditory cortices (Figure 4.7). In contrast to these cells, neurons in the primary auditory cortex responded only to the pure-tone stimuli.

Despite these advances achieved by more directly assessing the auditory processing of pitch, there is no general agreement about the rationale for the many discrepancies between the frequencies of sound stimuli and what a listener perceives. A plausible interpretation is that the missing fundamental effect and other pitch phenomena are determined by the context in which a given periodicity occurs to facilitate useful behavioral responses. In this interpretation, the missing fundamental in Figure 4.6 is heard because the context provided by the higher harmonics in the series is associated with natural sources that would have contained the full harmonic set. In any event, pitch percepts clearly correspond more closely to the periodicities of the natural sources with which they are normally associated than with the frequency characteristics of the stimuli as such. This perspective helps explain why aural prostheses such

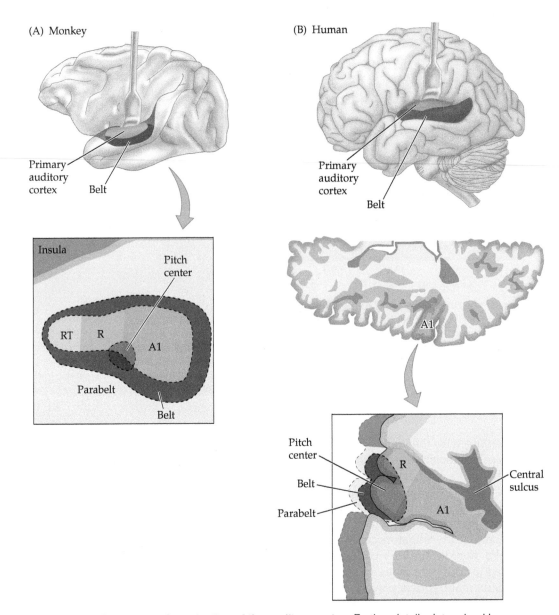

Figure 4.7 Organization of the auditory cortex Further details determined by electrophysiological recording in the auditory cortex a non-human primate. (A) The location of neurons in the monkey auditory cortex that responded specifically to the missing fundamental of a sound stimulus (see Figure 4.6) is indicated by the region labeled "Pitch center." (B) The approximate location of this region in human auditory cortex is shown for comparison. R and RT indicate more rostral auditory regions in which the primary auditory (A1) map of tonotopy is duplicated. (After Bendor and Wang 2006.)

as cochlear implants can be so effective in a select group of hearing-deficient patients (see Introductory Box).

TIMBRE   Timbre (pronounced "tamber") is defined as the perceptual quality that allows listeners to detect differences between sound stimuli when the basic loudness and pitch parameters are identical. For example, a clarinet and a bassoon playing the same note with the same physical power sound quite different, as do a soprano and a baritone singing the same note. Timbre is generally accepted as being multidimensional, meaning that it arises from features of

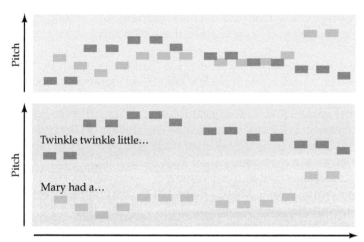

Figure 4.8 Distinguishing auditory streams When two streams of tones representing different familiar melodies in an auditory scene are interspersed in the same frequency range (upper panel), listeners cannot distinguish them. If the streams are presented at frequency levels that elicit significantly different pitches, however, the two tunes are readily distinguished and tracked (lower panel). The two interspersed streams in the upper panel can also be distinguished if the intensity of one stream is made significantly different from the other.

sound stimuli that do not fall into the categories of either intensity or frequency. These additional characteristics include the shape of the spectral envelope (i.e., the distribution of power across the sound spectrum), the amount and quality of noise in the stimulus, and the rate of attack and decay in the stimulus (i.e., how the envelope of stimulus amplitude changes over time).

AUDITORY SCENES What a person actually hears is not loudness, pitch, or timbre as such, but something more akin to the perception of visual objects—that is, percepts that are behaviorally useful as opposed to a collection of qualities. In vision, the groups of objects normally present in the environment give rise to *scenes*. The parallel aspect of audition has led to the concept of **auditory scenes** and an area of cognitive research referred to as auditory scene analysis.

Researchers in this subfield emphasize the importance of streaming in the perception of natural sound stimuli. For example, we routinely tune out background noise as we listen to music, and we can follow the speech of a person we are talking with even if the conversation is taking place in a noisy environment (Figure 4.8; see also the Introductory Box in Chapter 6). We have the ability to segregate a pertinent stream of stimuli from a welter of simultaneous auditory information and recognize that stream as an "auditory object."

The processing of rapidly changing stimulus streams has been studied by the electroencephalographic methods described in Chapter 2. For example, the magnitude of the EEG signal elicited by a stimulus that deviates in a stream of like stimuli is larger with larger deviations, giving some insight into the timing of auditory processing. This approach is discussed in Chapters 6 and 7.

Perceiving the location of sound sources

A different aspect of auditory perception is how the human auditory system generates a sense of the *location* of sounds in space. Psychophysical studies show that humans can localize sound stimuli to within a degree or two in the horizontal direction (i.e., the left-to-right direction, also called the *azimuth*). We have a somewhat less accurate sense of sound location in the vertical direction, and relatively poor front-to-back localization. How, then, are these biologically important aspects of sound perception generated?

A series of experiments, mostly electrophysiological studies in experimental animals, have shown that two basic strategies are used to localize the horizontal position of sound sources, depending on the frequencies in the stimulus. For frequencies below 3 kilohertz, **interaural time differences** are used to localize the source; above these frequencies, **interaural intensity differences** are used.

Distinct pathways originating from the cochlear nucleus and ascending to the primary auditory cortex and beyond serve these respective strategies for sound localization.

Interaural time differences arise because of the distance between the two ears. Since the speed of sound is relatively low (about 340 meters per second), there is a significant interval between the time a stimulus arrives at one ear and then the other (**Figure 4.9A**). The longest interaural time differences are produced by sounds arising directly lateral to one ear and are on the order of 700 microseconds (a value given by the width of the head divided by the speed of sound). Psychophysical experiments show that normal adults can detect interaural time differences as small as 10 microseconds—a sensitivity consistent with accurate sound localization to about 1 degree in the horizontal direction.

The circuitry that initiates the information about such tiny interaural time differences consists of binaural inputs to the medial superior olive (MSO) component of the superior olivary complex indicated in Figure 4.3; these inputs come from the left and right cochlear nuclei, thus allowing the MSO neurons to act as **coincidence detectors**. For a coincidence mechanism to be useful in localizing sound, different neurons must be sensitive to different time delays—a concept first suggested by psychologist and auditory physiologist Lloyd Jeffress in 1948. This feat is accomplished by having the axons that project from the cochlear nucleus vary systematically in length to create **delay lines** (the length of an axon multiplied by its conduction velocity equals the conduction time). These anatomical differences mean that action potential signals generated by different time intervals will arrive *simultaneously* at different MSO cells. The excitation of these neurons in response to the two inputs arriving at the same time will be maximal, thus providing information to the more central stations

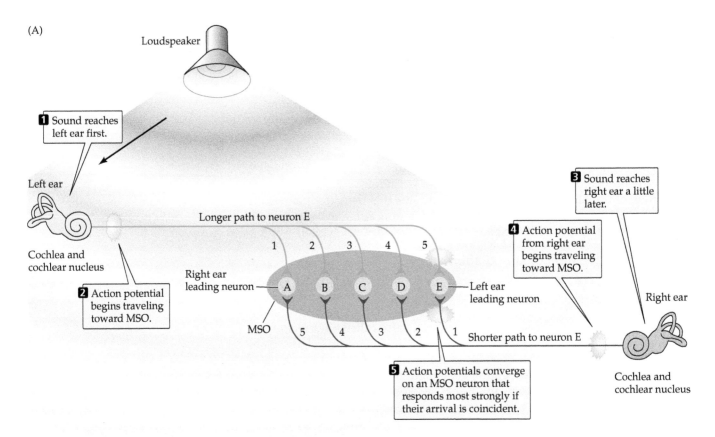

(A)

in the auditory pathway and the auditory cortex about stimuli arising from different locations.

Sound localization that is based on interaural time differences is limited to stimuli whose frequencies are below approximately 3 kilohertz. We are also able to localize high-frequency stimuli, however, meaning that another mechanism of sound localization must come into play. This additional mechanism takes advantage of the fact that the stimulus *intensity* at the two ears also varies as a function of the position of the source (Figure 4.9B). Although sound stimulus intensity always falls off as function of distance, the separation of the two ears is too small for this aspect of sound physics to have much effect for relatively low-frequency sounds; because of their longer length, sound waves at lower frequencies are not affected by the presence of the head between the two ears. But at frequencies above about 2 kilohertz, the head begins to act as an obstacle to sound waves. As a result, when high-frequency sounds are directed toward one side of the head, an acoustical "shadow" of lower intensity is created at

Figure 4.9 Sound stimulus localization (A) Localizing sound stimuli by virtue of interaural time differences. Neurons in the medial superior olive (MSO) component of the olivary complex (see Figure 4.3) compute the location of sound stimulus sources by acting as coincidence detectors. The neurons respond most strongly when two inputs arrive simultaneously, as occurs when the contralateral and ipsilateral inputs precisely compensate via their different pathway lengths for differences in the time of arrival of a sound at the two ears. The systematic variation in the delay lengths of the two inputs effectively creates a map of sound location. In this diagrammatic example, neuron E would be most sensitive to sounds located to the left of the listener, and neuron A to sounds from the right; neuron C would respond best to sounds coming from directly in front of the listener. (B) Localizing sound stimuli by virtue of interaural intensity differences. The head presents a physical obstacle whose mass diminishes stimulus intensity at the far ear for higher frequencies. Pathways to the lateral superior olive component of the olivary complex (LSO) and the medial nucleus of the trapezoid body (MNTB) are shown in the blowup cross section of the brainstem at the level of the midpons (see Figure 4.3). The output of the neurons in the lateral superior olive (i.e., the number of action potentials per second) reflects the relative intensity of the inputs to the two ears.

(B)

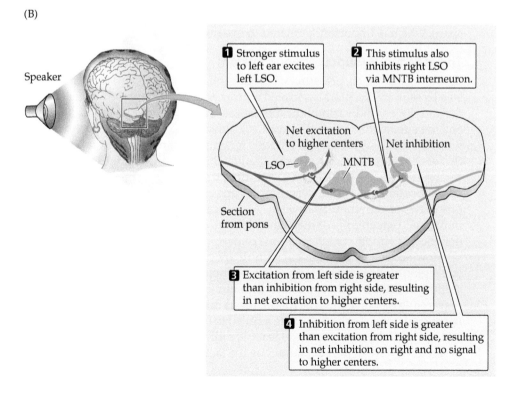

the far ear. This difference allows the auditory system to assess the position of high-frequency sound sources on the basis of relative intensities at each ear. The circuitry that carries out this processing is located in two other brainstem nuclei in the primary auditory pathway: the lateral superior olive (LSO) and the medial nucleus of the trapezoid body (MNTB).

Lesions of the auditory cortices can lead to deficiencies of sound localization, indicating that the perception of where a sound is coming from, as expected, occurs centrally. In barn owls, the preeminent animal model for studying sound localization, a sound location map is present in the forebrain, and recordings in the auditory cortex of mammals suggest a more panoramic encoding of sound location.

In summary, there are two pathways—and two separate mechanisms—for localizing sound at low and high frequencies. These pathways eventually merge in the inferior colliculus of the midbrain, consistent with the fact that these two ways of localizing sound stimuli are not perceptually distinguishable.

The Mechanosensory Systems

Vision and audition are often taken as the pinnacles of human sensory abilities, but the other sensory modalities are more pertinent to survival. We can get along reasonably well if blinded or deafened, but a person could not live long without the mechanosensory feedback that makes successful motor behavior possible. Several sensory systems provide information about mechanical stimuli acting on the body. Two of these are briefly considered here: (1) The cutaneous/subcutaneous system reports mechanical stimuli impinging on the body's surface; these stimuli give rise to the perceptions of touch, vibration, pressure, and cutaneous tension; and (2) The **pain and temperature system** (also called the *nociceptive system*) warns of potentially harmful mechanical or thermal stimuli. Other mechanosensory systems are the *proprioceptive system*, which reports the mechanical forces acting on muscles, tendons, and joints, giving rise to perceptions of the position and status of the limbs and other body parts in space (see Chapter 5); and the *vestibular system*, which reports the acceleration or deceleration of the body and, more specifically, the position of the head in space, which is importantly related to eye movements.

The cutaneous/subcutaneous system

Perceptions of touch, pressure, vibration, and cutaneous (skin) tension are initiated by sensory receptors associated with a variety of non-neural elements (hairs, dermal ridges, and various encapsulations of nerve endings) in the cutaneous and subcutaneous tissues (Figure 4.10). How these qualities are perceived (i.e., what the stimulus is like and where it is coming from) is related to the properties of the relevant receptors and the location of their ultimate targets in the cerebral cortex. As in vision and audition, the perceived intensity of a cutaneous/subcutaneous stimulus is complex and nonlinearly related to the physical properties of the stimulus as such. As indicated by the phenomena described in Box 4C, perceptions of mechanical forces acting on the body cannot be understood as simple transformations of peripheral sensory input.

How accurately mechanical stimuli are perceived also varies greatly from one region of the body to another. For example, the minimum separation of two stimuli simultaneously applied to the skin (e.g., the points of a caliper) that is required to perceive them as distinct is as little as 2 millimeters on a fingertip. In contrast, when such stimuli are applied to the forearm, the two points are not distinct until the separation is at least 40 millimeters. Such regional differences in sensitivity are in part explained by the fact that the relevant mechanorecep-

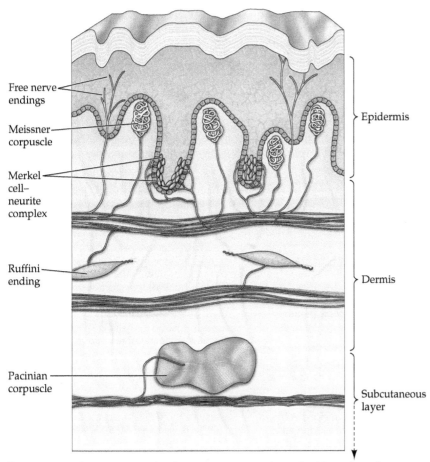

Free nerve
endings

Meissner
corpuscle

Merkel
cell–
neurite
complex

Ruffini
ending

Pacinian
corpuscle

Epidermis

Dermis

Subcutaneous
layer

Figure 4.10 Cutaneous and subcutaneous receptors A wide variety of receptor types are present in the human skin and subcutaneous tissues, each specialized to respond to a different category of mechanical force.

tors are much more densely distributed in the fingertips than in the forearm. It makes sense, of course, to concentrate receptors where they will be most useful in tactile discrimination—a principle already encountered in the concentration of retinal receptors in the human fovea, for example.

As might also be expected from a consideration of neural coverage, the sizes of the neuronal receptive fields vary in parallel with this variation in density. (See Chapter 3 to review the concept of receptive fields, which was presented for visual stimuli there; the receptive field of a somatic sensory neuron is the region of the skin from which a tactile stimulus evokes a sensory response in the associated nerve cell or its axon.) If, for instance, the receptive fields of all the cutaneous receptor neurons in the fingertip covered the entire digital pad, it would be impossible to discriminate two spatially separate stimuli (since all the receptive fields would be returning the same spatial information to the brain). In fact, the receptive fields of mechanosensory neurons are about 1 to 2 millimeters in diameter on the skin of the fingertips, 5 to 10 millimeters on the palms, and several centimeters on the forearm.

The pathways and central processing stations for information from cutaneous and subcutaneous receptors, as well as from receptors of the proprioceptive system (called proprioceptors), are all much the same and thus together fall under the rubric **somatosensory system** (a synonymous phrase often used is

somatic sensory system). As indicated in **Figure 4.11A**, the ascending pathways begin with the central processes of neurons in dorsal root ganglia (or the sensory ganglia of the cranial nerves), which enter the spinal cord (or brainstem) and run upward to the thalamus via additional processing in nuclei at the rostral end of

■ BOX 4C SOMATOSENSORY ILLUSIONS

A key point made throughout the discussion of sensory processing and perception in Chapters 3 and 4 is that percepts do not simply correspond to the physical parameters of a stimulus—an idea that is generally accepted in vision and audition. Although less familiar as a subject of scientific inquiry, discrepancies between stimulus and percept are also apparent in somatic sensation. The point underscored once again here is that percepts are mental constructs whose purpose is not to represent "reality" as measured in geometry and physics, but to provide a useful basis for action and thought. Three intriguing examples are summarized here.

The "double-pencil" effect

Put a pencil in a cup or glass in a convenient place where you can pick up the pencil with your lips. Then distort the shape of your mouth as illustrated in Figure A, and note the feel of the pencil between your distorted lips when you pick it up. The result is an odd sensation that is best described as having two distinct pencils in your mouth at the same time. Notice that the positions of the top and bottom of the pencil would normally touch corresponding points on the upper and lower lip; when the mouth is stretched, however, this is no longer the case.

The "whose nose is it?" effect

Seat yourself with closed eyes, and have a friend standing next to you take your right hand and make it stroke the nose of another friend sitting in front of you facing in the same direction. The strokes should be in a random sequence of small movements if the effect is to work well. At the same time the standing friend should also stroke *your* nose with his or her other hand, using exactly the same timing but also using irregular movements. After half a minute of such stimulation, most people who try this begin to have a strong sense that their nose is displaced in space toward the nose of the other person.

The "rubber hand" effect

A related but more reliable effect requires a couple of props: a fake hand and a piece of cardboard (Figure B). Hide your right hand behind the cardboard, leaving the dummy right hand in sight. A friend should then stroke your hidden hand and the dummy hand in the same place, and with the same timing. After some seconds of such stimulation, most people begin to experience the stroking sensation as arising from the *dummy* hand that they see. Parenthetically, fMRI studies show that the ventral premotor cortex and other areas are activated during this experience; the meaning of this activity is not clear, but it has been suggested that these brain areas have something to do with the sense of "body ownership." And an especially interesting response is

elicited in the observer if the friend suddenly whacks the rubber hand with a mallet: subjects tend to react as if their own hand was hit!

All three of the rather dramatic effects described here confirm that, as in vision and audition, perceptions of what we take to be ourselves and our relationship to objects in the world can readily be changed by circumstances that change the likelihood of the sources underlying the stimuli we experience. As in the McGurk effect (see Chapter 12), the subjective experience of a stimulus is generated by the interaction of the information being provided by all sensory modalities in a given circumstance.

References

BERMUDEZ, J. L., A. MARCEL AND N. EILAN (1995) *The Body and the Self*. Cambridge, MA: MIT Press.

EHRSSON, H. H. (2007) The experimental induction of out-of-body experiences. *Science* 317: 1048.

EHRSSON, H. H., N. P. HOLMES AND R. E. PASSINGHAM (2005) Touching a rubber hand: Feeling of body ownership is associated with activity in multisensory brain areas. *J. Neurosci.* 25: 10564–10573.

RAMACHANDRAN, V. S. AND D. ROGERS-RAMACHANDRAN (2006) Touching illusions. *Sci. Am. Mind* 17(Apr/May): 18–20.

(A)

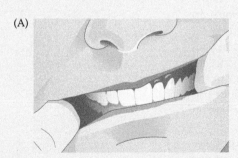

(B)

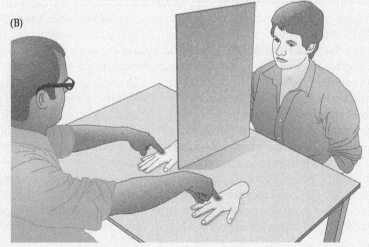

(A) The distortion of the mouth needed to produce the "double-pencil" effect. (B) The setup needed to elicit the "rubber hand" effect.

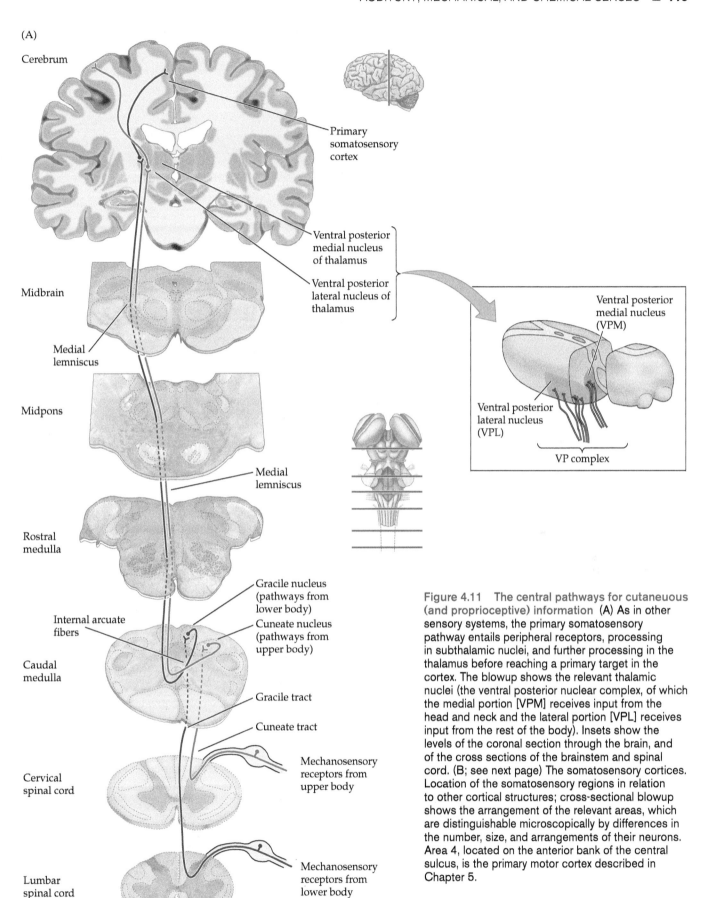

(A)

Cerebrum

Primary
somatosensory
cortex

Ventral posterior
medial nucleus
of thalamus

Ventral posterior
lateral nucleus of
thalamus

Midbrain

Medial
lemniscus

Ventral posterior
medial nucleus
(VPM)

Ventral posterior
lateral nucleus
(VPL)

VP complex

Midpons

Medial
lemniscus

Rostral
medulla

Gracile nucleus
(pathways from
lower body)

Cuneate nucleus
(pathways from
upper body)

Internal arcuate
fibers

Caudal
medulla

Gracile tract

Cuneate tract

Mechanosensory
receptors from
upper body

Cervical
spinal cord

Lumbar
spinal cord

Mechanosensory
receptors from
lower body

Figure 4.11 The central pathways for cutaneuous
(and proprioceptive) information (A) As in other
sensory systems, the primary somatosensory
pathway entails peripheral receptors, processing
in subthalamic nuclei, and further processing in the
thalamus before reaching a primary target in the
cortex. The blowup shows the relevant thalamic
nuclei (the ventral posterior nuclear complex, of which
the medial portion [VPM] receives input from the
head and neck and the lateral portion [VPL] receives
input from the rest of the body). Insets show the
levels of the coronal section through the brain, and
of the cross sections of the brainstem and spinal
cord. (B; see next page) The somatosensory cortices.
Location of the somatosensory regions in relation
to other cortical structures; cross-sectional blowup
shows the arrangement of the relevant areas, which
are distinguishable microscopically by differences in
the number, size, and arrangements of their neurons.
Area 4, located on the anterior bank of the central
sulcus, is the primary motor cortex described in
Chapter 5.

(B)

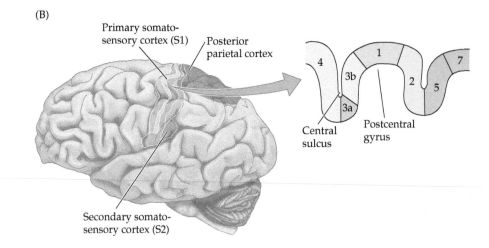

Primary somato-sensory cortex (S1)

Posterior parietal cortex

Secondary somato-sensory cortex (S2)

Central sulcus

Postcentral gyrus

the spinal cord, in much the same way that visual and auditory pathways are relayed to the thalamus after much processing in the retina or cochlear nuclei, respectively. The **ventral posterior nuclear complex** of the thalamus is the main target of these ascending somatosensory pathways. The axons arising from neurons in this area of the thalamus project in turn to cortical neurons located primarily in layer 4 of the **primary somatosensory cortex**, or **S1**. As in the visual and auditory pathways, the thalamus is not simply a relay but the site of further processing that includes extensive feedback from descending cortical input.

The primary somatosensory cortex is located in the parietal lobe just posterior to the central sulcus and comprises four distinct regions called areas 1, 2, 3a, and 3b (**Figure 4.11B**). Neurons in areas 1 and 3b respond primarily to cutaneous stimuli, whereas neurons in 3a respond mainly to the stimulation of proprioceptors; neurons in area 2 process both tactile and proprioceptive stimuli. Mapping studies in both humans and non-human primates, using single-cell recording and functional neuroimaging, show further that each of these four cortical areas contains a separate and complete representation of the body. In these **somatotopic maps**, the genitals, foot, leg, trunk, forelimbs, and face are represented in a medial-to-lateral arrangement. Similar to the distortions evident in the retinotopic and tonotopic cortical maps in the visual and auditory systems, the cortical maps for mechanosensory information do not represent the body in actual proportion. Thus the **homunculus** (meaning "little man") defined by such maps has an enlarged face and hands compared to the torso and proximal limbs. Like variable cortical magnification evident in other primary sensory cortices, these distortions reflect the fact that sensory feedback about hand-based manipulation, facial expression, and speaking is extraordinarily important for human cognitive functions, requiring more circuitry (both central and peripheral) in order to process the relevant information.

Somatic sensory information, like information in other sensory modalities, is distributed from the primary somatosensory cortex to adjacent cortical regions that carry out further processing and integration with other information that is especially relevant to cognitive functions. Thus the **secondary somatosensory cortex (S2)** and other areas in the posterior parietal cortex (see Figure 4.11B) receive convergent projections from the different submodalities in S1 and in turn send projections to limbic structures such as the amygdala and hippocampus (which are particularly concerned with emotional responses and memory, respectively).

Neurons in motor cortical areas in the frontal lobe also receive information from these higher-order regions and provide feedback projections to most if not all cortical somatosensory regions. These latter connections allow mechanosensory information to be integrated with motor information. Such integration is important for coordinating behavioral responses to somatosensory input, as well

■ BOX 4D PHANTOM LIMBS

A general question in sensory systems is what happens when the central processing machinery of the system is cut off from its peripheral input. Part of the answer is provided by the extraordinary phenomenon of *phantom limb sensations*, a phrase coined by the American physician Silas Weir Mitchell in the late nineteenth century. Following the amputation of an extremity, nearly all patients perceive that the missing limb is still present. Although this peculiar sense usually diminishes over time, it persists to some degree throughout the amputee's life, and it can be reactivated by injury or other perturbations near the amputation site.

These phantom sensations are not limited to amputated limbs; phantom breasts following mastectomy, phantom genitalia following castration, and phantoms of the entire lower body following spinal cord transection have all been reported (Figure A). Phantom sensations are also common after local nerve block for surgery. During recovery from brachial plexus anesthesia, for example, it is not unusual for the patient to experience a phantom arm that is perceived as whole and intact, but displaced from the real arm. When the real arm is viewed, the phantom appears to "jump into" the arm and may emerge and reenter intermittently as the anesthesia

wears off. Children born without limbs (from the effects of a mother having taken thalidomide during pregnancy, for example) have phantom sensations, even though the limb never developed.

A substantial number of amputees also develop *phantom pain*, which can be a very serious clinical problem. This unfortunate consequence of amputation is usually described as a tingling or burning sensation in the missing body part, but in some individuals the sensation is experienced as a stronger pain that the patients find increasingly debilitating. Phantom pain is one of the more common causes of chronic pain syndromes, which are notoriously difficult to treat. Ablation of the ascending pathways, portions of the thalamus, or even primary sensory cortex does not generally relieve the discomfort felt by these patients.

An imaginative cognitive approach to relieving phantom pain was introduced by Vilayanur Ramachandran, a neurologist and cognitive neuroscientist. Using an apparatus that provides the patient with a mirror image of the intact limb in place of the amputated limb (Figure B), Ramachandran has been able to provide some relief for a subset of these patients by having them perceptually associate the normal sensations with the intact mirror image that is seen in this circumstance as the missing limb. This therapeutic approach, odd though it may seem, shows again how readily our body image and the sensations related to it can be affected

by the information arising from other sensory modalities in unusual circumstances.

Sensory phantoms indicate that the central stations for processing somatic sensory information are not simply passive recipients of peripheral signals arising from mechanical stimuli, but active participants in the generation of percepts. This evidence of the active, and to some degree independent, role of the central stations of sensory systems in the generation of percepts is consistent with evidence in vision and audition that percepts are not simply transforms of peripheral input.

References

CRAIG, A. D., E. M. REIMAN, A. EVANS AND M. C. BUSHNELL (1996) Functional imaging of an illusion of pain. *Nature* 484: 258–260.

KOLB, L. C. (1954) *The Painful Phantom*. Springfield, IL: Charles C. Thomas.

MELZACK, R. (1989) Phantom limbs, the self and the brain (the D. O. Hebb Memorial Lecture). *Canad. Psychol.* 40: 1–14.

MELZACK, R. (1990) Phantom limbs and the concept of a neuromatrix. *Trends Neurosci.* 14: 88–92.

RAMACHANDRAN, V. S. AND S. BLAKESLEE (1998) *Phantoms in the Brain*. New York: Morrow.

SOLENEN, K. A. (1962) The phantom phenomenon in amputated Finnish war veterans. *Acta Orthop. Scand. Suppl.* 54: 1–47.

(A) Some phantoms experienced by war veterans after limb amputations. The amputated areas are demarcated by dashed lines; the colored areas indicate the regions of the most vivid sensations. (B) Apparatus used by Ramachandran to relieve phantom pain by conflating normal and phantom sensory input. The patient shown has his amputated right limb in the right-hand portion of the box, but he sees the missing hand as being intact in the mirror image he perceives. When he moves his intact left hand he experiences movement of the phantom that corresponds to the mirror image; such training can sometimes alleviate phantom pain. (A after Solonen 1962.)

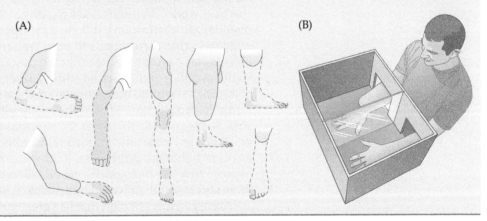

(A) (B)

as for other cognitive functions, such as directing attention to stimulus sources (e.g., moving the head and eyes to identify the source of a tactile stimulus). Unexpected perceptions (including pain) that arise when the somatosensory cortex is no longer connected to the periphery are described in **Box 4D**.

The pain system

A quite different mechanosensory system concerns the perception of **pain**, which is broadly defined as the sensations elicited by mechanical forces or thermal effects that are harmful to the body's integrity. Since alerting the brain to the dangers implied by noxious stimuli differs substantially from informing it about somatic sensory stimuli that are not in themselves harmful (although of course they may signify something in the environment that could be harmful), it makes sense that a special system be devoted to the perception of dangerous mechanical forces (as well as thermal energy) acting on the body.

The perception of pain is initiated by *free nerve endings* in the skin and deeper tissues (see Figure 4.10). These nerve endings are called **nociceptors**, from the Latin *nocere*, "hurt." Like other somatosensory receptors, nociceptive nerve endings arise from cell bodies in dorsal root ganglia (or the analogous ganglia associated with the brainstem) that send one axonal process to the periphery and the other into the spinal cord or brainstem (**Figure 4.12**). The projections that carry information initiated by non-nociceptive temperature-sensitive neurons follow the same anatomical route to the central nervous system, and thus are typically included in a discussion of pain pathways.

The spinal level processing nuclei for pain lie in the dorsal horns of the spinal cord at or near the entry of the peripheral nerves rather than in the caudal medulla. The major targets of the ascending pain and temperature axons are, like the targets of other mechanosensory axons, located in the thalamus. The somatosensory nuclei of the thalamus receive the bulk of these axons, and these neurons project in turn to the primary somatosensory cortex. The generally similar cortical targets for noxious and other mechanosensory stimuli are presumably responsible for the ability to consciously locate painful stimuli and to judge their intensity. Parallel projections to the reticular formation of the medulla, pons, and midbrain are responsible for the strong but largely unconscious autonomic activation that pain elicits; and projections to other areas, such as the anterior cingulate cortex, mediate emotional reactions to pain (see Chapter 10).

The perceptual quality of pain is particularly important from a cognitive standpoint because it so clearly confirms the idea that somatic sensory percepts are mental constructs, not simply translations of sensory stimuli that represent the "real world" in the relevant regions of the brain. Although all perceptual qualities are abstractions, it is easier to appreciate that there is nothing in the real world that corresponds to *pain*. We are intuitively inclined to think that objects can have properties that we describe as brightness or color, or that sound qualities exist in sound stimuli in some objective sense, but the idea that objects or the stimuli they produce are themselves imbued with pain makes no sense. A consideration of pain thus makes it easier to appreciate that although objects are tangible things in the external world, *perceptual qualities*, painful or otherwise, exist only in our brains. Like pain, perceptual constructs such as color, lightness, brightness, loudness, and pitch have evolved in humans because they are biologically useful, allowing us to generate behavior that is more successful than would be possible without these perceptual qualities.

Another aspect of pain that has great medical and economic importance is the underlying neuropharmacology. Analgesics, both prescribed and over-the-counter, are among the most widely used (and abused) medications of any kind, and the relief of pain is one of the central goals of clinical practice. Neurons in the regions of the dorsal horns and brainstem that process pain information have receptors for opioid analgesics (responding to drugs such as morphine), and other neurons in the primary pain pathway secrete endogenous opioids (i.e., morphine-like molecules produced by the body itself). These facts explain

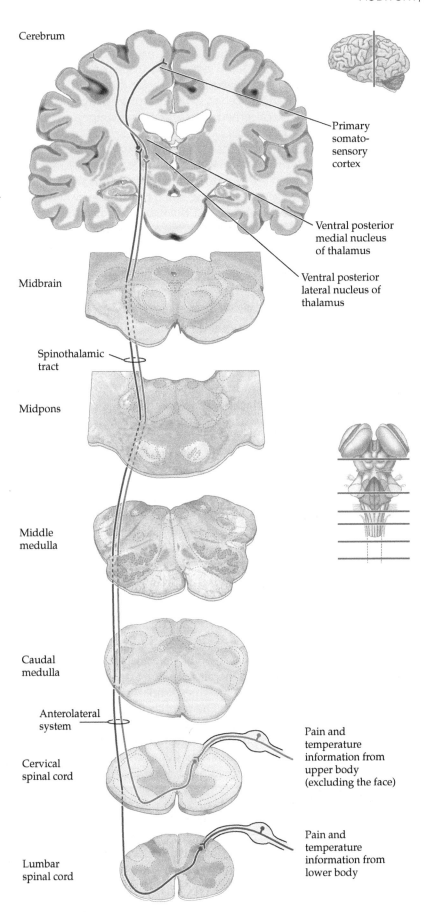

Cerebrum

Primary somato-sensory cortex

Ventral posterior medial nucleus of thalamus

Ventral posterior lateral nucleus of thalamus

Midbrain

Spinothalamic tract

Midpons

Middle medulla

Caudal medulla

Anterolateral system

Cervical spinal cord

Pain and temperature information from upper body (excluding the face)

Lumbar spinal cord

Pain and temperature information from lower body

Figure 4.12   The pain pathway Like the mechanosensory systems for tactile and proprioceptive information, the primary pain pathway entails peripheral receptors, processing in subthalamic nuclei, and thalamic processing before reaching the primary somatosensory cortex.

the efficacy of analgesic drugs that bind to opioid receptors, and the actions of opioid antagonists such as naloxone that are used to treat addiction to opioids such as heroin. This rapidly evolving knowledge of neuropharmacology and pain physiology also suggests possible explanations for the modulation of pain by hypnosis, acupuncture, and placebos. Cognitive processing elsewhere in the brain—including systems concerned with attention, memory, emotion, and reasoning—presumably affects these biochemical interactions in the pain pathway, with marked consequences on the subjective experience of pain that follows.

Especially germane to understanding pain in cognitive terms is the effect of context on pain perception. Physicians have long noted the difference between the objective reality of a painful stimulus and the subjective response to it. During World War II, anesthesiologist Henry Beecher and his colleagues made a detailed study of this phenomenon. They found that soldiers suffering from severe battle wounds often experienced little or no pain; indeed, many of the wounded expressed surprise at this odd dissociation. Beecher concluded that the perception of pain depends on the *context* in which potentially painful stimuli are experienced. Trauma to a soldier injured on the battlefield carries with it the benefit of being removed from further danger; a similar injury in a domestic setting presents quite a different set of circumstances (loss of work, financial liability, and so on). Such observations not only confirm that the perception of pain is a mental construct, but that the constructs are subject to extraordinary modulation by other sensory and cognitive factors.

A more specific example is the **placebo effect**, defined as a physiological response following the administration of a pharmacologically inert medication or treatment. The word *placebo* is Latin for "I will please," and the placebo effect has a long history of use (and misuse) in medicine. In one classic study of analgesia, fully 75 percent of patients suffering from postoperative wound pain reported relief after an injection of an inert saline solution. The researchers who carried out this work noted that the responders were indistinguishable from the nonresponders in both the apparent severity of their pain and their psychological makeup. In another study, medical students were given one of two different pills—one said to be a sedative and the other a stimulant. In fact, both pills contained only inert ingredients. Of the students who received the "sedative," more than two-thirds reported that they felt drowsy, and students who took two such pills felt sleepier than those who had taken only one. Conversely, a large fraction of the students who took the "stimulant" reported that they felt less tired. About a third of the group also reported side effects ranging from headaches and dizziness to tingling extremities and a staggering gait! Only 3 of the 56 students studied reported that the pills had no appreciable effect.

A common misunderstanding about the placebo effect is that patients who respond to a therapeutically meaningless reagent are not really suffering pain, but are just imagining it. This is not the case. The placebo effect in postoperative patients suffering pain can be blocked by naloxone, a competitive antagonist of opiate receptors, illustrating a neuropharmacological basis for the pain relief experienced. Moreover, recent neuroimaging studies show that the brain regions that are pharmacologically responsive to opioid analgesics (e.g., the anterior cingulate cortex and regions of the brainstem) are also active in response to a nominally analgesic placebo (Figure 4.13). Even more remarkably, the efficacy of medication, whether pharmacologically active or not, is influenced by factors such as cost (a more expensive product generates higher expectations). Although the mechanisms by which the perception of pain is modulated are only beginning to be understood, the placebo effect is quite real in terms of cognitive neuroscience.

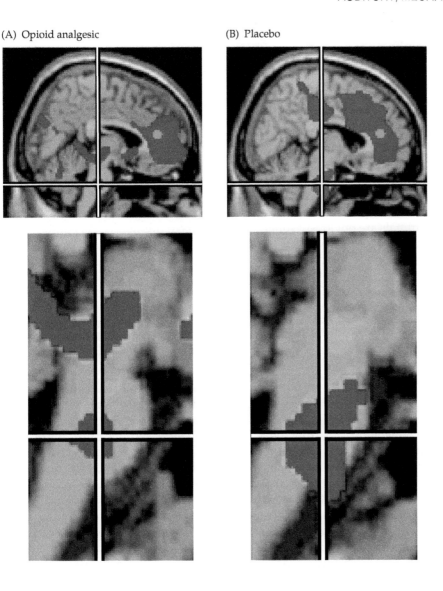

(A) Opioid analgesic

(B) Placebo

Figure 4.13 Brain activity in response to a placebo The regions activated in this fMRI study show that many of the same brain regions are active in response to the administration of an opioid analgesic (A) and to the administration of a placebo (B), thus showing the physiological basis of the placebo effect. The blue dot indicates the location of the anterior cingulate cortex. Crosshairs identify the same region of the brainstem in all panels. (From Petrovic et al. 2002.)

The Chemosensory Modalities

There are also several sensory systems that generate perceptions in response to chemical stimuli: the **olfactory system**, the **gustatory system**, and the **trigeminal chemosensory system**, each of which influences cognitive functions. The olfactory system detects airborne molecules and generates the percepts generally called **odors**. The gustatory system responds to ingested (primarily water-soluble) molecules and generates the percepts we call **tastes**. The trigeminal chemosensory system (so called because the cranial nerve that serves it has three branches) generates percepts elicited by noxious substances that come into contact with the skin or mucous membranes of the nose and mouth—the sensations elicited by chili peppers, for example. These latter percepts have not been given a class name, but they are irritating sensations that in some cases can be quite strong, even painful.

The importance of what we smell, taste, or sense as chemical irritation for cognitive functions is evident in everyday experience: these sensations can have dramatic effects on what we attend to, what we remember, our social interactions, our emotions, the decisions we make, and much more.

The olfactory system

The events leading to the perception of odors begin in the **olfactory epithelium**, a sheet of olfactory receptor neurons and supporting cells that lines approximately half of the human nasal cavity (**Figure 4.14A**). Cellular protrusions called cilia extend from the receptor neurons into the layer of mucus that lines the nasal cavity, where they are exposed to odorant molecules in the air that dissolve in the mucus layer. The ability to detect particular odors is the result of receptor proteins in the membranes of the cilia. Each receptor neuron expresses only a single receptor protein on its ciliary surfaces (out of an estimated total of about 650 such proteins that are coded by the relevant gene family in humans). Olfaction is often considered the least acute of the human senses, and a number of animals are obviously superior to humans in this ability. As pointed out by some skeptics, however, our performance might compare more favorably with that of animals like dogs if we went around with our noses to the ground.

Neurons that express the same receptor protein are distributed in a specific manner across the olfactory epithelium, and their axons project via the olfactory nerve to specific subsets of neuronal clusters called **glomeruli**, located in the **olfactory bulb** (**Figure 4.14B**). As in other sensory systems, this topographical arrangement of central projections in the olfactory bulb is referred to as a *map*. The coding scheme for olfactory information also has a temporal dimension: sniffing, for example, is a periodic event that elicits trains of action potentials and synchronous activity in populations of neurons. As indicated, the glomerular circuitry in the olfactory bulb processes olfactory information from the nasal receptors before relaying their output to the brain.

The axons arising from the olfactory bulb form a bundle called the **olfactory tract** that projects to several central stations, including the olfactory tubercle, the entorhinal cortex, and portions of the amygdala (**Figure 4.14C**). The major target of the olfactory tract is the three-layered **pyriform cortex** in the ventromedial aspect of the temporal lobe near the amygdala and the entorhinal cortex. Neurons in the pyriform cortex project in turn to several thalamic and hypothalamic nuclei, the hippocampus, the amygdala, and the orbitofrontal cortex. Thus, information about odors readily reaches a variety of forebrain regions, allowing olfactory cues to influence involuntary visceral and homeostatic behaviors (i.e., behaviors that control body physiology), as well as the cognitive systems mediating emotion, attention, and memory, among others. The pyriform cortex is analogous to the primary sensory cortices in vision, audition, and somatic sensation, and the adjacent areas indicated in Figure 4.14C are analogous to the higher-order processing regions in these other systems. Interestingly, functional MRI combined with pattern analysis shows that perceptual ratings of odor quality track particular fMRI patterns.

Humans can detect many substances at tiny concentrations (nanomolar or less). Moreover, minimal changes in molecular structure can lead to large perceptual differences when tested in the laboratory. The molecule D-carvone, for instance, smells like caraway seeds, whereas its stereoisomer L-carvone (a molecule identical except in its "handedness") smells like spearmint. Most naturally occurring odors—the smell of a flower, the aroma of cut grass, or less attractive odors that can be strongly aversive—are elicited by a combination of odorant molecules, even though they are typically experienced as a single smell.

Subliminal olfactory information can also be influential, suggesting that olfactory information could have subtle influences on processes of which we are largely unaware. Interest in this possibility was triggered by a study carried out several decades ago by behavioral psychologist Martha McClintock, then an undergraduate at Wellesley College. She reported in her senior thesis

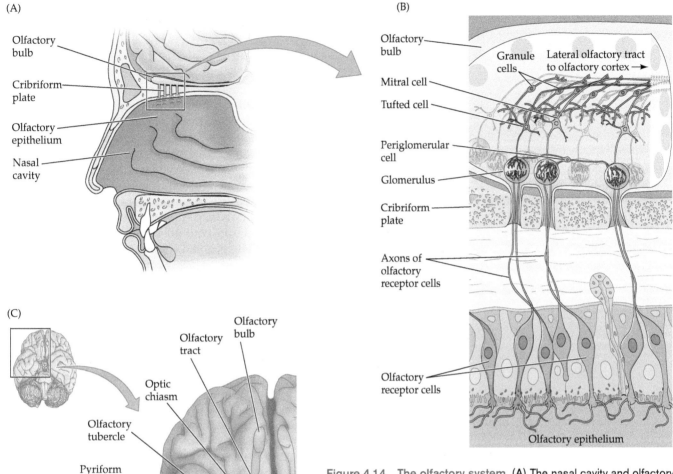

Figure 4.14 The olfactory system (A) The nasal cavity and olfactory epithelium. (B) Organization of the olfactory bulb and the formation of the olfactory tract in relation to the receptor cells in the olfactory epithelium. (C) Pathway from the olfactory bulb to the pyriform cortex, which is the primary target of the projections from the bulb. Note the close association of the pyriform cortex with the amygdala (a key structure in emotional processing) and the entorhinal cortex (a key structure in processing certain kinds of memories). The olfactory tract sends information to both of these structures, which can thus be affected by the processing that leads to the perception of odors.

that after several months of living together, the 135 women housed in her dormitory tended to have synchronized menstrual cycles. (The finding was later published.) McClintock went on to suggest that this effect is mediated by olfaction, since volunteers who had been exposed to the odorants in gauze pads from the underarms of women at different stages of their menstrual cycles also tended to have synchronized menses.

McClintock's work is often cited in discussions of the possible existence and nature of human **pheromones**. Pheromones are biochemical signals produced by various animal glands and are used as a means of social communication in a number of non-human species. Reproductive and other behaviors in rodents and other animals are determined in part by such signals; it is well established, for example, that species-specific pheromones determine a variety of social, reproductive, and parenting behaviors in mice. The role of pheromones in human behavior, however, remains speculative (and controversial).

The taste system

The taste system generates percepts derived for the most part from water-soluble molecules that interact with receptors in epithelial specializations on the tongue called **taste buds** (Figure 4.15A). Taste cells embedded in the taste buds produce information about the identity, concentration, and pleasant or unpleasant (*hedonic*) quality of the substance—all pertinent to the cognitive determination of whether something should be eaten, and how pleasing the sensation will be if the item is consumed (Figure 4.15B). At a more basic physiological level, this information also prepares the gastrointestinal system to receive food by causing salivation and swallowing (or gagging and regurgitation if the substance is noxious). Information about the temperature and texture of food is relayed from the mouth and pharynx via sensory receptors from the trigeminal and other sensory cranial nerves to the thalamus and somatosensory cortices.

The innervation of taste cells arises from neurons in cranial nerve ganglia. The initial target of these axons is the **nucleus of the solitary tract** in the brainstem, which is also the main target of afferent visceral sensory information related to the sympathetic and parasympathetic divisions of the visceral motor system (i.e., the system that innervates the body's organs). Interneurons connecting the different regions of this nucleus integrate gustatory and visceral information. Such interactions make good sense, since humans and other animals must quickly recognize if they are eating something unpalatable, and respond accordingly by gagging and spitting it out.

Axons from the gustatory component of the solitary nucleus project to the ventral posterior complex of the thalamus, where they terminate in the medial half of the ventral posterior medial nucleus (Figure 4.15C). The primary cortical target of these neurons is the anterior **insula** in the temporal and frontal lobes. As in other sensory systems, there is also a secondary taste area for higher-order cortical processing; this region is in the caudolateral orbitofrontal cortex, where neurons respond to combinations of visual, somatosensory, olfactory, and gustatory stimuli. When a given food is consumed to the point of satiety, some orbitofrontal neurons in non-human primates diminish their activity in response to the tastant, suggesting that this cortical region is involved in the motivation to eat (or not to eat) particular foods. Finally, reciprocal projections connect the nucleus of the solitary tract to the hypothalamus and amygdala. These two-way projections presumably influence hunger, satiety, and other homeostatic states associated with eating. This overall arrangement is thus relevant to much the same range of cognitive functions as is the olfactory system.

People perceive a wide variety of taste qualities, including sweet, salty, bitter, sour, astringent (cranberries and tea), pungent (spices such as ginger and curry), fatty, starchy, and various metallic tastes, to name but a few. As in the case of odors, this superabundance of perceptual qualities is difficult to classify in the relatively simple way that the perceptual qualities in vision, audition, and somatic sensation are categorized. As in olfaction, the sensory experiences engendered by the different tastes do not have a one-to-one correspondence with specific molecules. Tastes, like odors, typically derive from complex chemical mixtures. Moreover, quite different compounds can elicit the same general taste sensation. For instance, perceptions of sweet are elicited by saccharides (glucose, sucrose, and fructose), organic anions (saccharin), amino acids (aspartame, or NutraSweet), L-phenylalanine methyl ester, and proteins (monellin and thaumatin).

To complicate matters further, taste responses vary significantly among individuals. For example, 30 to 40 percent of the U.S. population cannot taste the bitter compound phenylthiocarbamide (PTC), but can taste molecules such as quinine and caffeine that also produce bitter sensations. This particular

(A)

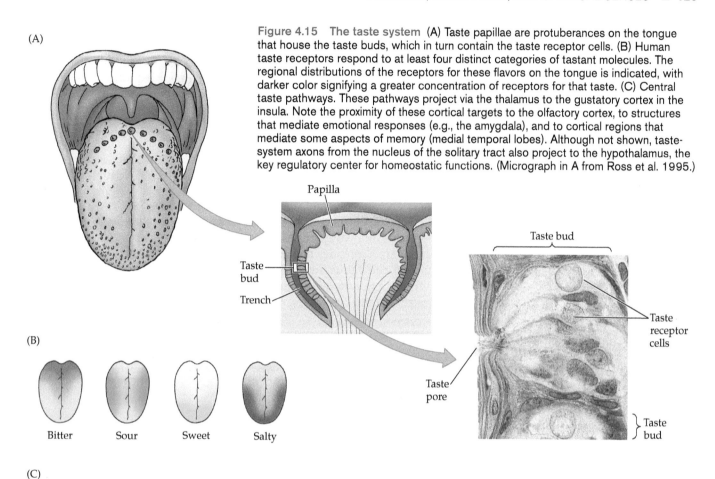

Figure 4.15 The taste system (A) Taste papillae are protuberances on the tongue that house the taste buds, which in turn contain the taste receptor cells. (B) Human taste receptors respond to at least four distinct categories of tastant molecules. The regional distributions of the receptors for these flavors on the tongue is indicated, with darker color signifying a greater concentration of receptors for that taste. (C) Central taste pathways. These pathways project via the thalamus to the gustatory cortex in the insula. Note the proximity of these cortical targets to the olfactory cortex, to structures that mediate emotional responses (e.g., the amygdala), and to cortical regions that mediate some aspects of memory (medial temporal lobes). Although not shown, taste-system axons from the nucleus of the solitary tract also project to the hypothalamus, the key regulatory center for homeostatic functions. (Micrograph in A from Ross et al. 1995.)

Papilla

Taste bud

Taste bud

Trench

Taste receptor cells

Taste pore

Taste bud

(B)

Bitter   Sour   Sweet   Salty

(C)

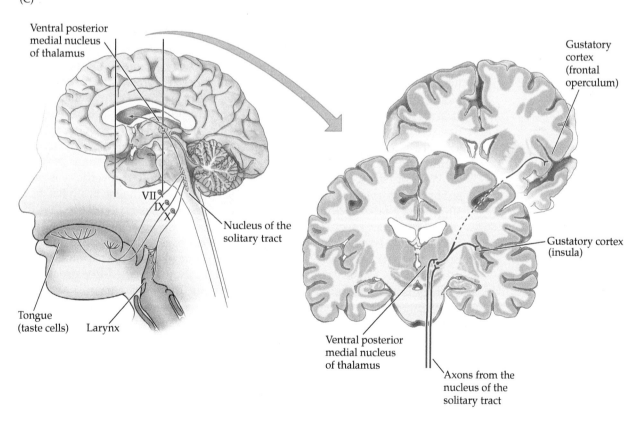

Ventral posterior medial nucleus of thalamus

VII
IX
X

Nucleus of the solitary tract

Tongue (taste cells)   Larynx

Gustatory cortex (frontal operculum)

Gustatory cortex (insula)

Ventral posterior medial nucleus of thalamus

Axons from the nucleus of the solitary tract

difference among individuals is the result of a single autosomal gene with a dominant (tasters) and a recessive (nontasters) allele for the PTC receptor. People who are extremely sensitive to PTC and its analogs, called *supertasters*, actually have more taste buds than normal and tend to avoid certain foods, such as grapefruit, green tea, and broccoli, all of which contain bitter-tasting compounds.

These perceptual observations in olfaction and taste accord with evidence in other sensory systems that underscore the difficulty of relating subjective experiences to the physical characteristics of the relevant stimuli, which in this case are airborne or water-soluble molecules.

Trigeminal chemosensation

The third system that responds to chemicals in the environment is the trigeminal chemosensory system. The trigeminal system consists of nociceptive neurons and their axons in the trigeminal ganglion and its nerve (cranial nerve V) and, to a lesser degree, includes nociceptive neurons whose axons run in the glossopharyngeal and vagus nerves (cranial nerves IX and X). These neurons and their endings in the mouth, nasal cavity, and lips are activated by chemicals classified as irritants, including air pollutants (e.g., sulfur dioxide), ammonia ("smelling salts"), ethanol (liquor), acetic acid (vinegar), carbon dioxide (in soft drinks), menthol (in various inhalants), and capsaicin (the compound in chili peppers that elicits their characteristic "hot" sensation). The corresponding percepts alert the organism to potentially harmful chemical stimuli that have been ingested or respired, or have come in contact with the face, and are thus closely tied to the pain system described earlier.

Some Final Points about Sensory Systems

Coding and labeled lines

Much recent work in olfaction has focused on the idea that the peripheral receptors are the starting point for specifically labeled lines that extend through the central stations of the system, thus determining the basic strategies of central processing and the ensuing percepts. A key advance came in the early 1990s with the discovery of genes that code for olfactory receptors. This research was pioneered by neuroscientists Richard Axel, Linda Buck, and other collaborators at several institutions. Subsequently, Axel and Buck, among others, showed that receptor neurons expressing a particular receptor often project to specific glomeruli in the olfactory bulb of mice. Similar studies have been carried out identifying the genes and receptor proteins in the gustatory system.

Work pursuing the appealing possibility that this initial specificity is present in the central olfactory and gustatory stations of the mouse brain have not supported a labeled-line coding scheme. So far, there is no evidence that the projections from specific glomeruli in the olfactory bulb have generated a correspondingly specific pattern in the pyriform cortex, and the nature of olfactory processing at this next level remains unclear. From what studies of processing in other primary sensory cortices (V1, A1, and S1) show, a labeled-line processing strategy is also unlikely in these other systems. In the primary visual cortex, for example, the same cortical neurons process information about a variety of stimulus features, and notions of labeled lines in V1 have long since been abandoned (although the broader concept of streams for different perceptual properties is still very much in play, as described in Chapter 3).

The malleability of sensory circuitry

Another issue of obvious importance in cognitive neuroscience, as well as in clinical practice, is the malleability, or *plasticity*, of the neural circuitry in sensory systems. When a particular region of a cortical sensory map is destroyed following a stroke, for instance, to what extent can another region be expected to take over the missing function? Conversely, when a normal individual uses a portion of the sensory cortex to an unusual degree (such as in becoming a highly trained musician or learning a second language), how does cortical organization change as a result?

A series of influential experiments on the plasticity of the visual system carried out by neurophysiologists David Hubel and Torsten Wiesel in the 1960s and 1970s showed relatively little plasticity of connections in the primary visual cortex of cats and monkeys after the first few weeks (cats) or months (monkeys) of life. If, for example, they removed one eye from a newborn kitten (or sutured one eye shut at birth), substantial rearrangement of cortical connections was apparent both in anatomical assessments of connectivity and in the receptive-field properties of the affected cortical neurons. However, when the same procedures were carried out in adult animals, there was little evidence of reorganization, in keeping with the clinical observation that when the equivalent of this sort of deprivation occurs in human infants (e.g., neonatal cataracts, in which the lenses of a newborn's eyes are opaque) and is not corrected early, later correction fails to prevent a permanent visual deficit.

It was therefore surprising when Michael Merzenich and his colleagues reported experiments in the somatosensory system of adult monkeys that gave a different result. When a digit was amputated, recordings from the relevant cortical region showed that the neurons that would normally have been responsive only to the amputated digit could now be activated by tactile stimuli applied to the adjacent fingers (**Figure 4.16A**). Moreover, augmented use of a given set of digits over a period of several months in a normal monkey caused the topographically related areas of the primary somatosensory cortex to expand

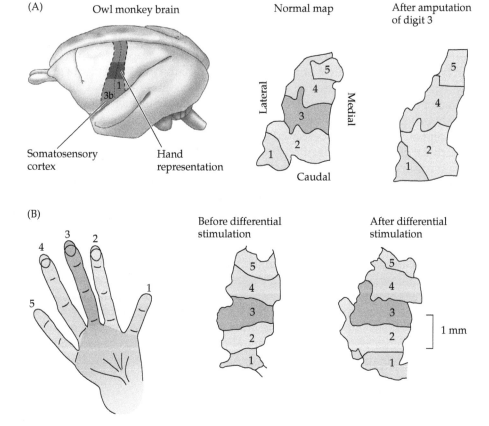

Figure 4.16 **Plasticity of the somatosensory cortex** (A) Reorganization of the primary somatosensory map in a monkey following amputation of a digit several weeks earlier. Numbers in the cortical maps correspond to the areas activated by stimulation of the indicated digits. (B) Expansion of the regions of the map representing digits 2 to 4 following several months of augmented activity of these digits by a specific task that required their use. (After Jenkins et al. 1990.)

significantly when mapped in the same way (Figure 4.16B). Observations of this sort are not possible in humans, for obvious reasons, but studies of individuals with a particular sensory skill obtained through years of practice appear to confirm such activity-dependent neural plasticity. Accomplished musicians, for example, show greater activation of the relevant cortical regions of the right hemisphere than do musically naïve subjects (see Box 4B).

Given these seeming differences in malleability between the visual and somatic sensory systems, visual physiologist Charles Gilbert and his group reexamined the plasticity of the visual system using experimental methods that were more like those that Merzenich had used to study the somatic sensory system. They destroyed small regions of the retina in a cat or monkey using a laser beam—a lesion similar in principle to the amputation of a digit. Much as had been observed in the primary somatosensory cortex, the topographical cortical region that would normally have responded to the damaged area of retina now responded to stimulation of adjacent retinal regions—a change similar to the effect illustrated in Figure 4.16A.

The most reasonable conclusion based on this and other evidence is that sensory cortices are capable of a great deal of reorganization in early life, when neural connections must adapt to a body that is changing rapidly as a result of postnatal growth and when learning about the world is especially important. Plasticity diminishes with maturation, but it is not lost altogether. Thus, the effects of damage will cause some changes in functional connectivity, and practice of a specific skill will be apparent in the greater overall activation of the region of cortex habitually stimulated during the exercise of that talent. Much clinical evidence, however, together with the classic experiments of Hubel and Wiesel (and now many others), indicates that cortical plasticity in adults is relatively limited, leading to permanent deficits after brain damage and progressively less facility learning new skills as humans and other animals age (as adults struggling to learn music for the first time, or a second language, know all too well).

Awareness of sensory stimuli

A potentially confusing fact is that so many sensory stimuli and the behaviors they elicit *don't* generate conscious perceptions. Examples are the changes in body posture based on proprioceptive stimuli, the eye movements elicited by vestibular stimuli, and the complex gastrointestinal responses elicited by olfactory or gustatory stimuli. The sensory processing of such stimuli is obviously influential, indeed vital, though it occurs without awareness. Since the concept of "unconscious percepts" is a contradiction in terms, how then should we think of and categorize behaviors that routinely (or just sometimes, as in vision or audition) occur unconsciously?

One approach to this problem is to classify unconscious behavioral responses as "simple reflexes" that are different from and/or less important than the behavioral responses correlated with sensory perceptions, which are by definition conscious. This tack, however, is unwarranted by what we now know from neuroscience. There is no evidence that the relevant stimulus-response pathways are any more or less "simple" by anatomical or physiological criteria than the pathways and processing stages that generate conscious experiences. In fact, the same pathways and central processing stations must be involved.

Thus, sensory processing does not necessarily lead to percepts, which are probably far less important in determining the majority of human behaviors than most of us assume. The problem of consciousness—its basis and its importance—remains a vexing one in cognitive neuroscience, and is taken up in Chapter 7.

The representation of sensory percepts

A final question is how sensory percepts (or their unconscious equivalents) are represented in the brain. That is, exactly what *are* sensory percepts in neurobiological terms? Although the answer is a matter of ongoing debate, there is consensus on at least some general points. First, there is widespread agreement that percepts arise from the activity of populations of neurons in the relevant regions of the primary sensory and association cortices. Indeed, there seems to be no real alternative to this conclusion. Second, much of the electrophysiological evidence indicates that individual neurons respond to multiple stimulus attributes; thus there is no simple linkage between stimulus features and the activity of particular neurons. And third, the responsiveness of cortical sensory neurons and the resulting perceptual qualities are related to stimulus properties in a nonlinear and often counterintuitive way (see Chapter 3 for examples in vision).

This evidence is inconsistent with the intuition that percepts are generated by neurons simply analyzing and encoding the features of objects, and that their purpose is to represent the world in the same veridical way as do the instruments of physics and chemistry. An alternative is that the neuronal activity underlying percepts reflects an operational rather than analytical link between sensory stimuli and the objective world, instantiated in sensory processing circuitry according to the success or failure of behavior over evolutionary and individual time (see Box 3C).

Summary

1. The primary auditory pathway begins with receptors (hair cells) in the basilar membrane that respond to local pressure changes. This information is processed in the cochlear nuclei, additional nuclei in the brainstem, the inferior colliculus in the midbrain, and the medial geniculate nuclei of the thalamus before being sent on to the primary auditory cortex (A1).

2. The major perceptual qualities in audition are loudness, pitch, and timbre. Loudness is the perception elicited by sound intensity; pitch is the perception elicited by periodic variations in the power of sound stimuli; and timbre is the perception of differences in the qualities of sound sources when their intensities and frequencies are the same.

3. The higher-order processing of sound stimuli that gives rise to auditory percepts occurs in the belt areas of auditory cortex adjacent to A1, which are generally analogous to the extrastriate cortical areas in the visual system. These areas are especially responsive to auditory stimuli that have biological significance, such as speech.

4. The responses to mechanical forces acting on the body are generated by the somatic sensory system. The cutaneous/subcutaneous component of this system generates the perceptions of touch, pressure, and vibration that arise from mechanical stimulation of receptors in the cutaneous and subcutaneous tissues.

5. A distinct pain system generates noxious percepts that alert us to mechanical or thermal stimuli that are potentially harmful.

6. Responses to chemicals in the environment are generated by the olfactory system, the gustatory system, and the trigeminal chemosensory system.

7. In olfaction, responses to airborne molecules that interact with receptors in the nasal cavity lead to the perception of odors. Gustation results when soluble molecules interact with receptors primarily on the tongue, leading to the perception of tastes. The trigeminal system responds to noxious chemicals that find their way into the nose and mouth, generating percepts usually described as irritating; as such, the trigeminal system is closely related to the pain system.

8. All three chemosensory systems ultimately provide information to regions of the brain that are closely tied to autonomic and emotional responses, including the reticular formation, the entorhinal cortex, the insula, and the amygdala.

9. Although we are inclined to equate sensory perceptions with conscious awareness, the processing elicited by most sensory stimuli and the responses to them never reach this level.

Additional Reading

Reviews

ALAIN, C. AND S. R. ARNOTT (2000) Selectively attending to auditory objects. *Front. Biosci.* 5: 202–212.

BARNES, S. J. AND G. T. FINNERTY (2010) Sensory experience and cortical rewiring. *Neuroscientist* 16:186–198.

BASBAUM, A. I., D. M. BAUTISTA, G. SCHERRER AND D. JULIUS (2009) Cellular and molecular mechanisms of pain. *Cell* 139: 267–284.

BEECHER, H. K. (1946) Pain in men wounded in battle. *Ann. Surg.* 123: 96.

BENDOR, D. AND X. WANG (2006) Cortical representations of pitch in monkeys and humans. *Curr. Opin. Neurobiol.* 16: 391–399.

BLACKWELL, B., S. S. BLOOMFIELD AND C. R. BUNCHER (1972) Demonstration to medical students of placebo response and non-drug factors. *Lancet* 1: 1279–1282.

BRANDT, T. (1991) Man in motion: Historical and clinical aspects of vestibular function. *Brain* 114: 2159–2174.

BUCK, L. B. (2000) The molecular architecture of odor and pheromone sensing in mammals. *Cell* 100: 611–618.

DARIAN-SMITH, I. (1982) Touch in primates. *Annu. Rev. Psychol.* 33: 155–194.

DUBNER, R. AND M. S. GOLD (1999) The neurobiology of pain. *Proc. Natl. Acad. Sci. USA* 96: 7627–7630.

FIELDS, H. L. AND A. I. BASBAUM (1978) Brain stem control of spinal pain transmission neurons. *Annu. Rev. Physiol.* 40: 217–248.

GOLDBERG, J. M. AND C. FERNANDEZ (1984) The vestibular system. In *Handbook of Physiology*, Section 1: *The Nervous System*, Vol. 3: *Sensory Processes*, Part 2, J. M. Brookhart, V. B. Mountcastle, I. Darian-Smith and S. R. Geiger (eds.). Bethesda, MD: American Physiological Society, pp. 977–1022.

GRIFFITHS, D. G. AND J. D. WARREN (2004) What is an auditory object? *Nat. Rev. Neurosci.* 5: 887–892.

HUDSPETH, A. J. (2008) Making an effort to listen: Mechanical amplification in the ear. *Neuron* 59: 530–545.

KAAS, J. H. (1990) Somatosensory system. In *The Human Nervous System*, G. Paxinos (ed.). San Diego, CA: Academic Press, pp. 813–844.

KAAS, J. H. AND T. A. HACKETT (2000) Subdivisions of auditory cortex and processing streams in primates. *Proc. Natl. Acad. Sci. USA* 97: 11793–11799.

KING, A. J. AND I. NELKEN (2009) Unraveling the principles of auditory cortical processing: Can we learn from the visual system? *Nat. Neurosci.* 12: 698–701.

LAURENT, G. (1999) A systems perspective on early olfactory coding. *Science* 286: 723–728.

LINDEMANN, B. (1996) Taste reception. *Physiol. Rev.* 76: 719–766.

MERZENICH, M. M., G. H. RECANZONE, W. M. JENKINS AND K. A. GRAJSKI (1990) Adaptive mechanisms in cortical networks underlying cortical contributions to learning and nondeclarative memory. *Cold Spring Harb. Symp. Quant. Biol.* 55: 873–887.

MOORE, C. I., S. B. NELSON AND M. SUR (1999) Dynamics of neuronal processing in rat somatosensory cortex. *Trends Neurosci.* 22: 513–520.

NELKEN, I. (2002) Feature detection by the auditory cortex. In *Integrative Functions in the Mammalian Auditory Pathway*, D. Oertel, R. Fay and A. N. Popper (eds.). Springer Handbook of Auditory Research, Vol. 15. New York: Springer, pp. 358–416.

NELKEN, I. (2008) Processing of complex sounds in the auditory system. *Curr. Opin. Neurobiol.* 18: 413–417.

NELKEN, I., A. FISHBACH, L. LAS, N. ULANOVSKY AND D. FARKAS (2003) Primary auditory cortex of cats: Feature detection or something else? *Biol. Cybern.* 89: 397–406.

PETROVIC, P., E. KALSO, K. M. PETERSSON AND M. INGVAR (2002) Placebo and opioid analgesia: Imaging a shared neural network. *Science* 295: 1737–1740.

PLACK, C. J. AND R. P. CARLYON (1995) Loudness perception and intensity coding. In *Hearing*, B. C. J. Moore (ed.). New York: Academic Press, pp. 123–160.

RAUSCHECKER, J. P. AND B. TIAN (2000) Mechanisms and streams for processing of "what" and "where" in auditory cortex. *Proc. Natl. Acad. Sci. USA* 97: 11800–11806.

READ, H. L., J. A. WINER AND C. E. SCHEINER (2002) Functional architecture of auditory cortex. *Curr. Opin. Neurobiol.* 12: 433–440.

SCHREINER, C. E., H. L. READ AND M. L. SUTTER (2000) Modular organization of frequency integration in primary auditory cortex. *Annu. Rev. Neurosci.* 23: 501–529.

SHEPARD, R. (1999) Pitch perception and measurement. In *Music, Cognition, and Computerized Sound: An Introduction to Psychoacoustics*, P. R. Cook (ed.). Cambridge, MA: MIT Press, pp. 149–166.

SKRABANEK, P. AND J. MCCORMICK (1990) *Follies and Fallacies in Medicine*. New York: Prometheus.

SMITH, E. C. AND M. S. LEWICKI (2006) Efficient auditory coding. *Nature* 439: 978–982.

WEINBERGER, N. M. (2004) Specific long-term memory traces in primary auditory cortex. *Nat. Rev. Neurosci.* 5: 279–290.

WINKLER, I. (2007) Interpreting the mismatch negativity (MMN). *J. Psychophysiol.* 21: 60–69.

ZUBIETA, J.-K. AND S. CHRISTIAN (2009) Neurobiological mechanisms of placebo responses. The year in Cognitive Neuroscience 2009, *Ann. NY Acad. Sci.* 1156: 198–210.

Important Original Papers

ALAIN, C., S. R. ARNOTT, S. HEVENOR, S. GRAHAM AND C. L. GRADY (2001) "What" and "where" in the human auditory system. *Proc. Natl. Acad. Sci. USA* 98: 12301–12306.

ALAIN, C., S. R. ARNOTT AND T. W. PICTON (2001) Bottom-up and top-down influences on auditory scene analysis: Evidence from event-related brain potentials. *J. Exp. Psychol. Hum. Percept. Perform.* 27: 1072–1089.

BEECHER, H. K. (1946) Pain in men wounded in battle. *Ann. Surg.* 123: 96.

BENDOR, D. AND X. WANG (2005) The neural representation of pitch in primate auditory cortex. *Nature* 436: 1161–1165.

BLOOD, A. J., R. J. ZATORRE, P. BERMUDEZ AND A. C. EVANS (1999) Emotional responses to pleasant and unpleasant music correlate with activity in paralimbic brain regions. *Nat. Neurosci.* 2: 382–387.

BUCK, L. B. (2000) The molecular architecture of odor and pheromone sensing in mammals. *Cell* 100: 611–617.

BUCK, L. AND R. AXEL (1991) A novel multigene family may encode odorant receptors: A molecular basis for odor recognition. *Cell* 65: 175–187.

CREUTZFELDT, O. AND G. OJEMANN (1989) Neuronal activity in the human lateral temporal lobe. *Exp. Brain Res.* 77: 490–498.

FLEISCHMANN, A. AND 10 OTHERS (2008) Mice with a "monoclonal nose": Perturbations in an olfactory map impair odor discrimination. *Neuron* 60: 1068–1081.

FLETCHER, H. AND W. A. MUNSON (1933) Loudness: Its definition, measurement, and calculation. *J. Acoust. Soc. Am.* 5: 82–108.

GILBERT, C. D. AND T. N. WIESEL (1992) Receptive field dynamics in adult primary visual cortex. *Nature* 356: 150–152.

GLAVE, R. D. AND A. C. M. RIETVELD (1975) Is the effort dependence of speech loudness explicable on the basis of acoustical cues? *J. Acoust. Soc. Am.* 58: 875–879.

HUBEL, D. H. AND T. N. WIESEL (1970) The period of susceptibility to the physiological effects of unilateral eye closure in kittens. *J. Physiol.* 206: 419–436.

HUBEL, D. H., T. N. WIESEL AND S. LeVAY (1977) Plasticity of ocular dominance columns in monkey striate cortex. *Philos. Trans. R. Soc. Lond. B* 278: 377–409.

JEFFRESS, L. A. (1948) A place theory of sound localization. *J. Comp. Physiol. Psychol.* 41: 35–39.

JENKINS, W. M., M. M. MERZENICH, M. T. OCHS, E. ALLARD AND T. GUIC-ROBLES (1990) Functional reorganization of the primary somatosensory cortex of owl monkeys after behaviorally controlled tactile stimulation. *J. Neurophysiol.* 63: 82–104.

JOHANSSON, R. S. (1978) Tactile sensibility of the human hand: Receptive field

characteristics of mechanoreceptive units in the glabrous skin. *J. Physiol.* (Lond.) 281: 101–123.

KNUDSEN, E. I. AND M. KONISHI (1978) A neural map of auditory space in the owl. *Science* 200: 795–797.

LADEFOGED, P. AND N. P. McKINNEY (1963) Loudness, sound pressure, and subglottal pressure in speech. *J. Acoust. Soc. Am.* 35: 454–460.

LAURENT, G. (1999) A systems perspective on early olfactory coding. *Science* 286: 723–727.

LEWICKI, M. (2002) Efficient coding of natural sounds. *Nat. Neurosci.* 5: 356–363.

MALNIC, B., J. HIRONO, T. SATO AND L. B. BUCK (1999) Combinatorial receptor codes for odors. *Cell* 96: 713–723.

MERZENICH, M. M., R. J. NELSON, M. P. STRYKER, M. S. CYNADER, A. SCHOPPMANN AND J. M. ZOOK (1984) Somatosensory cortical map changes following digit amputation in adult monkeys. *J. Comp. Neurol.* 224: 591–605.

MIDDLEBROOKS, J. C., A. E. CLOCK, L. XU AND D. M. GREEN (1994) A panoramic code for sound location by cortical neurons. *Science* 264: 842–844.

MOMBAERTS, P. AND 7 OTHERS (1996) Visualizing an olfactory sensory map. *Cell* 87: 675–686.

NELKEN, I., Y. ROTMAN AND O. BAR YOSEF (1999) Responses of auditory-cortex neurons to structural features of natural sounds. *Nature* 397: 154–157.

PANTEV, C., M. HOKE, B. LUTKENHONER AND K. LEHNERTZ (1989) Tonotopic organization of the auditory cortex: Pitch versus frequency representation. *Science* 246: 486–488.

PIERCE, J. (1991) Periodicity and pitch perception. *J. Acoust. Soc. Am.* 90: 1889–1893.

RIEKE, F., D. A. BODNAR AND W. BIALEK (1995) Naturalistic stimuli increase the rate and efficiency of information transfer by primary auditory afferents. *Proc. Biol. Sci.* 262: 259–265.

ROTSCHILD, G., I. NELKEN AND A. MIZRAHI (2010) Functional organization and population dynamics in the mouse primary auditory cortex. *Nat. Neurosci.* 13: 353–360.

SCHOUTEN, J. F., R. J. RITSMA AND B. I. CARDOZO (1962) Pitch of the residue. *J. Acoust. Soc. Am.* 34: 1418–1424.

SCHWARTZ, D. A. AND D. PURVES (2004) Pitch is determined by naturally occurring periodic sounds. *Hearing Res.* 194: 31–46.

SMITH, E. AND M. S. LEWICKI (2006) Efficient auditory coding. *Nature* 439: 978–982.

STETTLER, D. D. AND R. AXEL (2009) Representations of odor in the piriform cortex. *Neuron* 63: 854–864.

VASSAR, R., S. K. CHAO, R. SITCHERAN, J. M. NUNEZ, L. B. VOSSHALL AND R. AXEL (1994) Topographic organization of sensory projections to the olfactory bulb. *Cell* 79: 981–991.

VON BÉKÉSY, G. (1960) *Experiments in Hearing.* New York: McGraw-Hill. (A collection of von Békésy's original papers.)

WALL, P. D. AND W. NOORDENHOS (1977) Sensory functions which remain in man after complete transection of dorsal columns. *Brain* 100: 641–653.

WIESEL, T. N. AND D. H. HUBEL (1965) Comparison of the effects of unilateral and bilateral eye closure on cortical unit responses in kittens. *J. Neurophysiol.* 28: 1029–1040.

ZAHORIK, P. AND F. L. WRIGHTMAN (2001) Loudness constancy varying with sound source distance. *Nat. Neurosci.* 4: 78–83.

Books

BARLOW, H. B. AND J. D. MOLLON (1989) *The Senses.* Cambridge: Cambridge University Press, Chapters 17–19.

BREGMAN, A. (1990) *Auditory Scene Analysis: The Perceptual Organization of Sound.* Cambridge, MA: MIT Press.

DOTY, R. L., ED. (1995) *Handbook of Olfaction and Gustation.* New York: Dekker.

FIELDS, H. L. (1987) *Pain.* New York: McGraw-Hill.

MOORE, B. C. J. (2012) *An Introduction to the Psychology of Hearing,* 6th Ed. London: Academic Press.

NEUHOFF, J. G. (2004) *Ecological Psychoacoustics.* San Diego, CA: Elsevier.

PLOMP, R. (2002) *The Intelligent Ear: On the Nature of Sound Perception.* Mahwah, NJ: Erlbaum.

ROSSING, T. D., R. F. MOORE AND P. A. WHEELER (2002) *The Science of Sound,* 3rd Ed. San Francisco: Addison-Wesley.

SIMON, S. A. AND S. D. ROPER (1993) *Mechanisms of Taste Transduction.* Boca Raton, FL: CRC Press, Chapters 2, 6, 9, 10, 12, 13, and 14.

WALL, P. D. AND R. MELZACK (1999) *Textbook of Pain,* 4th Ed. New York: Churchill Livingstone.

5

Motor Systems: The Organization of Action

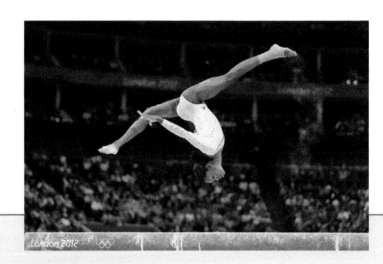

INTRODUCTION

Sensory systems provide the inputs to cognitive processes, and motor systems deliver the physical behavioral output that expresses cognitive goals. Thus, understanding the organization of motor systems is essential for understanding the organization of cognitive systems, which ultimately manifest perception, attention, emotion, and the consequences of decisions in action. All body movements are generated by the stimulation of skeletal muscle fibers by lower motor neurons whose cell bodies are located in the brainstem and spinal cord. Lower motor neuron activity is coordinated by interneurons in local circuits. Although such local circuits can produce simple reflexive movements on their own, they are governed by descending projections from upper motor neurons in the cerebral cortex and brainstem. These descending influences modulate the activity of local circuits to produce and coordinate complex sequences of movements that make up purposeful, goal-directed actions. This higher-order control of movement is mediated by upper motor neurons in the primary motor cortex and other premotor areas of the frontal and parietal lobes.

Neurons in motor cortex and premotor areas contribute critically to cognitive functions such as the planning and initiation of complex sequences of movements, the selection of behavioral goals for action, and the learning and remembering of new movement sequences. Thus, higher motor areas enhance the complexity and efficacy of behavior. All of these higher motor areas themselves are monitored and modulated by two other key motor systems—the cerebellum and the basal ganglia. Major functions of the cerebellum are to correct errors in ongoing movements and to learn new motor skills. Major functions of the basal ganglia are to gate motor commands and to facilitate simple forms of learning. The complex neural processing carried out by the basal ganglia and cerebellum also influences cognitive functions that are not directly expressed in motor activity, including motivation, emotion, and decision making.

■ INTRODUCTORY BOX APRAXIA

The importance of cognition for action is keenly apparent when the ability to plan movements or carry out motor programs is compromised. Such deficits are known as apraxias. *Apraxia*—Greek for "without act or deed"—is a loss of the ability to execute learned voluntary movements, especially complex sequences of movements, despite the motivation and physical capability to perform the actions.

Apraxias can take several forms. Ideomotor apraxia, for example, is an inability to voluntarily perform a learned action when presented with the appropriate objects, an inability to imitate what someone else is doing, or an inability to follow verbal instructions. An afflicted person might be unable to follow the command to wave goodbye, but able to properly wave when a familiar person leaves the room. Or she might be unable to pantomime combing her hair when given a comb and asked to pretend using it, but able to comb her hair when she wants to.

Ideational apraxia is the inability to carry out sequential tasks involving the use of tools or objects in the proper order. Patients with this form of apraxia might put on their shoes before putting on their socks or strike a candle against the side of a matchbox rather than striking a match and using it to light the candle.

A particularly vexing form of apraxia is verbal apraxia, which results in difficulty producing speech. Verbal apraxia can afflict both adults and children, the latter having potentially devastating consequences for learning and socialization.

Although the causes of apraxia remain largely unknown, ideational and ideomotor apraxia have been linked to damage of the parietal and premotor cortex, typically on the language-dominant side. Such damage can result from neurological insults such as stroke or ischemia, as in the case of ideomotor apraxia, or from the more diffuse degeneration that is associated with diseases such as Alzheimer's disease or Parkinson's disease. Unfortunately, the prognosis for apraxia is rather grim. Some recovery can be made with physical therapy or occupational therapy, particularly in younger patients, yet many people suffering from apraxia never recover and become dependent on communicative aids and assistive devices. Despite this rather bleak outlook, some people with apraxia, particularly children, do recover or adapt to the condition, especially in its milder forms.

References

GOLDENBERG, G. (2003) Apraxia and beyond: Life and work of Hugo Liepmann. *Cortex* 39: 509–525.

HALSBAND, U., J. SCHMITT, M. WEYERS, F. BINKOFSKI, G. GRÜTZNER AND H.-J. FREUND (2001) Recognition and imitation of pantomimed motor acts after unilateral parietal and premotor lesions: A perspective on apraxia. *Neuropsychologia* 39: 200–216.

HEILMAN, K. M., R. T. WATSON AND L. J. GONZALEZ-ROTHI (2007) Praxis. In *Textbook of Clinical Neurology*, 3rd Ed., C. G. Goetz (ed.). Philadelphia: Saunders Elsevier, pp. 55–64.

ZADIKOFF, C. AND A. E. LANG (2005) Apraxia in movement disorders. *Brain* 128: 1580–1597.

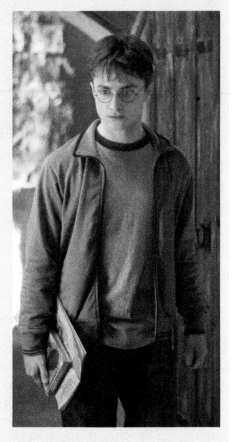

Example of mild apraxia. Actor Daniel Radcliffe, best known for his portrayal of the young wizard Harry Potter in the film series, struggles to tie his shoes because of a mild case of apraxia, sometimes referred to as dyspraxia.

Motor Control Is Hierarchical

Behavioral and theoretical studies of motor control strongly support a hierarchical model of the neural systems that organize action. The notion of hierarchical organization is vividly illustrated by the observation that complex movements, such as signing one's name, preserve distinctive features such as shape and style even when performed by different muscle groups. For example, the Russian physiologist Nikolai Bernstein asked people to sign their name with a pen held in the dominant (usually right) hand, and then with the pen attached near the wrist, elbow, or shoulder; with the pen attached to the right shoe; and even with the pen held in the mouth. Although penmanship was clearly sloppier and larger in scale under these decidedly unnatural conditions, the signature remained remarkably similar in overall form (**Figure 5.1**).

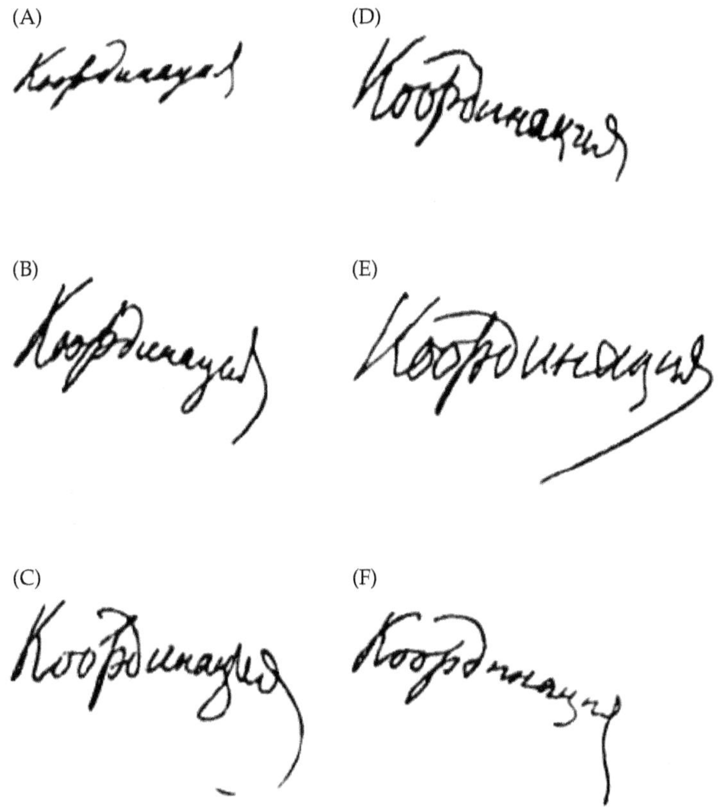

(A)

(D)

(B)

(E)

(C)

(F)

Figure 5.1   Behavioral evidence for motor programs
These signatures were made with a pen held in the right
hand (A), attached at the right wrist (B), attached at the
elbow (C), attached at the shoulder (D), attached to the
right shoe (E), and held in the teeth (F). Note the remarkable similarity in form retained by all the signatures. (From
Bernstein 1947.)

Such observations support the notion that complex behaviors are organized
at several levels. At the highest level are **motor programs**, which are sets of
commands to initiate a sequence of movements. Such motor programs are
distinguished by the fact that they are more or less ballistic, in the sense that
they do not strictly depend on incoming sensory information. Moreover, as
demonstrated by Bernstein's handwriting experiment, motor programs are
independent of the actual muscle groups used to carry them out. Finally, motor
programs originate within the central nervous system itself, rather than arising
directly from sensory signals from the periphery.

By contrast, at the lowest level of the motor control hierarchy are elementary
behavioral units that directly activate muscles. As described in the remainder
of this chapter, a variety of intermediate processing levels intervene between
motor programs and the elementary units of motor control. Such intermediate
processing in the motor system translates motor programs into the precisely
coordinated sequences of motor neuron activation and suppression that are
needed to generate the patterns of muscle contraction and relaxation responsible
for complex behavior.

Anatomical organization of motor systems

Hierarchical models of motor control can be loosely mapped onto neuroana-
tomically and neurophysiologically distinct elements of the central nervous
system. At a broad level, the neural circuits controlling skeletal movements
can be thought of as being made up of four distinct but interacting subsystems:
lower motor neurons in the spinal cord and brainstem; upper motor neurons
in the cortex and brainstem; the cerebellum; and the basal ganglia (**Figure 5.2**).

At the lowest level are circuits within the spinal cord and brainstem, composed of **lower motor neurons** and **local circuit neurons**. Lower motor neurons

Figure 5.2 Overall organization of the human motor system Four systems—upper motor neurons in the cortex and brainstem (blue), lower motor neurons in the spinal cord and brainstem (red), the cerebellum (green), and basal ganglia (brown)—make essential and distinct contributions to motor control.

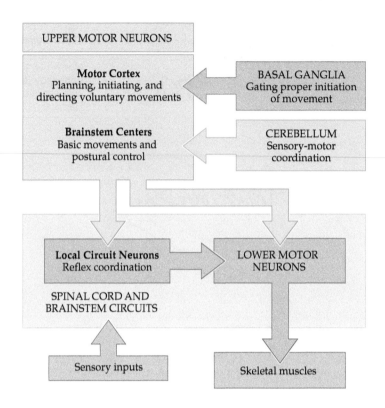

in the gray matter of the spinal cord and brainstem send axons out of the central nervous system to directly innervate skeletal muscle fibers, and they can be considered synonymous with the elementary behavioral units already mentioned. Lower motor neurons begin to fire action potentials immediately preceding contraction of the muscles they innervate; thus, their activity is directly correlated with movement of the relevant body part (Figure 5.3). Motor neurons involved in fine motor control, such as those used to move the fingers or control the position of the eyes, innervate far fewer muscle fibers than do motor neurons involved in gross movements of larger muscles, such as those used to move the legs during walking and running. Local circuit neurons, on the other hand, provide synaptic input to lower motor neurons and contribute to the local coordination of lower motor neuron activity. This is especially important for the coordination of reflexes engaged by rhythmic activities like walking and chewing (Box 5A).

At higher levels of the motor system, **upper motor neurons** in the cerebral cortex and brainstem provide descending control of local circuitry in the spinal cord and brainstem. The other two components of the motor system—the

Figure 5.3 Activity of lower motor neurons predicts muscle contraction and ultimately movement In the example here, the upper trace shows a recording from a lower motor neuron that innervates one of the eye muscles, causing the eye to rotate laterally. Note that the rate of action potentials is directly correlated with the amplitude and direction of the eye movement. (After Fuchs 1967.)

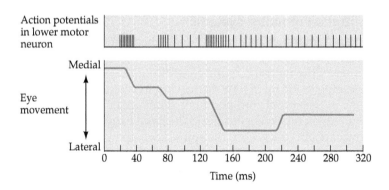

■ BOX 5A REFLEXES, CENTRAL PATTERN GENERATORS, AND RHYTHMIC BEHAVIORS

The fundamental unit of behavior is the reflex. Reflexes connecting the muscles to the spinal cord and then back to the muscles provide simple yet powerful mechanisms for controlling basic behavior (Figure A). Key components are local circuit neurons within the spinal cord that help connect incoming sensory information to appropriate motor neurons that enable movement. In fact, activation of the appropriate sets of local circuit neurons can generate complex patterns of muscle contraction and relaxation that result in rather sophisticated behavior. For example, the spinal cord (and brainstem) contains circuits capable of producing coordinated movements of the limbs with no input from the brain. Not surprisingly, these local circuits can also produce and sustain even more complex movements that are not simply reflexive responses to sensory inputs. Experimental work in a variety of animals has shown that rhythmic movements such as locomotion and swimming are actually produced by local spinal cord circuits known as central pattern generators.

Walking, to take a specific example, is a rhythmic behavior in which each foot moves from the stance phase, where it is in contact with the ground, to the swing phase, in which it is lifted and brought forward to begin the next stance phase. These phases of locomotion are associated with bursts of activity in extensor muscles during the stance phase and in flexor muscles during the swing phase (Figure B). Cats that have undergone surgical transection of the spinal cord anterior to the motor neurons controlling the hind limbs can nonetheless walk relatively normally on a treadmill. Their gait continues to follow the normal stance-swing-stance pattern, and the extensor and flexor muscles show coordinated bursts of activity typically associated with the stance and swing phases in normal animals (Figure C). Remarkably, cats with transected spinal cords can also adjust their walking speed when the treadmill is sped up or slowed down. When the sensory fibers entering the spinal cord via the dorsal roots are cut, however, the cat can continue to walk on the treadmill but can no longer adjust its gait or avoid obstacles.

These experiments, and others like them, demonstrate that the spinal cord and brainstem contain circuitry capable of controlling the timing and coordination

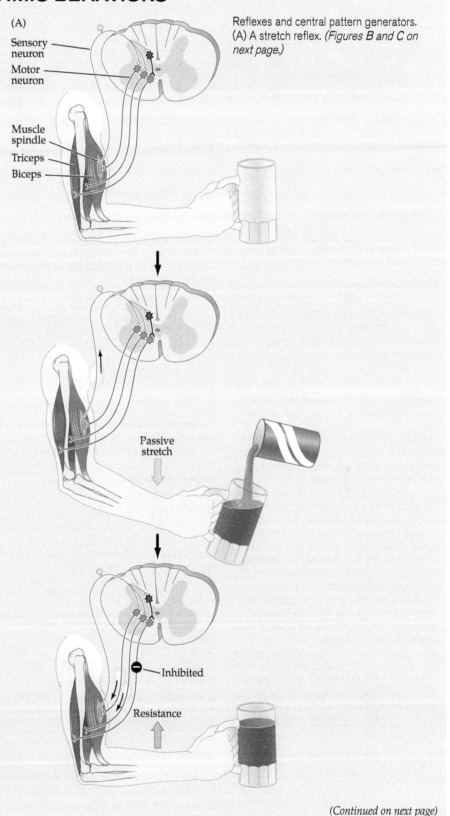

(A)
Sensory neuron
Motor neuron
Muscle spindle
Triceps
Biceps
Passive stretch
Inhibited
Resistance

Reflexes and central pattern generators. (A) A stretch reflex. *(Figures B and C on next page.)*

(Continued on next page)

■ **BOX 5A** *(continued)*

(B)

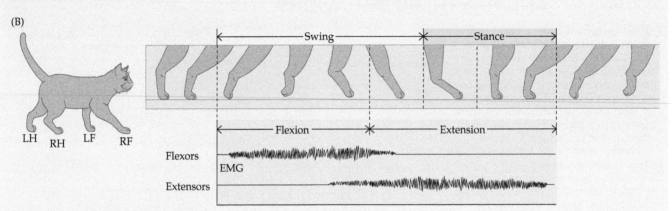

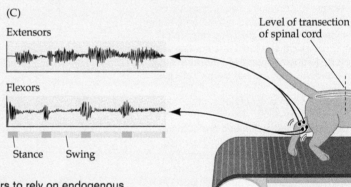

(B) A central pattern generator in the spinal cord. Electrical recordings from muscles in the legs of a cat show the relations of stance (foot planted), swing (foot lifted), and stance phases of locomotion. (C) After spinal cord transection, the hind limbs are still able to walk on a treadmill, and the reciprocal bursts of action potentials in the flexors and extensors during swing and stance phases are still evident. (After Pearson and Duysens 1976.)

of multiple muscles to produce complex rhythmic movements, that these circuits can respond to variations in the local physical environment such as obstacles, and that the needed processing can be performed in the absence of any input from higher brain centers.

Once evolution has generated a neural solution to a particular motor problem, the same mechanisms are often applied in new contexts to solve similar problems. Thus, central pattern generators, which evolved originally to mediate basic rhythmic functions such as swimming, walking, or swallowing, serve important roles in more complex, often cognitive, motor behaviors. For example, spoken language is arguably the most complex cognitive behavior generated by the brain, yet all human languages rely on the same basic motor processes for generating meaningful utterances (see Chapter 12). Verbal sequencing, much like the sequencing of other complex movement

patterns, appears to rely on endogenous central pattern generators instantiated in feedback loops between the cortex and basal ganglia that are quite similar to the sequences of neuronal activation in the spinal cord and brainstem central pattern generators considered here.

References

CALANCIE, B., B. NEEDHAM-SHROPSHIRE, P. JACOBS, K. WILLER, G. ZYCH AND B. A. GREEN (1994) Involuntary stepping after chronic spinal cord injury. Evidence for a central rhythm generator for locomotion in man. *Brain* 117(Pt. 5): 1143–1159.

FELDMAN, J. L., G. S. MITCHELL AND E. E. NATTIE (2003) Breathing: Rhythmicity, plasticity, chemosensitivity. *Annu. Rev. Neurosci.* 26: 239–266.

HUNT, C. C. AND S. W. KUFFLER (1951) Stretch receptor discharges during muscle contraction. *J. Physiol.* (Lond.) 113: 298–315.

LIDDELL, E. G. T. AND C. R. SHERRINGTON (1924) Reflexes in response to stretch (myotatic reflexes). *Proc. R. Soc. Lond. B* 96: 212–242.

MARDER, E. AND D. BUCHER (2001) Central pattern generators and the control of rhythmic movements. *Curr. Biol.* 11: R986–R996.

PEARSON, K. G. AND J. DUYSENS (1976) Function of segmental reflexes in the control of stepping in cockroaches and cats. In *Neural Control of Locomotion*, Vol. 18, R. Herman, S. Grillner, P. Stein, and D. Stuart (eds.). New York: Plenum, pp. 519–537.

cerebellum and basal ganglia—modulate the activity of upper motor neurons in order to make "online" corrections in response to perturbations in ongoing movements and to help initiate goal-directed movements, respectively. The localization of motor programs remains an active area of investigation.

(A) Lateral view

Premotor cortex Supplementary motor cortex Primary motor cortex

Medial view

Supplementary motor cortex Primary motor cortex

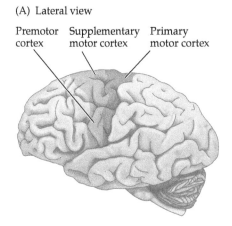

Figure 5.4 Upper motor neuron pathways (A) The primary motor cortex and premotor cortical areas. The primary motor cortex is located in the precentral gyrus. The motor and supplemental premotor areas are more rostral in the frontal lobe. (B) Descending pathways from the primary motor cortex. Pathway to the spinal cord and the lateral corticospinal tract in cross section.

Cortical Pathways for Motor Control

As we saw in the preceding discussion, the spinal cord and brainstem contain circuitry capable of generating an array of complex motor behavior. These subcortical systems serve animals with limited behavioral repertoires quite well, but in primates and other animals in which evolution has favored more demanding behaviors, the brain has evolved correspondingly complex higher motor centers capable of initiating and coordinating the local circuits and lower motor neurons that generate movements more directly.

Descending projections from the cerebral cortex to brainstem and spinal cord originate from upper motor neurons within the **primary motor cortex** and the adjacent **premotor cortical areas**, including the **premotor cortex** and **supplementary motor cortex** (Figure 5.4; see also the Appendix). In addition to having anatomical differences, the primary motor cortex is distinguished from other premotor areas by the very low intensity of current needed to evoke movements by electrical stimulation. The fact that low electrical current intensities applied to primary motor cortex can evoke movements indicates that the upper motor neurons of this area have relatively direct access to local circuit neurons and lower motor neurons in the brainstem and spinal cord.

The axons of the upper motor neurons in the primary motor cortex that

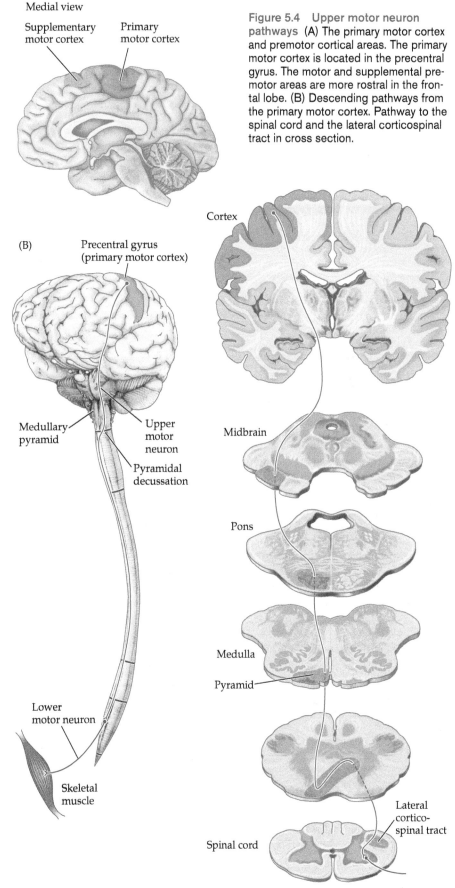

(B)

Precentral gyrus (primary motor cortex)

Medullary pyramid

Upper motor neuron

Pyramidal decussation

Lower motor neuron

Skeletal muscle

Cortex

Midbrain

Pons

Medulla

Pyramid

Spinal cord

Lateral cortico-spinal tract

■ BOX 5B MOTOR CONTROL OF FACIAL EXPRESSIONS

The neural control of facial expressions provides a fascinating and instructive example of how upper and lower motor neurons are coordinated to generate useful behavior, and how some aspects of emotion play into the generation of facial movements. The muscles of facial expression, including those that elevate the corners of the lips in a smile and raise the eyebrows in surprise, are under the direct control of lower motor neurons in the facial nerve nucleus in the pons. The projections of these lower motor neurons to the facial muscles via cranial nerve VII are strictly unilateral. Thus, damage to upper motor neurons in the facial nucleus or to the nerve itself causes unilateral paralysis of the muscles of facial expression on that side (Figure A). In contrast, the upper motor neurons that initiate and coordinate voluntary facial expressions reside in the primary motor cortex.

A particularly common, and usually reversible, form of such facial paralysis known as Bell's palsy is caused by inflammation of the facial nerve. Notably, the upper motor neurons controlling the inferior facial muscles project to the contralateral pons, and the upper motor neurons controlling the superior facial muscles project bilaterally. Thus, damage to the portion of the primary motor cortex corresponding to movements of the face results in weakness of the inferior facial muscles on the opposite side, but movements of the superior facial muscles are spared.

A second motor pathway more closely linked to emotion contributes to largely involuntary facial expressions. This pathway originates in premotor areas in the prefrontal cortex and basal ganglia, projects to the hypothalamus, and then continues to the brainstem reticular formation, ultimately targeting the facial motor nuclei in the pons. Activation of this pathway by an emotional experience evokes involuntary facial expression, such as the smile produced upon hearing a joke. Damage to this multisynaptic "extrapyra-

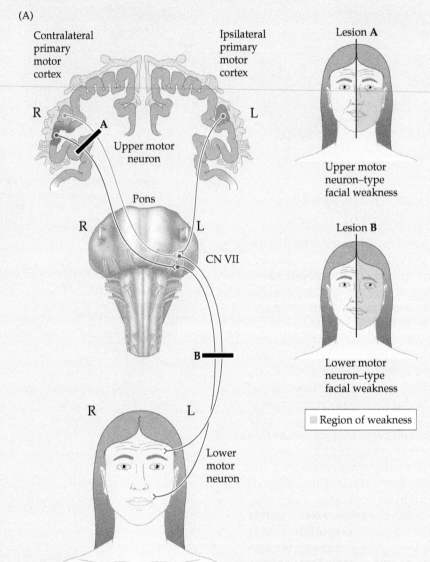

(A)

Voluntary and emotional control of facial expression. (A) Anatomical circuit controlling voluntary facial expression. Lower motor neurons in the pons project to the muscles of the upper and lower face. Upper motor neurons projecting to the pons are unilateral for the lower face, but bilateral for the upper face. A unilateral lesion to the facial nucleus in the pons results in complete paralysis of the face on the same side, whereas a unilateral lesion in the lateral part of the primary motor cortex results in paresis of the lower face on the opposite side due to bilateral projections serving the upper facial muscles.

innervate neurons in the brainstem, such as those controlling the muscles of facial expression (Box 5B), branch off at appropriate levels, and those continuing to the spinal cord coalesce and descend through the **medullary pyramids** (so named for their triangular appearance) in the pyramidal tract. The majority of corticospinal fibers cross the midline, or *decussate*, at the caudal end of the medulla and enter the lateral corticospinal tract in the spinal cord (see Figure

■ BOX 5B *(continued)*

(B)

| | Pyramidal (volitional) smile | Duchenne (emotional) smile |

Volitional facial paresis

Emotional facial paresis

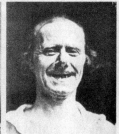
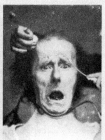

(C)

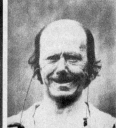

(B) Voluntary and emotional paresis of the face. Lesions to the face representation in primary motor cortex lead to unilateral weakness in smiling on command (left). Lesions to the emotional pathway for facial expression lead to an inability to smile in response to a joke, while voluntary smiling remains intact (right). (C) Duchenne de Boulogne's pioneering study of "faradization," or electrical stimulation, of the facial muscles. The patient in the photographs had lost sensation in the face and thus did not feel the effects of stimulation. Compare the stimulated "smile" (second from left) with the emotional smile (third from left).

midal" pathway (the voluntary pathway is referred to as the pyramidal pathway because it travels in the pyramids in the caudal medulla) renders patients unable to spontaneously express emotions in the face, although they can still produce symmetrical voluntary facial expressions (Figure B). Conversely, patients with damage to upper motor neuron pathways have difficulty voluntarily moving the muscles of the lower part of the contralateral face but nonetheless can smile, frown, or cry normally in response to emotional stimulation.

These distinctions between the pathway for voluntary facial expression and spontaneous, emotional facial expression were first described by the French neurologist and physiologist G. B. A. Duchenne de Boulogne, who photographed subjects producing facial expressions in response to direct electrical stimulation of the muscles and in response to emotional stimulation (Figure C). Duchenne de Boulogne demonstrated that some facial muscle groups, such as the orbicularis oculi, can be activated involuntarily only by subjective emotional experience—an expression known as the Duchenne smile. A forced or voluntary smile does not activate this muscle group, thus appearing strained and unnatural. The distinctions between voluntary and emotional facial expression pathways are often painfully obvious in the contrived facial expressions worn when we are less than sincere.

References

BLUMENFELD, H. (2002) *Neuroanatomy through Clinical Cases.* Sunderland, MA: Sinauer.

DARWIN, C. R. (1572) *The Expression of the Emotions in Man and Animals.* London: Murray.

DUCHENNE DE BOULOGNE, G. B. A. (1562) *Mécanisme de la Physionomie Humaine.* Cambridge: Cambridge University Press.

5.4B), and they terminate within the gray matter of the cord at levels appropriate to the distal muscles that they serve. A small minority of corticospinal fibers remain uncrossed, forming the medial or ventral corticospinal tract; these axons terminate within the medial spinal cord gray matter on both sides (after crossing through the spinal cord commissure). These medial corticospinal projections, as suggested by the loci of their targets, are involved in control of the midline (proximal) musculature (**Figure 5.5**).

Organization of the primary motor cortex

Early studies conducted in the late nineteenth century showed that electrical stimulation of the primary motor cortex in the precentral gyrus on one side of the primate brain evokes muscle contractions on the opposite side of the body. This apparently topographical organization of the primary motor cortex was

Figure 5.5 **Organization of the lower motor neurons in a cross section of the cervical spinal cord** Motor neurons innervating proximal muscles (i.e., those closest to the shoulder) are located medially (close to the midline); those innervating distal muscles (toward the digits) are located laterally (to the right or left).

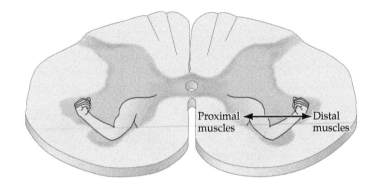

confirmed shortly after the start of the twentieth century by Charles Sherrington, who showed that stimulating adjacent regions of the precentral gyrus in apes elicited movements of adjacent contralateral body parts. The presence of a topographical map of body musculature in the primary motor cortex was further verified in humans by Sherrington's student Wilder Penfield, who, as a neurosurgeon in the 1930s, systematically stimulated different brain regions in human patients. Such motor maps revealed with direct electrical stimulation of the brain are also evident in the blood oxygenation level–dependent (BOLD) response when subjects are asked to move their lips, finger, thumb, elbow, or foot (Figure 5.6).

As in the sensory maps described in Chapters 3 and 4, these motor maps define a distorted representation of the body. A disproportionately large area of the lateral primary motor cortex was devoted to the lips, tongue, and hands; and a much smaller area of the dorsal and medial primary motor cortex was devoted to the lower extremities and genitalia (Figure 5.7). Thus, the amount of cortical space devoted to motor function corresponds to the capability of that area to exercise fine motor control, and it underscores the principle that more sophisticated processing is always reflected in a greater allocation of cortical space.

Figure 5.6 **Moving different body parts activates different parts of the primary motor cortex in humans** Human subjects lay on their back in an fMRI scanner with their eyes closed, while their heads and proximal limbs were secured in order to minimize involuntary movements. Subjects were asked to perform the following movements in succession: elevate the foot at the ankle, flex and extend the right elbow, make a fist with the right hand, tap the right thumb and index finger together, make a fist with the left hand, and purse the lips. The BOLD signal revealed neural activation most laterally for the lips, most medially for the foot, and in between for movements of the hands and fingers—in good accordance with the motor maps generated by intracranial electrical stimulation in human surgical patients. (After Lotze et al. 2000.)

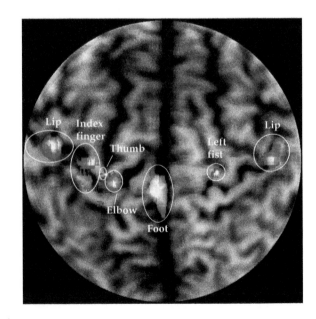

(A)

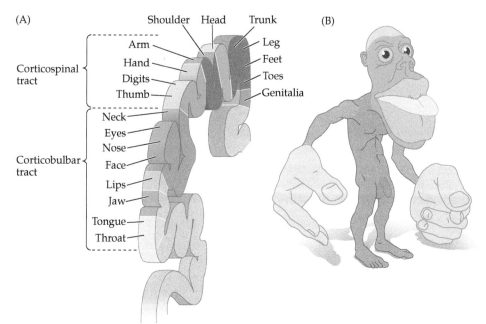

Figure 5.7 The distorted map of the body's musculature in the primary motor cortex (A) The primary motor cortex (M1) is located just in front of the brain's central sulcus. Regions controlling motor responses in different parts of the body are shown here in relative size and sequence. (B) The proportions of the homunculus show the parts of the body relative to their represented size in the primary motor cortex. (After Breedlove et al. 2007.)

Movement maps in the primary motor cortex

Especially pertinent to understanding how cognitive functions relate to the generation of motor behavior is the long-standing debate about the role of these motor maps in producing movement. The question centers largely on whether the activity of neurons in these motor maps specifies what to do (a motor command) or how to do it—the particular patterns of muscle activity necessary to generate the forces required for a particular movement.

Early studies in monkeys using low-intensity electrical stimulation suggested that the primary motor cortex might contain a map of individual muscles. However, later electrical stimulation studies in monkeys confirmed reports by Penfield and Sherrington that activation of some portions of the primary motor cortex evokes coordinated, multijoint movements (Figure 5.8). This observation is what would be expected, given that descending projections from the primary

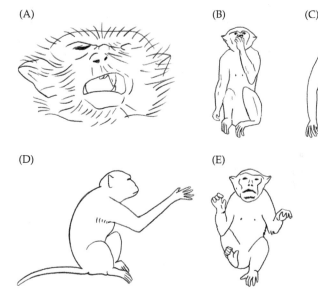

Figure 5.8 Complex movements evoked by stimulation of the primary motor cortex in the monkey Each drawing represents the animal's posture at the end of the stimulation. (A) Defensive-like posture of face. (B) Hand to mouth. (C) Manipulation-like shaping of fingers and movement of hand. (D) Outward reach with hand open, as if shaping to grasp. (E) Climbing- or leaping-like posture involving all four limbs. (After Graziano 2006.)

(A)

Implanted recording electrode

Juice reward delivery

Response button (target)

Restraint chair

Wrist restraint

(B)

Recording from cortical motor neuron

Record

Cortical motor neuron spike

Spinal motor neuron

Muscle activity

Spike-triggered muscle activity

Time (ms)

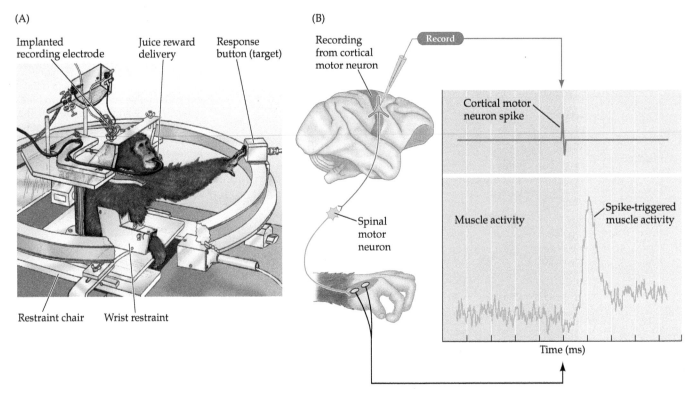

Figure 5.9 Determining the role of cortical motor neurons in generating movements (A) Experimental setup for recording from monkey primary motor cortex neurons in relationship to reaching. (B) As indicated in the diagram and sample recording, neurons in the primary motor cortex fire before movements occur. Movement onset is defined by the increase in the activity of the muscles in the electromyogram (EMG). (A after Evarts 1981; B after Porter and Lemon 1993.)

motor cortex target mainly local circuits in the brainstem and spinal cord rather than the lower motor neurons themselves.

Electrophysiological recordings from single neurons in the primary motor cortex of monkeys have largely supported the conclusion that movements and not muscles are represented in motor maps. In the late 1960s, neuroscientist Edward Evarts and his colleagues pioneered the technique of implanting electrodes in the motor cortex of monkeys that had been trained to reach toward cued targets in order to receive rewards (Figure 5.9A). The electrical signals generated by neurons were then compared to the muscle fiber action potentials recorded from the arm muscles, as well as to recordings of the direction and force generated by the arm during movement (Figure 5.9B). Evarts's group found that most neurons in the primary motor cortex fired action potentials in relation to a subset of movements, and that the firing rate corresponded to the changes in force generated by the muscles during movement. Moreover, many of these neurons began to discharge before the movements themselves were initiated, suggesting that their activation did not cause movement directly.

Commands to move the eyes are generated in a similar set of circuits comprising the **frontal eye fields** in the cortex and the superior colliculus in the midbrain, which then project to the brainstem reticular formation, which organizes and coordinates activation of the extraocular muscles by lower motor neurons in the brainstem (as discussed earlier). These and other observations are all consistent with the idea that higher motor centers, including the primary motor cortex and the frontal eye fields, provide both motor command signals that engage lower-level circuits to produce coordinated movements and signals that indicate, to some degree, how forceful these movements should be. That is, these upper motor neurons specify both what to do and how to do it.

Coding Movements by the Activity of Neuronal Populations

The motor maps discussed in the previous section are essentially gross anatomical descriptions of how the motor system is organized, but how these maps are related to coordinated movements is not entirely clear. The relatively coarse tuning of neurons in the primary motor cortex and other higher movement centers presents a problem for understanding how the brain generates a particular movement. Although the work described in the previous section provided evidence that maps specify movements, the direction and amplitude of a movement cannot be predicted with any precision from the activity of single neurons, which are often activated during a wide array of different movements.

One solution to this problem is the idea that the activity of hundreds or perhaps thousands of neurons is averaged in computing the desired movement. Early work focused on maps of eye movements because the oculomotor system, by virtue of its simplicity, is a useful model for sorting out the principles governing more complex movements. Movements of the eyes are also under the control of higher movement centers, although the organization of these pathways is distinct from that of higher pathways that control limb movements.

The study of eye movements is facilitated by the fact that the local circuits in the brainstem coordinating eye movements are under the direct control of neurons in the **superior colliculus**, an easily accessible layered structure in the midbrain. Electrical stimulation in the intermediate and deep layers of the superior colliculus in monkeys produces coordinated gaze shifts, and single neurons in these layers fire action potentials just before the rapid, ballistic eye movements known as **saccades** begin (Figure 5.10A). Moreover, electrical stimulation at any site evokes a saccade with a particular direction and

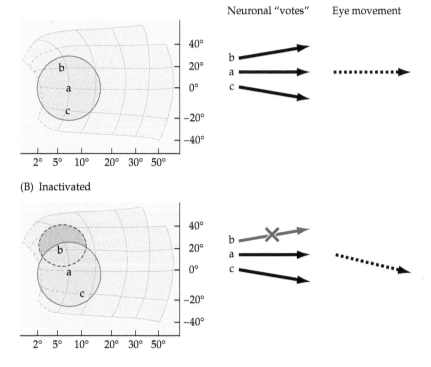

Figure 5.10 Population coding (A) Topographical map showing eye movements in the superior colliculus. Movement amplitude is coded in increasing steps from left to right, and movement direction is coded on the vertical axis. The light purple region is the zone of neurons activated preceding a movement 5 degrees to the right of the zone marked "a." (B) Pharmacological inactivation of the zone centered on "b" (red circle) in a monkey results in a shift in the weighted average of collicular activity, as well as the endpoint of the eye movement. (After Lee et al. 1988.)

Figure 5.11 Population vectors in the primary motor cortex Each line indicates the direction and amplitude of an arm movement decoded from the activity of a population of neurons recorded in the primary motor cortex. The time of the trials proceeds from bottom to top; S indicates the cue for movement, and M indicates the onset of movement. Movement in direct response to a cue results in immediate generation of a population vector specifying the movement. Delayed movement evokes a population vector specifying the movement hundreds of milliseconds before movement onset. (After Georgopolous et al. 1986.)

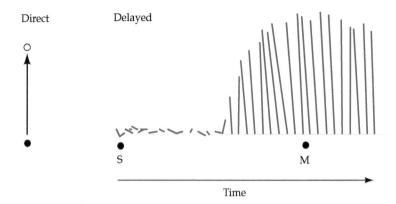

amplitude, whereas stimulation at nearby sites evokes saccades with slightly different vectors. Thus, the superior colliculus contains a topographical map of eye movements, much like the topographical maps of skeletal movements in the primary motor cortex (see Figure 5.7A).

Each superior colliculus neuron is thought to vote for its range of movements, with the weight of the vote cast determined by how strongly the neuron fired. The weighted votes would then be averaged across the population to arrive at the vector for the desired movement. To test this idea, small portions of the map of eye movements in the superior colliculus were reversibly inactivated in monkeys trained to look toward visual targets for fruit juice rewards. Following inactivation, eye movements were systematically biased away from the inactivated portion of the collicular map, as would be expected if movements were specified by the weighted average of the activity of all the neurons in the superior colliculus (Figure 5.10B). This experiment provided the first functional support for the notion that the brain achieves precise movements by averaging together the activation of large populations of coarsely tuned neurons.

The idea that precise movements are encoded by averaging the activity of many coarsely tuned neurons has been extended to the primary motor cortex. Neurons in the primary motor cortex are broadly tuned to generate a range of movement directions and amplitudes, firing strongly for some movements but weakly or not at all for others. A vector representing the weighted average of activity across the population of neurons in the motor cortex as a function of time (Figure 5.11) specifies the impending movement well in advance of any activity in the muscles. This observation supports the idea that the primary motor cortex encodes intended movements by the vector average of activity across the active neuronal population.

Planning Movements

Although many movements are more or less automatic in response to a sensory stimulus, other actions are planned in advance and their initiation held off until the circumstances are appropriate for their execution. For example, when monkeys are cued to reach toward a target but are forced to delay initiation of the reach, neurons in the primary motor cortex become active before the movement is initiated. Anticipatory activation of neurons during arm movement planning has been observed in a number of premotor areas as well, including the premotor, supplementary motor, dorsolateral prefrontal, and parietal cortices.

In the case of visual orienting movements, such activity is seen in the frontal and supplementary eye fields, and in the dorsolateral prefrontal and lateral parietal cortices. Planning-related activity in premotor areas typically persists when movement cues are removed and ceases when monkeys are cued to stop

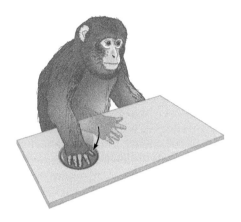

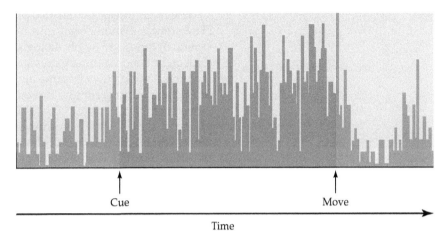

Cue   Move

Time

Figure 5.12   Evidence of anticipatory activity as a correlate of movement intention in the premotor cortex The histogram shows neuronal firing as a function of time in a monkey cued to reach toward a target after a delay (red). Neuronal activity continues from the cue until the movement, suggesting a neural correlate of the intention to reach toward the target.

planning the movement, thus suggesting a role in intention (Figure 5.12). One indication of the functional role of these premotor areas is that planning-related neuronal activity typically begins even earlier in these areas than in the primary motor cortex (or the superior colliculus for saccades).

These observations support the idea that motor areas are hierarchically organized, with premotor areas providing more abstract planning information related to behavioral goals, which is then translated into the intention to perform specific movements in the primary motor cortex (and the superior colliculus for visual orienting movements). Thus, higher motor areas appear to serve a functional role in specifying the motor program discussed earlier. Motor intention signals in the primary motor cortex are then translated by downstream local circuits in the brainstem and spinal cord into neural activity that specifies the patterns of muscle contraction necessary to accomplish the intended movements.

Scalp recordings from humans (see Chapter 2) have tended to confirm this hierarchical organization of movement planning. When subjects are asked to voluntarily generate a movement—for example, lifting a finger at a time of their choosing—EEG recordings from medial frontal electrodes show a pronounced negative wave that begins up to several seconds in advance of the actual movement. This **readiness potential** initially begins bilaterally over premotor areas, but later it becomes enhanced over the primary motor cortex contralateral to the finger movement (Figure 5.13). Neuroimaging studies have identified the readiness potential with activation in premotor areas, particularly the supplementary motor areas. Interestingly, when premotor areas are damaged along with the primary motor cortex, patients are unaware of (or even deny) their inability to move—a phenomenon known as **anosognosia**, meaning "loss of awareness." This clinical observation provides additional evidence that the premotor cortex is the source of motor planning and intentional awareness.

Figure 5.13   Readiness potential These EEG recordings were taken from scalp electrodes over premotor and supplementary motor cortices in human subjects asked to voluntarily move a finger. EEG amplitude when subjects attend to their own movement (blue) increases several seconds in advance of the actual movement. EEG amplitude when subjects attend to the urge to move–the readiness potential (red)–is enhanced relative to the movement potential. Readiness potentials begin later in the contralateral primary motor cortex, consistent with a hierarchical progression of motor intention. (After Eagleman 2004.)

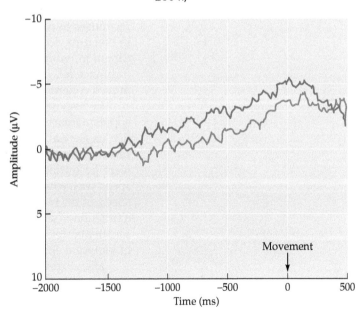

The readiness potential also provides a means of further exploring the role of awareness in motor planning. In a famous but controversial study conducted several decades ago by physiologist Benjamin Libet, subjects were asked to produce an uncued voluntary movement and then estimate (from a clock display) the time at which they became aware of the intention to move. EEG recordings indicated, not surprisingly, that estimates of the intention to move preceded the movement itself by about 200 milliseconds. However, readiness potentials over premotor areas clearly preceded subjects' awareness of when they intended to move. Although these results have a number of possible confounding factors, the study implies that conscious awareness actually follows the intention to move rather than preceding and thus causing it.

Selecting goals for action

At any given moment, several competing or alternative behavioral goals might be options for motor planning. For example, on approaching a stoplight that just turned yellow, a driver might either slow to stop, or accelerate to get through the intersection before the light turns red. The neural processes responsible for selecting a course of action to reach a goal (e.g., getting to the destination faster) and generating the relevant movement have come under increasing scrutiny as researchers have realized the importance of cognitive contexts for motor behaviors. Most such studies have focused on the processes that link sensory information to motor output.

Early electrophysiological studies in monkeys demonstrated that neurons in a variety of premotor areas where planning-related activity occurs respond to sensory cues used to guide movements. Moreover, these responses to sensory cues can be enhanced or diminished if the stimulus is made more or less likely to be the target of a movement. Subsequent work showed that such sensory-motor linkage is graded by the quality of information guiding the movement integrated over time. For instance, neurophysiologists William Newsome and Michael Shadlen provided evidence that neuronal responses in a number of premotor areas involved in saccadic eye movements are systematically related to the weight of sensory evidence favoring a particular movement. In these experiments, monkeys were trained to judge the net direction of motion in a field of moving dots and report this evaluation by shifting their gaze to a specific target if they judged the motion to be in one direction and a different target if they saw motion in the opposite direction (Figure 5.14A). Newsome and Shadlen systematically manipulated the quality of the evidence favoring responses to each target by changing the fraction of dots moving coherently in one direction or another. When about 50 percent of the dots moved in one direction, monkeys were nearly always correct in their responses; their performance fell to chance levels, however, when less than 5 percent of the dots moved coherently.

The responses of neurons in the posterior parietal cortex, frontal eye fields, supplementary eye fields, dorsolateral prefrontal cortex, and even superior colliculus were all found to be modulated by the strength of the motion stimulus favoring a particular eye movement response (Figure 5.14B). When monkeys were permitted to move their eyes as soon as they had made a decision, the speed with which neuronal activity in the parietal cortex increased matched the speed of the monkeys' eye movement responses. Similar graded responses as a function of stimulus quality have been reported in the higher-order somatosensory cortex and premotor areas in monkeys trained to report the frequency of vibration applied to the forearm by pushing a button.

Taken together, these studies imply that neurons in a number of premotor areas specify movements in a graded manner as sensory evidence is accumulated. This hypothesis was tested directly by applying microstimulation to

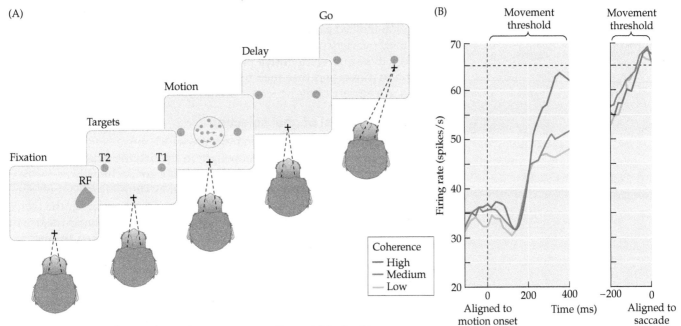

Figure 5.14 Dependence of a motor response on the weight of evidence
(A) Monkeys performed a visual discrimination task in which, by moving their eyes, they reported the direction of motion in a field of randomly moving dots. One target was in the response field (RF) of a neuron in the posterior parietal cortex; the other was in the opposite visual field. (B) The firing rate of neurons in posterior parietal cortex increased when monkeys viewed dots moving toward the target in the RF. The rate of increase over time was directly proportional to motion coherence, or the weight of evidence favoring an eye movement to the RF target. The relation between firing rate and motion coherence reflects the integration of motion over time. (After Roitman and Shadlen 2002.)

the frontal eye fields while monkeys performed the dot discrimination task illustrated in Figure 5.14A. Stimulation in this area evoked saccadic eye movements at short latencies, but the endpoints of the movements were systematically biased by the pattern of motion the monkeys saw (**Figure 5.15A**). Moreover, the amount of bias gradually increased as monkeys viewed the motion longer, as well as when the fraction of coherently moving dots was gradually increased (**Figure 5.15B**). When the locations of the movement targets were not revealed

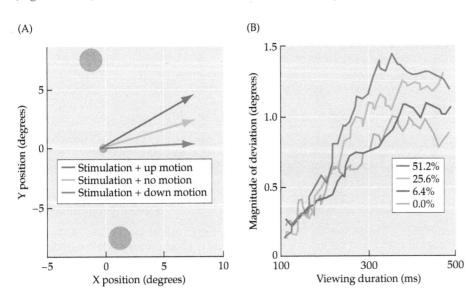

Figure 5.15 Graded conversion of sensory percepts into action
(A) Monkeys were trained to fixate centrally while observing motion stimuli that were moving either up or down, or that had no net motion. Microstimulation of the frontal eye fields evoked eye movements that were systematically biased by the direction of viewed motion, thus indicating that ongoing motor planning in this area is influenced by gradually accumulating motion information. (B) The magnitude of the deviation in stimulation-induced eye movements depended on both motion coherence of the stimuli and viewing duration. With higher motion coherence, the rate of deviation in eye position as a function of time increased, implying that the integration of sensory evidence over time favors a particular motor response. Each curve represents a particular percentage of dots moving coherently. (After Gold and Shadlen 2000.)

in advance of the dot stimulus, however, dot motion had very little effect on stimulation-evoked saccades.

All told, a variety of observations support the conclusion that motor preparation is a dynamic, competitive process linking sensory information to the intention to move, and that such processing entails the graded activation of neurons in a variety of higher-order premotor cortical (and subcortical) areas.

Motivational control of goal selection

Although sensory stimulation often indicates which movement should be produced (e.g., the response to the yellow light in the driving example described in the previous section), people must often select a goal primarily on the basis of additional, far more complex stimuli, as well as stored information about the likely state of the environment (in the yellow-light example, the factors indicating the relative need to get to the destination quickly that influence the significance of the stimulus). Indeed, when monkeys performed the moving-dot task illustrated in Figure 5.14, they reported their judgments not because of the stimulus per se, but because if they responded, they would receive squirts of fruit juice—highly desirable treats.

Although behavior is typically directed toward acquiring rewards and avoiding punishments, very little is understood about the mechanisms that guide the motor system to select goals that satisfy such biological motivations. This question was tackled directly in a series of studies by neurobiologists Paul Glimcher and Michael Platt designed to understand how internal motivations shape the responses of neurons in the posterior parietal cortex (Figure 5.16). They trained monkeys to choose between looking at two visually identical lights and then, across a series of trials, systematically varied either the probability or the amount of fruit juice reinforcement the monkeys received for looking at one light versus the other. Platt and Glimcher found that neurons in the posterior parietal cortex were sensitive to the **reward value** of shifting gaze to a particular target, which depended on both the probability and the magnitude of the juice reward associated with that target.

Neurons in a number of premotor areas, including the dorsolateral prefrontal cortex, supplementary eye fields, frontal eye fields, and posterior cingulate cortex have also been found to be sensitive to movement value. Further, fMRI studies of people choosing between movements of different value have found similar scaling of activation by movement value. In one study, scientists asked

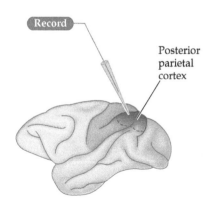

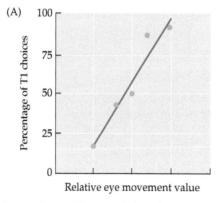

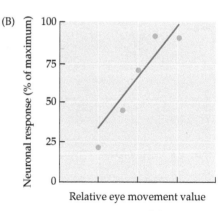

Figure 5.16 The sensitivity of premotor neurons to movement values (A) Monkeys choose to spend time looking at a particular target in direct proportion to the relative reward value of that action. (B) Neurons in the posterior parietal cortex respond in direct proportion to the relative reward value associated with an eye movement. (After Platt and Glimcher 1999.)

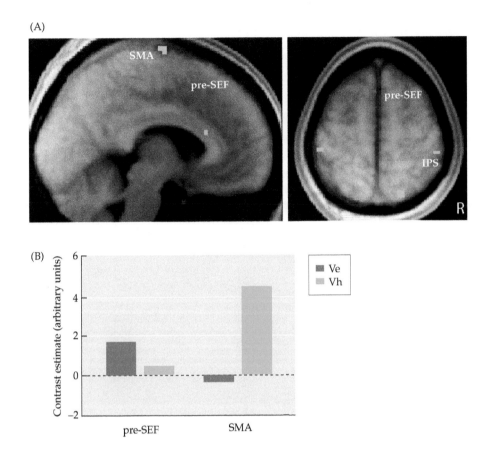

Figure 5.17 Action value signals in the human brain (A) Region of the supplementary motor area (SMA) showing correlations with action values for hand movement (Vh; green) and a region of presupplementary eye field (pre-SEF) showing correlations with action values for eye movements (Ve; red). IPS, intra-parietal sulcus. (B) Average sizes of the effects of eye movement value (red) and hand movement value (green) extracted from the SEF and SMA. The effects shown here were calculated from trials independent of those used to functionally identify the region of interest. Note that only Ve (but not Vh) modulates the signal in the pre-SEF, and that activity in the SMA shows the opposite pattern. (After Wunderlich et al. 2009.)

people to choose between an eye movement and a hand movement, each of which varied in value across trials. As expected, people generally tended to choose the more valuable option. Importantly, activity in the supplementary eye field (Figure 5.17) tended to vary with the value of the eye movement, whereas activity in the supplementary motor area tended to vary with the value of the hand movement, paralleling the findings from single-neuron recording studies done in monkeys. Together, these studies suggest that selecting a movement goal involves scaling neuronal responses associated with each possible movement by that movement's value, thereby biasing the motor system to produce a movement that best satisfies biological motivations such as acquiring rewards or avoiding punishments.

Sequential Movements and the Supplementary Motor Area

The discussion so far has focused on the selection and planning of a *single* movement. Clearly, however, the behavioral repertoire of humans and other animals normally consists of *sequences* of movements that together constitute meaningful behaviors that satisfy specific goals. Not surprisingly, regions of the frontal cortex are specialized to support the production of movement sequences. As a rule, the **supplementary motor area**, or **SMA** (also called area 6) is crucial for generating movements in the absence of explicit sensory cues, and the premotor cortex is especially important for the production of cued movements. When the SMA is ablated, monkeys can no longer perform well-learned movements and must instead rely on external cues to tell them which movement should be performed. The reverse is true for lesions of the premotor cortex, which selectively disrupt visually guided movements but do not affect

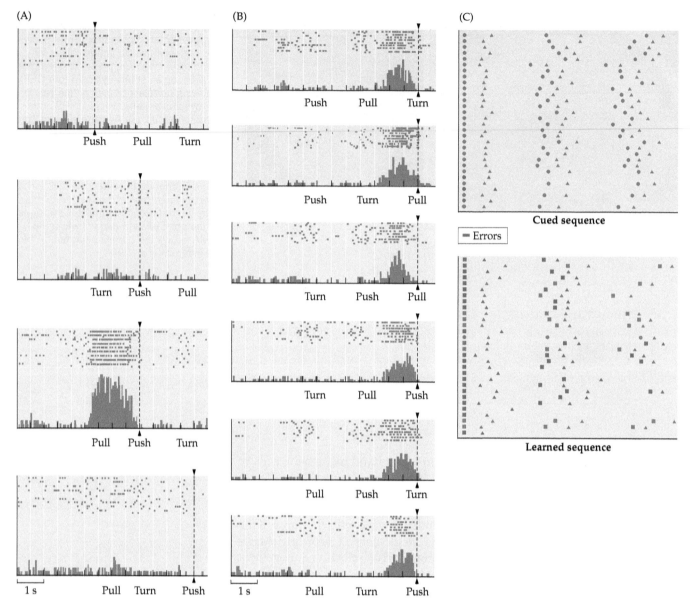

(A)

(B)

(C)

Figure 5.18 Neuronal responses mediating action sequences (A) The SMA neuron recorded here responds selectively to the sequence "pull, push, turn." (B) In this case, the SMA neuron responds selectively to the last movement in a sequence, independent of the type of movement required. (C) Pharmacological inactivation of the SMA causes errors in producing learned sequences but not explicitly cued sequences of movements. (After Tanji and Shima 1994.)

well-learned responses that can be made in the absence of sensory cues. These results suggest a functional dissociation between the premotor cortex and the supplementary cortex for producing cued and uncued movements, respectively.

A similar logic applies to the production of movement sequences, which requires the ability to generate action in the absence of external cues specifying each individual movement. In an important and revealing experiment, physiologist Jun Tanji and colleagues trained monkeys to make a sequence of arm movements based on a visual cue. For example, a red light might mean "push, pull, turn," whereas a green light might mean "turn, push, pull." Note that the visual cues specify which sequence of movements to make rather than cuing any single movement directly. Tanji and his group then recorded from SMA neurons while monkeys performed this sequence generation task.

Tanji's group found that many neurons in the SMA were selectively activated when a particular action embedded within a sequence was performed (Figure 5.18A). Moreover, many neurons responded only for a particular action sequence, irrespective of the type of movement (Figure 5.18B). For example, some neurons

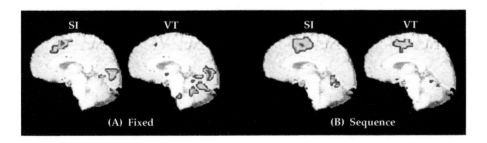

Figure 5.19 Activation of the human supplementary motor cortex when subjects intentionally generate sequences of finger movements These fMRI data were gathered from a single human subject asked to repeatedly touch index finger to thumb (A) or to generate a learned sequence of finger-to-thumb movements (B), cued either internally (SI) or by a visual stimulus (VT). (From Deiber et al. 1999.)

responded to the second movement in the sequence, whereas others responded to the third. These observations suggest that SMA neurons convey information needed to guide the production of a sequence of reaching movements. This supposition was confirmed when Tanji and colleagues reversibly deactivated the SMA by injecting muscimol, an agonist of the neurotransmitter gamma-aminobutyric acid (GABA), thus enhancing local inhibitory connections and silencing the output neurons. When the SMA was silenced in this way, monkeys were unable to perform sequences from memory (Figure 5.18C). Transcranial magnetic stimulation applied over the supplementary motor cortex in humans (see Chapter 2) also disrupts the production of manual sequences, in accord with the results in monkeys.

Activation of SMA neurons in monkeys by internally generated sequences of action is supported by neuroimaging studies in humans demonstrating preferential activation of the supplementary motor cortex during self-initiated finger movements, compared with visually triggered movements. Moreover, such modulations were even stronger when subjects generated sequences of movements rather than repeating the same movement over and over (Figure 5.19). Together, these observations support the conclusion that the supplementary motor area provides relatively abstract motor intention signals that control the internally guided production of sequences of actions, whereas the prefrontal cortex plays a more important role in the initiation and termination of movement sequences. The primary motor cortex then issues sequences of commands that activate pools of motor units in the brainstem and spinal cord to produce the desired movements.

Sensory-Motor Coordination

Another key issue in understanding motor control concerns the transformations needed to translate spatial and textural information gleaned from sensory inputs into appropriate motor commands. For example, shifting gaze to a visual target is a relatively trivial computational problem, mainly because the vector representing the locus of retinal stimulation relative to the fovea is aligned with the vector representing the amplitude and direction of an eye movement that directs the fovea to the target. This happy marriage of sensory and motor coordinates does not, however, apply to other sensory-guided movements. Thus, reaching toward a visible target such as a cup of coffee requires translating the retinal location of the target into a location anchored to the position of the hand.

To do this, the retinal vector must in some way be combined with information about the position of the eye in the head, the head's position with respect to the rest of the body, and the hand and arm relative to everything else. Similarly complex coordinate transformations are needed in order to look accurately in the direction of an auditory stimulus, scratch an itch, walk to a geographically challenging destination, or undertake innumerable other routine challenges that require translations from one or more frameworks to another. Thus, in

Figure 5.20 Deficits in visually guided reaching and grasping caused by parietal lesions (A) The reaching and grasping of objects is measured by electrodes hooked up to the subject's finger, thumb, and wrist. (B) Lines connect the precision grip made with thumb and forefinger for a patient with parietal lesion (R.V.) and a control subject. The optimal grasp crosses the center of mass of the object. (A after Goodale, http://psychology.uwo.ca/faculty/goodale/research/index.html; B after Milner and Goodale 1995.)

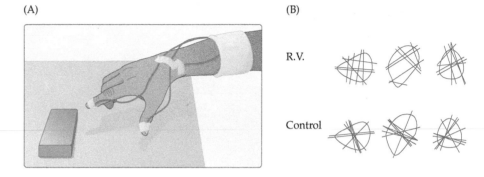

(A)

(B)

R.V.

Control

addition to selecting, planning, and initiating movements, neural mechanisms must use sensory information to compute the appropriate spatial coordinates for guiding movements.

Several lines of evidence suggest that the parietal cortex is crucial for sensory-motor coordination. In partial support of this idea, damage to the parietal cortex in humans can disrupt both reaching and saccades—a clinical syndrome known as **optic ataxia**. The spatial errors that arise from this condition reveal a failure to correctly integrate information about the locations of the eye, hand, and target. Disruptions in sensory-motor integration are also manifest when patients with parietal lesions attempt to grasp objects (Figure 5.20). Compared to control subjects without lesions, such patients fail to grasp objects accurately across their centers of mass. These errors invariably lead to difficulties in actually picking up objects—a deficit also found in monkeys following pharmacological inactivation of the parietal cortex.

The observation of such deficits following parietal damage, along with the observation that damage to the lateral temporal cortex typically disrupts object identification and naming (anosognosia), led neurobiologists Mel Goodale and David Milner to suggest that the dorsal visual stream may be particularly important for using vision to guide movement, whereas the ventral visual stream may be specialized for object identification (see Chapter 3). Endorsing this idea, patients with temporal lobe damage may have difficulty describing the orientation of a mail slot (i.e., vertical or horizontal) but no trouble putting an envelope into it, while patients with parietal damage typically have no trouble naming objects, despite finding it difficult to reach for and grasp them.

In sum, lesion data from human patients support the idea that the parietal cortex is a critical locus for the integration of visual, eye position, and limb position data necessary to produce coordinated movements of the eyes and hands. Note, however, that complex computations like transforming retinal coordinates into object-centered coordinates may not be made explicitly. Because the circuitry that enables complex motor behavior has evolved simply to associate complex inputs with complex outputs on the basis of evolutionary success, neuronal computations such as those underlying coordinate transformations may never be understood explicitly.

Initiation of Movement by the Basal Ganglia

The motor cortex (and for eye movements, the superior colliculus) comprises a more or less hierarchical set of circuits responsible for selecting, planning, and initiating sequences of movements that satisfy goals. At the same time, an important set of subcortical circuits in the **basal ganglia** appears to serve as a **gating** mechanism, inhibiting potential movements until they are fully

■ BOX 5C MOTOR SYSTEMS AND INTERVAL TIMING

In addition to the overall ability of the brain to adjust numerous functions to daily cycles of light and dark, it is essential for humans and other animals to keep time on much shorter scales, allowing them to anticipate predictable events that have biologically important consequences. Interval timing is the ability to keep track of time on the order of seconds to minutes, and nearly all aspects of human behavior require this sort of temporal judgment. Changing lanes on a highway, catching a ball, cooking an omelet, playing a musical instrument, and telling a joke all require accurate tracking of temporal intervals.

The dependency of such behaviors on timing suggests an intimate relationship between the initiation and coordination of action and the sense of time. In fact, interval timing appears to depend on neural circuits involved in the coordination and initiation of action, including the basal ganglia and its inputs from prefrontal cortex, and the cerebellum. For example, lesions of the basal ganglia (the substantia nigra, caudate, and putamen in particular) disrupt the ability of rats to reproduce temporal intervals by pressing a bar. Further, patients with damage to the basal ganglia (e.g., in Huntington's or Parkinson's disease) show increased variability in timing tasks in both millisecond and second ranges. Endorsing a role for basal ganglia function in interval timing is the observation that dopaminergic drugs systematically speed up or slow down the sense of the passage of time, as revealed by the behavior of humans or rats instructed to reproduce elapsed temporal intervals. Other brain regions involved in motor coordination also appear to be involved in timing. Patients with cerebellar damage perform various time production and discrimination tasks poorly when they receive no feedback about the accuracy of their responses.

The close link between timing and motor behavior is also evident in the buildup of activity in neurons in the lateral intraparietal area (LIP) when monkeys plan a saccadic eye movement at a specific time. LIP neurons typically ramp up their activity in anticipation of movement initiation, reaching a peak just at move-

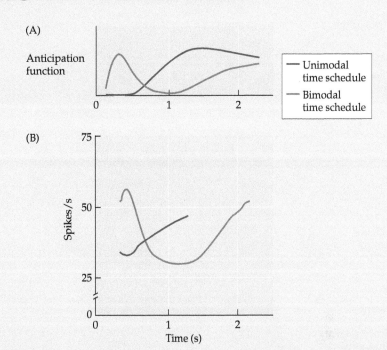

(A) Anticipation function

— Unimodal time schedule
— Bimodal time schedule

(B)

Timing signals in evolving motor commands. Monkeys waited for a "go" cue to initiate a saccadic eye movement to a target to receive a juice reward. In separate blocks of trials, the "go" signal was either unimodally distributed or bimodally distributed in time. (A) Behavioral anticipation functions computed from reaction times for the unimodal (purple) and the bimodal (red) time schedule, demonstrating that monkeys had an internal sense of when movements were most likely to be requested. (B) Average neural activity recorded during waiting period for the "go" signal under the bimodal (red) and the unimodal (purple) time schedule. (After Janssen and Shadlen 2005.)

ment onset (Figure A). When monkeys are confronted with different temporal dependencies, or hazard rates, between the onset of cues specifying where and when to move, the buildup of activity in LIP neurons anticipates the "go" cue, thus betraying the monkey's sense of elapsing time (Figure B). Such signals may be critical for initiating ballistic movements under time pressure—whether catching an insect to eat, swinging at a 90-mile-per-hour fastball, or flatpicking a guitar. Together, the behavioral and neurobiological evidence suggests that motor systems take advantage of the temporal structure of the environment to anticipate, initiate, and coordinate behavior and, further, that such processes may be responsible for our own subjective sense of time.

References

Behusi, C. V. and W. H. Meck (2005) What makes us tick? Functional and neural mechanisms of interval timing. *Nat. Rev. Neurosci.* 6: 755–765.

Ivry, R. B. (1996) The representation of temporal information in perception and motor control. *Curr. Opin. Neurobiol.* 6: 851–857.

Janssen, P. and M. N. Shadlen (2005) A representation of the hazard rate of elapsed time in macaque area LIP. *Nat. Neurosci.* 8: 235–251.

Jazayeri, M. and M. N. Shadlen (2010) Temporal context calibrates interval timing. *Nat. Neurosci.* 13: 1020–1026.

appropriate for the circumstances in which they are to be executed. By helping to coordinate movement timing, the basal ganglia also appear to play an important role in the subjective sense of time (Box 5C).

(A)

Cerebrum

Motor cortex

VA/VL complex of thalamus

Striatum { Caudate nucleus, Putamen }

Globus pallidus, external and internal segments

Subthalamic nuclei

Midbrain

Substantia nigra pars compacta

Substantia nigra pars reticulata

(B)

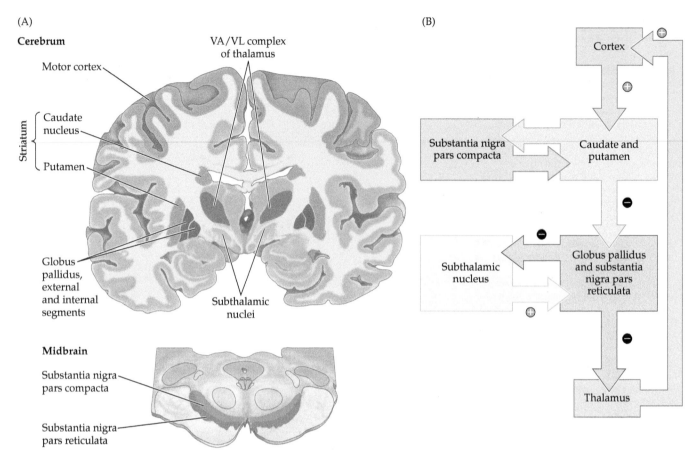

Figure 5.21 **The basal ganglia loop that starts and stops movements** (A) Coronal section through the human forebrain showing the principal components of the basal ganglia. The caudate and putamen (orange) are the zones receiving the main inputs to the basal ganglia. The globus pallidus (purple) provides the principal output, which projects to the ventral anterior and ventrolateral (VA/VL) nuclear complex of the thalamus, which in turn projects to the motor cortex. The substantia nigra pars reticulata in the midbrain serves as the output nucleus for the basal ganglia circuits controlling eye movements. (B) Pro-jections from the cortex excite neurons in the caudate and putamen, which then inhibit neurons in the globus pallidus and substantia nigra pars reticulata. This effect sup-presses tonic inhibition of the thalamus by the globus pallidus, thereby further exciting the cortex. The substantia nigra pars compacta provides modulatory dopaminergic inputs to the basal ganglia, and a circuit through the subthalamic nucleus serves a secondary role in releasing movement.

The basal ganglia are made up of three principal nuclei: the **caudate** and **putamen** (known collectively as the **striatum**), and the **globus pallidus** (Figure 5.21A). In addition, two other nuclei—the subthalamic nucleus and the substantia nigra pars compacta—make important contributions to basal ganglia function. Nearly all cortical areas project to the basal ganglia, principally through the caudate and putamen. The globus pallidus is the output nucleus of the basal ganglia and modulates the activity of cortical neurons via a relay through the thalamus. Activation of the caudate and putamen inhibits the globus pallidus, thereby releasing the thalamus and its cortical targets from tonic inhibition (Figure 5.21B). The net effect of basal ganglia activation is thus excitation of cortical neurons. The balance of excitatory and inhibitory effects of the basal ganglia releases and coordinates desired movements. Circuits projecting through the caudate to the **substantia nigra pars reticulata (SNr)** and on to the superior colliculus serve a similar braking function for saccades.

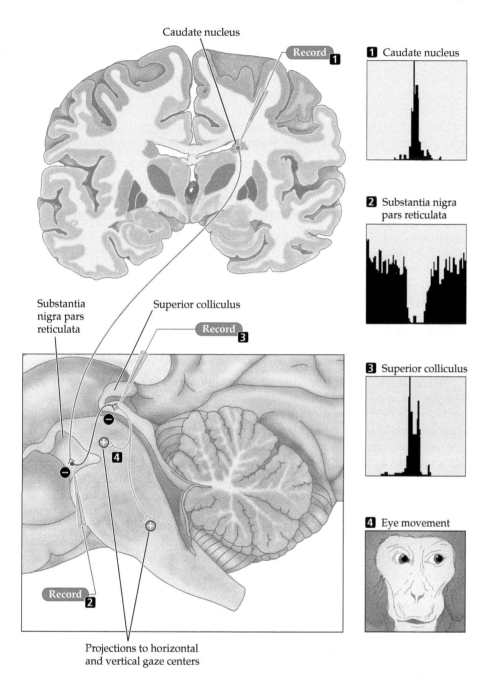

1 Caudate nucleus

2 Substantia nigra pars reticulata

3 Superior colliculus

4 Eye movement

Caudate nucleus

Record **1**

Substantia nigra pars reticulata

Superior colliculus

Record **3**

Record **2**

Projections to horizontal and vertical gaze centers

Figure 5.22 **The superior colliculus–basal ganglia relationship** Neurons in the caudate nucleus fire bursts of action potentials just before eye movement initiation (1). Immediately thereafter, neurons in the substantia nigra pars reticulata shut down (2), resulting in a burst of action potentials in the superior colliculus (3) and the production of an eye movement (4). (After Hikosaka and Wurtz 1989.)

The role of the basal ganglia in movement inhibition and initiation has been examined directly in monkeys trained to make eye movements to visible and remembered targets while recording from neurons in the SNr, the analogue of the globus pallidus output circuit for eye movements. In one study, SNr neurons fired tonically until just before saccade onset, when they abruptly ceased firing for the duration of the movement (Figure 5.22). At about the same time, neurons in the superior colliculus associated with the saccade began firing action potentials.

When the superior colliculus is released from tonic inhibition by injection of the GABA agonist muscimol into the SNr, monkeys cannot suppress unwanted saccades. These results indicate that one important function of the basal ganglia is to inhibit undesired movements and permit desired ones. More recent work, however, has suggested that this "braking function" is not all or none. When the rewards delivered for successful saccade performance are varied, neurons in the caudate nucleus show graded changes in firing rate that correspond to reward size. Similar reward-dependent modulations are apparent in the firing rates of SNr neurons. Thus, graded changes in the net activation of basal ganglia circuits may help ensure that biologically valuable movements are produced.

The importance of the basal ganglia for motor control and initiation is vividly evident in two relatively common neurological disorders: Parkinson's disease and Huntington's disease. In **Parkinson's disease**, the selective death of neurons in the substantia nigra pars compacta that use the neurotransmitter dopamine increases the excitatory tone of the direct pathway through the basal ganglia. Patients with Parkinson's show a marked disruption in the ability to initiate voluntary movement. In addition to the tremor at rest that is characteristic of this disease, these patients have difficulty generating purposeful movements and often show a slow, shuffling gait as a result. By contrast, when their movements are guided by more immediate sensory stimuli, such as marks on the floor that the patient is asked to step over, gait appears relatively normal. A primary treatment for Parkinson's disease remains supplementation of dopamine levels with L-dopa, a synthetic precursor to dopamine. This augmentation of dopamine function helps restore the ability of the basal ganglia to release tonic inhibition from the thalamus, thereby enhancing motor cortex excitability and improving motor function. Chronic treatment with the drug, however, can lead to cognitive problems.

In contrast to Parkinson's disease, **Huntington's disease** involves hereditary atrophy of the caudate nucleus. Patients with Huntington's typically have signs and symptoms that are the opposite of those seen in Parkinson's disease. They exhibit **choreiform** (dancelike) **movements** of the trunk and extremities that they are unable to control. They also suffer a gradual onset of psychotic thought patterns and eventually dementia. We can understand these symptoms by considering the net inhibitory effect of caudate projections through the indirect pathway described already. Damage to this pathway releases potential movements from inhibition, thus resulting in the production of unwanted actions.

Another basal ganglia syndrome, **hemiballismus**, ensues from unilateral damage to the subthalamic nucleus. This neurological insult causes choreiform movements of the contralateral limbs resembling those in Huntington's disease. Thus, electrophysiological, pharmacological, and neurological patient data all support the idea that a main function of the basal ganglia is to gate the production of movements directed to specific goals.

Basal Ganglia and Cognition

The motor deficits associated with basal ganglia dysfunction, tragically evident in Parkinson's and Huntington's diseases, lead inexorably to the conclusion that these structures play a critical role in gating movement. Some of the problems with these diseases and their treatment, however, seem explicitly cognitive, and recent neurophysiological and neuroimaging findings appear to confirm this implication. Anatomical studies have also demonstrated the existence of several nonmotor pathways through the basal ganglia, including a limbic or emotional channel and an associative or cognitive channel (Figure 5.23).

These separate pathways appear to serve distinct but related functions in emotion and cognition, and these roles are especially prominent in humans and other primates. According to this view, the same principles governing movement disinhibition in the motor pathway apply to emotional or cognitive processing in the limbic and associative channels. Each channel thus comprises a feedback loop beginning in the cortex, projecting through the basal ganglia, and ultimately providing excitatory feedback to the cortex. In this model, cortical

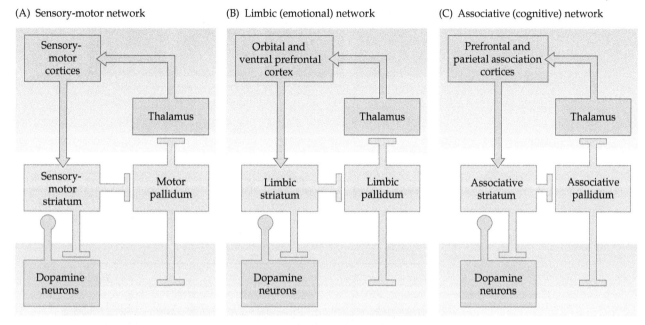

Figure 5.23   The motor model of basal ganglia contributions to emotion and cognition (A) The basal ganglia influence movement via a sensory-motor network from the cortex, through the basal ganglia and thalamus, and back to the cortex. This network disinhibits desired movements. (B) The basal ganglia contribute to emotional function via an analogous limbic network, beginning in orbital and ventral prefrontal cortex, projecting through the ventral or limbic striatum, through the thalamus, and back to the cortex. (C) The basal ganglia may contribute to cognitive function via a similar associative feedback loop between association cortex and the basal ganglia. The action of all three networks is enhanced by projections from midbrain dopamine neurons. (After Yin and Knowlton 2006.)

inputs to the basal ganglia serve as a source of potential variability in behavior, and the basal ganglia themselves contribute to the selection of behavior on the basis of prior outcomes.

This framework helps explain some of the nonmotor consequences of basal ganglia dysfunction. For example, animals with lesions of the basal ganglia, particularly the caudate and putamen, can perform movements but cannot perform or learn new actions to acquire rewards or avoid punishments. Patients with Parkinson's disease, who exhibit diminished basal ganglia functioning because of dopaminergic dysfunction, also show impairments in probabilistic classification tasks that require subjects to make predictions based on a series of cues. Similar impairments in learning and memory follow damage to prefrontal regions projecting to the associative basal ganglia pathway, and, as noted, one of the hallmarks of Huntington's disease is psychotic thought processes. The ability to produce learned sequences of movements is also disrupted in patients with damage to the basal ganglia, and this disruption is evident in both Parkinson's disease and Huntington's disease.

Neuroimaging studies have confirmed that the basal ganglia are activated when human subjects learn new movement sequences. In one typical study, subjects were asked to perform a task in which they were required to manipulate a joystick with the right hand (**Figure 5.24A**). During some blocks of trials, the mapping between the joystick movement and the direction of movement of a target cursor on a computer screen was shifted by 90 degrees. When brain activity was compared between blocks of trials requiring such motor

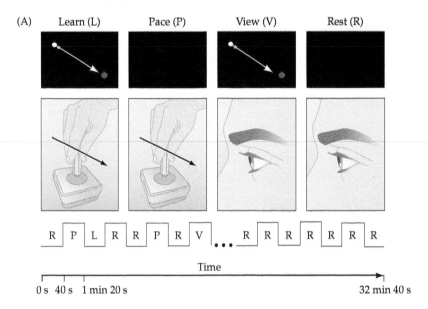

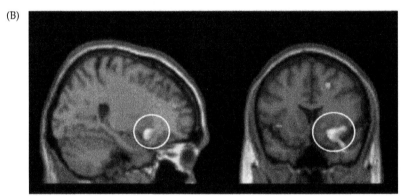

Figure 5.24 The contribution of the basal ganglia to motor learning (A) Human subjects grasped a joystick to move a cursor on a computer screen. In some blocks of trials ("Learn"), the direction of cursor movement and the direction of joystick movement were offset by 90 degrees. In other blocks of trials, subjects simply moved the cursor without feedback ("Pace"), watched the cursor move by itself ("View"), or rested ("Rest"). **(B)** Functional MRI activation during motor learning was strongest in the putamen (circled). (After Graydon et al. 2005.)

adaptation and blocks of trials in which movements were produced without visual feedback, the putamen was selectively activated (Figure 5.24B). These observations, and others like them, endorse the idea that the basal ganglia play a broad role in linking sensory events and motor actions, while also helping to suppress undesirable movements and to initiate movements that satisfy goals.

Neurophysiological studies in animals, as well as neuroimaging in humans, have also demonstrated that basal ganglia neurons are modulated by the anticipation of reward, thus linking this network to the adaptive modification of behavior based on outcomes—the computational basis of reinforcement learning (see Chapters 10 and 14). Such studies also suggest that addictive behavior could reflect the "hijacking" of this basal ganglia system by chemicals that activate receptors associated with reward. Specifically, cue-induced craving could ensue from the unconscious association of environmental cues present during drug consumption with pathological reward modulation of basal ganglia cognitive

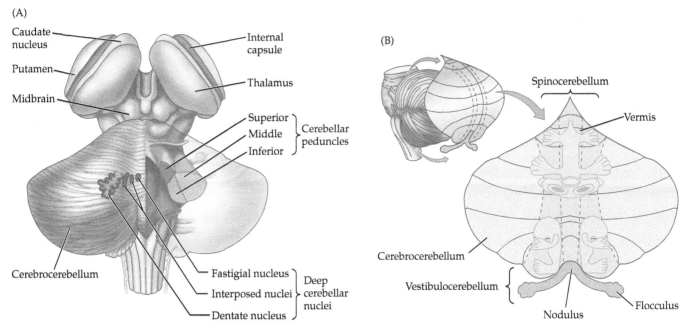

Figure 5.25 Organization of the cerebellum (A) The cerebellum consists of an outer cortex of neurons, deep nuclei, and large fiber tracts, known as *peduncles*, coursing in and out. Inputs to the cerebellum arrive via the middle and superior cerebellar peduncles, and the deep nuclei project out of the cerebellum via the inferior and superior cerebellar peduncles. **(B)** The cerebellar cortex can be divided into the spinocerebellum, which receives inputs from the spinal cord; the cerebrocerebellum, which receives inputs from the cerebral cortex via the pons; and the vestibulocerebellum, consisting of the flocculus and nodulus, which receives inputs from the vestibular nuclei. The spinocerebellum is organized topographically according to inputs from spinal cord neurons carrying proprioceptive information. In contrast with upper motor neurons of the cortex and basal ganglia, cerebellar circuits mediate movements of the ipsilateral musculature.

pattern generators. In any event, these and other studies hint at the powerful influence of the basal ganglia on a wide range of cognitive behavior.

Error Correction and Motor Coordination by the Cerebellum

Circuits within the brainstem help coordinate lower-level reflex circuits in the spinal cord and brainstem motor nuclei to make the anticipatory postural adjustments needed to accommodate movements, correct posture for ongoing changes in balance, and coordinate more complex multijoint movements. Supplementing the brainstem circuits that mediate these aspects of motor coordination, another specialized set of neural circuitry has evolved to provide additional control of sensory-motor interactions. The key component at the center of this circuitry is the **cerebellum**, a large, foliated structure that sits atop the pons in the brainstem (Figure 5.25). The cerebellum is responsible for online error corrections necessary to produce smoothly coordinated, skilled movements.

Exquisitely organized circuits of specialized neurons within the cerebellar cortex (Figure 5.26A) appear to compute the net error between ongoing motor commands issued by the motor cortex and the actual movements being produced. These error signals are relayed back to the frontal and parietal cortices via projections from the dentate nucleus (the deep nuclear output structure for

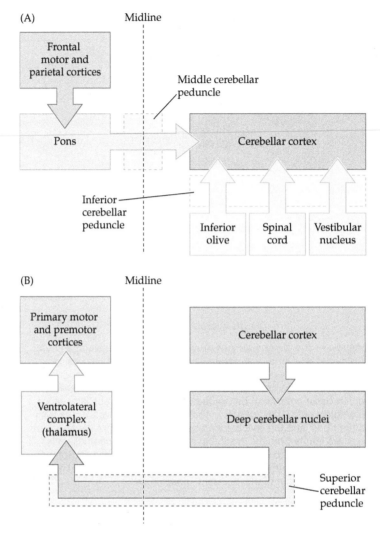

Figure 5.26 Cerebellar inputs and outputs These block diagrams illustrate the inputs (A) and major outputs (B) of the cerebellum.

the cerebrocerebellum) to the ventrolateral complex of the thalamus (**Figure 5.26B**). As a result, damage to the cerebellum causes an inability to perform smooth movements.

Lesions of the medial cerebellar vermis result in a condition known as *truncal ataxia* (uncoordinated, disorganized movement), which is characterized by a wide-based, unsteady gait similar to that of someone who has had too much alcohol to drink. Damage to the lateral cerebellum, on the other hand, disrupts the sensory coordination of limb movements and is known as *appendicular ataxia*. A useful clinical test of appendicular ataxia requires patients to point from their nose to the clinician's finger and back again (**Figure 5.27**). Patients with damage to the ipsilateral cerebellum show halting, uncoordinated movements of the hand and arm; this deficit is called **intention tremor** because it is evident only during voluntary movements. The jerky movements of appendicular ataxia appear to result from disruptions in the normal smooth compensation for ongoing errors in finger trajectory.

The role of the cerebellum in correcting ongoing errors in order to coordinate smooth movement extends to correcting errors during motor learning. In short,

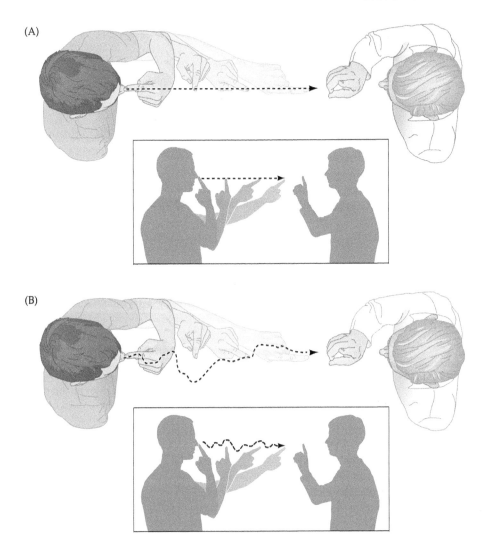

(A)

(B)

Figure 5.27 Cerebellar ataxia Patients are asked to point rapidly from the clinician's finger to their own nose and back again. (A) Normal subjects point smoothly and rapidly from nose to finger and back again. (B) Patients with cerebellar ataxia produce irregular, jerky movements, known as *intention tremor*, when reaching from nose to finger and back again. (After Blumenfeld 2010.)

lesions that damage the cerebellum disrupt the ability to learn new motor skills. Moreover, the cerebellum is activated during motor learning. When subjects are asked to track a target on a computer screen and the target randomly jumps to another position at the end of each trial, motor error during tracking is initially quite large but improves with practice (Figure 5.28). Activation in the cerebellum parallels this change in performance, peaking during initial learning and declining with improvement in performance.

Cerebellar Contributions to Cognitive Behavior

Traditionally, the cerebellum and its canonical circuitry have been considered a strictly motor structure providing error correction during motor acts and motor learning. With the advent of modern neuroimaging, however, it has become increasingly clear that the cerebellum contributes to cognitive processing

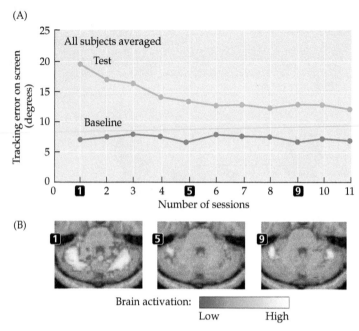

Figure 5.28 Changes in the cerebellum during motor learning (A) Subjects tracked a target on a computer screen using a mouse. During test sessions, the cursor was rotated 120 degrees about the center of the screen, thus requiring motor learning. In baseline sessions, the cursor remained unrotated. Improvements in the average performance of subjects over time in test sessions indicate motor learning. (B) The corresponding brain activation maps show significant activation in test sessions (decreasing from left to right) relative to baseline during learning. Activity in the cerebellum decreased with motor learning. (After Imamizu et al. 2000.)

as well. Portions of the cerebellum are activated during nonmotor learning, attention, timing, and verbal working memory tasks. Furthermore, recent neuropsychological studies of patients with cerebellar damage have reported deficits in speech, learning rates, timing, and working memory. Problems in orienting attention in autistic individuals have also been linked to abnormalities in the cerebellum.

Despite all this evidence, it is not clear how or why the cerebellum participates in cognitive functions. One proposal is that the computational power of the cerebellum as an efficient and accurate error correction device has simply been harnessed to serve cognitive functions that also require error correction (Figure 5.29). This model assumes that the cellular architecture repeated throughout the cerebellum can be used to perform the same computation on any set of inputs. For the motor system, these inputs would arise in the primary and premotor cortices, and the output would be a feedforward prediction of the sensory consequences of the impending movement. For cognitive tasks, the inputs would arise in the prefrontal cortex and specify intended cognitive operations, and the output would be the predicted cognitive consequences of the operation. Such predictions would then be compared against actual cognitive consequences, and the resulting error signals would be used to update both future cognitive operations and the internal models of their outcomes.

Support for this general class of models comes from the observation that, in addition to the heavy inputs from the motor and premotor cortices, the prefrontal cortex has massive connections to the cerebellum via the pontine nuclei. In fact, prefrontal inputs to the cerebellum in humans are at least as prominent as inputs from motor and premotor cortex. Moreover, prefrontal

(A)

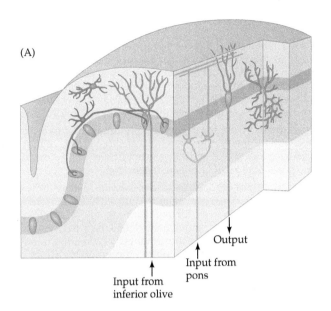

Output

Input from pons

Input from inferior olive

Figure 5.29 **Model of cerebellar contributions to cognition** (A) The canonical circuitry of the cerebellar cortex. Inputs to the cerebellar cortex arrive from the pons and inferior olive, a brainstem relay nucleus. (B) Model of cerebellar feedforward simulation and error correction of motor commands. The cerebellum computes the predicted sensory consequences of movement. The error between the predicted and actual consequences of movement is then fed back into the cerebellum to update future predictions. (C) The same model applied to cognitive processing. The cerebellum computes the predicted cognitive consequences of cognitive operations, and the error between predicted and actual cognitive outcomes is used to refine future predictions. (After Ramnani 2006.)

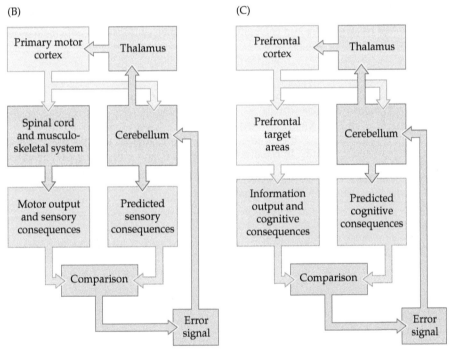

inputs to the cerebellum are more developed in humans than in non-human primates, and these differences parallel differences in cognitive complexity across species (see Chapter 15). Cognitive operations instantiated in prefrontal circuits feeding to the cerebellum might rely on the highly stereotyped cellular architecture of the cerebellum to provide fast, accurate, and automatic "simulations" of the output of these cognitive operations. This conjecture is supported by the observation that prefrontal circuits show reduced activation during the course of learning, whereas cerebellar circuits become more active. The cerebellum may thus provide another example in which neural circuitry originally adapted to one purpose is co-opted for another; that is, the circuitry for motor control (see Figure 5.29B) is co-opted for use in cognitive information processing (see Figure 5.29C).

Summary

1. Motor control is hierarchical. Lower motor neurons in the spinal cord and brainstem are the final common pathway for the motor commands that determine behaviors arising from skeletal muscle movements, and they are thus the effectors for many cognitive processes. Upper motor neurons in the primary motor cortex and cortical premotor areas issue motor commands that activate local circuits and lower motor neuron pools to achieve more specific behavioral goals.

2. Descending pathways from the motor and premotor cortices are important in planning and initiating voluntary, goal-directed sequences of movement, especially for learned motor skills. Of special relevance here, these circuits are sensitive to motivational goals that guide movement selection.

3. The motor and premotor cortices are under the modulatory influence of the basal ganglia and cerebellum. The basal ganglia control the initiation and stopping of movements and contribute to motor skill learning, the production of movement sequences, and the selection of movements that satisfy behavioral goals. The cerebellum acts further to coordinate movements by correcting unanticipated errors in ongoing motor processing in the motor and premotor cortices.

4. Acting together, the various motor circuits mediate production of the complex intrinsic and learned sequences of movement that are characteristic of human motor behaviors that express cognitive goals.

5. Damage to any of these motor control circuits results in specific disruptions in movement planning, initiation, or coordination. Damage to some of these circuits—the basal ganglia and cerebellum in particular—also causes deficits in a variety of cognitive functions.

Go to the **COMPANION WEBSITE**

sites.sinauer.com/cogneuro2e
for quizzes, animations, flashcards,
and other study resources.

Additional Reading

Reviews

ANDERSEN, R. A. AND H. CUI (2009) Intention, action planning, and decision making in parietal-frontal circuits. *Neuron* 63: 568–583.

BURKE, R. E. (1981) Motor units: Anatomy, physiology, and functional organization. In *Handbook of Physiology*, Section 1: *The Nervous System*, Vol. 2, Part 1, V. B. Brooks (ed.). Bethesda, MD: American Physiological Society, pp. 345–422.

COHEN, Y. E. AND R. A. ANDERSEN (2002) A common reference frame for movement plans in the posterior parietal cortex. *Nat. Rev. Neurosci.* 3: 553–562.

DUM, R. P. AND P. L. STRICK (2002) Motor areas in the frontal lobe of the primate. *Physiol. Behav.* 77: 677–682.

FIEZ, J. A. (1996) Cerebellar contributions to cognition. *Neuron* 16: 13–15.

GAHERY, Y. AND J. MASSION (1981) Coordination between posture and movement. *Trends Neurosci.* 4: 199–202.

GEORGOPOULOS, A. P., M. TAIRA AND A. LUKASHIN (1993) Cognitive neurophysiology of the motor cortex. *Science* 260: 47–52.

GRILLNER, S. AND P. WALLEN (1985) Central pattern generators for locomotion, with special reference to vertebrates. *Annu. Rev. Neurosci.* 8: 233–261.

HENNEMAN, E. AND L. M. MENDELL (1981) Functional organization of the motoneuron pool and its inputs. In *Handbook of Physiology*, Section 1: *The Nervous System*. Vol. 2, Part 1, V. B. Brooks (ed.). Bethesda, MD: American Physiological Society, pp. 423–507.

HIKOSAKA, O. (1991) Basal ganglia: Possible role in motor coordination and learning. *Curr. Opin. Neurobiol.* 1: 635–653.

PEARSON, K. (1976) The control of walking. *Sci. Am.* 235 (December): 72–86.

PESARAN, B. AND J. A. MOVSHON (2008) What to do or how to do it? *Neuron* 58: 301–303.

RAMNANI, N. (2006) The primate corticocerebellar system: Anatomy and function. *Nat. Rev. Neurosci.* 7: 511–522.

WOLPERT, D. M., J. DIEDRICHSEN AND J. R. FLANAGAN (2011) Principles of sensorimotor learning. *Nat. Rev. Neurosci.* 12: 739–751.

WOLPERT, D. M. AND M. S. LANDY (2012) Motor control is decision-making. *Curr. Opin. Neurobiol.*, in press.

YIN, H. H. AND B. J. KNOWLTON (2006) The role of the basal ganglia in habit formation. *Nat. Rev. Neurosci.* 7: 565–576.

Important Original Papers

BURKE, R. E., D. N. LEVINE, M. SALCMAN AND P. TSAIRES (1974) Motor units in cat soleus muscle: Physiological, histochemical, and morphological characteristics. *J. Physiol.* (Lond.) 238: 503–514.

CHANG, S. W. C., C. PAPADIMITRIOU AND L. H. SNYDER (2009) Using a compound gain field to compute a reach plan. *Neuron* 64: 744–755.

COSTA, M. AND S. J. H. BROOKES (1994) The enteric nervous system. *Am. J. Gastroenterol.* 89: S129–S137.

EVARTS, E. V. (1981) Functional studies of the motor cortex. In *The Organization of the Cerebral Cortex*, F. O. Schmitt, F. G. Worden, G. Adelman and S. G. Dennis (eds.). Cambridge, MA: MIT Press, pp. 199–236.

FETZ, E. E. AND P. D. CHENEY (1978) Muscle fields of primate corticomotoneuronal cells. *J. Physiol.* (Paris) 74: 239–245.

GEORGOPOLOUS, A. P., A. B. SCHWARTZ AND R. E. KETTNER (1986) Neuronal population coding of movement direction. *Science* 233: 1416–1418.

GRAZIANO, M. S., C. C. TAYLOR, T. MOORE AND D. F. COOKE (2002) The cortical control of movement revisited. *Neuron* 36: 349–362.

HENNEMAN, E., E. SOMJEN AND D. O. CARPENTER (1965) Excitability and inhibitability of motoneurons of different sizes. *J. Neurophysiol.* 28: 599–620.

HUNT, C. C. AND S. W. KUFFLER (1951) Stretch receptor discharges during muscle contraction. *J. Physiol.* (Lond.) 113: 298–315.

JANSEN, A. S. P., X. V. NGUYEN, V. KARPITSKIY, T. C. METTENLEITER AND A. D. LOEWY (1995) Central command neurons of the sympathetic nervous system: Basis of the fight or flight response. *Science* 270: 644–646.

LEE, D. L., W. H. ROHRER AND D. L. SPARKS (1988) Population coding of saccadic eye movements by neurons in the superior colliculus. *Nature* 332: 357–360.

LIDDELL, E. G. T. AND C. S. SHERRINGTON (1925) Recruitment and some other factors of reflex inhibition. *Proc. R. Soc. Lond. B* 97: 488–518.

PLATT, M. L. AND P. W. GLIMCHER (1999) Neural correlates of decision variables in parietal cortex. *Nature* 500: 233–235.

RESULAJ, A., R. KIANI, D. M. WOLPERT AND M. N. SHADLEN (2009) Changes of mind in decision-making. *Nature* 461: 263–266.

SELEN, L. P. J., M. N. SHADLEN AND D. M. WOLPERT (2012) Deliberation in the motor system: Reflex gains track evolving evidence leading to a decision. *J. Neurosci.* 32: 2276–2286.

SHADLEN, M. N. AND W. T. NEWSOME (1996) Motion perception: Seeing and deciding. *Proc. Natl. Acad. Sci. USA* 53: 625–633.

TANJI, J. AND K. SHIMA (1994) Role for supplementary motor area cells in planning several movements ahead. *Nature* 371: 413–416.

WALMSLEY, B., J. A. HODGSON AND R. E. BURKE (1978) Forces produced by medial gastrocnemius and soleus muscles during locomotion in freely moving cats. *J. Neurophysiol.* 41: 1203–1215.

WUNDERLICH, K., A. RANGEL AND J. P. O'DOHERTY (2009) Neural computations underlying action-based decision making in the human brain. *PNAS* 106: 17199–17204.

Books

ASANUMA, H. (1989) *The Motor Cortex.* New York: Raven.

BLESSING, W. W. (1997) *The Lower Brainstem and Bodily Homeostasis.* New York: Oxford University Press.

BRODAL, A. (1981) *Neurological Anatomy in Relation to Clinical Medicine,* 3rd Ed. New York: Oxford University Press.

GABELLA, G. (1976) *Structure of the Autonomic Nervous System.* London: Chapman and Hall.

GLIMCHER, P. W. (2005) *Decision, Uncertainty, and the Brain: The Science of Neuroeconomics.* Cambridge, MA: MIT Press/Bradford.

PENFIELD, W. AND T. RASMUSSEN (1950) *The Cerebral Cortex of Man: A Clinical Study of Localization of Function.* New York: Macmillan.

PURVES, D. AND 5 OTHERS (2012) *Neuroscience,* 5th Ed. Sunderland, MA: Sinauer.

SHERRINGTON, C. (1947) *The Integrative Action of the Nervous System,* 2nd Ed. New Haven, CT: Yale University Press.

6

Attention and Its Effects on Stimulus Processing

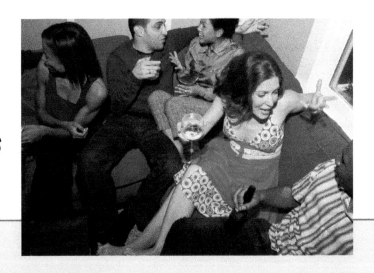

INTRODUCTION

During every waking moment, humans and other animals are bombarded with stimuli from multiple sensory modalities. At the same time, we are inundated by information from non-sensory sources, including ongoing emotions, memories, and trains of thought that arise as problems are encountered, solutions imagined, and decisions made. To navigate successfully in the real world, the neural resources available in a brain with finite processing capabilities must be efficiently directed to the aspects of this overwhelming information load that are likely to matter most from moment to moment. Attention is the name given to this broad cognitive function, which plays a fundamental role in virtually everything we do.

Before the development of modern methods for directly measuring brain activity, studies of attention were limited largely to the behavioral measures traditionally used in cognitive psychology. Nonetheless, by manipulating aspects of stimulus presentation and task instructions and then measuring behavioral response characteristics such as reaction time and accuracy, researchers were able to learn a great deal about attentional processing and the limits of attentional capacity, leading to the development of theoretical models of attention that remain influential today. Much additional insight about attentional mechanisms has been gained over the last few decades using modern methods of cognitive neuroscience, including the ability to directly assess the influence of attention on stimulus processing by measuring brain activity during attentional tasks.

This chapter begins with an overview of psychological studies of attentional phenomena and the cognitive models that have been derived from them, focusing on the key findings and conclusions about the influence of attention on stimulus processing that have been based on behavioral measures. It then describes studies that have used measures of neural activity to more directly assess the influence of attention on stimulus processing.

■ INTRODUCTORY BOX THE COCKTAIL PARTY EFFECT

A classic example of attention in the auditory modality experienced in everyday life is known as the cocktail party effect. This term refers to the phenomenon in which multiple conversations and other sounds are occurring simultaneously (such as at a cocktail party), yet a listener can selectively focus on one voice or conversation and effectively tune out the others. The cocktail party effect shows that even though multiple auditory stimulus streams enter the ears and nervous system concurrently, listeners can focus on and follow one particular stream. Moreover, assuming we stay focused, it is the attended stream that enters conscious awareness and that we can later remember. How is all this accomplished?

A particularly influential experiment that explored auditory attention in the face of competing streams was carried out by psychologist Colin Cherry in 1953 (see figure). In this study, two different streams of auditory information (two voices, each speaking a different passage) were presented to the left and right ears, respectively. The subject was instructed to attend to one of these inputs, immediately repeating its content (a task called *shadowing*). Such shadowing is demanding, requiring that subjects attend closely to one input while ignoring the other.

After the subjects had performed this task, Cherry tested them on their ability to report the content of the two vocal inputs. He found that they could accurately report the content of the attended stream, but very little from the unattended one. Indeed, the main feature of the unattended stream that most subjects could accurately report was whether the speaker was male or female. This sort of observation was interpreted as indicating that unattended inputs are filtered out at low levels of perceptual processing on the basis of very basic physical characteristics. Moreover, the study made clear that subjects cannot attend effectively to two input streams at the same time, illustrating a fundamental limitation of attentional processing capacity.

Studies that followed, however, showed that things are not so simple. For instance, a study a few years later showed that subjects tended to notice

An auditory shadowing study of selective attention. Subjects were presented with two verbal streams simultaneously—one to each ear—and asked to verbally shadow (i.e., immediately repeat) one of the streams. When tested later, they could accurately report the content of the attended stream but could report little of the unattended one. (Depiction of experiment from Cherry 1953.)

when their name was mentioned in an unattended auditory stream. Indeed, most of us have had the experience of attending to one conversation while effectively tuning out other simultaneous conversations, and suddenly noticing our name (or another personally important word or phrase, such as our hometown) being mentioned in one of those other conversations. Such observations indicate that at least some information in an unattended stream is being processed up to the level of semantic meaning, and is not being completely filtered out at a lower level.

From a more general standpoint, the ability to selectively focus attention on a single stream of sensory input varies across individuals. Some students, for example, are able to focus effectively on reading or on other types of study material regardless of what else is going on around them, whereas others find it

difficult to concentrate in noisy environments. Moreover, impairment of the ability to selectively focus attention is one of the major symptoms in pathological states such as schizophrenia and attention deficit hyperactivity disorder (ADHD). Individuals with these disorders have difficulty maintaining attentional focus on a particular stimulus input channel or specific task, and tend to be easily distracted by competing stimulation.

References

CHERRY, E. C. (1953) Some experiments on the recognition of speech, with one and with two ears. *J. Acoust. Soc. Am.* 25: 975–979.

MORAY, N. (1959) Attention in dichotic listening: Affective cues and the influence of instructions. *Q. J. Exp. Psychol.* 5: 56–60.

The Concept of Attention

The word **attention** is used in several ways in everyday discourse, as well as more formally in cognitive psychology and cognitive neuroscience. To complicate matters further, *attention* must be distinguished from other neuroscientific terms that are related to it but are not synonymous. A key distinction is the relationship of attention and arousal.

Global states, arousal, and attention

From a neural standpoint, the term **arousal** describes a global state of the brain. The broadest categorization of arousal is whether an individual is awake or asleep, although it may be more accurate to view neural arousal as falling along a continuum whose extremes are deep sleep and full wakefulness. Regardless, an individual who is asleep is not only less aroused than someone who is awake, but is obviously also much less attentive and reactive to external stimuli and events.

Even individuals who are awake, however, can clearly be operating at different levels of arousal or alertness. Describing someone as *alert* typically means that the person is fully awake, generally vigilant, and attending intently to the local environment. In contrast, people who are drowsy are less attentive to the events going on around them. This assessment is both intuitively clear and readily supported by behavioral testing data, which show slowed reaction times and reduced performance accuracy in cognitive tasks when people are drowsy.

The selective nature of attention

A key distinction between arousal and attention is that attention can be, and typically is, selectively focused. *Selective attention* refers to the allocation of processing resources to the analysis of certain stimuli or aspects of the environment, generally at the expense of resources allocated to other concurrent stimuli or aspects. Most research into the cognitive psychology and cognitive neuroscience of attention has been devoted to the study of selective attention, typically in the context of sensory processing.

A particularly widely studied example of selective attention in audition is the *cocktail party effect* (see Introductory Box), in which a listener can selectively focus on one voice or conversation and effectively tune out other simultaneously occurring ones. In vision, a classic example of selective attention is **visual spatial attention** (Figure 6.1), a phenomenon described in studies carried out by the German physicist and vision scientist Hermann von Helmholtz at the end of the nineteenth century. When Helmholtz briefly flashed arrays of letters on a screen and asked subjects to report the letter appearing at a particular location, he observed that if they steadily fixated their gaze on a particular point in the visual field but directed their **covert attention** to another region of the field (i.e., without moving the eyes), then the stimuli presented in the attended location could be reported much better than stimuli in the rest of the field. Such covert attention in vision is in contrast to **overt attention**, in which eye gaze is explicitly directed to a visual stimulus or location of interest.

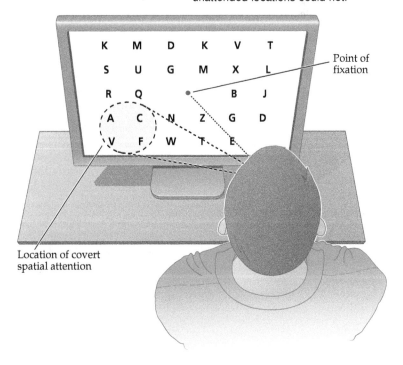

Figure 6.1 Studying visual spatial attention Selective attention to a subset of a visual scene enhances the processing of information from the attended portion at the expense of processing information from the rest of the scene. In the original experiment by Hermann von Helmholtz, subjects were briefly presented with an array of letters and asked afterward to recall the letters they had seen. Helmholtz observed that if a subject was asked to covertly attend to a certain area of the visual field away from fixation, then the items in the attended portion of the letter array could be accurately reported, whereas items in unattended locations could not.

Point of fixation

Location of covert spatial attention

Such findings have established that attention directed toward particular aspects of the environment generally leads to improved processing of the attended stimuli, but typically at the expense of the processing of other simultaneously presented information.

Behavioral Studies of Attention Capacity and Selection

As mentioned in Chapter 1, psychology in the first half of the twentieth century was dominated by the behaviorist approach. By the 1950s, however, an information-processing approach had taken root, providing a framework that allowed researchers to think of attention as adaptively maximizing the utility of limited processing resources. This way of thinking led to a series of experiments that investigated attentional capacity and its limits by testing the comprehension or retention of information by subjects placed in attentionally demanding situations in which there were competing information streams.

The level at which selection occurs

A major goal of these behavioral studies of information processing was to gain more insight into the stage or stages at which attention affects the processing of sensory input. During the development of this research, models of attention became divided into those proposing early levels of attentional selection and those proposing later levels. Models of **early selection** postulated that there is a low-level gating mechanism that can filter out or attenuate irrelevant information before the completion of sensory and perceptual analysis. In contrast, theories of **late selection**, at least the strong versions of such models, proposed that all stimuli are processed through the completion of sensory and perceptual processing before any selection occurs.

In the late 1950s, in an important step for the development of early-selection theories, psychologist Donald Broadbent published a paper asserting that attentional selection can occur very early in processing. More specifically, he proposed that sensory input can be gated at early sensory processing stages on the basis of fundamental physical characteristics of the stimuli (e.g., location in space, color, pitch, etc.), thereby determining which information proceeds to higher levels of analysis (Figure 6.2A).

The need to modify this simple gating model became apparent shortly thereafter because, as already mentioned, some information in an unattended auditory input channel, such as one's name, can reach the level of semantic analysis (see Introductory Box). Such findings led researchers in the early 1960s to propose a late-selection model, in which attentional filtering occurs relatively late in stimulus processing. According to such theories, all sensory stimuli are fully processed, in terms of both their physical characteristics and their possible higher-level meaning. In this view, it was not until after this higher-level processing was complete that attention exerted its influence and determined which input information entered consciousness or influenced behavior.

In the 1960s, psychologist Anne Treisman proposed another solution. She altered Broadbent's concept of an early-stage gate that is simply open or closed to be a more adaptable early-filtering system that could attenuate the inputs from concurrent sensory channels in a flexible manner (Figure 6.2B). In this model, some unattended semantic information reaches higher levels, although it might be substantially attenuated. Accordingly, in an unattended channel, only highly salient information (e.g., one's own name) would exceed the threshold to be selected, reach conscious awareness, and be reportable by the individual.

In the 1970s, other researchers concluded that an even better model to explain the various findings was one in which incoming information could be filtered at various levels of processing, depending on the needs for a particular task

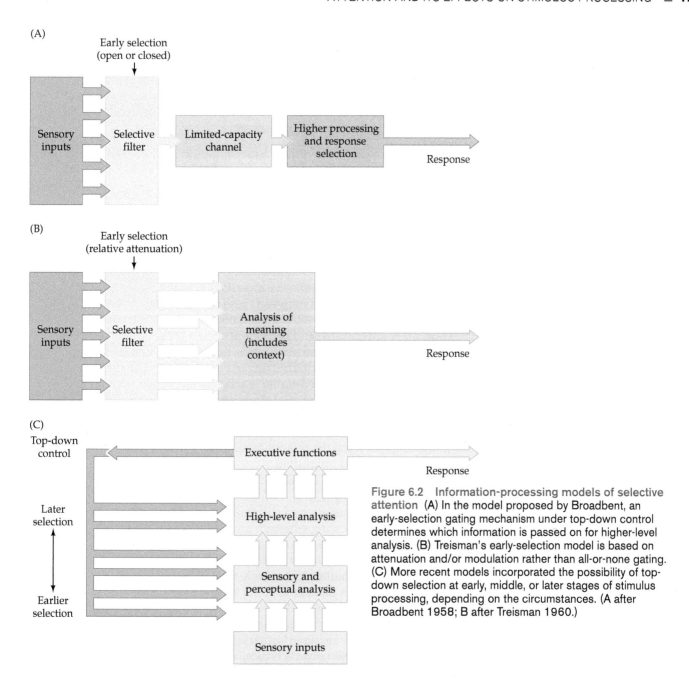

Figure 6.2 **Information-processing models of selective attention** (A) In the model proposed by Broadbent, an early-selection gating mechanism under top-down control determines which information is passed on for higher-level analysis. (B) Treisman's early-selection model is based on attenuation and/or modulation rather than all-or-none gating. (C) More recent models incorporated the possibility of top-down selection at early, middle, or later stages of stimulus processing, depending on the circumstances. (A after Broadbent 1958; B after Treisman 1960.)

or set of circumstances (Figure 6.2C). These models proposed that in some situations sensory information might be filtered out or selected at relatively early processing stages according to basic physical characteristics such as color or pitch. Under other circumstances, however, more complex aspects of the information in a stimulus, such as its semantic content, would be required to make the selection, which would then occur at a later stage. Forms of these hierarchical models, in which attention can influence processing at multiple levels, still hold sway for many attention researchers today.

In most of these psychological theories of attentional function, *early* and *late* have tended to refer to processing stage, with the more basic sensory analyses (e.g., analyses of the physical characteristics of stimuli) presumably being done early in the processing sequence, and more complex analyses (e.g., of stimulus meaning) not occurring until later stages. Some of these psychological theories also suggested a rough mapping of these processing stages onto the brain, with early processing presumably corresponding to basic analyses in the brainstem and lower-level sensory cortices, and late processing occurring in higher-level association cortices. Behavioral testing, however, cannot provide direct evidence for such ideas. The ways in which newer approaches have helped settle these questions about the levels and timing of attentional influence on stimulus processing are taken up later in this chapter.

Endogenously versus exogenously driven selective attention

Most of the behavioral observations described so far in this chapter entail *voluntary* attentional tasks. That is, to follow the instruction of an experimenter or to fulfill an intrinsic desire, subjects consciously direct attention to a particular aspect of the environment, such as to a specific voice or to a particular location in visual space. This type of attention is called **endogenous attention**. In contrast, numerous stimuli arising from events or conditions in our everyday environment attract attention automatically; such attention is called **exogenous attention** (also referred to as **reflexive attention**). A major distinction in attention research has thus been made between these two ways in which processing resources are induced to be directed toward objects or events in the environment.

Thus, more specifically, endogenous attention is the ability to voluntarily direct attention depending on one's goals, expectations, and/or knowledge. A good example is the voluntary directing of visual attention to specific locations in the visual field (as described earlier; see Figure 6.1). In one particularly useful paradigm for studying such spatial attention, subjects receive advance cues on each trial as to where in the visual field a stimulus is most likely to occur. These cuing paradigms, developed by psychologist Michael Posner and colleagues in the late 1970s, enabled the relative facilitation of processing due to attention to be characterized and quantified.

In the standard version of this paradigm, subjects maintain visual fixation on a central point during a series of trials (Figure 6.3A). Each trial begins with a centrally presented cue, such as an arrow pointing to the left or the right, or a letter or word cue, indicating where an upcoming target stimulus is most likely to occur. When the target appears, regardless of whether it occurs in the cued location, the subject must detect it or perform a discrimination task related to it, such as deciding whether it is a circle or an oval. In most of the trials (e.g., 80 percent) the target is presented at the validly cued location, but sometimes it is presented at the other (invalidly cued) location. Versions of these sorts of studies often also include trials with neutral cues (e.g., a double arrow or a neutral letter) that provide no information about the likely location.

In such cuing studies, subjects typically are faster to respond to validly cued targets than to invalidly cued ones (Figure 6.3B). In addition, relative to the neutral-cue condition, subjects respond more quickly to validly cued targets (reflecting the *benefits* of attention having been directed to the location where the target occurs) and more slowly to invalidly cued targets (reflecting the *costs* of attention having been directed to another location). Varying the cue-to-target interval in such experiments has shown that these behavioral attention effects can begin by about 300 milliseconds after the instructional cue and can be held for seconds afterward. The general interpretation of such studies is that the behavioral effects observed reflect the influence of attention on the processing of targets in the cued location. This facilitation has typically been interpreted as arising from attentional modulation of the relevant sensory processing, in accord with the early-selection models of attention already discussed.

Although we voluntarily direct attention to events that interest us because of behavioral goals and other intrinsic factors, it is more often the case that stimuli arising from the environment attract our attention involuntarily. These involuntary

(A)

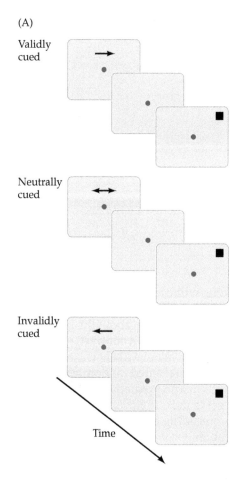

Validly cued

Neutrally cued

Invalidly cued

Time

(B)

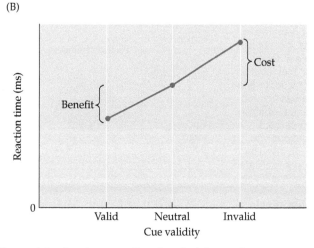

Figure 6.3 A cuing paradigm for studying endogenous visual spatial attention (A) In this paradigm, a centrally presented instructional cue indicates where a target will most likely be presented (validly cued), where it will be less likely to be presented (invalidly cued), or the cue can provide no information either way (neutrally cued). (B) Typical results show the benefits and costs in the reaction time for target detection after valid and invalid cuing, relative to the neutral-cue condition. (After Posner et al. 1980.)

shifts of attention, which define exogenous attention, occur continually during our waking lives as we navigate an ever-changing environment. Particularly salient stimuli, such as a loud noise, a flash of light, or a quick movement, tend to trump whatever we happen to be attending to at the moment. However, we are always attending to *something* (externally or internally) while we are awake, and all manner of stimulus characteristics and combinations can determine what attracts our attention at any given moment.

Like endogenous attention, exogenous attention has been studied in a variety of behavioral experiments. One commonly used approach also employs trial-by-trial cuing, but in this case a sensory cue such as a flash of light is presented at a particular location shortly before a target stimulus is presented either in that location or elsewhere (Figure 6.4A). In these circumstances, subjects are again quicker to respond to a target presented in the cued location compared to the uncued location, at least when the target comes very soon after the cue (Figure 6.4B, left half of graph). Subjects are also faster for validly cued targets than for targets following a neutral cue (e.g., when a light flash occurs at both locations), and slower for targets at invalidly cued locations than in the neutral-cue condition. As with endogenous attention, these effects can be conceptualized in terms of benefits and costs.

On the face of it, this sort of paradigm and the behavioral effects observed are similar to studies of endogenous cuing and their findings. In both instances, a cue induces a shift in the focus of attention that facilitates the sensory processing of stimuli in the attended region and diminishes the efficacy of processing elsewhere. Despite these similarities, however, endogenous and exogenous cuing have important functional differences. In endogenous cuing, information

Figure 6.4 Exogenously triggered (reflexive) attention (A) In this paradigm a brief flash is presented in one of two possible target locations, serving as an exogenous cue for a target that might follow at that location or at the other location. The occurrence of a target at the cued versus uncued location is random, with the probability at each location being 50 percent. (B) Shortly after the exogenous cue (green-shaded time period), stimulus processing at that location is facilitated, as indicated by faster response times to cued relative to uncued targets. At longer intervals (red-shaded time period), however, there is a decrement in performance for the cued targets, known as *inhibition of return*. (After Klein 2000; data from Posner and Cohen 1984.)

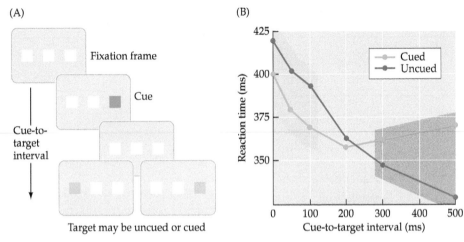

about the likelihood that the target stimulus will occur in the cued location is provided by prior knowledge (e.g., being informed where the target is likely to occur). If an instructional cue provides no information about the likely location of the target, there is no behavioral enhancement. In contrast, exogenous attention is not driven by any explicit information about a likely target location. That is, even if an exogenous cue (e.g., a flash) is presented randomly in the two possible locations from trial to trial, and thus has no predictive value for where a target will occur, the processing of a target in the cued location is nonetheless facilitated, presumably because the flash preceding the appearance of a target automatically draws attention to that location.

Endogenous and exogenous attentional cuing also differ in the time courses of their influence on target processing. For endogenously cued conditions, the improved processing of a validly cued target can begin by about 300 milliseconds after the cue and can last for some seconds afterward, or longer if subjects maintain their focus of attention on the instructed location. In contrast, exogenous cuing effects start earlier and are short-lived, beginning as early as 75 milliseconds after the cue and lasting only a few hundred milliseconds or so. Moreover, at still longer intervals (about 400 to 800 milliseconds after the cue), the effect of the target validity tends to reverse, with subjects actually responding somewhat more slowly to targets in the cued location (Figure 6.4B, right half of graph). This phenomenon, known as **inhibition of return**, is not observed with endogenous cuing. Although the cause of this inhibition is not understood, it has been suggested that it may promote the exploration of new, previously unattended places or objects in the environment by slowing the return of attention to recently attended ones. In any event, it is clear that the pattern of effects on behavioral task performance differs between attentional shifts that are triggered endogenously and those that are driven by exogenous factors.

Neuroscience Approaches to Studying Attention

Cognitive psychologists have schematically represented the cognitive architecture of attention generally along the lines depicted in Figure 6.2C, at least with regard to its role in allocating resources for sensory and perceptual processing. In this conception, higher levels of the system are able to modulate stimulus processing at various lower levels. In translating such a scheme to a neuroscience framework, studies of attention have tended to be approached from two major perspectives: (1) investigating how the neural processing of stimuli are modulated by attention under different circumstances; and (2) determining the sets of higher-level control regions of the brain that coordinate this modulation, and the mechanisms by which they do so.

Studying the neural effects of attention on stimulus processing

Much of attention research has focused on the first of the two main aspects just noted—namely, assessing the effects of attention on stimulus processing. It is logical to hypothesize that attentional modulation of stimulus processing would be reflected in dynamic alterations of the neural activity evoked by stimuli in particular regions of the brain. For sensory systems, this means modulation at one or more levels of the various sensory processing streams, represented generically by the thick yellow pathway arrows in Figure 6.5.

As described earlier, studies using measures of behavioral performance such as reaction time, accuracy, and verbal report have provided important insight into the brain's limited capacity to process information, as well as the role of attention in selectively allocating these limited processing resources. Behavioral studies, however, depend on relatively indirect approaches to these questions. The ability to measure brain activity while subjects (human or animal) are engaged in cognitive tasks has evolved rapidly in recent years (see Chapter 2). These methods have provided an unprecedented ability to directly assess the influence of attention on sensory and perceptual processing, thereby providing direct information on the timing, brain areas, and level at which attentional influences can occur under different circumstances.

Moreover, these approaches can reveal much about the neurobiological mechanisms of attentional effects on stimulus processing. For example, if attention affects the processing of a stimulus in the relevant sensory cortex, does it do so by simply enhancing the amplitude of the evoked response, by extending the duration of its processing with a brain area, by narrowing the tuning curves of the neurons involved (see Chapter 3), or by some other means? Regardless, the modulatory effects on stimulus processing presumably underlie the effects of attention on performance observed in behavioral studies. The rest of this chapter focuses on the effects of attention on stimulus processing using these neurally based techniques.

Studying the control of attention in the brain

Another main goal in studies of attention using brain-based methods is to understand the mechanisms by which these attentional modulations of stimulus processing are brought about and coordinated in the brain, and to examine the idea that specific sets of brain regions might work together as part of an overarching attentional control system (see Figure 6.5). As described in the next chapter, a number of studies, both in normal individuals and in patients, have

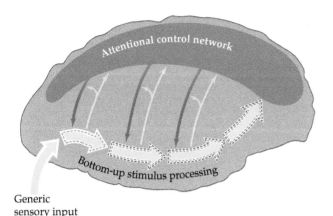

Generic
sensory input

Figure 6.5 Attentional functions in the brain In this schematic representation, the yellow arrows indicate a generic sensory input and processing system, and the blue region and arrows represent an attentional control network—broadly construed—and associated control signals. The dotted orange and red lines around the thick yellow processing arrows are meant to indicate modulation of the stimulus processing stream by the putative control network. The yellow and blue vertical arrows indicate interactions between the sensory processing and control networks at various levels.

indicated that some higher-level brain areas are indeed involved in attentional control, particularly relatively specific regions in the frontal and parietal cortices. This network of regions appears to carry out this attentional control function by means of top-down neural signals (descending blue arrows in Figure 6.5) that regulate stimulus processing at various levels in the sensory and association cortices. These proposed mechanisms for managing our attentional resources within a limited-capacity processing system are taken up in the next chapter.

Neural Effects of Attention on Stimulus Processing: Auditory Spatial Attention

As noted earlier, auditory selective attention is needed when two or more streams of auditory information are occurring simultaneously and processing resources need to be focused on one of them. In most natural circumstances, streams of auditory stimuli—such as verbal streams coming from different people in a room—are differentiated mainly by virtue of their respective sources being separated spatially. Studies in which auditory attention has been directed toward locations in space have shown effects on stimulus-evoked neural activity that are mostly similar to those involving selective attention to one ear versus the other. Thus, these studies are grouped together here as forms of auditory attention that are predominantly spatial.

Electrophysiological studies of the effects of auditory spatial attention

An important question, already touched on in this chapter, concerns the stage (or stages) of stimulus processing at which attentional mechanisms come into play. Event-related potentials (ERPs) that extract specific time-locked responses from the ongoing scalp EEG have been particularly informative in addressing this question because of their temporal precision (see Chapter 2). Figure 6.6 shows a typical ERP response to a brief tone stimulus, which can be broken down into three main phases.

During the first 10 milliseconds after the tone onset, a series of small waves known as **brainstem evoked responses** (**BERs**) is observed (**Figure 6.6A**). These very early latency waves in the auditory ERP reflect activity evoked in the auditory brainstem nuclei as the sound stimulus information reaches them along the afferent pathways (see Chapter 4). The next phase (10 to 50 milliseconds; **Figure 6.6B**) reflects mainly the early evoked

(A) Brainstem evoked responses

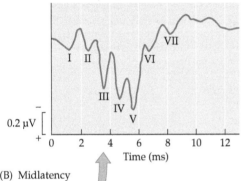

(B) Midlatency responses

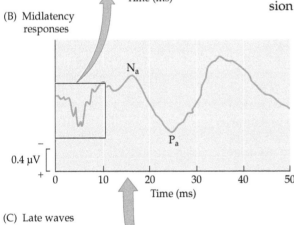

(C) Late waves

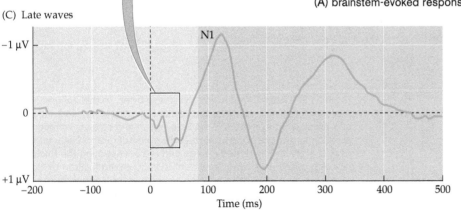

Figure 6.6 ERP response to a tone stimulus The average ERP in response to a simple tone stimulus can be divided into three phases: (A) brainstem-evoked responses (BERs) are the small waves in the first 10 milliseconds, which are numbered I–VII in roman numerals; (B) early cortical midlatency responses from 10 to 50 milliseconds, including waves N_a and P_a, which include initial activity in primary auditory cortex; and (C) slower-frequency cortical late waves from higher-order auditory areas, beginning with the large negative-polarity wave N1 peaking at 100 milliseconds. Note that negative (N) potentials are plotted upward, as is often the case in EEG and ERP research (see Chapter 2). µV = microvolts. (After Picton et al. 1974.)

activity in auditory cortex, as evidenced by intracranial recordings and ERP source analysis. This activity is followed by a set of longer-latency waves that continue for several hundred milliseconds (Figure 6.6C), reflecting extended activity in the secondary and association auditory cortices. Recording these responses while subjects are engaged in attentional tasks can provide insight into the timing and level at which attention affects auditory stimulus processing.

Analyzing the responses to spatially segregated auditory stimulus streams that are selectively attended (as in a dichotic listening task) reveals the usefulness of this approach (Figure 6.7A). In this paradigm, monaural tone pips are delivered to the left and right ears in random order, with an occasional deviant tone (e.g., slightly fainter or slightly different pitch) in each stream. On half of the trial blocks, the task is to attend closely to all the sounds in one ear to detect the occasional deviant stimulus in that ear, while ignoring all sounds to the other ear. In the other half of the blocks, the subjects attend to the other ear to detect targets there. In this **attentional stream paradigm**, introduced by cognitive neuroscientist Steven Hillyard and colleagues in the early 1970s, the stimuli are identical in both attention conditions; the only difference is the covert focusing of attention toward one input channel or the other. The ERP responses to the same physical stimulus when it was attended versus when it was unattended can then be compared.

Using this paradigm, Hillyard showed that a specific ERP component known as the **auditory N1** (a negative-polarity sensory wave occurring about 100 milliseconds after a sound) was larger when the tone stimulus was attended (Figure 6.7B). This increase of the N1 was observed for *all* stimuli in the attended ear (i.e., for both the nontarget stimuli and the deviant target stimuli). The relatively early timing led investigators to conclude that this effect provided neural evidence for an early-selection mechanism of attention.

Figure 6.7 Early and late selection during auditory attention (A) The auditory attentional stream paradigm is a means for studying the mechanisms of auditory selective attention. Asterisks indicate tones that deviate slightly from the rest of the stimuli in that stream in a particular feature, such as loudness or pitch. These tones serve as targets in the attended channel. **(B)** The effect of auditory attention on the N1 wave at 100 milliseconds in the auditory ERP is thought to reflect a relatively early attentional selection. **(C)** The P300 effect elicited only by detected targets in the attended channel is thought to reflect a late-selection process to distinct elements within the attended channel. μV = microvolts. (B,C after Hillyard et al. 1973.)

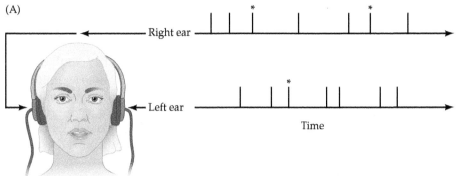

(A)

Right ear

Left ear

Time

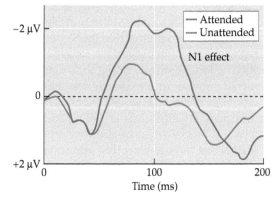

(B) Between auditory channels
     (early selection)

—2 μV

N1 effect

— Attended
— Unattended

0

+2 μV

0   100   200

Time (ms)

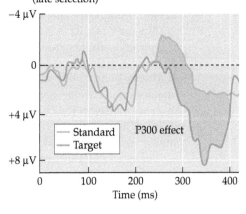

(C) Within auditory channel
     (late selection)

—4 μV

0

+4 μV

+8 μV

— Standard
— Target

P300 effect

0   100   200   300   400

Time (ms)

In addition to eliciting an enhanced N1, the detected deviant targets in the attended ear elicited a large, longer-latency, positive wave known as the **P300** or **P3**, peaking at about 300 to 450 milliseconds over posterior parietal areas (Figure 6.7C). This later separation of activity within the attended channel between the target and nontarget responses was proposed to reflect the late selection of the target occurring at longer latencies. These results thus provided neural evidence for both early and late selection during auditory attention.

The N1 enhancement just described can begin as early as 70 milliseconds after stimulus onset. The lack of an earlier attentional effect, however, suggested that all the earlier sensory processing, including early cortical processing from 20 to 70 milliseconds, is immune to attentional influence. To address the question of early attentional selection more closely, cognitive neuroscientist Marty Woldorff and colleagues used a version of the auditory attentional stream paradigm that required particularly strongly focused attention, while multiple phases of the auditory ERP response were acquired in parallel. Under these conditions, the brainstem evoked responses (BERs) remained unaffected (Figure 6.8A), thus arguing against any brainstem-level gating as a mechanism of selective auditory attention—a view that has been supported by various other studies. However, a slightly later effect was observed: an enhanced positive wave from 20 to 50 milliseconds for attended stimuli, preceding the longer-latency N1 enhancement (Figure 6.8B). Because the latency of this **P20–50 attention effect** coincided with the initial activity in auditory sensory cortex, it provided strong neural evidence that early attentional selection can occur at this stage of sensory processing.

Follow-up studies using the localizing capabilities of magnetoencephalography (MEG) indicated that the magnetic counterparts of both the P20–50 and the N1 attentional enhancement effects indeed derived from low-level auditory cortical areas on the lower bank of the Sylvian fissure, with the P20–50 effect likely arising from primary auditory cortex (Figure 6.8C) and the N1 effect from secondary auditory cortex (see Chapter 4). This combination of results thus established that attention can affect stimulus processing in the sensory cortices very early in the auditory input stream, thereby providing particularly strong support for early-selection models of attention.

Neuroimaging studies of the effects of auditory spatial attention

Compared to electrophysiological techniques, functional neuroimaging has been used considerably less for studies of auditory attention in humans. Several PET studies in the 1990s showed that attending versus not attending to auditory stimuli resulted in overall enhanced activity in the auditory cortical regions on the lower bank of the Sylvian fissure. Other studies using dichotic listening paradigms similar to the ones described in the preceding section showed that attending to input to one ear versus the other had a greater enhancing effect for activity in contralateral versus ipsilateral auditory cortex. Both of these results thus accord with the ERP and MEG studies already discussed in showing that auditory attention influences sensory processing activity in low-level auditory cortex.

The use of fMRI to study auditory attention has also been limited, especially compared with its extensive use in studies of visual attention (to be described shortly). A major reason has been that the rapid switching of the magnetic-field gradients in magnetic resonance imaging is acoustically noisy, thus tending to interfere with the processing of experimental auditory stimulation. However, improvements in fMRI methodology (e.g., somewhat quieter scanners) have enabled its more effective use for auditory studies, thus allowing its higher spatial resolution to be brought to bear on mechanisms of auditory attention.

For example, high-resolution fMRI scans have shown that attention tends to modulate activity in specific regions of the auditory cortex. In particular,

(A) No effect on attention on BERs

Central site (Cz)

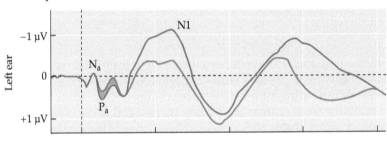

(B) P20–50 attention effect (20–50 ms)

Event-related potentials

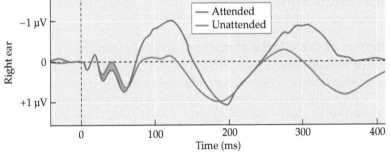

Attentional difference waves (attended minus unattended)

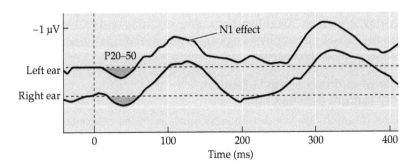

(C) MEG localization of P20–50 attention effect

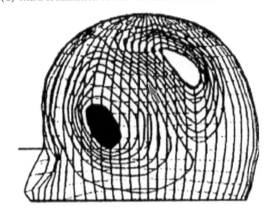

Figure 6.8 Early auditory attention effects during dichotic listening (A) Even during very strongly focused auditory spatial attention, no modulation of the brainstem-evoked potentials (BERs) in the first 10 milliseconds is observed. (B) However, an early cortical effect is reflected as enhanced activity from 20 to 50 milliseconds for attended relative to unattended tones (the P20–50 attention effect), providing particularly strong support for early-selection theories. (C) Using MEG, the P20–50 effect was indeed localized as a local dipolar source (red arrow) in primary auditory cortical areas on the lower bank of the Sylvian fissure, providing yet further support that attention can affect early sensory processing activity in the low-level sensory cortices. μV = microvolts. (A,B after Woldorff et al. 1987; C after Woldorff et al. 1993.)

Figure 6.9 **Effects of auditory attention on processing in the auditory cortical regions** In this fMRI study, the effects of attention were seen mainly in the auditory belt areas surrounding the primary auditory cortex. (A) Stimulus-dependent activation was observed in both the primary auditory cortex in Heschl's gyrus (HG) and the more lateral auditory belt areas in the superior temporal gyrus (STG). (B) Attention-related modulations were seen mainly in the more lateral belt areas and not in the primary auditory cortex. μV = microvolts. (From Petkov et al. 2004.)

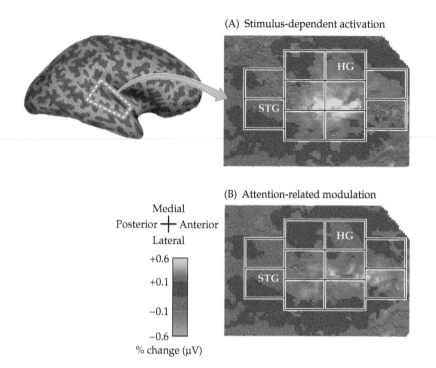

these neuroimaging studies have reported relatively little effect of attention on stimulus processing in primary auditory cortex, with the effects appearing mainly in the surrounding auditory belt areas (**Figure 6.9**). These effects in secondary auditory cortical areas most likely correspond to the large N1 ERP effect, described earlier, that is often observed in auditory attention studies. The earlier and considerably smaller P20–50 electrophysiological attention effect, which seems likely to derive from primary auditory cortex, may not last long enough or be large enough to produce a good fMRI signal.

Animal studies of the effects of auditory spatial attention

Relatively little neurally based research on auditory attention has been carried out in experimental animals, especially compared to studies of visual attention in animals, which will be described shortly. The reason is that such research must be performed in awake, behaving animals—typically monkeys—and it is generally harder to train them to carry out auditory attention tasks than visual ones. The research that has been done, however, accords with the ERP and imaging work, suggesting that similar attentional effects occur across species and can be observed at the level of single neurons. Electrophysiological studies of auditory attention in monkeys in simplified dichotic listening paradigms have indicated that attended stimuli produced larger single-unit responses in auditory cortex as early as 20 milliseconds after stimulus onset. These results fit well with the P20–50 electrophysiological effects observed in human dichotic listening studies (described earlier).

The effects of auditory spatial attention on auditory feature processing

Although the research described in the preceding sections demonstrated that attention to a spatially segregated auditory stimulus stream can increase the amplitude of evoked neural activity early in auditory processing, another question concerns the consequences of such enhancement for later processing stages. For example, does this early enhancement lead to improvements in perceptual discriminability of stimuli in the attended stream of input relative to that in the unattended stream? If so, one would predict a greater differentiation in neural processing between stimulus types having different feature characteristics in an attended versus an unattended auditory stream.

In pursuing this issue in a dichotic listening paradigm with occasional deviant stimuli (similar to that shown in Figure 6.7A), another ERP component, called the **mismatch negativity (MMN)**, has been especially useful. Deviant auditory stimuli in a stream of otherwise identical sounds produce a negative wave peaking at about 150 to 200 milliseconds after the deviant stimulus. This MMN effect, first reported by cognitive neuroscientist Risto Näätänen and colleagues in the late 1970s, is elicited by deviations in any basic auditory feature (e.g., pitch, intensity, location), and source analysis has indicated that it derives mainly from auditory cortex. Moreover, the MMN becomes larger as the feature deviation increases, and the minimal degree of deviation that produces this neural response is about the same as for the perceptual threshold for discriminating the deviant.

Näätänen theorized that this response reflects the outcome of a series of processes in which a template of the standard repeated stimulus, including all its features, is established and stored in the brain. Each auditory stimulus is automatically compared to this template; if the stimulus does not match the template in any of its fundamental sensory features, a mismatch response is triggered and reflected in the MMN wave. Accordingly, the MMN has been used as a marker of the successful discrimination of the relevant auditory feature, with its amplitude reflecting the extent or quality of the feature discrimination (i.e., the discrimination of the deviant from the standard stimuli).

Early studies of the MMN reported that it was elicited when subjects were not explicitly attending to the auditory stimuli, and that the amplitude of this feature deviance effect was not affected by attention. These observations were interpreted as suggesting that the processes causing the MMN (auditory feature analysis, template making, comparison processes, and ultimately the mismatch activity) were all strongly automatic and not subject to attentional influence. However, later fast-rate ERP and MEG studies invoking more focused attention showed that the MMN amplitude was actually substantially lower within an unattended channel relative to an attended one (Figure 6.10).

These results indicate not only that attention can modulate the overall amplitude of early neural responses elicited by auditory stimuli, but that this early modulation leads to a large later effect on auditory feature analysis, and thus that auditory feature analysis is indeed susceptible to attentional influence. On the other hand, some MMN is elicited even in a strongly ignored auditory channel, indicating that some feature analysis is automatically performed for all auditory input, as proposed by Näätänen. This evidence accords with the commonsense idea that although it is valuable to allocate more processing resources to the sensory input of

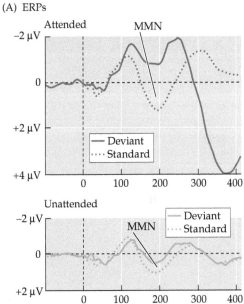

(A) ERPs

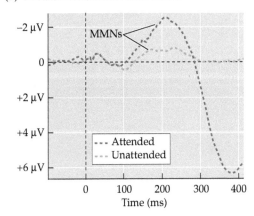

(B) Deviance-related difference waves

Figure 6.10 Effects of attention on auditory feature processing as reflected by the mismatch negativity ERP component (A) These overlays of the ERPs elicited by the feature-deviant stimuli and the standard (nondeviant) stimuli in the attended and unattended auditory streams show that the mismatch negativity (MMN), which typically appears as increased negative-wave activity between 150 and 220 milliseconds in response to the feature-deviating stimulus, is significantly larger in the attended condition. (B) The overlay of deviance-related difference waves (deviant ERP minus nondeviant ERP for the two attention conditions) shows strong effects of auditory attention on the MMN, and thus on auditory feature discrimination. μV = microvolts. (After Woldorff et al. 1991.)

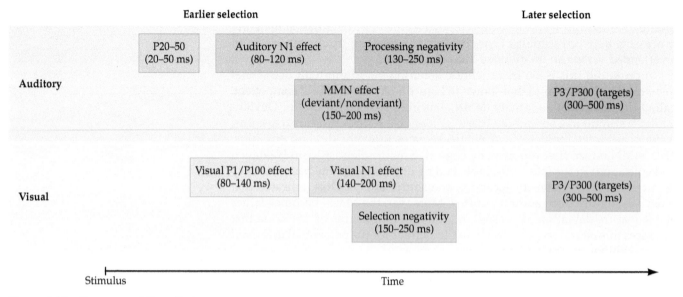

Figure 6.11 Summary of the effects of attention on ERPs The major effects of auditory and visual attention on various ERP components.

greatest interest at each moment, it would be ill advised to completely turn off the processing of other inputs that might indicate the sudden occurrence of a new, biologically important stimulus elsewhere.

Figure 6.11 summarizes the main ERP effects of auditory attention, along with the various corresponding ERP effects of visual attention that will be discussed next.

Neural Effects of Attention on Stimulus Processing: Visual Spatial Attention

As in audition, recordings of brain activity can be used to examine how attention influences stimulus processing during visual attention tasks. Historically, studies of visual attention have concentrated on spatial paradigms, reflecting the fact that vision is particularly spatial in nature.

Electrophysiological studies of the effects of visual spatial attention

As with auditory attention, ERPs in response to visual stimuli can be especially informative about the timing of attentional effects. Figure 6.12A shows a typical visual ERP response to a stimulus in one visual field (the right visual field in this example), recorded from a site over the left occipital cortex. The first prominent wave is the visual P1, or P100, a positive wave peaking at about 100 milliseconds over occipital sites contralateral to the visual field of the stimulus (consistent with the crossing projection of visual information; see Chapter 3). The visual P1 derives mainly from neural activity in the low-level extrastriate visual cortical areas (V2, V3, V4), with some contribution on its earliest portion from primary visual cortex (V1). The P1 wave is followed by the visual N1 component, which peaks about 180 milliseconds after the stimulus and is thought to reflect sensory processing activity in a combination of extrastriate and parietal visual areas.

As in the dichotic listening experiments described earlier, streams of visual stimuli can be presented to two (or more) locations in the visual field. In this sort of paradigm subjects typically attend to a stream of stimuli at one location or another to detect occasional target stimuli in that stream (Figure 6.12B). Evoked brain activity to the same physical stimuli can then be analyzed for differences as a function of whether the stimuli were attended or unattended.

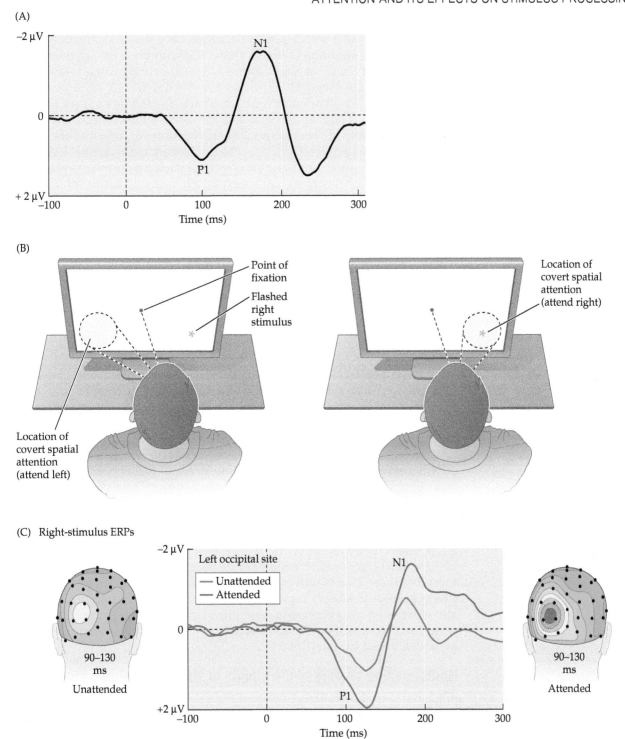

Figure 6.12 Effects of visual spatial attention on ERP responses to visual stimuli (A) Recorded over the left occipital lobe to a light flash in the right visual hemifield, this ERP shows the visual P1 and N1 components peaking at 100 and 180 milliseconds, respectively. (B) In this paradigm for investigating the effects of visual spatial attention, the subject is attending to a location either in the right visual field or in the left visual field for unilaterally presented visual flash stimuli on that side, and ignoring stimuli on the other side. (C) Representative ERPs elicited by right-field stimuli when attended versus unattended are shown here, along with the corresponding topographical distributions on the scalp at the latency of the P1 peak. Attention enhances the amplitude of the sensory P1 component, with little change in waveform or scalp distribution. Such an effect is consistent with the conclusion that attention induces a gain enhancement in the responses to stimuli occurring in an attended region of space. μV = microvolts.

ERP studies using such a stream paradigm have shown distinctive effects of visual spatial attention on early visual ERP components—in particular, enhancement of the P1 at about 100 to 120 milliseconds, often followed by an enhanced N1 at about 180 milliseconds (Figure 6.12C). For a unilateral visual stimulus, the P1 attention effect typically appears as a simple increase in amplitude (i.e., a larger positive wave), consistent with it reflecting a simple change in the "gain" of the underlying sensory processing activity—that is, the same neural areas being activated, but more strongly when attended. As with the analogous auditory studies, this effect has been interpreted as reflecting an early-selection mechanism that boosts the early activity elicited by attended stimuli in the visual sensory cortices. Additional studies have indicated that these effects reflect an enhancement of activity specifically in extrastriate visual cortex rather than in primary visual cortex (see the next section).

ERPs have also been examined in endogenously cued attention paradigms to examine brain activity elicited by targets as a function of whether they were validly or invalidly cued. The electrophysiological effects are similar to those in visual stream experiments, with validly cued targets (which are presumably more attended) producing larger P1 and N1 responses relative to invalidly cued targets, thus correlating with the faster behavioral responses, while also delineating the processing level of the attentional influence. A similar approach with exogenously cued attention showed that the enhanced processing of validly cued targets (again as reflected in faster reaction times) at short cue-target intervals were also associated with enhanced P1 and N1 components. Thus, for both endogenously and exogenously cued spatial attention, the effects on the sensory pathways appear to entail a modulation of relatively early sensory processing activity in visual sensory cortex.

Although these various early effects on visual sensory processing are typically observed with visual spatial attention, additional attentional selection and influence can occur at later stages of processing in these paradigms. More specifically, the detected targets within an attended visual stimulus stream (relative to the nontargets in that stream) evoke the long-latency P300 ERP response, closely analogous to the response elicited for auditory targets within an attended auditory stream, discussed earlier (see Figure 6.7C). The similarity of these late target-specific responses *across* sensory modalities supports the view that these effects reflect a late attentional selection, beyond any early effects in specific sensory regions. Other types of late-selection processes are also observed during other visual attention circumstances, such as during the widely studied attentional blink that occurs within a single stream of rapidly presented visual stimuli (Box 6A).

Neuroimaging studies of the effects of visual spatial attention

The effects of visual spatial attention have also been extensively studied with hemodynamically based functional neuroimaging techniques such as PET and fMRI (see Chapter 2). An early influential study along these lines used PET imaging (along with ERP recordings; see next section) in an attentional stream paradigm like that described in the previous section. Subjects were presented with bilateral stimuli in the upper visual field and asked to attend to either the left or the right half of the stimuli for the occurrence of occasional targets on that side. Given the crossed anatomical organization of the human visual system, if visual attention affected stimulus processing at early sensory levels, then the effects of attention should also follow this organization. That is, relative to passively viewing bilateral stimuli, attending to the left side of the stimuli should cause increased activity in right occipital cortex, whereas attending to

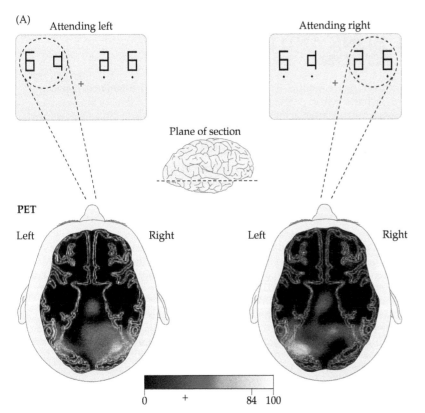

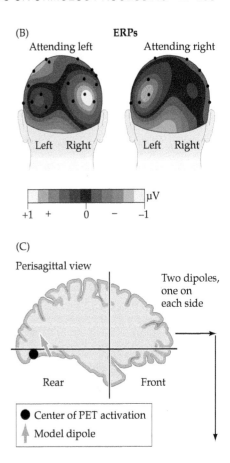

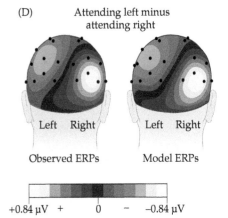

Figure 6.13 **Effects of visual spatial attention in visual cortex** In parallel studies using PET and ERP recordings, subjects were presented with bilateral stimuli in the upper visual field. In different trials they attended to either the left or the right side of the screen (or, as a control, viewed the stimuli passively). (A) PET images show that the lateralized spatial attention enhanced activity in the contralateral ventral occipital cortex. (B) Corresponding ERP effects on the P1 at 100 milliseconds show enhanced activity over contralateral occipital scalp. (C,D) Source analysis of the P1 attention effect, facilitated by combining the PET and ERP data, indicates that model dipoles in the locations of the PET activation foci fit the observed ERP distributions quite closely. μV = microvolts. (From Heinze et al. 1994.)

the right side should increase activity in the left occipital cortex. As Figure 6.13 shows, this is exactly the pattern found in the neuroimaging data.

Recall from Chapter 3 that the low-level visual cortical regions, both primary (V1) and extrastriate (V2, V3, V4), are retinotopically organized much more fully than just to represent the contralateral visual field. For example, the sensory regions representing the upper visual fields are in ventral contralateral occipital cortex inferior to the calcarine sulcus, whereas the lower visual fields are represented in dorsal contralateral occipital cortex, superior to the calcarine sulcus. In the PET study just described, the attention-related enhancement of neural activity was not only contralateral but located in ventral occipital regions, in agreement with the attention being directed to the stimuli in the upper visual field. In later studies, this retinotopic organization of the effects of spatial attention was more fully and precisely demonstrated by first delineating the early visual areas with an fMRI mapping technique before performing a visual spatial attention study in the same subjects. This approach showed that visual spatial attention directly enhances stimulus processing in the specific portions

■ BOX 6A THE ATTENTIONAL BLINK AND LATE ATTENTIONAL SELECTION

Many of the studies outlined in this chapter describe how attention can affect stimulus processing at relatively early stages and anatomically low levels of the sensory pathways. However, other studies have indicated that, in some circumstances, attentional selection happens at later times and at higher anatomical levels. An intriguing example of higher-level late selection comes from findings related to the **attentional blink**, a phenomenon discovered through a paradigm developed in the early 1990s.

In the attentional blink paradigm, stimuli are presented in rapid sequence in a single stream (typically about 8 to 11 per second), with the task to detect or discriminate occasional target stimuli in the stream (e.g., a digit among a series of letters; Figure A). The main behavioral finding in these studies is that shortly after detection of one target item (T1), the ability to detect a second target (T2) in the series is reduced. By varying the lag times of the second target relative to the first (i.e., changing the number of intervening nontarget stimuli), experimenters have shown that the ability to detect the second target is impaired when it occurs between 150 to 450 milliseconds after a detected initial target (Figure B). This effect was termed *attentional blink* because it seemed that while someone is engaged in discriminating a target, there is a brief deficit in the ability to devote sufficient processing resources to detect a second target. It was inferred that this deficit results from attentional capacity limitations at some level of the system, perhaps a processing bottleneck while in a target discrimination stage.

The attentional blink is different from the limitations indicated during most of the stimulus selection processes described in the text, in which attention was focused on particular speakers, spatial locations, or stimulus features, which resulted in a reduced allocation of attention to other inputs, locations, or features. In the attentional blink there is only one stream of stimuli, and all the stimuli in that stream occur in a spatially attended location, are relevant, and are attended. The phenomenon nonetheless adds to the evidence that attending to one thing—whether a target in a stream of stimuli, the selection of a response, or a particular location or source—impedes the ability to attend to something else at the same time.

(A)

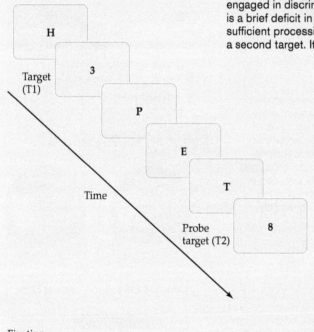

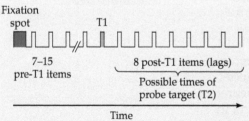

(B)

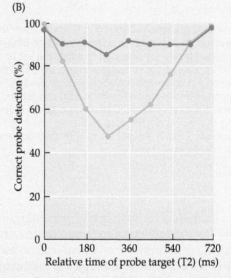

The attentional blink. (A) Paradigm: Stimuli are presented in a rapid stream (here, about 11 per second) in which occasional target stimuli (T1 and T2) are to be detected. (B) Typical behavioral results: When one target occurs alone, it is detected very well (blue line). When a second target (T2) follows a first target (T1) within approximately 150 to 450 milliseconds, the ability to report the occurrence of the second target (green line) is reduced. (A,B after Raymond et al. 1992.)

of the low-level visual sensory areas that represent the particular attended region of space (**Figure 6.14**).

In agreement with the ERP observations discussed in the previous section (see Figure 6.12), most early neuroimaging studies found robust effects of visual attention on stimulus processing in relatively low-level extrastriate visual cortical

■ **BOX 6A** *(continued)*

To understand the level of processing reached by a target occurring during the attentional blink, cognitive neuroscientist Steve Luck and colleagues designed a series of experiments that looked at the components of ERPs elicited by the second target when it occurred at different lag times relative to the first target. In particular, they analyzed the ERPs elicited by the second target when it occurred in the "blink" period after the first target and was less likely to be reported, compared to when it occurred at the nonblink lag times and thus could consistently be reported. The results showed that the sensory ERP components elicited by the second target—the P1 at 100 milliseconds and N1 at 180 milliseconds—did not differ as a function of whether the target occurred during the blink period (Figure C, orange and green lines). This observation is in sharp contrast to studies of

visual spatial attention, in which attention strongly modulates the amplitudes of the P1 and N1 sensory ERP components.

Next, Luck's group structured an experiment to ask whether the second target elicited a semantically related wave, known as the N400, that is generated when subjects attend to and process words, occurring at about 300 to 500 milliseconds (see Chapter 12). When the second target occurred during the blink period and was less likely to be reported, it nonetheless elicited a robust N400 of similar size to that elicited by target words occurring outside the blink period (Figure C, red line). Thus, even when the second target could not be reported, the information in the stimulus seemed to have been processed up through the level of semantic analysis. In particular, the attentional selection appeared to be occurring after semantic analysis

but before a stage of conscious detection and awareness (see Figure C, blue line, for the P300 component related to conscious target detection), or at least before a stage of encoding and storage that would enable later verbal reporting.

On the other hand, a more recent study reported that increasing the task difficulty for detecting the first target decreased the N400 response to the secondary target words occurring during the blink time period. These findings would suggest that during a full attentional blink the stimuli are not so fully processed, at least with regard to processing at the level of semantic analysis. Regardless, the early sensory ERP waves consistently seem to be fully intact, even when the attentional blink occurs and the words cannot be reported. Thus, during the circumstances of the attentional blink the attentional selection clearly happens at a considerably later stage of processing than during other types of attention, such as visual spatial attention.

References

GIESBRECHT, B., J. L. SY AND J. C. ELLIOT (2007) Electrophysiological evidence for both perceptual and postperceptual selection during the attention blink. *J. Cogn. Neurosci.* 19: 2005–2018.

LUCK, S. J., E. K. VOGEL AND K. L. SHAPIRO (1996) Word meanings can be accessed but not reported during the attentional blink. *Nature* 383: 616–618.

RAYMOND, J. E., K. L. SHAPIRO AND K. M. ARNELL (1992) Temporary suppression of visual processing in an RSVP task: An attentional blink? *J. Exp. Psychol. Hum. Percept. Perform.* 18: 849–860.

VOGEL, E. K., S. J. LUCK AND K. L. SHAPIRO (1998) Electrophysiological evidence for a postperceptual locus of suppression during the attentional blink. *J. Exp. Psychol. Hum. Percept. Perform.* 24: 1656–1674.

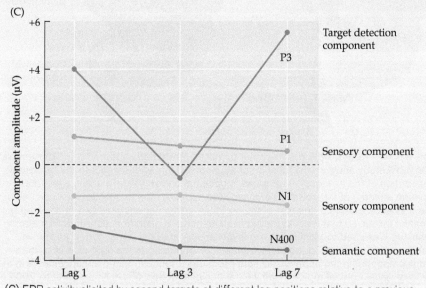

(C) ERP activity elicited by second targets at different lag positions relative to a previous target: Neither the P1 nor the N1 sensory component elicited by the second target—nor the longer-latency semantically related N400 wave—differed as a function of whether the target occurred during the blink period. The only component affected was the even later P3 wave associated with conscious detection. Thus, these data suggest that the second target was processed up through the level of semantic analysis, even when it could not be detected or reported very well. μV = microvolts. (C after Vogel et al. 1998.)

areas (e.g., V2, V3, V4) but not in primary visual cortex. More recent neuroimaging studies, however, have shown that strongly focused visual attention can also influence stimulus processing at the level of V1, although typically more weakly. Moreover, in accordance with these effects, other fMRI studies have shown that the trial-to-trial variations in the level of activity evoked in V1 by

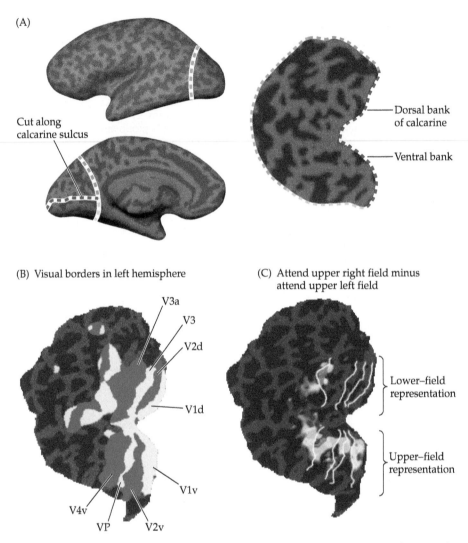

Figure 6.14 Retinotopic organization of visual spatial attention effects An example of an fMRI study showing the location of attention effects with respect to the retinotopic organization of the low-level visual areas in occipital cortex. (A) MRI scans were used to create a model of the cortex as a convoluted surface; from this model the occipital lobe was separated from the rest of the cortex by computer analyses and "cut" along the calcarine sulcus so that it could be laid flat with minimal distortion. (B) An fMRI mapping technique was used to identify the low-level sensory areas of visual cortex, as shown by the alternating colors. d, dorsal; v, ventral. (C) Attending to the right side of bilateral stimuli presented in the upper visual field produces attention-related enhancements in the low-level visual cortical region in left ventral occipital cortex. (From Noesselt et al. 2002.)

a visual stimulus during a difficult visual detection task correlated with the likelihood of detecting and/or perceiving the visual stimulus on each trial.

Neuroimaging studies have also reported effects of visual spatial attention on stimulus processing at even lower anatomical levels of the visual system, including in the lateral geniculate nucleus, the main thalamic relay station in the primary visual pathway from retina to visual cortex (see Chapter 3). Note, however, that fMRI alone cannot determine the timing of any of these effects, whether in thalamus, V1, or extrastriate regions. Resolving this issue using noninvasive brain activity measures generally requires a combination of methods, as described in the next section.

Other neuroimaging studies have investigated the influence of visual spatial attention on processing a stimulus when it occurs by itself compared to occurring in the context of distracting stimuli. For example, fMRI studies have revealed that when multiple stimuli are presented simultaneously in the visual field, their cortical representations in the areas concerned with object recognition in the temporal lobe tend to interact competitively, with each inhibiting activations by the others. Directing attention to one of the stimuli, however, counteracts the suppressive influence from nearby stimuli, and thus may help filter out distracting irrelevant information in cluttered visual scenes. These sorts of mutually suppressive interactions between competing stimuli, along with the role that attention plays to bias processing toward the one that is being attended, has been termed **biased competition**.

Combining electrophysiological and neuroimaging studies of visual spatial attention

The PET and fMRI studies described in the previous section indicated the areas of visual cortex, and thus the anatomical levels in the visual system, at which the processing of visual stimuli is influenced by visual spatial attention. Because of the sluggishness of hemodynamically based imaging signals, however, these methods do not provide information on the timing of these effects (see Chapter 2). Both EEG and MEG techniques provide timing information, but they have substantially coarser spatial resolution. Thus, the combining of these methods has obvious advantages. For example, the PET visual attention study described earlier also recorded ERPs in the same paradigm. In addition to showing enhanced PET activation in the expected regions of visual cortex, this study revealed an enhanced P1 sensory ERP component at 100 milliseconds over occipital scalp contralateral to the direction of attention (see Figure 6.13B). Moreover, source modeling of the P1 enhancement placed it close to the focus of the PET activation in ventral contralateral occipital cortex (see Figure 6.13C,D). Later, combined-methodology studies of visual spatial attention directed within the lower visual field showed that both the PET attention effect and the P1 attention effect originated in the dorsal contralateral occipital cortex, thus both following the retinotopic organization of the visual sensory pathways. This pattern of results therefore supports the view that visual spatial attention affects the sensory processing of visual stimuli not only in low-level visual cortical areas, but also early in the sensory processing sequence.

Other studies have indicated that attention can also have an effect at *longer* latencies on sensory processing activity, but in the lower-level sensory cortices. The pattern of these effects suggests a **reentrant process**, in which attention-related activity returns to the same low-level sensory areas that were initially activated in the ascending pass through the system, presumably reflecting enhanced late processing of the stimulus information in those areas (Box 6B).

Animal studies of the effects of visual spatial attention

Visual attention has also been studied to great advantage in awake, behaving animals with single-unit recording techniques. The findings, mostly in macaque monkeys, provide details of the effects of attention in the visual cortices at the local circuit level that are not possible with scalp recording or noninvasive neuroimaging. As described in Chapter 3, the key information derived from single-unit studies in the visual cortices is typically related to the neuronal receptive fields. In general, visual cortical neurons fire strongly only if a stimulus is presented within the cell's receptive field, and if the stimulus has the specific characteristics to which the cell is tuned. Once a sensory neuron is located for recording and its receptive field characterized, the animal's attention can be

■ BOX 6B ATTENTION-RELATED "REENTRANT" ACTIVITY

As noted in the text, studies have provided evidence of effects of spatial attention that are temporally early in the processing stream, as well as in anatomically "early" (i.e., low-level) cortical regions in the sensory systems. One example is the extrastriate P1 effect during visual spatial attention. Such effects can be explained in terms of attention modulating the activity evoked in these sensory cortices during the initial ascending flow of sensory information. However, spatial attention can also enhance later stimulus-evoked activity, at about 250 milliseconds, with a similar overall scalp distribution but of polarity opposite that of the P1 (see figure). This N2 effect localizes to the same occipital cortical regions that are activated and enhanced with attention in the P1 latency. These observations suggest attention-related *reentrant* processes in which there is a "return" of attention-related activity to the same low-level sensory cortical areas, but at longer latencies.

Whereas these N2 late reentrant effects of attention occur in extrastriate visual cortex, fMRI studies have also shown attention effects in V1. However, relatively little evidence of early-latency effects of attention in V1 has been observed with ERPs, with the earliest effect typically observed being the extrastriate P1 effect described in the text. This pattern of findings led to the hypothesis that the fMRI attentional enhancement in V1 may reflect a longer-latency reentrant effect that is not picked up by ERP recording. In agreement with this idea, a later study specifically provided MEG evidence for longer-latency attentional effects in V1 occurring at about 225 to 250 milliseconds.

Attention-related reentrant activity in visual cortex. Subjects were presented with bilateral stimuli, and the task was to covertly attend to either the left or the right side of the stimuli. These topographical maps reveal the time sequence of differential ERP activity from 0 to 400 milliseconds for attending to the left versus attending to the right of the bilateral stimuli. The subtraction shows that the enhanced activity contralateral to the direction of attention occurs in two phases: an early phase at about 100 milliseconds (the P1 effect, as described in the main text) and a later phase at about 250 milliseconds (an N2 effect). Both of these attention effects were localized to extrastriate areas in contralateral dorsal occipital cortex identified in a matching PET study (corresponding to the visual cortical representation of the lower visual field). The late effect presumably reflects the reentrance of attention-related activity to the same early visual areas that were also modulated earlier by attention during the initial feedforward sweep through the ascending pathways. μV = microvolts. (From Woldorff et al. 2002.)

Single-unit recording studies in monkeys have also shown late attention-related activity in early visual areas, including V1. For example, in a study of the effects of attention on stimulus processing in visual cortex, effects were found at the level of V1, as well as in extrastriate visual cortex. Importantly, the V1 attention effects were relatively late (after 300 milliseconds), following those in V2 and V4, and well past the initial feedforward activation of V1. Thus, these results fit well with the attention-related reentrant effects in the human electrophysiological studies.

The functional role of such attention-related feedback in low-level sensory regions is not clear. One possibility is that the first ascending volley through the system, even when enhanced by prestimulus focused attention, may provide only a relatively coarse first "look" at the stimulus input. The reentrant activity would presumably enable more finely tuned analyses after some interaction with higher brain areas. The reason that late attention effects might extend back to V1 in some cases and not others could be the greater need to extract more detailed information for tasks that are more demanding, such as when stimuli are closely spaced. Various computational models based on these ideas have been developed.

References

MARTÍNEZ, M. AND 9 OTHERS (1999) Involvement of striate and extrastriate visual cortical areas in spatial attention. *Nat. Neurosci.* 2: 364–369.

MEHTA, A. D., I. ULBERT AND C. E. SCHROEDER (2000) Intermodal selective attention in monkeys. I: Distribution and timing of effects across visual areas. *Cereb. Cortex* 10: 343–358.

NOESSELT, T. AND 8 OTHERS (2002) Delayed striate cortical activation during spatial attention. *Neuron* 35: 575–587.

WOLDORFF, M. G., M. LIOTTI, M. SEABOLT, L. BUSSE, J. L. LANCASTER AND P. T. FOX (2002) Temporal dynamics of the effects in occipital cortex of visual-spatial selective attention. *Cogn. Brain Res.* 15: 1–15.

manipulated to investigate the effects on the neuron's firing rate and pattern in response to stimuli.

Cognitive neuroscientists Jeff Moran and Robert Desimone reported more than 25 years ago that spatial attention could indeed modulate neuronal responses in visual cortex, and that the influence depended on how the attended location, the stimulus features, and the cell's receptive field were related (Figure 6.15). Recall that sensory neurons are typically rather selective about the stimuli to which they respond. Certain stimuli (i.e., those with particular features—e.g., horizontal bars) are especially effective at activating a visual sensory neuron when they fall within its receptive field, whereas other stimuli without that feature (e.g., vertical bars) are rather ineffective.

■ **BOX 6B** (continued)

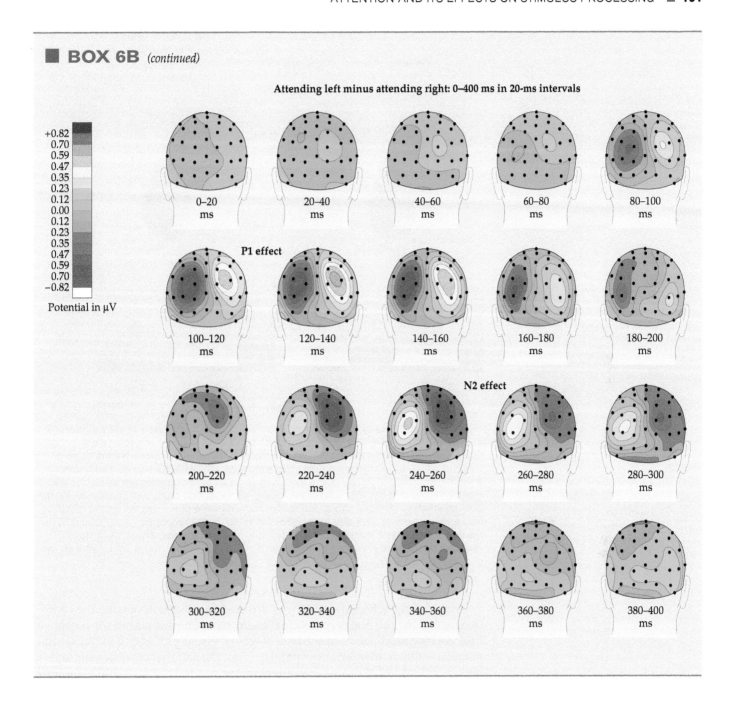

In this seminal study, monkeys were trained to attend to stimuli at one location in the visual field and ignore stimuli at another while the activity of single cells was recorded from visual area V4. Before each block of trials, the monkeys were cued where to attend—an approach similar to paradigms in human studies. When an effective sensory stimulus and an ineffective sensory stimulus were both presented within a cell's receptive field, and the effective stimulus was attended, the cell fired strongly. If the ineffective sensory stimulus was attended, however, the cell gave a much weaker response, even though the effective stimulus was also being presented within its receptive field. This result indicated that neuronal responses depend on the locus of attention *within* the receptive field, at least in V4 neurons.

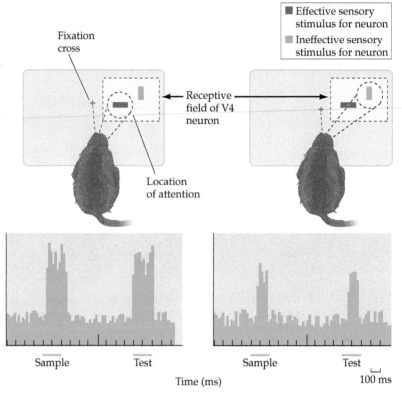

Figure 6.15 Effects of visual spatial attention on the firing rates of single neurons in area V4 At the attended location (circled), two stimuli—sample and test—were presented sequentially; the monkey had to discriminate whether they were the same or different. Irrelevant stimuli were presented simultaneously with the sample and test but at a separate location in the receptive field. Stimuli could either be effective stimuli for the neuron (red bars in this example) or ineffective stimuli (green bars; see Chapter 3). When both an effective stimulus and an ineffective stimulus were presented within the receptive field and the monkey attended to the effective stimulus, the responses were robust. When the monkey attended to the ineffective stimulus, however, the responses were much reduced, despite the presence of an effective stimulus in the receptive field. (After Moran and Desimone 1985.)

Importantly, when attention was directed to a location outside the receptive field of the cell, the response to the effective stimulus within the receptive field was *not* modulated. In the later stages of visual processing in the ventral pathway—that is, in inferior temporal cortex—the pattern was different. At this higher-order level of processing, attention modulated the neuronal responses even if the ignored stimulus was far away from the attended one, presumably because at this level the receptive fields are much larger (see Chapter 3).

In contrast to the modulations observed in extrastriate cortical regions, there were no effects on stimulus processing in primary visual cortex (V1) in these initial studies. However, subsequent studies showed that this lack of a V1 effect may have been due to the small size of the receptive field of V1 relative to the size of the stimuli used. In accordance with this view, small attentional modulations of V1 neuronal responses were observed when relevant and distracting stimuli were placed very close to one another.

In another key study, the orientation tuning curves (i.e., the tuning curves for lines of different orientations) of neurons in both V4 and V1 were assessed as a function of whether the stimuli were presented in a spatially attended location. Enhanced activity with attention was observed in both areas, although the enhancement was substantially larger in V4. Notably, however, the stimulus

Figure 6.16 **Effects of attention on the tuning curves of single neurons** In this study of single-unit firing in visual area V4 in monkeys, spatial attention had no effect on the width or shape of the tuning curve (here, for line orientation), but rather enhanced responses to all stimulus orientations, consistent with a multiplicative scaling mechanism. (After McAdams and Maunsell 1999.)

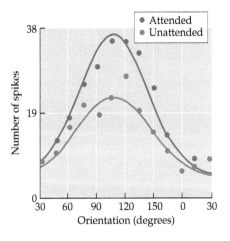

selectivity, as measured by the relative width of the orientation tuning curve, was not systematically altered by attention (Figure 6.16). That is, the modulatory effects of spatial attention consisted of a simple multiplicative scaling of the responses at all stimulus orientations (i.e., the response amplitudes at all stimulus orientations increased by the same multiplicative factor). Although a number of studies have shown attention effects with this multiplicative pattern, other studies have suggested that, under some circumstances, attention can sharpen the tuning of a neuron's responses (or the tuning across the neuronal population).

Another important effect shown at the neuronal level is that spatial attention increases *contrast sensitivity* (Figure 6.17). Specifically, in these studies visual stripes of different luminance values were presented inside the receptive field with different degrees of contrast while monkeys attended to a location either within the receptive field or outside of it. The largest increases in firing rate were in response to contrasts in the lower and middle portions of the dynamic range of the neuron, where amplification would be more useful. Moreover, attention increased the likelihood of eliciting a neuronal response near the contrast threshold level.

Other work has focused on the influence of attention on oscillatory electrical activity in the brain (i.e., neuroelectrical fields varying at a particular

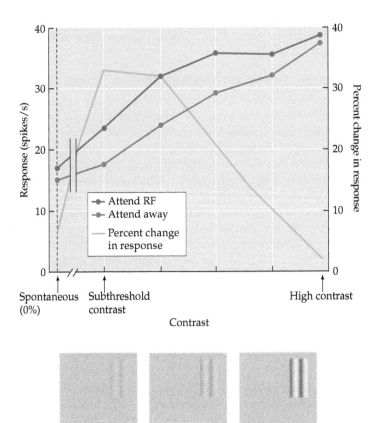

Figure 6.17 **Spatial attention increases the contrast sensitivity of V4 neurons** The influence of spatial attention on neuronal responses (spikes/s) in monkey V4 was plotted as a function of the contrast of the eliciting stimuli in the neuron's receptive field (RF). The monkey's task was to attend either to the location of the stimulus inside the RF or to a location outside the RF in order to detect target gratings at those locations. The visual contrast of the gratings was varied across a wide range (examples shown at bottom). The red trace shows the response to stimuli occurring in the RF when attention was directed to that location, and the blue trace shows the responses to those same stimuli occurring in the RF when attention was directed to a different location. The percent increase of the responses when attending within versus outside the RF is shown in the green trace. Spatial attention increased the neuronal responses, but proportionally more strongly at lower and middle contrast levels, where it would presumably be more useful. (After Reynolds et al. 2000.)

frequency or set of frequencies), and the mechanisms that such influences may reflect. In one such study, neuronal activity was recorded in V4 while monkeys directed their spatial attention to behaviorally relevant visual stimuli and ignored nearby distracters. Neurons sensitive to a particular stimulus showed increased synchronization of their action potential spiking with oscillatory activity in the gamma-band frequency range of the local field potentials (35 to 70 hertz)—that is, spiking during only certain phases of the field potentials—when the stimulus was attended relative to when it was not. Other studies have shown that behavioral responses are faster when there is strong gamma-band synchronization in the neurons activated by the relevant stimulus, and slower when there is strong gamma-band synchronization among the neurons sensitive to distracters, suggesting that these neural oscillatory effects are related to successful selection of the relevant stimulus.

Still other research has uncovered attention-related interactions between different frequency bands of the local field potentials in the sensory cortices (i.e., intracranial EEG). These interactions include those known as phase-amplitude coupling, wherein the amplitude of higher-frequency oscillations varies with the phase of lower-frequency oscillations (e.g., short bursts of high-frequency gamma-band waves that occur only during the peaks of ongoing lower-frequency oscillations, rather than at other phases of the lower-frequency waves). For example, recent studies have indicated that when stimuli in an attended stream of stimuli are presented with some temporal regularity, the lower-frequency oscillations of the local field potentials, along with the accompanying bursts of higher-frequency activity, tend to synchronize with the regularly occurring stimulus presentations. This synchronization seems to play a role in the selective attention process, perhaps by rhythmically aligning the excitability of the cortical neurons with the temporally predictable occurrences of the attended stimuli.

In sum, the results from single-unit and local field potential studies in experimental animals underscore the influence of visual spatial attention on the sensory processing of stimuli at low levels of the system, while at the same time providing important details about the characteristics of these effects at the neuronal and local circuit levels.

The effects of visual spatial attention on visual feature processing

As described earlier, the processing of auditory features in a spatially unattended channel (versus a spatially attended one) can be studied using the mismatch negativity (MMN) ERP as an index of low-level auditory sensory processing. In a similar way, the processing of the visual features of a stimulus occurring at an unattended visual location can also be examined using brain activity measures. Moreover, such processing in the unattended location can be studied as a function of the processing demands at the attended location. For instance, as described in Chapter 3, area MT+ in the lateral occipital lobe is a key brain region for processing the motion of visual stimuli. In a neuroimaging study that focused on fMRI activity in this brain region as a gauge, the perceptual load of a task in the center of the visual field was manipulated (easy versus hard task) while task-irrelevant moving stimuli were presented in the peripheral visual field (Figure 6.18). The key finding was that more activity was elicited in area MT+ by these task-irrelevant peripheral moving stimuli during the easy central-vision task compared to the difficult one.

This result was interpreted to mean that, when subjects had only an easy task to attend to in one spatial location (less **perceptual load**), more processing capacity was available for stimuli in unattended locations, leading to fuller processing of the stimulus features of those unattended-location stimuli (in this case, motion-related features). In contrast, when the task was more difficult, fewer resources were available for the concurrent peripheral stimuli, resulting

(A)

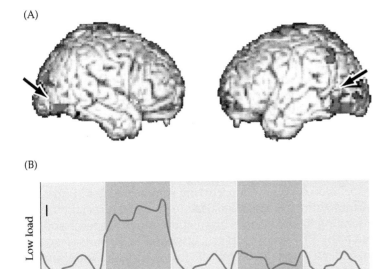

(B)

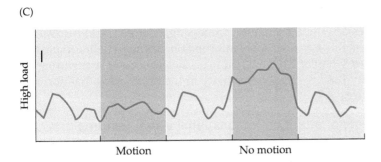

Figure 6.18 Effects of attention on visual feature processing at unattended locations In this fMRI study, subjects performed either an easy task (low load) or a difficult task (high load) in central vision while task-irrelevant motion stimuli either were or were not presented peripherally. (A) These functional images show the enhanced activity in motion-processing area MT+ (arrows) due to the irrelevant peripheral motion during the low-versus high-load central-task condition. (B,C) Time courses of the average activity levels in MT+ in the different load conditions show greater activity to the irrelevant peripheral motion during the low-load central task (B) and not during the high-load central task (C). The small black vertical bar on the left side of each graph indicates a 0.1 percent fMRI signal change. (After Rees et al. 1997.)

in less processing of the sensory features of those other stimuli. These results again underscore the capacity limitations for processing sensory stimuli and the role of attention in allocating those resources.

Neural Effects of Attending to Nonspatial Stimulus Attributes

The studies of attention effects on stimulus processing discussed so far have focused on paradigms in which attention is directed to different locations in visual space or to spatially segregated auditory input streams. However, attention can also be directed toward the nonspatial attributes of stimuli, such as the pitch of auditory stimuli, or the color or motion of visual stimuli.

The neural effects of attention to nonspatial auditory features

In audition, an obvious nonspatial quality that might be attended is pitch (see Chapter 4). Attending to this aspect of sound stimuli is biologically useful because pitch in vocalizations provides information about body size, gender, emotional state, and, in many languages, the meanings of words (see Chapter 12). By the same token, attending selectively to pitch can also be useful in discriminating auditory streams, either for speech sources or in other circumstances.

Studies of attention to auditory features such as pitch have been carried out using streams of auditory stimuli while brain activity is measured with ERPs. Instead of attending to stimuli in one ear or one spatial location, subjects attend to a stream of stimuli of a particular pitch (e.g., high tones in a randomly presented sequence of high and low tones) to detect an infrequent deviant sound in that stream (e.g., a slightly fainter high tone). The ERPs to the sounds are then compared on the basis of whether they were in the attended-pitch stream or not.

One effect of attention observed in this paradigm is a prolonged negative wave, often called a **processing negativity**, that begins somewhat after the N1 component, the sensory component at 100 milliseconds. Thus, the effects of feature-based auditory attention on stimulus processing generally start later than those observed in studies of spatial auditory attention, and they do not include an enhancement of the N1 sensory component or of the earlier P20–50 wave. They do seem, however, to reflect attentional enhancements of activity in the auditory association cortices, but occurring somewhat later in time.

Functional neuroimaging has also been used to study featural auditory attention, such as attending to tonal versus linguistic features of speech sounds. For example, in an early PET study, subjects attended to streams of speech sounds to perform either a phonetic comparison (comparing the vowels in two consonant-vowel-consonant nonwords) or a tonal comparison (comparing the pitches of the same stimuli). Whereas attending to the phonetic features activated left frontal and parietal areas associated with language processing, attending to the tonal aspects resulted in greater activity in right frontal regions (**Figure 6.19**). These results are in line with neuropsychological studies showing that left-hemisphere lesions impair semantic processing, whereas right-hemisphere lesions impair the ability to extract tonal information that helps define a speaker's emotional state (see Chapter 12). Thus, these results indicate that attending to a particular auditory feature enhances activity in the brain areas that normally process that feature.

The neural effects of attention to nonspatial visual features

The neural effects of attending to nonspatial features of visual stimuli have also been studied. For example, visual streams that differ in a single feature (e.g., red color versus blue) can be presented in random order at a single spatial

Figure 6.19 Effects of attention to auditory features These averaged PET subtraction images superimposed on averaged MRI horizontal slices at different inferior-superior levels in the brain show significant increases in focal cerebral blood flow between conditions. (A) Passive listening to noise minus a baseline condition of silence yielded significant activations bilaterally in Heschl's gyri. (B,C) Passive listening to speech minus passive listening to noise in these slices shows significant bilateral activation in the superior temporal gyrus anterior to Heschl's gyri (B), in the left inferior frontal cortex (B and C), and in the left posterior temporal area (C). (D,E) Phonetic task versus passive listening to speech in these slices shows activation increases in language-processsing regions (see Chapter 12) known as Broca's area in the left frontal lobe (D) and Wernicke's area within the left superior parietal lobe (E). (F) Pitch task versus passive listening to speech produced significant activity in the right prefrontal cortex. (From Zatorre et al. 1992.)

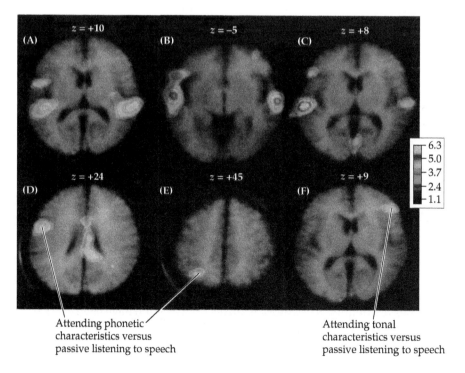

Attending phonetic characteristics versus passive listening to speech

Attending tonal characteristics versus passive listening to speech

(A) (B)

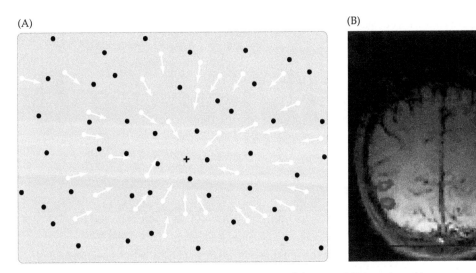

Figure 6.20   Effects of attention to a visual feature (A) In this fMRI study, subjects were presented with superimposed patterns of stationary dots and moving dots, and the task was to attend to either the stationary or the moving dot pattern. (B) Attending to the moving dot patterns enhanced activity in motion-processing area MT+. (From O'Craven et al. 1997.)

location, the task being to attend to only those stimuli with a certain feature (e.g., red) in order to detect occasional targets within that color series. ERPs elicited by the nontarget stimuli when they are attended can then be compared to the ERPs elicited by the same stimuli when a different color is attended. The hallmark of these feature attention effects is a sustained negative wave, often called a **selection negativity**, over posterior (parieto-occipital) scalp beginning about 150 milliseconds after the stimulus. Analogous to the *processing negativity* in auditory feature attention (see the previous section), this effect thus begins later than visual spatial attention effects, and it does not include an enhancement of the sensory-evoked P1 and N1 occipital components, the modulations of which appear to be specific for spatial attention.

Attention to nonspatial visual stimulus attributes has also been examined using functional neuroimaging. An early PET study by cognitive neuroscientist Maurizio Corbetta and colleagues in the early 1990s had subjects attend to the form, color, or motion of visual stimuli. Relative to a baseline condition, enhanced activity was seen in regions of visual cortex that corresponded to the feature selectively attended. That is, attending to the color of the stimuli enhanced activity in regions associated with color processing (V4), attending to the motion of the stimuli activated the motion-processing area MT+, and attending to the form of the stimuli activated lateral occipital areas associated with form processing (see Chapter 3). Studies using fMRI have extended these findings to a wide range of visual features and to higher spatial resolution (Figure 6.20). As in spatial attention studies in which attending to specific locations in the visual field enhanced activity in the regions of visual sensory cortex that represent that location in space, attention to stimulus features enhances activity in the regions of visual cortex that specifically process the feature being attended.

Single-unit recordings in monkeys have also contributed to understanding this aspect of attention. In an influential study of feature attention in monkeys, activity was recorded from single neurons in motion area MT+ while moving stimuli were occurring both within and outside the cell's receptive field (Figure 6.21). The key finding was that attending to motion occurring *outside* a cell's receptive field that had that cell's preferred motion direction increased the

(A)

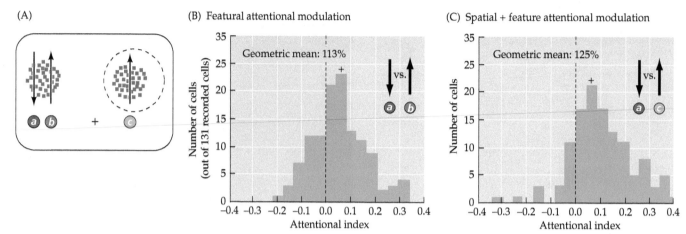

(B) Featural attentional modulation

(C) Spatial + feature attentional modulation

Figure 6.21 Feature attention in monkeys (A) The stimulus in the receptive field of the neuron that was recorded from (dashed circle) always moved in the cell's preferred direction (motion *c*), whereas the stimulus outside the field could move in either the same direction (*b*) or the opposite direction (*a*). Monkeys attended to either *a* or *b* motion in various spatial locations to detect changes in speed or direction. (B) Attending *outside* the receptive field to motion in the *preferred* versus the nonpreferred direction of the cell (*b* versus *a*, in this example) induced a higher firing rate in the cell, reflecting an increased response to the preferred-direction motion occurring within its receptive field, even though it was not task relevant and was not being attended. Specifically, the histogram categorizes 131 recorded cells as a function of an attentional index, for which positive values reflect increased responses when the attended stimulus moved in the preferred-motion direction of the cell. The histogram is shifted to the right, indicating an increased response when the attended stimulus outside the receptive field moved in the cell's preferred direction. (C) In addition, spatial attention–attending to a preferred stimulus *within* the receptive field versus attending to a nonpreferred stimulus outside the receptive field (*c* versus *a*)–shifts the histogram even farther to the right, reflecting additional enhancement of the firing rate. (After Treue and Martinez-Trujillo 1999.)

neuron's firing to task-irrelevant motion in the same direction occurring inside its receptive field, even though the motion inside the receptive field was task-irrelevant. This feature-based attention enhanced the amplitude of the tuning curve in a multiplicative way (simple enhancement of the responses), without affecting its width, similar to the effects described earlier for spatial attention.

Because of the similarity of these attentional effects in both spatial and feature-based attention, they were linked together in a framework termed the **feature similarity gain model**. In this model, the attentional modulation of the amplitude (i.e., the *gain*) of a sensory neuron's response depends on the similarity of the features of the currently relevant target and the feature preferences of that neuron. The results also suggested that neural representations of stimuli in parts of the visual field with no relevance to the task (but with feature similarity to the targets in an attended location) can be modulated by feature-based attention. Such influence of featural attention broadly across the visual field in turn suggests that this mechanism could be useful in **visual search** tasks (e.g., searching for a friend in a green sweater in one location will enhance sensitivity to green across the visual field).

The effects of visual attention to objects

Just as attention to stimulus features such as color, form, or motion modulates sensory processing in the regions of visual cortex that process those features, attention to objects modulates stimulus processing in the regions of visual cortex that specifically process objects as categorical entities. As described in Chapter 3 in the discussion of how different types of visual objects are processed, certain regions of higher-level visual cortex along the fusiform gyrus in the inferior occipital and temporal lobes are relatively specialized for processing faces, whereas a more medial and anterior temporal lobe area is relatively specialized for the processing of houses and buildings.

In an fMRI study of object-based attention, spatially overlapping, partially transparent faces and houses were presented, and attention was directed to the faces; as a result, activity increased in the face-sensitive areas of cortex (the fusiform face area [FFA] in ventral occipital cortex). Conversely, attending to the houses increased activity in a house-sensitive area. Note that spatially overlapping object stimuli were employed so that attention to location could not be used to separate the objects, thus allowing the effects to be validly attributed to object-based attention. Another fMRI study revealed that attending to faces in a series of face and scene images increased activity in the FFA relative to passive viewing, whereas ignoring the faces to attend to the scenes decreased activity in the FFA to a level below that of the activity during passive viewing (Figure 6.22). Such results suggest mechanisms involving both enhancement of activity for attended stimuli and suppression of activity for ignored stimuli.

Object-based attention has been investigated further in studies asking how attention increases the efficiency of information processing. For instance, in addition to causing increased neural firing rates (as mentioned already),

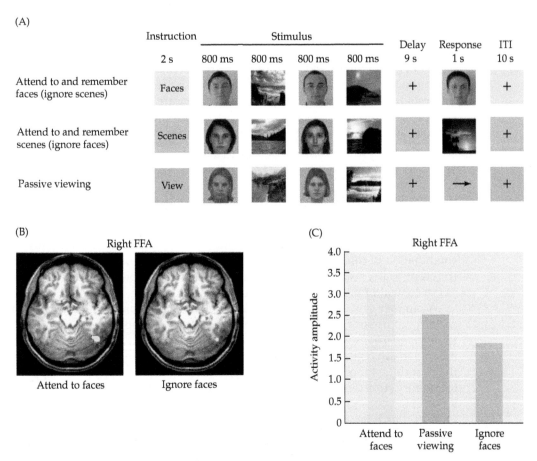

Figure 6.22 Attention to objects (A) Participants were presented with a series of images of faces and scenes, while they attended to the faces (in order to try to remember them later), attended to the scenes to remember those (and ignored the faces), or just passively viewed the stimuli. **(B,C)** Activity in the face-sensitive fusiform face area (FFA) in ventral occipital cortex was higher when attending to faces relative to just passively viewing stimuli, but lower than passive viewing when ignoring the faces. ITI = intertrial interval. (After Gazzaley et al. 2005.)

attention could increase the selectivity of the neural population representing an object stimulus. For example, it has been shown that a region of the lateral occipital lobe in humans is heavily involved in the analysis of visual objects. To further investigate these processes, researchers have used fMRI to measure the influence of attention on the selectivity in this region as a function of the angle at which an object is viewed. Attention to objects increased not only the neural responses overall in this region, but also their selectivity as a function of the viewing angle, suggesting that attention under these circumstances can increase the specificity of the neural population representing an attended object.

Single-unit studies in both monkeys and humans have suggested that some neurons can be particularly sensitive to certain objects and less sensitive to others. Moreover, attention to certain objects over others can specifically modulate the responses of those neurons. In one study recording single neurons in human patients, participants were provided with ongoing feedback as to the relative level of activity of these selectively sensitive neurons. By attending specifically to certain objects in the visual scene, in conjunction with this single-cell biofeedback, the participants were able to selectively enhance the activity of these neurons.

Object-based attention has also been studied in the context of how visual image features of an object are linked together into one unified percept. For example, in a combined MEG-fMRI study subjects attended to one of two superimposed transparent surfaces composed of dot arrays moving in opposite directions. When the surface moving in the attended direction displayed an irrelevant color feature change, neural activity within a color-selective region of visual cortex increased rapidly. Such an increase did not occur, however, when the irrelevant color change was in the unattended surface. This effect suggests that when certain features of an object are attended, the attentional enhancement tends to spread across the object's features to encompass the other features of the object, even if they are task-irrelevant.

Neural Effects of Attention across Sensory Modalities

Most studies of attention have been carried out within a single sensory modality. However, sensory stimuli arising from natural objects typically possess features in several sensory modalities. Thus, attention must be continually active in allocating resources to the stimulus information in the sensory modality or combination of modalities that are of particular importance at each moment. In recent years, studies have increasingly focused on how attention operates in the context of multisensory contexts and stimulation.

A number of studies have provided evidence for **supramodal attention** in certain circumstances, such as within the domain of spatial attention. The term *supramodal* refers to cognitive processes that are invoked jointly across modalities (in contrast to *modality-specific*, which refers to a cognitive process that is unique for one specific modality). Consider, for example, what happens to auditory stimulus processing when visual attention is directed to a particular location in space to facilitate the processing of visual stimuli presented there. ERP studies have shown that the sensory components elicited by auditory stimuli are enhanced when they occur in a visually attended location, even when they are task-irrelevant. Correspondingly, the sensory ERP responses to task-irrelevant visual stimuli are enhanced when they occur in a location being attended for auditory stimuli. Similar results have been observed between the visual and tactile modalities, as well as between tactile and auditory modalities.

Complementary studies using fMRI have indicated that these enhanced responses to stimuli in the task-irrelevant modality include increased activity at relatively low-level processing areas in the sensory cortices. The biological value of this supramodal linkage during spatial attention is easy to understand: if important stimuli pertinent to one modality are arising from a particular location, stimulus information from another modality arising from the same location is also likely to be important.

Other studies have investigated how attention can spread across modalities. Specifically, when stimuli from two different modalities occur close together in time, attention to the stimulus in one of the modalities will tend to spread to encompass the concurrently occurring stimulation in another modality. Moreover, this spread of attention appears to be related to the tendency of the brain to link together simultaneously occurring stimulation from different modalities into a multisensory object. Such multisensory spreading of attention parallels the within-vision findings, mentioned earlier, showing that attention to one feature of a multifeature visual object can spread across the visual object to enhance processing of the other features of that object. In the multisensory cases, the spreading of attention seems even able to spread across space to encompass concurrent stimulation in another modality arising from a different spatial location, which may be the basis of the ventriloquism phenomenon described in Chapter 3.

Finally, another influence of multisensory attention concerns the integration of sensory information from different modalities when an entire multisensory phenomenon is relevant and attended. In the real world, multisensory information needs to be integrated perceptually into more or less coherent wholes (e.g., a barking dog, a talking person, a bouncing ball). The predominant view until recently was that such **multisensory integration** is mostly preattentive and relatively automatic. However, recent studies indicate that most multisensory integration effects, including those that occur relatively early in processing and within low-level sensory cortices, are enhanced when the entire event or object is attended. In sum, attention has an extensive reach, affecting the neural processing of stimuli at multiple levels and in a variety of ways, including the integration of stimulus features that cross modality boundaries.

Summary

1. Attention is a vital cognitive function that plays a fundamental role in virtually everything we do. It was initially studied by cognitive psychologists using behavioral measures such as reaction time, discrimination accuracy, and the ability to report the content of attended versus unattended stimulus streams. This early work established that attention is limited in its capacity, confirming the intuition that it is difficult to attend to more than one thing at a time, and that when people are asked to do so, their performance deteriorates.

2. A major distinction in attention research has been between the ways that processing resources are induced to be directed toward locations or stimuli in the environment. Endogenous attention is the ability to voluntarily direct attention according to one's goals, expectations, or knowledge. Exogenous (or reflexive) attention consists of attention triggered by particularly salient stimuli in the environment. Both lead to enhanced processing of the location and/or stimuli toward which attention has been directed.

3. The ability to ascertain how, when, and where attention operates in the central nervous system is limited using behavioral measures alone. Understanding of both the psychological and the neural mechanisms of attention has been greatly advanced by combining behavioral approaches with cognitive neuroscience methods, including the direct recording of brain activity while humans or other animals are engaged in attentional tasks.

4. Electrophysiological studies in both humans and experimental animals have shown that the effects of auditory and visual *spatial* attention on stimulus processing can begin at the early cortical processing stages in the ascending sensory pathways—in humans as early as 20 milliseconds in audition and 70 milliseconds in vision, consistent with early selection theories of information processing. Corresponding neuroimaging studies have shown that spatial attention specifically

enhances stimulus processing activity in the sensory cortical areas that process the attended region of space.

5. Attention can also be directed toward *nonspatial* attributes of stimuli, such as their feature attributes (e.g., pitch or color) or object characteristics. Such nonspatial attention tends to influence stimulus processing activity somewhat later in time than does spatial attention. Like spatial attention, feature and object attention enhances stimulus-evoked activity in the sensory cortical regions specifically involved in the processing of that particular stimulus attribute.

6. Under some circumstances, such as during the attentional blink, attention influences stimulus processing only at later stages, involving higher levels of analysis in non-sensory cortical regions. More generally, attention effects can also occur at later phases of processing in a reentrant way, influencing stimulus-evoked activity in low-level sensory cortical regions, but at later stages of processing.

7. Single-unit studies in experimental animals have provided insight into the details of attentional effects on stimulus processing at the cellular level. Neurons fire at higher rates when the location of the stimulus in space is attended and/or the when stimulus attributes to which they are tuned are attended. Attention to a stimulus feature in one location tends to enhance the processing of that feature for all stimuli in the visual field.

8. Recent studies have increasingly focused on how attention operates in multisensory contexts, rather than just within a single sensory modality. A particularly key finding is that attention is important for facilitating the integration of stimulus information from several modalities into a multisensory perceptual whole.

Go to the **COMPANION WEBSITE**

sites.sinauer.com/cogneuro2e
for quizzes, animations, flashcards, and other study resources.

Additional Reading

Reviews

DESIMONE, R. AND J. DUNCAN (1995) Neural mechanisms of selective visual attention. *Annu. Rev. Neurosci.* 18: 193–222.

DRIVER, J. (2001) A selective review of selective attention research from the past century. *Br. J. Psychol.* 92: 53–78.

KASTNER, S. AND L. G. UNGERLEIDER (2000) Mechanisms of visual attention in the human cortex. *Annu. Rev. Neurosci.* 23: 315–341.

LUCK, S. J., G. F. WOODMAN AND E. K. VOGEL (2000) Event-related potential studies of attention. *Trends Cogn. Sci.* 4: 432–440.

MAUNSELL, J. H. R. AND S. TREUE (2006) Feature-based attention in visual cortex. *Trends Neurosci.* 29: 317–322.

SHAMMA, S. A., M. ELHILALI AND C. MICHEUYL (2011) Temporal coherence and attention in auditory scene analysis. *Trends Neurosci.* 34: 114–123.

TALSMA, D., D. SENKOWSKI, S. SOTO-FARACO AND M. G. WOLDORFF (2010) The multifaceted interplay between attention and multisensory integration. *Trends Cogn. Sci.* 14: 400–410.

Important Original Papers

BECK, D. M. AND S. KASTNER (2005) Stimulus context modulates competition in human extrastriate cortex. *Nat. Neurosci.* 8: 510–516.

CERF, M. AND 6 OTHERS (2010) On-line voluntary control of human temporal lobe neurons. *Nature* 467: 1104–1108.

CORBETTA, M., F. M. MIEZIN, S. DOBMEYER, G. L. SHULMAN AND S. E. PETERSEN (1991) Selective and divided attention during visual discriminations of shape, color, and speed: Functional anatomy by positron emission tomography. *J. Neurosci.* 5: 2383–2402.

DEUTSCH, J. A. AND D. DEUTSCH (1963) Attention: Some theoretical considerations. *Psychol. Rev.* 70: 80–90.

DE WEERD, P., M. R. PERALTA III, R. DESIMONE AND L. G. UNGERLEIDER (1999) Loss of attentional stimulus selection after extrastriate cortical lesions in macaques. *Nat. Neurosci.* 2: 753–758.

FRIES, P., J. H. REYNOLDS, A. E. RORIE AND R. DESIMONE (2001) Modulation of oscillatory neuronal synchronization by selective visual attention. *Science* 291: 1560–1563.

GAZZALEY, A., J. W. COONEY, K. McKEVOY, R. T. KNIGHT AND M. D'ESPOSITO (2005) Top-down enhancement and suppression of the magnitude and speed of neural activity. *J. Cogn. Neurosci.* 17: 507–517.

HEINZE, H. J. AND 11 OTHERS (1994) Combined spatial and temporal imaging of brain activity during visual selective attention in humans. *Nature* 372: 543–546.

HILLYARD, S. A., R. F. HINK, V. L. SCHWENT AND T. W. PICTON (1973) Electrical signs of selective attention in the human brain. *Science* 182: 177–180.

HOPFINGER, J. B., M. H. BUONOCORE AND G. R. MANGUN (2000) The neural mechanisms of top-down attentional control. *Nat. Neurosci.* 3: 284–291.

KASTNER, S., P. DE WEERD, R. DESIMONE AND L. G. UNGERLEIDER (1998) Mechanisms of directed attention in the human extrastriate cortex as revealed by functional MRI. *Science* 282: 108–151.

LAKATOS, P., G. KARMOS, A. D. MEHTA, I. ULBERT AND C. E. SCHROEDER (2008) Entrainment of neuronal oscillations as a mechanism for attentional selection. *Science* 320: 110–113.

LAVIE, N. (1995) Perceptual load as a necessary condition for selective attention. *J. Exp. Psychol. Hum. Percept. Perform.* 21: 451–468.

MACALUSO, E., C. D. FRITH AND J. DRIVER (2000) Modulation of human visual cortex by crossmodal spatial attention. *Science* 289: 1206–1208.

McADAMS, C. J. AND J. H. R. MAUNSELL (1999) Effects of attention on orientation-tuning functions of single neurons in macaque cortical area V4. *J. Neurosci.* 19: 431–441.

MORAN, J. AND R. DESIMONE (1985) Selective attention gates visual processing in the extrastriate cortex. *Science* 229: 782–784.

MOTTER, B. C. (1993) Focal attention produces spatially selective processing in visual cortical areas V1, V2, and V4 in the presence of competing stimuli. *J. Neurophysiol.* 70: 909–919.

O'CRAVEN, K. M., P. E. DOWNING AND N. KANWISHER (1999) fMRI evidence for objects as the units of attentional selection. *Nature* 401: 584–587.

PETKOV, C. I., X. KANG, K. ALHO, O. BERTRAND, E. W. YUND AND D. L. WOODS (2004) Attentional modulation of human auditory cortex. *Nat. Neurosci.* 7: 658–663.

POSNER, M. I., C. R. R. SNYDER AND B. J. DAVIDSON (1980) Attention and the detection of signals. *J. Exp. Psychol. Gen.* 59: 160–174.

REES, G., C. D. FRITH AND N. LAVIE (1997) Modulating irrelevant motion perception by varying attentional load in an unrelated task. *Science* 278: 1616–1619.

REYNOLDS, J. H. AND D. HEEGER (2009) The normalization model of attention. *Neuron* 61: 168–185.

REYNOLDS, J. H., T. PASTERNAK AND R. DESIMONE (2000) Attention increases sensitivity of V4 neurons. *Neuron* 26: 703–714.

SAENZ, M., G. T. BURACAS AND G. M. BOYNTON (2002) Global effects of feature-based attention in human visual cortex. *Nat. Neurosci.* 5: 631–632.

SCHOENFELD, M. A. AND 6 OTHERS (2003) Dynamics of feature binding during object-selective attention. *Proc. Natl. Acad. Sci. USA* 100: 11806–11811.

TOOTELL, R. B. AND 6 OTHERS (1998) The retinotopy of visual spatial attention. *Neuron* 21: 1409–1422.

TREISMAN, A. (1960) Contextual cues in selective listening. *Q. J. Exp. Psychol.* 12: 242–248.

TREUE, S. AND J. C. MARTINEZ TRUJILLO (1999) Feature-based attention influences motion processing gain in macaque visual cortex. *Nature* 399: 575–579.

WOLDORFF, M. G., S. A. HACKLEY AND S. A. HILLYARD (1991) The effects of channel-selective attention on the mismatch negativity wave elicited by deviant tones. *Psychophysiology* 28: 30–42.

WOLDORFF, M. G. AND 6 OTHERS (1993) Modulation of early sensory processing in human auditory cortex during auditory selective attention. *Proc. Natl. Acad. Sci. USA* 90: 8722–8726.

YANTIS, S. AND J. JONIDES (1990) Abrupt visual onsets and selective attention: Voluntary versus automatic allocation. *J. Exp. Psychol. Hum. Percept. Perform.* 16: 121–134.

ZATORRE, R. J., A. C. EVANS, E. MEYER AND A. GJEDDE (1992) Lateralization of phonetic and pitch discrimination in speech processing. *Science* 256: 846–849.

Books

HUMPHREYS, G., J. DUNCAN AND A. TREISMAN, EDS. (1999) *Attention, Space and Action: Studies in Cognitive Neuroscience.* Oxford: Oxford University Press.

NÄÄTÄNEN, R. (1992) *Attention and Brain Function.* Hillsdale, NJ: Erlbaum.

PARASURAMAN, R., ED. (1998) *The Attentive Brain.* Cambridge, MA: MIT Press.

POSNER, M. I. (1978) *Chronometric Explorations of Mind.* Hillsdale, NJ: Erlbaum.

WRIGHT, R. D. AND L. M. WARD (2008) *Orienting of Attention.* New York: Oxford University Press.

7

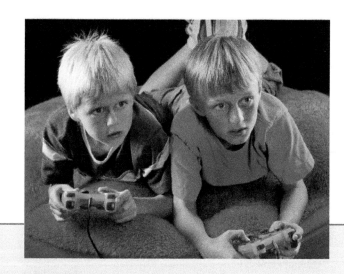

The Control of Attention

INTRODUCTION

In the previous chapter we introduced the idea that the cognitive systems view of attention can be translated into a neuroscience framework as shown schematically in Figure 6.5. We also noted that, within this framework, the study of attention can be approached from two major perspectives: (1) investigating the ways in which stimulus processing is modulated by attention in different circumstances; and (2) determining the sets of higher-level regions of the brain that control and coordinate this modulation, and the mechanisms by which they do so. Chapter 6 focused on the first of these perspectives, describing studies of how attention affects the processing of sensory stimuli, both neurally and behaviorally. The present chapter focuses on the processes and mechanisms by which these modulatory effects on stimulus processing are controlled, examining in particular the evidence for an overarching system or set of systems that allocates and coordinates attention generally.

As with most other cognitive functions, the relevant insights into the control of attention have come from complementary clinical and basic research, using a variety of methods. The findings from clinical observations suggest a preeminent role of regions of the parietal and frontal cortices in attentional control. Monitoring brain activity in normal subjects and in animals carrying out attentional tasks has confirmed the importance of these regions in attentional control and provided insight into how such control is exercised. These findings have led in turn to the development of models of attentional control that propose modulation by networks of interacting brain areas. Further experiments testing the interactions between brain areas predicted by these models have supported these general ideas. Finally, the relation of attention and attentional control to the overall level of brain activity and mental alertness leads naturally to the difficult issue of the neural basis of consciousness, which is also discussed in this chapter.

■ INTRODUCTORY BOX HEMISPATIAL NEGLECT SYNDROME

A relatively common brain lesion that results in striking attentional deficits arises from damage to the right inferior parietal lobe (Figure A), most often because of a stroke. Such lesions, first described in the 1940s by the British neurologist Russell Brain, cause deficits in spatial attention to the left side of personal and extrapersonal space (i.e., the side contralateral to the lesion). The most obvious characteristic of patients with right parietal lesions is that they tend to ignore stimuli in their left visual field. For example, a patient with such a **hemispatial neglect** syndrome may fail to notice another person approaching from the left, but will notice when someone approaches from the right. Similarly, when shown a picture with three horizontally aligned objects (on the left, middle, and right) and asked what objects they see, such patients typically fail to report the object on the left.

Depending on the extent and severity of the lesion, when an object in the left visual field is specifically pointed out, patients then tend to report being able to see it. Thus, the impairments in hemispatial neglect syndrome are quite different from the visual deficit that follows a lesion in the visual cortex (see Chapter 3). Patients with visual cortical lesions are effectively blind in specific corresponding parts of the contralateral visual field (the blind area of the visual field is called a *scotoma*). In contrast, the underlying problem in neglect syndrome appears to be an attentional deficit, not a sensory deficit; the patients can apparently *see* stimuli in the left visual field, but they tend not to notice them or be able to orient their attention to them effectively.

The left-sided neglect evident in these patients can be demonstrated clinically by one of several simple tests. In the single-line bisection test (Figure B), patients are asked to mark the center of

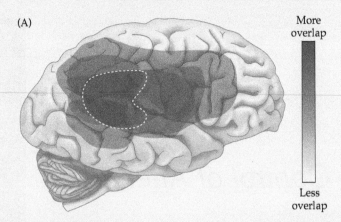

(A)

More overlap

Less overlap

Left hemispatial neglect syndrome lesions. This composite diagram shows the distribution of right-hemisphere damage in eight patients with left hemispatial neglect. The degree of overlap of damaged brain areas across patients is indicated by shading level. Although some of the lesions include parietal and frontal lobes, as well as parts of the temporal lobe, the region most commonly affected is in the right inferior parietal lobe (dashed line). Clinical tests of left hemispatial neglect caused by damage to the right inferior parietal lobe. The performance in the single-line bisection test (B) and the line cancellation test (C) shown here is characteristic of neglect patients. (D) An example of a visual copying task as performed by a hemineglect syndrome patient. (E) A clock face drawn from memory by a neglect patient. (A after Heilman and Valenstein 1985; B,D from Posner and Raichle 1994; C from Blumenfeld 2010; E from Grabowecky et al. 1993.)

a horizontal line. Patients with neglect tend to discount the left side of the line, and thus their estimate of the center is displaced to the right. In the line cancellation test (Figure C), the patient is asked to draw a line through each of a number of lines scattered across a page; in this test, patients cancel lines mainly on the right-hand side of the page. In addition, the left-sided neglect is not limited to ignoring objects in their left hemispace; patients with this syndrome also tend to ignore the left sides of objects *wherever* they are in visual space. For example, if asked to draw a copy of an object, these patients tend to draw only its right side (Figure D). Such patients even tend to

ignore the left side of their visual imagery and memory. So, if asked to draw a clock from memory, they are likely to draw half a clock, sometimes remembering to include all 12 numbers in the drawing, but placing all of the numbers to the right (Figure E).

More detailed behavioral assessments of hemispatial neglect elicit what is referred to as *extinction*. This phenomenon is revealed when a neurologist stands in front of the patient with arms outstretched and moves a finger on either the right or the left hand. If a finger on either side is moved by itself, the patient generally reports the presence of the moving finger correctly, presumably

Clinical Evidence for Brain Regions Involved in Attentional Control

Well before the advent of modern techniques that directly measure brain activity during attentional tasks, clinical data from patients showed that when certain areas in the parietal and frontal cortices are damaged, the ability to direct attention is markedly compromised. As described in the Introductory Box, the most common lesion that results in attentional deficits arises from damage to the right inferior parietal lobe. As noted, damage to this region causes striking

■ INTRODUCTORY BOX (continued)

(B) "Bisect the line"

(C) "Cancel the lines"

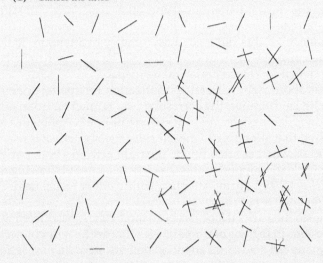

(D) "Copy this picture of a house"

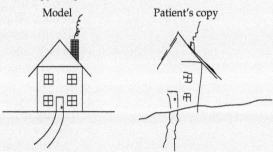

Model Patient's copy

(E) "Draw a clock"

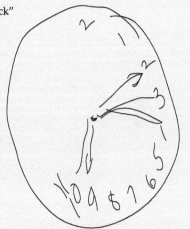

because a moving stimulus is a particularly strong attractor of attention, even for these patients. If both fingers are moved at the same time, however, the patient typically reports seeing only the one on the right. This test suggests that the normal competition between the stimulus inputs from the two sides is now dominated by the right visual field, which "extinguishes" the input from the left. Extinction emphasizes again that the underlying problem is an attentional deficit, not a sensory deficit.

Although attentional neglect is typically most obvious in vision, the deficit can also be observed in other sensory modalities. For example, many patients seem to be less aware of the left side of their own bodies. This deficit is reflected by the tendency of such patients to shave or apply makeup on only the right side of their face, or to be concerned about aspects of their clothes only on the right side of their body. Thus, the attentional deficits in hemispatial parietal neglect syndrome appear to involve **supramodal** attentional mechanisms (see Chapter 6). The breadth of the attentional deficits caused by damage to the parietal lobe indicates that this brain region plays a critical role in the control and allocation of attention.

References

BLUMENFELD, H. (2010) *Neuroanatomy through Clinical Cases*, 2nd Ed. Sunderland, MA: Sinauer.

GRABOWECKY, M., L. C. ROBERTSON AND A. TREISMAN (1993) Preattentive processes guide visual search: Evidence from patients with unilateral visual neglect. *J. Cogn. Neurosci.* 5: 288–302.

HEILMAN, H. AND E. VALENSTEIN (1985) *Clinical Neuropsychology*, 2nd Ed. New York: Oxford University Press.

POSNER, M. I. AND M. E. RAICHLE (1994) *Images of Mind*. New York: Scientific American Library.

deficits in spatial attention to the left side of space (the side contralateral to the lesion), with effects evident across sensory modalities. Although left parietal lesions can lead to right-sided versions of these effects, they tend to be milder and more subtle.

This pattern of clinical findings implies that the parietal cortex, particularly on the right, is involved in attentional control. An obvious question, then, is why the neglect exhibited in such patients is generally limited to lesions of the right parietal lobe. One theory holds that the right parietal lobe specifically controls attention to both left and right sides of space, whereas the left parietal lobe controls attention mainly to the right. If so, then attention to the right side of personal or extrapersonal space would be controlled by both parietal lobes, whereas attention to the left would be controlled primarily by the right parietal lobe. This asymmetry would explain why loss of function in the right parietal lobe, but not generally the left, results in an asymmetrical pattern of attentional deficits. Another possible reason for this right-hemispheric asymmetry in humans for spatial attention is the evolutionary development of hemispheric specialization, with the left hemisphere becoming more specialized for language (see Chapter 12) and the right for attentional and other functions. Consistent with this view, non-human primates, which have very limited language function, show little evidence for this right-sided asymmetry of attention. Rather, damage in non-human primates to the inferior parietal lobe in either hemisphere causes an orienting deficit for the contralateral hemispace.

While these ideas about right parietal specialization for spatial attention would explain the clinical findings, the corresponding human neuroimaging results in normal individuals have been equivocal on this point. Although a few studies have suggested that attending to the left side of space activates mainly the right parietal cortex, whereas attending to the right activates both parietal cortices, most have not clearly supported this dissociation, instead showing that both hemispheres are activated during attention within either visual field. The reason for this discrepancy is not clear.

Although damage to the parietal lobe has been most clearly associated with neglect syndrome, lesions in regions of frontal cortex that are heavily connected with the parietal regions can also cause attention deficits. In particular, lesions to the frontal eye fields disrupt the ability both to initiate eye movements toward targets in the visual field opposite the lesion, and to direct attention toward that side. As a general rule, unilateral frontal lesions tend to have a greater effect on the more overt aspects of attention, such as the ability to direct eye movements toward the contralateral hemispace.

Another brain lesion that has striking effects on attention is bilateral damage to the dorsal posterior parietal and lateral occipital cortex, leading to a disorder known as **Balint's syndrome** (Figure 7.1). Damage of this sort, however, presents quite a different clinical picture and an even more debilitating deficit. First characterized by the Hungarian physician Rezso Balint, the signature of

Figure 7.1 Balint's syndrome lesions The lesion in Balint's syndrome is typically located in posterior parietal and lateral occipital cortex bilaterally. (From Friedman-Hill et al. 1995.)

Lateral views

Occipital view

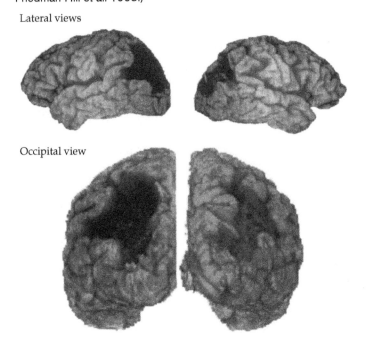

Coronal MRI

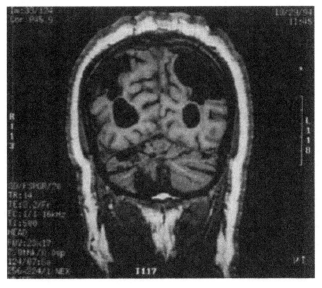

(A) "How many colors do you see?"

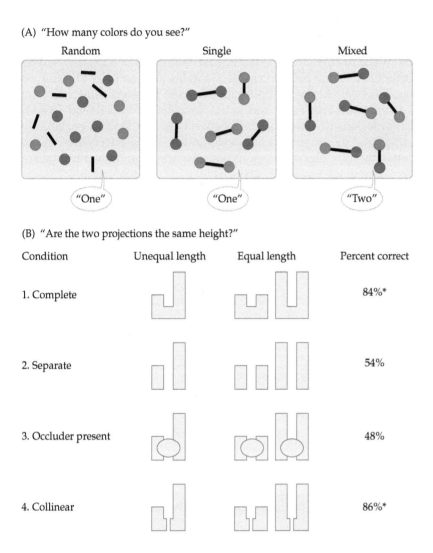

Figure 7.2 Simultanagnosia in Balint's syndrome (A) The inability of patients with Balint's syndrome to perceive or attend to more than one object at a time prevents them from noticing more than one color in the displays shown in the left and middle panels. If the blue and red circles are connected to form single objects (right panel), however, the patients are able to report both colors, indicating that the deficit lies in the inability to attend to multiple objects rather than in a failure to attend to multiple qualities. (B) Similarly, when patients are asked to compare the lengths of two nearby rectangles, their performance is near chance (50 percent correct) if the objects are separated, but they perform much better if the components are connected as part of the same object. The asterisk denotes performance statistically better than chance. (A after Humphreys and Riddoch 1993; B after Cooper and Humphreys 2000.)

this syndrome is threefold: (1) *simultanagnosia*, the inability to attend to and/or perceive more than one visual object at a time; (2) *optic ataxia*, the impaired ability to reach for or point to an object in space under visual guidance; and (3) *oculomotor apraxia*, difficulty voluntarily directing the eye gaze toward objects in the visual field with a saccade.

Simultanagnosia is the deficit most closely associated with Balint's syndrome. With this symptom, if a neurologist holds up two different objects and asks patients what they see, they report seeing only one object or the other but not both, even if the objects are right next to each other. In contrast to hemispatial neglect syndrome, with Balint's syndrome the relative positions of the objects within the patient's visual field do not matter. If the unseen object is jiggled to attract attention, patients will then say they see it, but they will have lost the perception of the first object. Moreover, when patients with Balint's syndrome are presented with an array of randomly distributed objects, half of which are of one color and half of another color, they report seeing just one color or the other, but not both (Figure 7.2A, left and middle). But if the differently colored items are attached so that each object contains both colors, patients then report seeing both colors in the array (Figure 7.2A, right). Similarly, these patients have trouble perceiving and comparing the lengths of two nearby rectangular bars unless they are connected as parts of the same overall object (Figure 7.2B). Thus, patients with Balint's syndrome can attend to more than one stimulus quality or stimulus part, but only when the parts are embodied in the same object.

Lesions in the brainstem can also impair attentional control. When the superior colliculus, which plays a critical role in the generation of saccadic eye movements, has been damaged, both monkeys and humans show a slowing of saccade latency to a target stimulus in the contralateral visual field. In addition, collicular lesions slow the shifting of covert visual attention, particularly attention triggered by exogenous or novel stimuli. These effects are thought to be mediated by collicular interactions with the attention-related frontal and parietal cortical regions already discussed.

Such collicular-cortical interactions are apparent in the so-called *Sprague effect*, in which the hemispatial neglect induced by a parietal lesion in humans can be mostly nullified by a lesion of the superior colliculus on the other side. The proposed explanation is that the parietal lesion–induced neglect is not from the cortical damage itself, but from the lesion causing an imbalance of activity between the two parietal lobes in attentional control. According to this theory, a lesion of the contralateral colliculus helps to restore the appropriate balance, because of its connectivity to the parietal lobe on the same side. Regardless, this effect underscores a role of the superior colliculus in attentional control, including via functional interactions with attentional control regions in the cortex.

Control of Voluntary Attention

The clinical observations described in the previous section imply that the cortical deficits from damage to parietal and frontal regions are related to attentional control rather than to sensory processing. Accordingly, tasks involving attentional orienting and control in normal subjects would be expected to elicit changes in neural activity in these areas. Both imaging and electrophysiological studies have shown that this is indeed the case.

Activation in frontal and parietal cortex during endogenous attentional tasks

One of the first functional neuroimaging studies that specifically investigated the voluntary orienting of attention was a PET experiment carried out in the early 1990s by cognitive neuroscientist Maurizio Corbetta and colleagues. Subjects were required to switch attention repeatedly from one location to another in either the left or the right visual field to detect a target. Relative to a baseline task in which attention was maintained but not switched, the attentional shifting elicited enhanced activity in regions of posterior parietal and superior frontal cortex. Other studies confirmed that tasks that involve the voluntary orienting of attention (relative to baseline tasks that do not) typically increase activation in regions of a frontoparietal network, as well as regions of the insular cortex and the anterior cingulate cortex. These findings thus support the view that these regions play a role in attentional control.

Delineating the role of the frontoparietal network in the control of attention

A major limitation of the early neuroimaging studies examining attentional control derives from their dependence on a blocked design (see Chapter 2)—here, in particular, comparing blocks of trials in which participants are performing an attentional task to blocks of trials in which they are not. A more definitive approach for isolating brain activity related to attentional control is to use attentional cuing paradigms in conjunction with event-related recordings of the brain activity. As discussed in Chapter 6, the classic cuing paradigm for studying voluntary attention contains an instructional cue (e.g., an arrow pointing to the left or the right), followed shortly after by a target stimulus (see Figure 6.3). Most of the time (typically about 75 percent), the target occurs at the cued location, but sometimes it occurs at the uncued one.

Behavioral studies using this paradigm have shown that targets at the cued versus the uncued location are detected faster and more accurately, and neurophysiological studies have demonstrated corresponding enhancements of sensory responses. An advantage of the cuing paradigm for studying the neural mechanisms underlying attentional control is that it separates the point in time at which subjects are instructed by the cue to direct their attention to a specific spatial location or sensory feature from the point in time at which the target stimulus occurs (and thus when the allocation of attention may affect processing of the target). If the brain responses elicited by the attention-directing cue can be separated from those associated with the processing of the target, it should be possible to differentiate the neural activity related to attentional control from other processes.

Using fMRI to study cued attention in this way initially proved challenging, however, because the sluggishness of the BOLD fMRI response (described in Chapter 2) results in substantial overlap of cue- and target-related activity when these events occur in close succession. One way that fMRI researchers got around this problem was simply to slow down the entire cued-attention task. For example, in an early study using this approach, subjects were cued with a centrally presented arrow to attend to either the left or the right side of a computer screen for an upcoming bilateral target display. To address the overlap of the cue and target fMRI responses, most trials had a rather long cue-target interval (about 9 seconds) and the research focused on only those trials, which allowed investigators to extract and compare the event-related fMRI responses to the cues and to the targets. Such studies found cue-triggered responses in the dorsolateral prefrontal cortex, inferior parietal cortex, and medial frontal cortex (Figure 7.3).

Although such slow-rate event-related fMRI studies enable the separation of cue-related and target-related processing, the slow rate introduces some other limitations (e.g., subjects not orienting very fully, the invocation of extensive working memory processes, subject boredom). More advanced methods have since been developed that allow separate extractions of cue- and target-related activity at somewhat shorter cue-target intervals (typically about 2 to 3 seconds). These studies have confirmed the presence of cue-triggered effects in the frontal and parietal cortices under these circumstances, while more finely delineating the brain areas associated with attentional control.

Other event-related approaches have further characterized the functional roles of different portions of the fronto-parietal network and neighboring regions. In one study, for

(A) Responses to instructional cues

Attend left 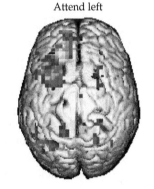 Attend right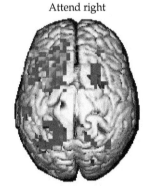

(B) Responses to targets

Attend left 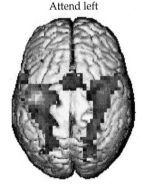 Attend right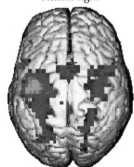

Figure 7.3 Dissociation of cue- and target-triggered responses in a slow-rate, cued spatial-attention paradigm Subjects in this fMRI study were presented with central cues instructing them to attend to a location in the left or the right visual field to discriminate a target stimulus that would follow. On most trials, the cue-target interval was about 9 seconds, thus reducing the overlap of the cue and target event-related fMRI responses and allowing the responses to be separately extracted and compared. (From Hopfinger et al. 2000.)

Figure 7.4 Nonspatial switching of attention activates medial parietal regions Subjects in fMRI studies were presented with two spatially overlapping streams of stimuli while they attended to one stream or the other. Cuing stimuli embedded in the stream indicated a switch point at which the subject either continued to attend to that stream ("stay") or switched to attend to the other stream ("switch"), depending on the embedded cue. In (A), subjects switched attention between features (color attribute versus motion attribute). In (B), subjects switched attention between object categories (faces versus houses). (A from Liu et al. 2003; B from Serences et al. 2004.)

(A) Switching attention between different visual features (switch versus stay)

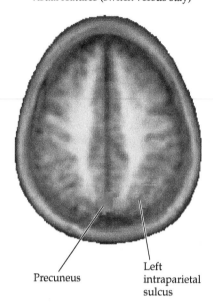

Precuneus   Left intraparietal sulcus

(B) Switching attention between different object categories (switch versus stay)

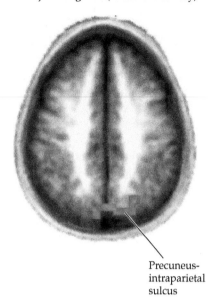

Precuneus-intraparietal sulcus

example, subjects were asked to attend to one of two rapidly presented streams of stimuli on the left and right of fixation, and the occurrence of specific cues within the attended stream signaled the subjects either to switch attention to the other stream or to stay and continue attending to the same stream. A comparison of the event-related fMRI responses to "switch" versus "stay" cues activated regions in the parietal portions of the frontoparietal network, although with relatively little contribution from the frontal regions compared to the central-cuing experiments already described. The reason for the reduced frontal activity may be that both the switch and the stay conditions involve a new deployment of attention that invokes frontal activity, which would thus be subtracted out in the comparison.

Studies using these sorts of switch and stay paradigms have also been used to study nonspatial attention. These studies have shown that parietal regions are also activated when switching attention between two types of visual features (color attributes versus motion attributes) or between two types of visual objects (faces versus houses; Figure 7.4). With nonspatial attentional switches, however, the switch-specific parietal activations tend to be somewhat closer to the midline than with switches of visual spatial attention, suggesting a possible subregion specificity of these parietal areas for different types of attentional control.

Ascertaining the temporal flow of brain activations underlying attentional control

The sluggishness of the fMRI signal means that this technique provides little information about the timing and sequence of the activations of regions involved in attentional control. To investigate the temporal characteristics of activity in these components, some recent studies have combined data from parallel ERP and fMRI studies using identical visual spatial attentional cuing paradigms. In addition, some such studies have included additional control trials, such as those beginning with cues that instructed subjects *not* to shift attention on that trial, so that the activity specific for attentional orienting could be more specifically delineated.

As shown in Figure 7.5A, the ERPs indicate that the attention-directing cues and the control cues elicit similar activity in the first 350 milliseconds,

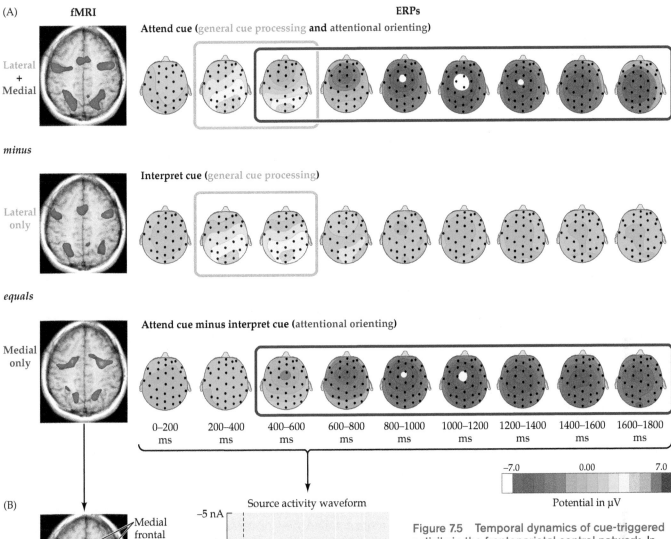

Figure 7.5 Temporal dynamics of cue-triggered activity in the frontoparietal control network In this combined fMRI-ERP study, subjects were given either a centrally presented instructional cue to shift attention to the left or right ("attend cue") to detect a possible upcoming target there, or a control cue indicating that no shift of attention was required on that trial ("interpret cue"). (A) In the fMRI study, a contrast between the interpret-cue responses (second row) and the attend-cue responses (first row) revealed that the more medial portions of the frontoparietal cortex were specifically involved in attentional orienting, and the more lateral areas with general cue processing. Corresponding contrasts of the ERP data show that attend-cue and interpret-cue instructions elicited similar general cue-processing activity in the first 350 milliseconds, followed by a sustained negative wave over frontal, central, and parietal scalp lasting hundreds of milliseconds that was associated with attend cues only. μV = microvolts. (B) Using the fMRI activations to facilitate the analyses, source modeling of the ERP orienting-specific control activity showed that the frontal regions of the medial orienting network were activated 200–300 milliseconds earlier than the parietal regions. nA = nanoamperes. (After Woldorff et al. 2004; Grent-'t-Jong and Woldorff 2007.)

presumably reflecting general processing and interpretation of the cue, which the parallel fMRI data showed to be associated with the more lateral portions of the frontoparietal network. Subsequently, however, the attention-directing cues (but not the control cues) elicited a sustained, orienting-specific negative-polarity ERP wave that was linked to fMRI activity in the more medial portions of the frontoparietal network, including the frontal eye fields and intraparietal sulcus. Moreover, analyses of this orienting-specific activity indicated an earlier contribution from these frontal regions than from the parietal ones (Figure 7.5B). The initiation of the orienting-specific activity by the frontal regions during voluntarily directed (endogenous) attention is consistent with a role proposed more generally for the

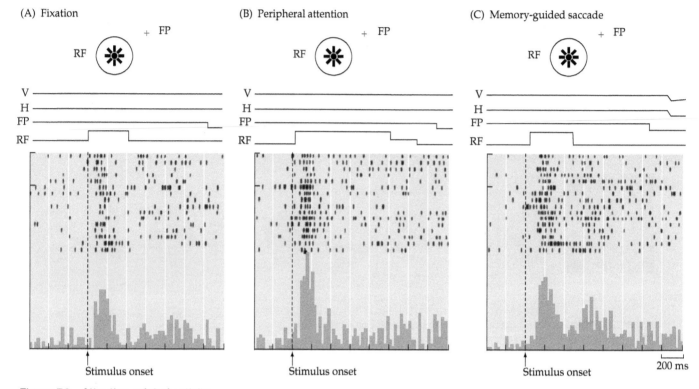

(A) Fixation

(B) Peripheral attention

(C) Memory-guided saccade

Stimulus onset

Stimulus onset

Stimulus onset

200 ms

Figure 7.6 Attention-related activity in parietal neurons In this study, an electrode was placed in the lateral intraparietal (LIP) area of a macaque monkey and used to record action potentials from single neurons, shown here as peristimulus histograms aligned with stimulus onset (see Figure 2.5). (A) Neuronal firing was recorded in response to a stimulus occurring in the receptive field of the neuron while the monkey was engaged in a fixation task. (B) Covertly attending to the stimulus resulted in an increase in the firing rate of the neuron in response to the stimulus occurrence relative to the rate in the fixation task. (C) When the monkey needed to respond to the target by making a delayed saccade to the target location according to memory of that location, there was an additional increase in firing rate just before the saccade. FP, fixation point; H, horizontal eye channel; RF, receptive field; V, vertical eye channel. (After Colby et al. 1996.)

frontal cortex of keeping track of task goals and controlling and coordinating other regions to help accomplish those goals (see Chapter 13).

Single-neuron recordings in frontal and parietal cortex during attentional control

Single-unit recordings in frontal and parietal areas in non-human primates have provided a more detailed view of attentional control processes at the neuronal level. A number of electrophysiological studies of attention in monkeys have focused on recordings from neurons in a region of the posterior parietal cortex called the lateral intraparietal (LIP) area (located in the intraparietal sulcus, IPS) and in the frontal eye fields in the dorsal frontal cortex. These two regions in the monkey appear to roughly correspond functionally to the parietal and frontal areas in humans where neuroimaging studies have shown activity related to attentional control.

Neuronal firing patterns in LIP have implicated this region in planning an eye movement (saccade) to a relevant target in the visual field, as well as in the covert focusing of attention toward that location (Figure 7.6). For example, the firing rates of some LIP neurons to a stimulus in their receptive field is greater when the monkey is required to make a saccade to a target location rather than to just fixate on the center of the screen. Moreover, the stimulation of neurons in LIP can trigger eye movements to a location in the contralateral visual field. The response of LIP neurons is also enhanced, however, when the monkey attends to the stimulus but does not move its eyes toward it, or when the task requires delaying the saccade to the target location. These results have been interpreted to mean that the enhancement is not due to saccade generation per se, but rather to the allocation of attention to the spatial location of the target in the neuron's receptive field.

Similar increases of neuronal activity occur in LIP during fixation tasks in which the monkey can predict the onset and location of a behaviorally significant stimulus; these increased levels of background firing during the period before stimulus onset are analogous to the activity triggered by attention-directing cues in the human neuroimaging described in previous sections. Thus, the activity of LIP neurons is modulated by factors that are associated not with sensory processing or motor planning, but rather with attentional or other cognitive factors.

Other studies have suggested that stimulus *salience* (i.e., how much a stimulus stands out from its surroundings) is a key determinant of this enhanced activity observed in LIP neurons. The salience could derive from stimulus-driven factors (e.g., the sudden onset of a stimulus) or relevance to a specific behavioral goal. Indeed, it has been suggested that the LIP may have a topographically organized salience map of the environment that is influenced by both stimulus-driven and endogenous factors.

The frontal eye fields (FEF), the area in the dorsal frontal cortex shown in human neuroimaging studies to be involved in attentional control, as described earlier, are also known to be involved in the control of saccadic eye movements. For example, microstimulation of specific regions in the FEF in monkeys triggers saccades to specific locations (called *saccade movement fields*) in the contralateral visual field. The combination of saccade-related activity and attentional control activity in the FEF has contributed to the development of the **premotor theory of attention**, which posits that shifts of attention and preparation of goal-directed action are closely linked because they are controlled by shared sensory-motor mechanisms. Moreover, the premotor theory claims more specifically that the saccade-related circuitry mediates covert visual spatial attention.

Nonetheless, the neurons in FEF may have attentional control functions that are distinguishable from saccade-planning processes. For example, like LIP neurons, recordings in FEF show enhanced activity not only when the monkey is about to make a saccade to a neuron's saccade movement field, but also when an attended or otherwise relevant target stimulus appears at that location. Moreover, both visually responsive neurons and saccade-related movement neurons have been found in the FEF, and the activity of these neurons has been examined during tasks in which the response is a lever press rather than a saccade. The results indicate that when attention is allocated to a visual target under these circumstances, enhanced activity is observed in the visually responsive neurons, but not in the saccade-related neurons (**Figure 7.7**). Such observations imply that FEF neurons give rise to attentional control signals that are independent of explicit saccade command or saccade preparation activity from the same brain region.

Some recent studies have also investigated the timing of the single-unit neuronal responses in the frontal and parietal regions. For example, in a study directly examining the coordination of attentional control (**Figure 7.8**), neuronal signals were recorded from both prefrontal and parietal regions simultaneously while monkeys were engaged in several different visual tasks, one of which induced attentional shifts

Figure 7.7 Attention-related activity in frontal eye field neurons Average activity from FEF neurons was recorded during search tasks involving a manual response. (A) Neuronal activity aligned with the time of the search array presentation. (B) The same data aligned with the time of the manual lever response. The responses of target-selective visually responsive neurons and the responses of movement (i.e., saccade-related) neurons are shown separately. Orange lines plot the average activity on trials in which the target landed in the response field; purple lines, the activity on trials in which only distracters landed in the response field. For the visually responsive neurons there was a clear target-related effect; for the movement neurons, however, the target-related and distracter-related activity levels were nearly identical. (After Thompson et al. 2005.)

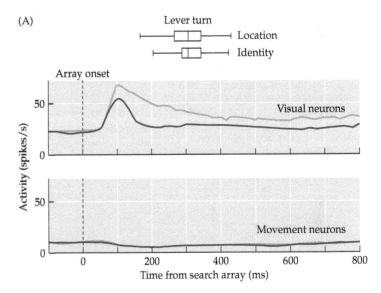

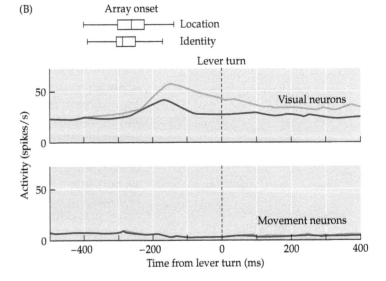

Figure 7.8 Temporal sequence of single-unit activity in frontal and parietal attentional control regions (A) Monkeys were trained to perform a match-to-sample task, in which they were rewarded for making a saccade to the target, while single-unit neuronal activity was recorded concurrently from both frontal and parietal attentional control regions: lateral prefrontal cortex (LPFC); frontal eye fields (FEF), and lateral intraparietal area (LIP). In one condition, the targets were different enough from the distracters that the target could be identified quickly by bottom-up feature detection (pop-outs). In the other condition, the target was similar enough to the distracters that finding it required a conjunction search and thus top-down attentional control. (B) Each of the three curves plotted in each of the graphs here shows cumulative spiking activity over time in different brain regions. The *y*-axis plots the level of statistical significance of the spiking activity during the trials differing from the baseline period between trials. The *x*-axis marks time, with time 0 corresponding to the saccade onset. In the bottom-up condition (left graph), the first area to differ from baseline was the parietal area LIP, about 160 milliseconds before the saccade, followed by the frontal LPFC and FEF regions. In the top-down condition (right graph), the pattern was reversed: FEF and LPFC preceded LIP. (After Buschman and Miller 2007.)

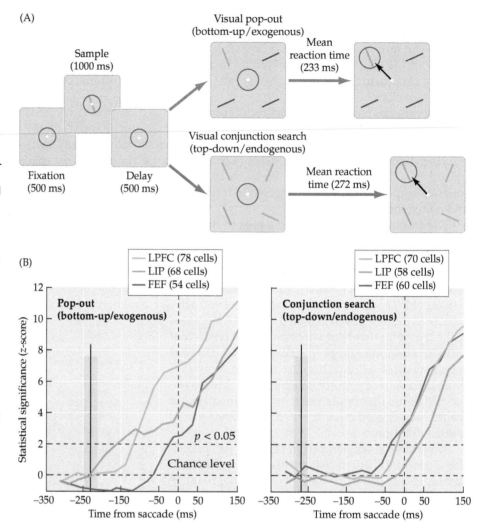

in a more volitional, or top-down, fashion (i.e., endogenously). Under these circumstances, the frontal neuron activity reflected the target location prior to the parietal activity (Figure 7.8B, right panel). These single-unit results suggest a frontal-then-parietal sequence of activity during endogenous attentional control and are thus roughly consistent with the temporal cascade of processing inferred from the combined ERP-fMRI studies in humans described earlier (see Figure 7.5B).

Preparatory activation of sensory cortices during attentional control

Although neurons in frontal and parietal cortex are consistently activated during attentional tasks, an important question is how activity in these higher-level regions could lead to enhanced stimulus processing in the sensory cortices. Some insight into this issue has also been provided by cued-attention fMRI studies. For example, when subjects are directed to attend to a particular visual-field location while expecting the onset of a visual stimulus there, activity increases not only in the frontal and parietal cortices, but also in the extrastriate cortex. This attention-related increase of activity in visual cortex in the absence of visual stimulation was interpreted as reflecting a "preparatory bias" due to top-down neural signals from the frontoparietal control network that favor the attended location.

This idea has been extended in other cued-attention studies. Figure 7.9A (bottom) shows the contralateral attention-related enhancement of target processing in one such study, similar to the stimulus-processing enhancement described in Chapter 6. However, these same regions showed enhanced contralateral activation in response to the attention-directing instructional cues *before* the targets actually appeared (Figure 7.9A, top). Thus, although this enhanced activity occurs in sensory cortex, it does not reflect attentional effects on target stimulus processing, because the stimulus has not yet been presented. Rather, it appears to reflect a preparatory activation of visual sensory areas due to top-down influences from the frontoparietal cortices by attention, which is thought to then lead to a modulation of the stimulus-evoked activity when the expected stimulus input appears.

Figure 7.9 Preparatory biasing activity in visual sensory cortex during spatial attention tasks (A) This fMRI study of humans performing visual spatial attention tasks shows that engaging the attentional control network by providing attention-directing cues leads to enhanced activity in contralateral visual sensory cortex prior to—or even in the absence of—a visual target. The sensory cortex activity elicited by the targets themselves closely corresponds to the pretarget biasing activity elicited by the cues. (B) Single-unit recordings in awake, behaving monkeys show that attention to a location in space increases the background firing of V4 neurons that have receptive fields (RFs) in that location. (C) Pretarget biasing of sensory cortex triggered by attention-directing cues is also seen with ERPs (a negative-polarity wave termed *biasing-related negativity*), which also provide timing information for this effect in humans. µV = microvolts. (A from Hopfinger et al. 2000; B after Luck et al. 1997; C after Grent-'t-Jong and Woldorff 2007.)

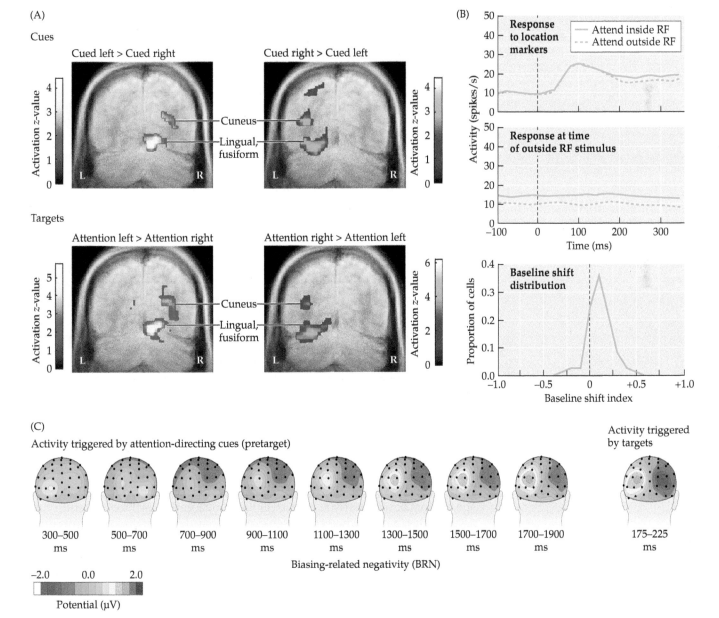

A simple but intuitive metaphor for this preparatory process might be turning up the volume on the radio because an important announcement is expected, facilitating interpretation of the message when it comes. Indeed, other fMRI studies have reported analogous prestimulus preparatory effects in auditory cortex during cued auditory attention paradigms, supporting the view that this activation reflects a more general attentional control mechanism.

Electrophysiological studies have also found evidence that attention can elicit preparatory activity. For example, in a single-unit spatial attention study in monkeys structured like the human visual attention studies, a sustained level of enhanced background firing rates was observed in neurons in the extrastriate visual cortical regions that process the stimuli to be attended. This enhanced background firing was separable from the attention-related enhancement of the transient responses evoked by attended stimuli, but presumably helped lead to the evoked-response enhancement for the attended stimuli when they occurred (Figure 7.9B). ERP and EEG studies in humans also have shown pretarget preparatory activity in the sensory cortical regions in cuing paradigms, while also indicating that its onset follows in time the onset of the control-related activity in frontal and parietal cortex (Figure 7.9C). Moreover, the amplitude of this prestimulus activity has been shown to correlate with the amplitude of the sensory-evoked responses to the attended target stimuli when they occur, as well as with the behavioral detectability of those targets.

Other prestimulus changes that have been observed in the sensory cortices following an attention-directing instructional cue are changes in oscillatory brain activity, particularly in the alpha band (8 to 12 hertz) of the EEG (see Chapter 2). Activity in this band is inversely related to attention, increasing when subjects are drowsy or less alert. These modulations have also been found to be brain-region specific. For example, during cued visual attention tasks similar to those described earlier in the chapter, alpha-band activity tends to be reduced over occipital cortex contralateral to the direction of visual attention, often with corresponding increases over ipsilateral occipital cortex. These changes have been interpreted as reflecting another type of preparatory activity in specific areas of sensory cortex for the processing of expected upcoming stimulus input, with decreased alpha power contralaterally reflecting increased excitability of occipital areas specific to the target location, and increased alpha power ipsilaterally reflecting active inhibition of irrelevant areas.

Control of Exogenously Induced Changes in Attention

Most experimental work on attentional control has focused on voluntary attention in response to instructional cues. As described in Chapter 6, however, attentional shifts can also be triggered exogenously by salient stimuli in the environment, such as a loud sound or a sudden movement. Indeed such stimulus-driven shifts of attention occur very often in everyday life.

Attentional shifts triggered by sudden stimulus onsets

As with voluntary attentional orienting, the shifts of attention triggered by salient or sudden stimuli also result in enhanced detection and discrimination of stimuli that occur shortly afterward at the same location as the cuing stimulus. As noted in Chapter 6, however, such exogenously driven attentional shifts tend to ensue more quickly than with endogenous attention and to be reflexive in nature —that is, triggered even if the cuing stimulus does not predict the occurrence of a subsequent stimulus at that location. Exogenously triggered shifts of attention, particularly to a specific location in space, also result in enhanced evoked activity in the corresponding regions of sensory cortex in response to stimuli that occur shortly afterward in that location.

The control mechanisms for these exogenously triggered attentional shifts have also been studied using approaches in which brain activity associated with the triggered orienting of attention is recorded, although there have been far fewer such studies. The results suggest that some of the same frontal and parietal control regions that are implicated in the control of endogenous attention are also activated by exogenously triggered attentional control, although the temporal sequences of the activations of these areas appear to differ.

More specifically, as mentioned earlier, neurons in the FEF were activated prior to those in LIP under conditions eliciting endogenous attention (see Figure 7.8B, right panel). In contrast, under conditions in which the inducement of attentional control was exogenously triggered, this sequence was reversed, with the parietal neurons activated prior to the frontal neurons (see Figure 7.8B, left panel). Some recent EEG studies in humans suggest a similar reversal of sequence (parietal before frontal) under exogenously triggered attentional circumstances. In addition, the monkey intracranial data suggest that the electrophysiological synchrony between the frontal and parietal areas is stronger in lower oscillatory frequencies during endogenous attention and in higher frequencies during exogenously triggered attention. These various results suggest that attentional control activity in the frontal and parietal cortices may occur in different sequences in different attentional circumstances, and may involve different neural processes, including the induction of neuronal synchrony at different frequencies.

Attentional reorienting activates a ventral frontoparietal system

As described earlier in the discussion of studies of endogenously cued attention, validly cued targets (i.e., targets that occurred in the location the instructional cue had indicated was most likely) were not only detected better and/or faster, but elicited larger responses in visual cortex, presumably because of preparatory attentional signals from frontal and parietal control regions. By contrast, responses in more inferior regions of the right hemisphere, particularly near the right temporoparietal junction (TPJ), where the inferior lateral parietal lobe abuts the posterior temporal lobe, were more strongly activated by *invalidly* than validly cued targets (Figure 7.10). On the basis of these results, the investigators reasoned that on invalidly cued trials, subjects first oriented their attention to the cued location and then had to reorient attention to another location when

Figure 7.10 **Activation of the right temporoparietal junction during reorienting of attention** In an event-related fMRI study of visual spatial attention, subjects were presented with cues instructing them to shift attention to a location on a particular side of the screen to detect a target that was more likely to occur there (80 percent chance; validly cued) versus the other side (20 percent chance; invalidly cued). (A) The functional map comparing the fMRI responses to invalidly and validly cued targets shows greater activity in the right TPJ for invalidly cued targets, suggesting involvement of this area in the reorienting of attention to unexpected events. (B) The event-related fMRI response waveforms show that this increased activity is elicited for both left and right invalidly cued targets. R IPL, right inferior parietal lobule; R STG, right superior temporal gyrus. (After Corbetta et al. 2000.)

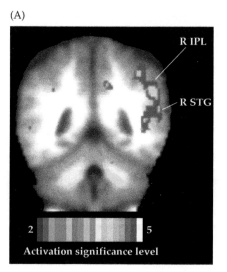

(A)

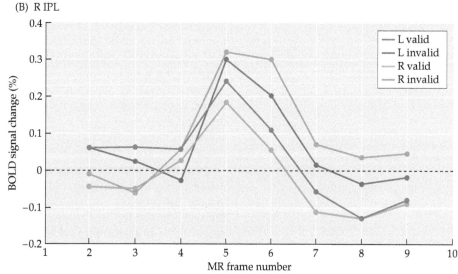

(B) R IPL

the target appeared there. The increased activity in the right TPJ was interpreted as reflecting this stimulus-triggered shift of attention.

It was further reasoned by researchers that if these TPJ areas are involved in responding to shifts of attention toward new stimuli occurring in the environment, then they should also be activated by infrequent targets in a stream or by other infrequently occurring novel stimuli. These predictions have been roughly borne out in other neuroimaging studies, further supporting the role of the right TPJ, along with similarly functioning areas in the right ventral frontal lobe, in the triggering of stimulus-driven shifts of spatial attention. As described in the next section, it has been proposed that these areas might be activated first in detecting a salient stimulus, which would then invoke control activity in the dorsal frontoparietal control network.

Single-unit recording studies in non-human primates lend additional support to this interpretation. In particular, neurons in the inferior lateral parietal cortex in the monkey respond more strongly to target stimuli occurring at unattended than attended locations, roughly mirroring the human neuroimaging findings in the TPJ. In addition, neurons in this area appear to encode the location of stimuli that differ in some distinctive way from the background (e.g., "pop-out" stimuli, described in the next section).

Visual Search

Another domain of attention that has become a research topic in its own right is **visual search**, the process of inspecting a complex scene for something of particular interest. For example, we may be looking for a friend in a crowd of people and having a tough time finding that person. We may then remember that our friend is wearing a green sweater and refine our search strategy by looking around for green items. If only a few people are wearing green, the friend might easily be found by this search. But if a lot of people are wearing green (e.g., if it is St. Patrick's Day in Boston), we might need a different strategy.

Behavioral studies of visual search

The processes underlying visual search have been studied by many investigators since initial work on this subject by psychologist Anne Treisman and colleagues in the 1980s. Such experiments typically employ a task in which an array of multiple items is presented and, as in the example of the friend in the crowd, subjects must find a particular item in the array. The item being searched for is referred to as the *target*, and the other items in the array as *distracters*. Manipulating the characteristics of the target and distracters allows the strategies used in visual search to be identified. For example, the array presented to subjects might consist of *T*s and *O*s, each of which could be green or orange. If the task is to detect a green item and all the rest of the items are orange, the search is easy and the target is quickly found. Indeed, the target appears to "pop out" of the array (Figure 7.11A, left panel). Detecting a *T* in an array of *O*s is similarly easy and fast (Figure 7.11A, right panel). Rapidly detected target stimuli such as these, which possess a single featural difference from the distracters in the visual array, are called **pop-out stimuli**.

In visual searches for pop-out stimuli, it does not matter much how many distracters are in the array: if the time it takes to detect the target is plotted against the number of distracters, the resulting function is essentially flat (as the red line plotted in Figure 7.11C illustrates). Such results suggest that the detection of pop-out items does not require sequential shifts of attention to individual items, but rather is accomplished by taking in the whole array more or less at once and processing all the items in parallel. In this sense, the salient

(A) Pop-out search

Find a green letter

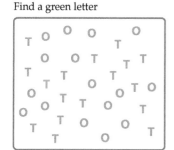

Find a *T*

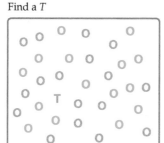

(B) Conjunction search

Find a green *T*

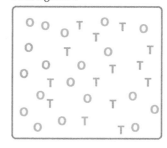

(C)

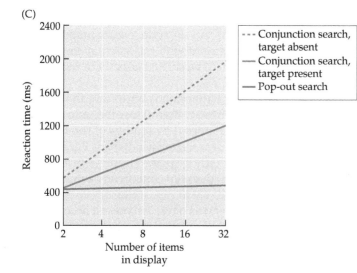

- - - Conjunction search, target absent
—— Conjunction search, target present
—— Pop-out search

Figure 7.11 Attention in visual search paradigms
(A) Each of these two examples of search arrays contains a pop-out target (one green item among orange items on the left, one *T* among Os on the right). (B) In this search array the target (a green *T*) is defined by a conjunction of two features (being green and being a *T*), each of which is present separately in various of the distracters but not together in any of them.
(C) This idealized plot shows response times as a function of the number of distracters in a pop-out search as in (A) or a conjunction search as in (B). Pop-out searches are quick, and the reaction times do not vary with the number of distracters, suggesting that the search is done in a parallel fashion—taking in the array as a whole and rapidly finding the one item with a single distinguishing feature. In contrast, conjunction searches are slower, and the reaction time increases linearly as a function of the number of distracters, suggesting a serial search process. In accord with this interpretation, a conjunction search in which the target is absent (and the subject presses the appropriate button when convinced of its absence) takes substantially longer. (After Treisman and Gelade 1980.)

nature of the pop-out target (e.g., the only green item among orange ones, or the only *T* among Os) tends to attract attention to that location and item more or less automatically.

In contrast, detection of a target item defined by a *conjunction* of features shows different characteristics. For example, consider trying to find a green *T* in a display like the one in **Figure 7.11B**, which contains both *T*s and *O*s and both green and orange items. Even if the display contains only one target (e.g., only one green *T*), that target is neither the only green item among orange ones nor the only *T* among Os. Thus, it does not pop out and is not easily found. Therefore, in contrast to pop-out targets, the speed of finding a **conjunction target** increases linearly with more distracters (**Figure 7.11C**).

Theoretical models of visual search

The behavioral pattern in visual searches for conjunction targets suggests that a focused form of attention is required to find the target. For finding targets under such circumstances, then, it is thought that attention must be serially directed to the various items individually to determine which has the feature combination of interest. Accordingly, the increased reaction time as a function of the number of distracter items is presumably due to the time required to perform this process for more items. Moreover, if subjects have to press one button when the target is present in a display and another when the target is absent, the slope of the search function is greatly increased, differing by about a factor of two (see Figure 7.11C). One explanation that has been proposed for this pattern is that on target-absent trials, attention has to be explicitly directed to every item in the display to determine that none has the right conjunction of features. In contrast, in target-present trials, on average only half of the items need to be scrutinized before the target is found, thereby yielding a search function with roughly half the slope as in target-absent trials.

These sorts of results led Treisman and colleagues to a model of visual attention known as **feature integration theory**, which conceptualizes the perceptual system as being organized as a set of feature maps. In vision, these maps would represent characteristics such as color, form, motion, or texture, each map providing information about the locations in the visual field of that particular feature. According to this theory, the processing in these feature maps is done early and in parallel, consistent with results showing that searches for an item with a unique feature are not influenced by the number of distracters. In contrast, in conjunction searches information from separate feature maps must be compared or combined in some way, consistent with the fact that conjunction searches take longer and require attention to be shifted serially to the various items in the array.

This model also proposed that focused attention is important in resolving the **binding problem**, how perceptual features are bound together into coherent representations of objects. This idea is supported by studies of the tendency of subjects to report **illusory conjunctions** of features in a display. For example, subjects might report seeing a red *O* in a briefly displayed multi-item array that contains red items and *O*-shaped items but does not contain any actual red *O*s. The key finding is that subjects are more likely to report illusory conjunctions among unattended items than among attended ones. This result accords with the idea that focused attention shifted serially to each item in turn is required to find the conjunction, and that focused attention helps bind the different features of an object into a coherent whole.

An important caveat about these models of visual search is that they imply a dichotomy between the search characteristics for detecting stimuli that "pop out" and stimuli that do not. Other research, however, has indicated that there is not such a clear dichotomy in processing visual search stimuli. With some stimulus features, for example, the search functions have a fairly shallow slope but are not completely flat, indicating a modest dependence on the number of distracters. In addition, searches for certain types of target items in displays can initially require a degree of serially shifted attention, but after extensive training the same searches can show the relatively flat search functions characteristic of pop-out stimuli. These observations suggest a more complex arrangement in which attention and its influence on sensory processing are more flexible than the initial versions of the feature integration model suggested.

Other models of search have been proposed to deal with these limitations. One such model is known as **guided search**. In this scheme, proposed by psychologist Jeremy Wolfe, two basic components determine the allocation of attention: an activation map driven by stimulus factors, and an activation map driven by top-down influence from higher-level factors and behavioral goals. In this conception, visual inputs are first filtered by different feature-tuned subsystems to generate the sorts of maps suggested in feature integration theory. The activation intensity of items within each stimulus-driven feature map is taken to depend on the local difference of the item in that feature dimension relative to neighboring areas in the visual field—a concept similar to what have been termed **saliency maps** in other models. The intensity associated with each item in the various top-down activation maps is further postulated to depend on prior knowledge, with items that share more similar feature values to the searched-for target tending to be more strongly activated. Together, the bottom-up and top-down activation maps form a general activation map that reflects the probability of the target presence across the search space. The combined map then guides the search, in that attention is first allocated to the highest value within the general activation map, and then reallocated to the second-highest activation value if the highest value is not the target, and so on. This allocation and reallocation of attention is proposed to then continue until the target is found (or the viewer determines that a target is not present).

Neural processes underlying visual search

Although more limited in number, other studies have investigated the brain events underlying visual search. For example, event-related fMRI studies have shown that most of the areas of dorsal frontal and parietal cortex implicated in endogenous attentional control are also active during visual search. Moreover, the activity in these areas falls off once the target is found, consistent with the view that these areas play a role in these search processes. Adding to this evidence, single-unit recordings in monkeys show that neurons in the inferior parietal cortex near the temporoparietal junction (TPJ) appear to code the location of distinctive (pop-out) stimuli in the visual field, consistent with the fMRI activation findings. In addition, when searching for a pop-out target in an array, frontal eye field (FEF) neurons discriminate between targets and distracters, regardless of whether the monkey makes a saccade to the target or just shifts attention covertly, and distracters produce larger responses in both FEF and LIP neurons when they are more similar to the searched-for target. Thus, these activation patterns may in part reflect the neural implementation of so-called salience maps that have been proposed on the basis of behavioral studies.

The neural underpinnings of visual search, particularly for pop-out stimuli, have also been studied with ERPs and MEG (see Chapter 2). When an array of stimuli is presented containing a pop-out item as a target, a negative wave peaking at about 250 milliseconds is evoked over the parietal and occipital regions contralateral to the pop-out location (Figure 7.12). This so-called **N2pc wave** has been used in numerous experiments to study the temporal characteristics of attentional shifting during visual search tasks. Some of these studies have included determining the speed of attentional shifting during visual search. In one study, for example, subjects needed to detect and shift attention first to a pop-out item of one color on one side of the visual field, and then to a pop-out item of a different color on the other side. These processes were reflected first by an increased negative wave (an N2pc) peaking at 250 milliseconds contralateral to the first pop-out, followed shortly after (100 milliseconds later) by an increased negative wave on the other side, presumably reflecting the temporal characteristics of these switching processes.

ERP and MEG source analyses of the N2pc activity have suggested that it derives from a combination of activity in the contralateral parietal and ventral occipitotemporal cortices. Thus, this activity may reflect both the control processes related to the shifting and focusing of attention (e.g., processing

(A) Pop-out condition

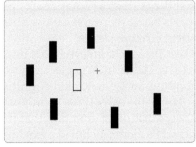
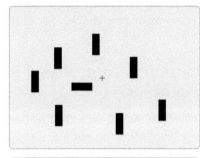

(B)
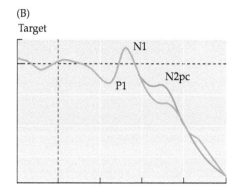
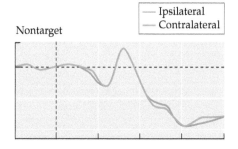
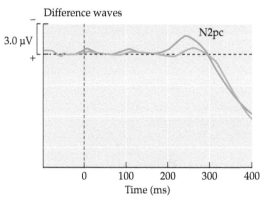

Figure 7.12 Neural processes related to the coordination of visual search The N2pc ERP response to target pop-out stimuli in a visual array is shown. The detection of a pop-out target in an array (A) elicits an enhanced negative wave over contralateral parietal and occipital scalp regions (B), reflecting the shift of attention to that location. In (B), the top panel shows the contralateral and ipsilateral ERP responses when the pop-out was the target to be detected, the middle panel shows the corresponding ERPs when the pop-out was not the target, and the bottom panel shows the difference waves between these. In the term *N2pc*, N stands for "negative," 2 for the second large negative peak, p for "posterior," and c for "contralateral." μV = microvolts. (After Luck and Hillyard 1994.)

in the parietal cortex) and the ramifications of that switch on processing in visual sensory cortex. In any event, this neural activity provides a useful high-temporal-resolution marker for studying mechanisms of attentional shifting in complex visual scenes.

Attentional Control as a System of Interacting Brain Areas

Taken together, the studies described thus far in this chapter make clear that, like other complex cognitive functions, attentional control is mediated by a network of brain regions and not by a single region. Accordingly, it is useful to look at these areas as components of a system that work together, with different parts being recruited for the different types of attentional functions under different circumstances.

Over the years, investigators have viewed such a system in different ways. Clinical evidence from neglect syndromes and findings from single-unit studies in non-human primates led cognitive neuroscientist and neurologist Marcel Mesulam in the early 1980s to propose a large-scale brain network for the control and coordination of attention that included regions in the frontal and parietal cortices. His model included a frontal component (the frontal eye fields, premotor cortex, and prefrontal cortex), a parietal component (superior parietal lobe), and a limbic component (cingulate cortex). The frontal component was proposed to convert strategies for attentional shifting into specific motor acts, the parietal component to provide a dynamic representation of salient events in multiple frames of references and to compute strategies for attentional shifting, and the limbic component to compute the "motivational relevance" of external events and maintain the "level of effort" of executing attentional tasks. Mesulam's model also identified the reticular formation in the lower brainstem as important in modulating overall arousal.

In the early 1990s, incorporating PET neuroimaging data, psychologist Michael Posner and cognitive neuroscientist Steve Petersen proposed that the brain regions involved in attentional control can be divided into two main systems: An anterior attentional system (in which the anterior cingulate cortex in the midline frontal cortex played a key role) was thought to be important for monitoring the environment and detecting the occurrences of target stimuli. The posterior system—comprising the posterior parietal lobe, the superior colliculus in the midbrain, and a part of the thalamus known as the pulvinar—was proposed to be involved in orienting to visual locations. Later versions of this model, endeavoring to incorporate subsequent fMRI and neurotransmitter data, postulated an organization made up of three systems: (1) an *alerting system* of frontal and parietal regions, particularly in the right hemisphere, related to the cortical distribution of the brain's norepinephrine system; (2) an *orienting system* associated with superior parietal and frontal regions and the temporoparietal junction (TPJ), along with the superior colliculus and pulvinar, modulated mostly by the neurotransmitter acetylcholine; and (3) an *executive system* associated with the anterior cingulate and lateral prefrontal cortex, characterized mainly by dopaminergic activity.

Probably the most influential model of attentional control today was proposed by cognitive neuroscientists Maurizio Corbetta and Gordon Shulman in 2002. Incorporating findings from human neuroimaging studies, these researchers suggested that the cortical control of attention can be divided into two main systems that carry out different functions but interact extensively (Figure 7.13). One system, consisting of parts of the intraparietal cortex and superior frontal cortex, was taken to be involved in preparing and applying goal-directed (endogenous) selection of relevant stimuli and responses. As already noted, a

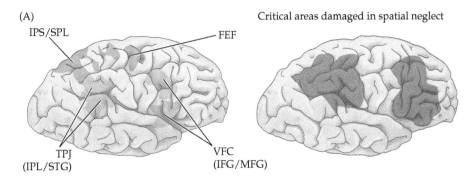

(A)

IPS/SPL

FEF

Critical areas damaged in spatial neglect

TPJ
(IPL/STG)

VFC
(IFG/MFG)

(B) Top-down control

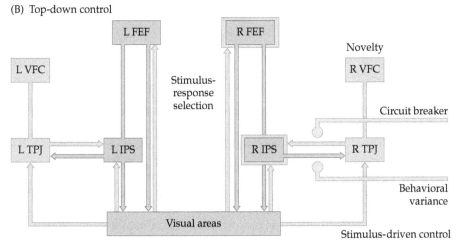

L FEF

R FEF

Novelty

L VFC

R VFC

Stimulus-
response
selection

Circuit breaker

L TPJ

L IPS

R IPS

R TPJ

Behavioral
variance

Visual areas

Stimulus-driven control

Figure 7.13 A combined endogenous-exogenous model of attentional control (A) The attentional control network in this model is functionally segregated into two interacting systems. The left panel shows a dorsal frontoparietal network controlling endogenous shifts of attention (blue), and a right ventral system responsible for reorienting and the exogenous capture of attention (orange). The right panel indicates the areas that cause neglect syndrome when damaged, which are proposed to match the ventral network better. (B) In this model, the dorsal IPS-FEF network is proposed to be involved in the top-down control of visual processing (blue arrows), and the TPJ-VFC network to be more involved in stimulus-driven control (orange arrows). The IPS and FEF are also modulated by stimulus-driven control. Connections between the TPJ and IPS can interrupt ongoing top-down control when unattended salient stimuli are detected. FEF, frontal eye field; IFG/MFG, inferior frontal gyrus/middle frontal gyrus; IPS/SPL, intraparietal sulcus/superior parietal lobule; IPL/STG, inferior parietal lobule/superior temporal gyrus; TPJ, temporoparietal junction; VFC, ventral frontal cortex. (After Corbetta and Shulman 2002.)

number of cuing studies using neuroimaging techniques have implicated these areas in endogenous attentional control. The other system, consisting of the TPJ and ventral frontal cortex, mainly on the right, was proposed to be specialized for the detection of behaviorally relevant stimuli, particularly unexpected or highly salient stimuli that trigger attentional orienting in a more exogenous way. Moreover, after detection of such events, these areas were supposed to act as an alerting system or "circuit breaker" to signal and recruit activity in the dorsal frontal and parietal regions, which would then direct neural processing resources to these novel triggering events and to the location where they occurred. Thus, this proposal incorporates interactions between exogenous (i.e., stimulus-driven) and endogenous mechanisms of attentional control.

One interpretation based on this model is that the actual attentional orienting is accomplished by the more dorsal frontal and parietal regions (FEF and IPS), although their activation may be initiated in different ways. In exogenously triggered attention, for example, activation would be initiated by signaling from the right-sided ventral system (e.g., the right TPJ) that had picked up a particularly salient stimulus. In contrast, during endogenous attentional shifting in response to an instructional cue or a behavioral goal, the processing is presumably funneled in from other higher-level brain regions. For example, the input could come from the more lateral frontal and parietal regions that have been implicated in interpreting the meaning of an instructional cue (see Figure 7.5A) and in making a decision on the basis of a complex set of external or internal processes. The idea would be that, regardless of how the attentional-orienting control circuits of the dorsal network (i.e., FEF and IPS) are activated, they would implement the attentional control by sending signals to appropriately bias or otherwise prepare the sensory cortical regions that need to process the upcoming (or ongoing) stimuli (see Figure 7.9).

Corbetta and Shulman also proposed that the deficits seen in neglect syndrome are more related to the right-sided ventral exogenous system than to the more dorsal system. Probably the main reason for this proposal is that neglect, at least in humans, is much more apparent with right-sided lesions, and the exogenously triggered activation of the ventral system also tends to be more apparent in the right hemisphere than in the left. These researchers have also argued, however, that the area of parietal damage that most consistently leads to neglect is actually somewhat more inferior than previously thought (see Figure 7.13A), closer to the right TPJ, which is the region implicated during exogenously triggered reorienting of attention in neuroimaging studies, as described earlier (see Figure 7.10). On the other hand, the right TPJ (and right ventral frontal cortex) is activated by sudden stimuli in both visual fields. Why damage to these areas does not cause orienting problems for stimuli in *both* visual fields is not explained by this model.

Interactions between Components of the Attentional System

The idea that attentional control depends on several interacting networks of brain regions that work together as interacting systems to enhance neural processing in sensory and other brain regions has naturally led to studies specifically investigating the functional interactions between these areas. For example, the temporal sequence of activation described earlier for endogenous visual attention (see Figure 7.5) suggests that cue interpretation and decision processes are first performed in the lateral frontoparietal regions of the dorsal network, which may then project information into the more medial portions of the network that specifically mediate attentional orienting (FEF and IPS).

Within these more medial components of the network, the actual attentional orienting appears to be initiated by the frontal component (FEF), joined shortly later by activity in the IPS in the parietal lobe, and the two together then bias processing in the appropriate sensory cortices. As mentioned already, both combined ERP-fMRI recordings in humans and single-unit recordings in monkeys suggest this frontal-then-parietal functional sequence during top-down (endogenous) attention (see Figures 7.5B and 7.8B).

In addition to these observations of temporal sequences of control-related brain activity, other data have provided direct evidence for causal links between the components of these systems. For example, it has been shown that, during auditory selective attention, patients with damage to one side of the prefrontal cortex have reduced attention-related modulations of the early sensory processing for auditory stimuli received by the contralateral ear. These results suggest that the frontal cortex is required for such attention-related modulations in the sensory cortex, in accord with the view that the frontal cortex provides the signal that helps accomplish the observed modulations of sensory activity.

Similarly, applying low-amplitude transcranial magnetic stimulation (TMS; see Chapter 2) to the frontal cortex on one side increases activity in the visual cortex ipsilateral to the stimulated frontal lobe and enhances behavioral performance in discriminating stimuli in the contralateral visual hemifield. On the other hand, a strong, presumably disruptive, TMS pulse applied to the right parietal lobe can produce neglect-like symptoms in normal subjects. Again, these findings support the idea that regions in a frontoparietal network are critical for coordinating and modulating the sensory cortices to process stimulus input optimally (or at least more efficiently).

Related work in non-human primates is consistent with this interpretation. Low-level focal microstimulation in the frontal eye fields of monkeys (Figure

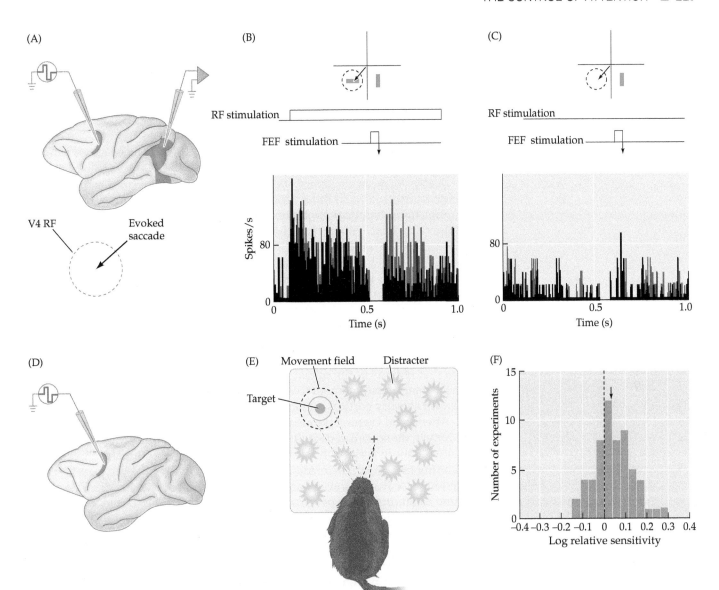

Figure 7.14 Effects of frontal eye field microstimulation on neuronal responses in V4 and on covert attention (A–C) Microstimulation of sites within the FEF, below the threshold for eliciting a saccade, was carried out while the visual stimulus responses of single V4 neurons were recorded in monkeys performing a fixation task. (A) The stimulating electrode was positioned so that suprathreshold stimulation would evoke a saccade into the receptive field (RF) of the V4 cell under study. (B) This example shows the effect of subthreshold FEF microstimulation on the response of a single V4 neuron to an oriented bar presented in the cell's receptive field. The mean response during control trials is shown in black; the enhanced response arising from the FEF microstimulation, in red. (C) In contrast, on trials in which the visual stimulus was presented outside the receptive field of the V4 neuron, no enhancement is seen. (D–F) In another study, subthreshold microstimulation in FEF was carried out while the monkey's performance in a covert attention task was measured. (D) To study the effects on covert attention, a microelectrode was positioned in the FEF to evoke saccades to a fixed location with respect to the center of gaze ("movement field"). (E) Monkeys performed an attention task in which they had to detect the transient dimming of a visual stimulus (target) at the movement field location corresponding to the FEF microstimulation site. The attention task was performed with and without subthreshold stimulation of the FEF site just prior to dimming of the target stimulus. (F) Subthreshold microstimulation increased the monkey's sensitivity to the target change (i.e., the relative sensitivity distribution was shifted to the right). This effect was observed only when the target was within the movement field of the cells being recorded. (After Moore et al. 2003.)

7.14A–C) enhances the evoked responses to visual stimuli of neurons in V4 that have the corresponding receptive fields. On the other hand, microstimulation in the FEF suppresses the stimulus-evoked responses of V4 neurons with noncorresponding receptive fields. In addition, low-level stimulation in the FEF also improves target discrimination performance of attended targets in the relevant spatial location of the visual field (Figure 7.14D–F). These findings imply that the dorsal frontoparietal network exerts modulatory control over stimulus processing in the sensory cortices, and thus over concomitant behavioral performance. Other studies investigating the relationship between oscillatory top-down signals from frontal cortex to visual cortical regions and the neuronal spiking in those visual regions have further supported this view.

Additional support for the interactive roles proposed for these various components of the attentional control systems is an fMRI study showing that trial-by-trial variations in reaction time during a visual attention task were correlated with variations in the fMRI activity in regions of the attentional control system. In particular, attentional lapses (trials with slower reaction times) were found to be reflected by reduced activity *prior* to the stimulus trial in the dorsal anterior cingulate and dorsal prefrontal regions that have been implicated in controlling attention. This pretrial decrease in frontal activity was then followed after the stimulus occurrence by reduced activity in the relevant areas of visual cortex. This temporal pattern thus also supports the idea that regions of the dorsal frontoparietal network regulate attention and performance from moment to moment by modulating processing in the task-relevant sensory cortical regions.

Attentional lapses have also been characterized by concurrent increases in activity in the so-called **default-mode network**, a set of brain areas that become relatively more active when someone is *not* engaged in an attentionally demanding task (Box 7A). In addition, increased stimulus-evoked activity in the right inferior frontal gyrus and the right temporoparietal junction have been found to predict better performance on the *next* trial. This effect could reflect stimulus-triggered reorienting activity in the right-sided ventral exogenous system proposed by Corbetta and Shulman, possibly providing the hypothesized interrupt signal for the dorsal system and a mechanism for recovery following a transient waning of attentional focus. These patterns of activation as a dynamic function of attention and performance endorse the view that attentional control is mediated by functional interactions between components of these postulated attentional networks.

Generality of Attentional Control Systems

An important question about attentional systems and attentional control concerns their generality. For example, are the same dorsal frontal and parietal regions that are widely implicated in visual attentional control also used for attentional orienting in other sensory modalities? And are the control regions that shift visual attention to features or objects the same as those invoked for visual spatial attention? Even more generally, do these regions, or at least some of them, reflect a central executive control system that directs attentional resources throughout the brain? And do these same regions control attention directed to mental processes such as thoughts, feelings, desires, and plans that are not directly related to environmental stimuli?

Neuroimaging studies suggest provisional answers to some of these questions. Some portions of these attentional control circuits, for example, appear to be general and others more specific. Thus, many of the same regions of dorsal frontal and parietal cortex implicated in visual spatial attention are also active in

■ BOX 7A **THE DEFAULT-MODE NETWORK**

On the basis of neuroimaging studies, neuroscientist Marcus Raichle and colleagues proposed a *default* level of activity in many regions of the brain, a baseline level from which cognitive tasks induce increases of activity. Conversely, studies by this group and other researchers have shown that certain brain regions, including the posterior cingulate cortex, the ventral anterior cingulate cortex, and the medial prefrontal cortex, consistently show *greater* activity during resting states than during the processing of specific cognitive tasks. When the activity during a baseline or rest condition is subtracted from the activity during cognitive tasks, relative decreases of activity (generally called *deactivations*) are observed in these areas.

Because cognitive tasks induce activation increases in other brain areas carrying out the relevant processing, this finding led to the proposal that these regions constitute a network supporting a default mode of brain function that is engaged in the *absence* of any particular cognitive task (Figure A). Further supporting the hypothesis that these areas constitute a network, analysis of the functional connectivity of these areas (i.e., how much their activity co-varies across time; see Chapter 2) has shown strong coupling during the resting state (Figure B).

From the standpoint of understanding attentional control, analyses of the functional connectivity between the components of this default-mode network and the components of the frontoparietal network activated during attentional tasks (see text) found significant *inverse* correlations of activity during rest. Such results suggest that these may be complementary networks—the attentional control systems being activated for demanding cognitive tasks, and the default-mode network being activated when the brain is "idling."

Single-unit recordings in monkeys have supported these inverse activation patterns for the default-mode network. For example, neurons in the posterior cingulate cortex, a posterior brain region considered to be part of the default-mode network, show changes in firing rates that closely match the fMRI activation patterns observed in humans. In particular, their fluctuations are anticorrelated with activity in dorsal parietal regions associated with the attentional control network

(A)

(B)

Default-mode network activity is anticorrelated with frontoparietal attentional control regions. (A) Functional MRI data were collected from a subject at rest, and one part of the default-mode network, the posterior cingulate cortex (PCC), was chosen as a seed region to help identify other parts of the network. The time course of activity in the seed region was correlated with every other part of the brain, and those correlation coefficients are shown plotted on an inflated representation of the brain surface. Using this simple method, the rest of the default-mode network shows up as warm-colored, indicating a similar activity profile as that of the PCC, whereas areas of the frontoparietal attentional control network show up in cooler colors, indicating an anticorrelation with the PCC. (B) Functional MRI activity time courses over one run are plotted from two regions of the default-mode network (PCC and medial prefrontal cortex, or MPF) and from one region of the attentional network (intraparietal sulcus, or IPS). The time courses clearly show that when activity in one network goes up, activity in the other goes down. (After Fox et al. 2005.)

and predict lapses in attention and the ability to switch from one task to another. Moreover, neuroimaging studies also have shown abnormal activity patterns in the default-mode network in several major neurological and psychiatric disorders, including being less active in autism and more so in schizophrenia.

The obvious question is what purpose neural activity in a default-mode network serves; that is, why should these regions be active if and when the brain is doing nothing in particular? Although activity in the default-mode network might be re-

(Continued on next page)

■ **BOX 7A** *(continued)*

lated to the mind simply "idling," another possibility is that this network is activated when attention is inwardly focused, the "standard" attentional control system being activated primarily when a subject is focused on events and stimuli in the external environment.

Whatever this network does, its activation pattern is evident in monkeys as well, so it presumably evolved to carry out a relatively basic function. Whereas sorting out the functions of these postulated networks will require much more work, the inverse relationship of activity in the default-mode network and in the dorsal frontoparietal attentional control network

during focused attention suggests that these complementary systems play an overarching interactive role in systemwide brain function related to attentional and cognitive control.

References

Fox, M. D., A. Z. Snyder, J. L. Vincent, M. Corbetta, D. C van Essen and M. E. Raichle (2005) The human brain is intrinsically organized into dynamic, anticorrelated function networks. *Proc. Natl. Acad. Sci. USA* 102: 9673–9678.

Hayden, B. Y., D. V. Smith and M. E. Platt (2009) Electrophysiological

correlates of default-mode processing in macaque posterior cingulate cortex. *Proc. Natl. Acad. Sci. USA* 106: 5948–5953.

McKiernan, K. A., J. N. Kaufman, J. Kucera-Thompson and J. R. Binder (2003) A parametric manipulation of factors affecting task-induced deactivation in functional neuroimaging. *J. Cogn. Neurosci.* 15: 394–408.

Raichle, M. E., A. M. MacLeod, A. Z. Snyder, W. J. Powers, D. A. Gusnard and G. L. Shulman (2001) A default mode of brain function. *Proc. Natl. Acad. Sci. USA* 98: 676–682.

auditory attentional-orienting tasks, although the locus of the neural activation for the latter tasks appears to be more medial and dorsal. Other findings have indicated that switching attention between different object types or features also elicits activity near some of the same regions in parietal cortex implicated in visual spatial attention orienting tasks, although also somewhat more medially (see Figure 7.4).

Studies of the parietal cortex and its activation patterns in a wide range of cognitive tasks have suggested a role in executive control more generally. Similarly, portions of the FEF, lateral PFC, and other nearby frontal cortical regions show activation during a variety of attentional and cognitive control tasks, in accord with the view that the frontal cortex is a key player in executive control more generally, such as in keeping track of task goals and coordinating processes in other brain areas. For example, various portions of the frontoparietal control network, along with midline prefrontal regions such as the anterior cingulate cortex, appear to be invoked for attentional and cognitive control purposes in the face of conflicting stimulus input, such as during the well-known color-naming Stroop task (see Chapter 13). In addition, some of these same areas have also been implicated as being involved in working memory (see Chapter 13), as well as in the retrieval of long-term memories (see Chapter 9).

Finally, note that these broader ideas about the attentional control networks are mainly based on studies of covert attention, most often in the context of vision—that is, tasks in which the subject attends to a particular region of the visual field but without moving the eyes to fixate that location. In the real world, however, we typically move our eyes to a location or an object that interests us, or that has otherwise attracted our attention. This link between eye movement and attention implies that the control of eye movements is likely closely related to the control of covert attentional shifts, as mentioned earlier. In support of this idea, the control circuits for saccadic eye movements show considerable overlap with the control circuits for covert attention (Figure 7.15). Indeed, because of the extensive overlap of brain regions serving these functions, it has been hypothesized that the covert visual attentional control system may have evolved as a useful adjunct to the system already in place underlying the control of eye movements and overt attentional orienting.

In summary, current evidence suggests that the attentional control systems make use of many of the same brain areas for the same general purposes of

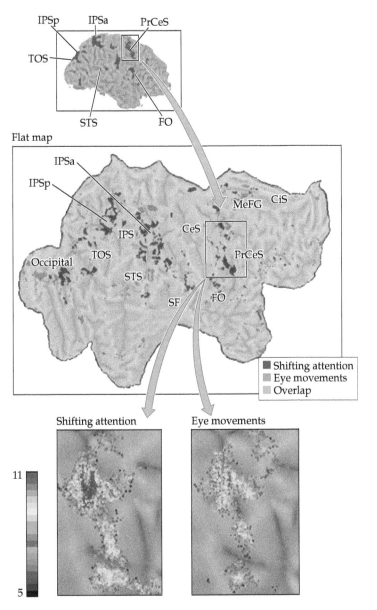

Figure 7.15 Covert versus overt attentional networks Functional MRI activation during covert attentional (red) and overt eye movement (green) shifts to different stimulus locations is shown for one subject. The functional data are projected onto both a three-dimensional (top) and a flattened two-dimensional (middle) representation of the subject's brain. The enlargements in the bottom panel show the activity in cortical regions in and around the precentral sulcus (PrCeS), near what is thought to be the equivalent of the FEF in humans. Considerable overlap (shown in yellow) is observed in frontal, parietal, and temporal regions, indicating a close functional relationship between the neural systems for shifting attention and for shifting eye gaze to spatial locations. It has been suggested that this overlap might reflect a covert attentional system that, during the course of evolution, co-opted the circuits already in place for saccadic eye movement control. CeS, central sulcus; CiS, cingulate sulcus; FO, frontal operculum; IPS, intraparietal sulcus; IPSa, anterior IPS; IPSp, posterior IPS; MeFG, medial frontal gyrus; SF, Sylvian fissure; STS, superior temporal sulcus; TOS, transverse occipital sulcus. (From Corbetta et al. 1998.)

allocating and regulating processing resources, but with the specific patterns of their activation varying as a function of the particular task at hand.

Attention, Levels of Arousal, and Consciousness

Any consideration of attentional systems leads to questions about the continuum of arousal with which we are all familiar, and in turn to the knotty problem of consciousness and its neural basis. Human beings spend each 24-hour cycle that defines a day in a variety of brain states. About a third of our lives is spent in the several stages of sleep, a state that (except possibly for periods of dreaming) would seem to be clearly unconscious. Even when we are fully awake, however, our awareness of the world around us and of our internal state in terms of thoughts, feelings, hopes, and desires varies greatly. These different brain states range from fully vigilant attention, through inattentiveness, drowsiness, and ultimately sleep; each of these states reflects different levels of consciousness in the sense of wakefulness, which is in turn a prerequisite to consciousness.

What follows is a brief review of how the brain regulates changes from alert wakefulness to deep sleep, the bearing this physiological regulation has on consciousness, and some clinical observations relevant to the neural underpinnings of consciousness and perceptual awareness.

Sleep and wakefulness

Sleep is not simply the result of diminished brain activity or of a shutting off of sensory input, but is characterized by a distinctive set of brain states. Humans descend into sleep in a succession of *stages* defined by electroencephalographic criteria (Figure 7.16). The control of these different states of consciousness is now fairly well understood as a result of many years of electrophysiological, anatomical, and pharmacological work. Observations dating from the 1940s showed that electrically stimulating a group of neurons that lies near the junction of the pons and midbrain causes wakefulness and arousal. Thus, wakefulness—or consciousness in this particular sense—is based on dedicated, active, neural mechanisms.

(A)

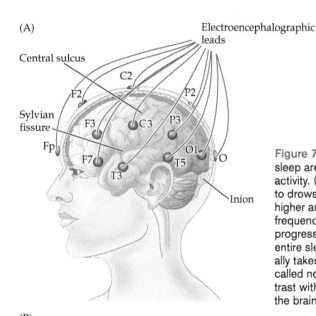

Figure 7.16 **The stages of sleep** (A) Levels of wakefulness and sleep are usually monitored by electroencephalographic (EEG) activity. (B) The changes from alert wakefulness through boredom to drowsiness are indicated by shifts toward lower frequencies and higher amplitudes of the recorded signal. This pattern of lower-frequency and higher-amplitude waves continues throughout the progressive loss of consciousness that falling asleep entails. The entire sleep sequence from drowsiness to deep (stage IV) sleep usually takes about an hour. The descending stages into deep sleep are called non-rapid eye movement (non-REM) sleep. These stages contrast with periods of rapid eye movement (REM) sleep, a time when the brain again becomes active and most dreaming occurs.

(B)

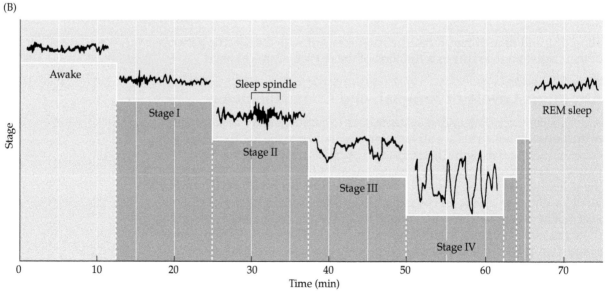

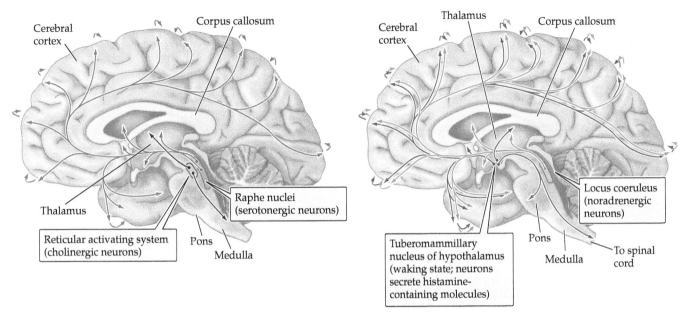

Figure 7.17 Brain activity in sleep and wakefulness Increased levels of activity of cholinergic neurons in the reticular activating system are the primary cause of wakefulness, and their relative inactivity is the cause of physiological unconsciousness. Other brainstem nuclei involved in this complex regulatory scheme are noradrenergic neurons of the locus coeruleus and serotonergic neurons of the raphe nuclei. Both monoaminergic and cholinergic systems are active during the waking state (see Table 7.1). The neurons of the tuberomammillary nucleus produce the histamine-containing molecule orexin and are active during the awake state (which explains why antihistamines make people drowsy).

Investigators now generally agree that the sequence of human brain states illustrated in Figure 7.16 is generated by a collection of nuclei in the central region of the brainstem that is involved in the regulation of arousal—a region called the **reticular activating system**. The most important of these controlling elements are the cells in the cholinergic nuclei of the pons-midbrain junction, the noradrenergic cells of the **locus coeruleus**, and the serotonergic neurons in the **raphe nuclei** (Figure 7.17; Table 7.1). The activity of these brainstem nuclei modulates the degree of consciousness over the day on a continuum from alert wakefulness to deep sleep. These nuclei are in turn controlled by circadian clocks

Table 7.1 Brainstem Nuclei That Regulate Sleep and Wakefulness

BRAINSTEM NUCLEI RESPONSIBLE	NEUROTRANSMITTER INVOLVED	ACTIVITY STATE OF THE RELEVANT BRAINSTEM NEURONS
Wakefulness		
Cholinergic nuclei of pons-midbrain junction	Acetylcholine	Active
Locus coeruleus	Norepinephrine	Active
Raphe nuclei	Serotonin	Active
Tuberomammillary nuclei	Orexin (histamine)	Active
Non-REM sleep		
Cholinergic nuclei of pons-midbrain junction	Acetylcholine	Decreased
Locus coeruleus	Norepinephrine	Decreased
Raphe nuclei	Serotonin	Decreased
REM sleep on		
Cholinergic nuclei of pons-midbrain junction	Acetylcholine	Active
Raphe nuclei	Serotonin	Inactive
REM sleep off		
Locus coeruleus	Norepinephrine	Active

in the suprachiasmatic nucleus in the hypothalamus, which are entrained to the light-dark cycles that define day and night.

Consciousness

Although being awake is clearly a prerequisite to being conscious in the sense of being aware of the world and the self, these functions are not equivalent. Definitions of **consciousness** thus refer to at least three different aspects or meanings of the term:

1. A physiological meaning that describes consciousness in terms of the brain state we think of as **wakefulness**; this definition entails understanding the nature of brain activity that distinguishes wakefulness from sleep, and from unconscious states such as anesthesia or coma.

2. A more abstract meaning refers to a subjective **awareness** of the world, a brain state that must have a more subtle signature than wakefulness, since one can be awake and yet be unaware of some or even most aspects of the external and internal environments.

3. A meaning that refers to **self-awareness**, a term that defines consciousness in the sense of being aware of oneself as distinct from other selves in the world.

The latter two meanings of consciousness refer not to the neuroanatomical and physiological bases of wakefulness, but to the deeply puzzling ability we all have to be subjectively aware of the world and of ourselves as actors in it. Whereas consciousness as wakefulness and its physiological basis fits easily in the conventional framework of neurobiology, consciousness as awareness or self-awareness raises more difficult and contentious philosophical issues, and it has been far more difficult to pursue with the techniques of cognitive neuroscience or, for that matter, with any other methods.

Investigating consciousness is further complicated by the fact that being *aware* is not the same as being *self*-aware: one can imagine an animal that is aware of sensory data without having the integrated sense of a separate self that humans possess. Indeed, as described in Chapter 15, this sense takes some time to emerge even in developing humans. Laboratory animals such as rats and pigeons seem aware of the world, or at least of stimuli in it, but whether they are self-aware seems unlikely. By contrast, some non-human primates seem to be both aware of the world and (at least to some degree) aware of themselves as participants in it, although the level, or even existence, of such awareness is controversial.

Going further down the scale of brain (or nervous system) complexity, very simple animals presumably lack awareness altogether, at least in any conventional sense. Indeed, the most neurally simple animals presumably operate as automatons, although it is not clear which taxonomic level marks this distinction. Moreover, it is important to note that even in the human nervous system most neural processing is largely automatic, operating below the threshold of awareness. Think, for example, of all the homeostatic neural mechanisms that ensure your well-being in innumerable ways even as you read this sentence and ponder its significance.

Neural correlates of consciousness in normal subjects

These daunting issues notwithstanding, a number of neuroscientists, including some cognitive neuroscientists, have sought to address the basis of consciousness by ferreting out a signature of the neural processing that occurs when we are aware of something (e.g., a visual stimulus) compared to when we are not (e.g., presentation of the same stimulus under circumstances in which it does not elicit a reportable percept). Historically, the list of notable scientists who took up the mystery of consciousness includes electrophysiologist John Eccles, physicist Roger Penrose, cell biologist Gerald Edelman, and molecular biologist Francis Crick. All received Nobel Prizes for seminal work in their respective fields before seeking to understand consciousness, which they saw as the ultimate challenge in biology.

Although none of these giants succeeded in achieving the breakthroughs they hoped for, they generated several interesting theories based on quantum mechanics, information theory, and even the structure of neuronal microtubules. More importantly, their work prompted many neuroscientists to think more about this fascinating issue.

Along more conventional lines, recent studies of both normal subjects and patients with various pathological conditions have shed some light on this challenge. Most such work has, for practical reasons, been done in the context of visual perception, but the results tend to be assumed to apply to other sense modalities. In normal subjects, the most common approach has been to assess the nature and location of neural activity while a particular sensory percept shifts in and out of awareness. By asking the subject (or experimental animal) to report these perceptual transitions (verbally, by a button press, or on a touch screen), the investigator can compare neural activity that occurs during awareness of a stimulus to activity when the subject is unaware of the stimulus.

Some of the most widely used paradigms for this sort of study are binocular rivalry, the attentional blink, perceptual aftereffects, and visual masking (see Chapters 3 and 6). In most such paradigms, the stimulus remains unchanged and thus serves as its own control.

An especially attractive paradigm has been **binocular rivalry** (Figure 7.18). As described in Chapter 3, binocular rivalry refers to the fact that when a particular stimulus is presented to one eye while a discordant stimulus is presented to the other, the visual perception is of either one stimulus or the other, and it alternates back and forth every few seconds; there is only transient blending of both eye views. Using human subjects or monkeys trained to report what they are seeing at any given moment, electrophysiological or fMRI methods have been used to assess the changes in brain activity that occur when there is a switch of conscious content. For example, when the monocular inputs are faces and houses, recordings of fMRI activity show increases in the fusiform face area of the temporal lobe when a face is seen (see Chapter 3), and in the parahippocampal place area when houses are seen (see Figure 7.18). In similar paradigms, single neurons in monkeys in the visual cortex tend to show increased activity when the animal is perceiving the view of one eye but not the other.

A different fMRI paradigm with the same aim of probing activity changes in the low-level visual cortical regions during perception versus its absence takes advantage of visual aftereffects (see Chapter 3). For example, orientation aftereffects can be induced by exposing subjects to a series of lines (referred to as *gratings*) in a particular orientation (say, 45 degrees) for a minute or two; following this exposure, "neutral" line stimuli (vertical lines) are perceived for a number of seconds as being slightly tilted in the direction opposite the angle of the inducing exposure. The same inducing stimulus can be presented without awareness by masking it during the presentation. One can then ask whether lack of awareness of the inducing stimulus abolishes the aftereffect. It does not, implying that the low-level visual cortical neurons sensitive to orientation (see Chapter 3) are just as active when subjects are aware of the inducing stimulus as when they are not.

This lack of effect has been further confirmed in non-human primates by examining the activity of depth-sensitive (disparity-tuned) neurons in V1 that are active in response to stereoscopic stimuli. Again, little or no difference in activity is apparent when the monkeys indicate behaviorally that they

Figure 7.18 **Visual perception during binocular rivalry** Functional MRI study of brain activity as a function of the reported perception of the subjects. (A) Face images and house images were first presented at separate times (to both eyes) in order to localize regions in the brain particularly responsive to faces (fusiform face area, FFA) and to houses (parahippocampal place area, PPA). (B) Binocular rivalry paradigm. Face images and house images were then presented simultaneously and continuously, faces to the left eye and houses to the right eye. Even though the physical stimulus was not changing, the perception under these circumstances alternates every few seconds or so between perceiving the face and perceiving the house. (C) Time-locked, averaged fMRI activity in the FFA and PPA as a function of the reported perception by the subjects. When the face stimulus was the one being perceived, fMRI activity increased in the FFA and decreased in the PPA; when the house input was the one being perceived, the activity pattern reversed. The subsequent flip of activity that occurs somewhat later in time derives from the perceptual switch back a few seconds later. (After Tong et al. 1998.)

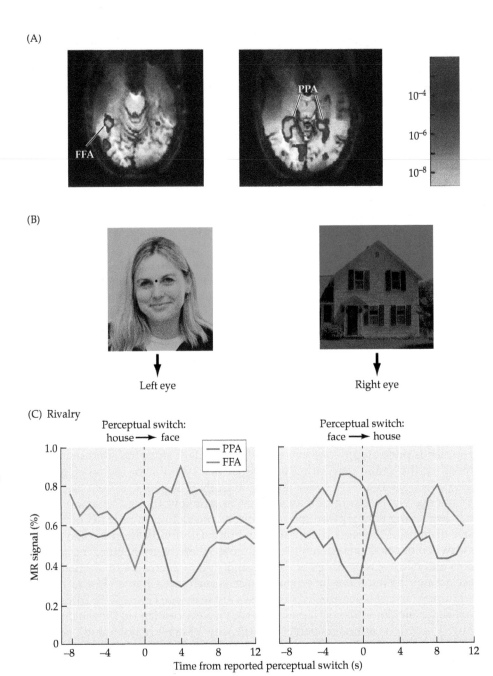

experienced a perception of depth compared to when they do not. In short, studies of activity in at least the earliest stages of visual cortical processing have not led to any clear hallmark of visual awareness.

It may help in rationalizing these somewhat confusing results to distinguish lower-order visual processing from higher-order visual processing in the visual association cortices. Recall from Chapter 3 that the higher-order visual areas are broadly divisible into a ventral stream running to the temporal lobe that is concerned with the recognition of visual stimuli (the "what" pathway), and a dorsal stream that is more concerned with stimulus location and spatial relations (the "where" pathway). It has been argued that correlations of neural activity with stimulus awareness in monkeys tend to increase as recording sites move away from V1 along the ventral pathway, toward the temporal lobe.

This interpretation accords with the majority of the studies mentioned in the preceding discussion, and with additional human fMRI studies testing this idea.

Another point is that the activity in some other cortical regions not generally thought of as visual is also correlated with visual awareness. Thus, other neuroimaging studies in humans have shown that perceptual changes in binocular rivalry and other bi-stable image paradigms are associated with activity in frontal and parietal cortical regions (i.e., they show altered activity in these cortical regions that is time-locked to the subjects' reports of the perceptual changes). As described earlier in the chapter, these regions have been implicated in changes in attentional control. Consistent with this evidence, other perceptual effects such as "pop-out" of a visual stimulus, or the awareness of a previously missed stimulus feature, are also correlated with activity changes in frontal and parietal areas. Transient functional disruption of processing in these areas by TMS also disturbs perception in normal subjects. Disturbances in perception following damage to these higher-level brain regions further confirm that they are somehow involved in perceptual awareness and consciousness, although their roles in these phenomena remain unclear.

Another idea concerning possible neural mechanisms underlying perceptual awareness involves a longer-latency return of activity back to the relevant sensory processing regions, but much later in time than the initial feedforward cascade. This longer-latency activity, termed **reentrant** or **recurrent** neural activation, has been proposed as an important underpinning of perceptual awareness. Because of the sluggishness of the fMRI BOLD signal, this method is unable to delineate such recurrent activity. EEG studies, however, have suggested that recurrent activity in visual processing regions correlates with reported awareness of an attended visual stimulus, although the tightness of the link between the activity and awareness is still unsettled.

Considered together, this evidence is consistent with the generally accepted idea that perception is based, at least in part, on altered activity of populations of cortical neurons in the regions of the association cortices that process the relevant stimulus, integrated with information arising from contextual influences and activity in higher-level brain areas. With respect to vision, the observed correlations described here suggest that activity in the visual association cortices is probably *necessary* for visual awareness, and that reentrance of activity in these areas may be particularly important. However, extrastriate activity does not appear to be a *sufficient* cause of stimulus awareness, and no clear defining neural signature of visual awareness has yet been discerned.

Neural correlates of consciousness in pathological conditions

Clinical evidence, some of it discussed already in other contexts in previous chapters, is also germane to understanding the neural basis of awareness and consciousness. A pathological phenomenon of particular interest in this regard is **blindsight**, most thoroughly studied over the last 40 years by psychologist Larry Weiskrantz and his colleagues. As described in Chapter 3, patients with damage to the primary visual cortex are blind in the affected area of the contralateral visual field (recall that as a result of the visual system anatomy, V1 in the right occipital lobe processes information arising from the left visual field, and V1 in the left occipital lobe processes input from the right visual field).

Objects presented within the area of blindness in the visual field (i.e., the scotoma) are simply not seen, at least according to the patient's verbal reports. Nevertheless, when some blindsight patients are forced by the experimenter to make a response to simple stimuli presented within their scotoma, the responses are often significantly above chance performance. For instance, if patients are asked to guess whether a stimulus line within their scotoma is vertical or horizontal, they answer correctly much of the time, even though they claim to have seen nothing. Blindsight can also be simulated in normal individuals by transient inactivation of V1 through TMS applied over the occipital lobes. Although the TMS creates a temporary scotoma for a specific region of the visual field, the features of simple stimuli presented in the unseen region tend to be guessed correctly at levels well above chance.

Functional neuroimaging and electrophysiological studies of patients with blindsight show that the unseen stimuli elicit some activity in extrastriate regions past V1, implying that these cortical areas are needed for successful behavior in the absence of awareness. This evidence underscores the conclusion of the previous section that extrastriate activity may be necessary for awareness but is not sufficient. One proposed explanation of blindsight is that subcortical visual processing of the stimulus, or coarse subcortical input to extrastriate cortex that bypasses V1, influences the patient's guesses. This interpretation accords with other evidence that subliminal (unconscious) information processing influences behavior of all sorts.

Another example of neural pathology pertinent to understanding awareness is the experience of *split-brain patients* that was described in the context of language (see Chapter 12). When the corpus callosum is cut as a treatment for otherwise intractable epileptic seizures, direct communication between the right and left hemispheres is no longer possible. The perceptual consequences of this surgery, first studied by cognitive neuroscientists Roger Sperry and Michael Gazzaniga in the 1960s, have suggested that the divided hemispheres in these patients function relatively independently, and that awareness generated by neural processing in one hemisphere is largely unavailable to the other.

For example, when simple written instructions such as "laugh" or "walk" are presented visually to the left visual field—and thus to the right brain—of a split-brain patient, many subjects have enough rudimentary verbal understanding in the right hemisphere to execute the commanded action. However, when asked to report *why* they laughed or walked, they typically confabulate (i.e., make up) a response using the superior language skills in the left hemisphere—saying, for instance, that something the experimenter said struck them as funny, or that they were tired of sitting and needed to walk a bit. Thus, the same individual under these circumstances seems to harbor two relatively independent domains of perceptual awareness and consciousness. This evidence raises the provocative question of whether consciousness is really the unified function we take it to be, and what role the corpus callosum plays in engendering such unity.

Whereas blindsight and hemispheric division lead to circumstances in which patients are unaware of stimulus processing that nonetheless influences their behavior, it is also possible to be aware (or believe one is aware) of something that doesn't actually exist. Perhaps the most striking illustrations of this sort of phenomenon are the *phantom limb* experiences of amputees described in Chapter 4.

Recall that a common experience following amputation is the patient's subjective awareness of the missing arm or leg, even though the physical limb and its peripheral sensory input are absent. Although the interpretation of this bizarre condition is debated, the awareness of the missing limb and sensations arising from it (pain is especially problematic for some amputees) seem quite real to the patient, emphasizing that processing of peripheral information is an active process in which the cortex constructs the percepts we experience. Hallucinations and visual illusions make the same point. In keeping with the evidence discussed in Chapters 3 and 4, awareness of the world does not simply arise by virtue of direct central representations that are generated by peripheral sense organs. Recognition of this fact adds an additional challenge to the problem of understanding the bases of consciousness.

Another clinical pathological condition pertinent to consciousness is **coma**. *Coma* (Greek for "deep sleep") is the term applied to the brain state of individuals who have suffered brain injury that leaves them in a deeply unconscious state defined by apparent unresponsiveness to sensory stimuli. The condition typically involves compromised function of the brainstem and other deep brain structures, such that the normal interaction of these structures with the cerebral cortex is interrupted.

Coma can arise from varying degrees of brain damage, and the prognosis is often uncertain. Most comatose individuals recover consciousness within a few days or weeks as the compromised neurons and the circuits they contribute to gradually regain their functions. Impairment can persist for much longer, however, if neural damage is more profound. Some patients recover consciousness after months, although typically with residual effects, and extremely rare cases have been reported in which consciousness was regained after some years. This variability has led to social, religious, and political controversy over the point at which an unresponsive patient should be considered to be in a **persistent vegetative state**—a diagnosis that raises ethical issues about decisions concerning whether to withhold life support measures. This sensitive issue means there has been, and will continue to be, great interest in techniques that could contribute to better understanding of a given patient's prognosis.

Electroencephalography has long been fundamental to diagnosing *irreversible brain death*, which occurs when brain trauma is so severe that no EEG activity can be recorded (i.e., there is a flat electrical trace). More recently, functional neuroimaging has also been used to evaluate persistent vegetative state, sometimes with surprising results. For example, in one case the brain of a 23-year-old woman who had been uncommunicative for 5 months following a traffic accident was functionally imaged. Despite her condition, fMRI showed that her brain responded to simple verbal commands by generating appropriate patterns of activity (Figure 7.19).

These studies of clinical conditions pertinent to awareness have been both extraordinarily interesting and informative (split-brain studies) and/or clinically important (studies of persistent vegetative state), but they have not led to any clear conclusions about the neural bases of consciousness. To judge from studies of normal subjects, awareness of sensory stimuli entails a modulation of activity in the sensory cortices (more so in the higher-order association cortices),

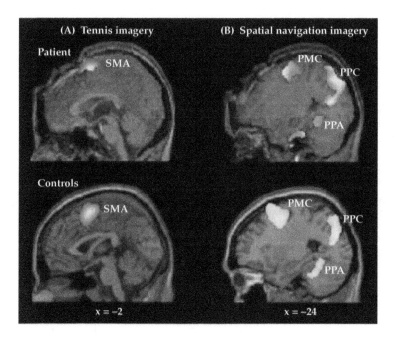

Figure 7.19 Purposeful brain responses in a patient in a persistent vegetative state In this study, fMRI was used to scan a patient who made no overt responses to external stimuli. (A) When she was asked to imagine playing tennis, however, her brain showed increased fMRI activation in the supplementary motor area (SMA) similar to that observed in normal control subjects. (B) And when she was asked to imagine walking around her house, her brain showed activity in the premotor cortex (PMC), posterior parietal cortex (PPC), and parahippocampal place area (PPA), again as in normal controls. (After Owen et al. 2006.)

as well as in frontal and parietal cortices that support attention and many other cognitive functions. However, the efforts to identify a neural basis for awareness and consciousness, and to gain an understanding of their relationship to attention, have not yet provided the sort of fundamental answers sought by many of the investigators in this field.

In the end, it may be that the phenomenon of consciousness is like the phenomenon of life. In centuries past, and up until the early decades of the twentieth century, some great philosophers and scientists sought a special property (often referred to as the *elan vital* or "life force," coined by the French philosopher Henri Bergson in 1907) that would distinguish living from nonliving matter. Today the concept of a life force is defunct; life is generally recognized as a descriptor that harbors no special non-physical mystery, its sufficient and necessary causes being largely understood. It is possible that the apparent mysteriousness of consciousness will also fade gradually away as cognitive neuroscientists understand more and more about the operation of neural networks—whether brains or simulated networks.

Summary

1. Given that paying attention elicits changes at many levels of the nervous system, an obvious question is whether there is an overarching control system (or systems) for the myriad attentional effects on stimulus processing that have been observed using behavioral, electrophysiological, and brain imaging methods.

2. Clinical data from patients indicate that when certain areas in the parietal and frontal cortices are damaged, the ability to direct and allocate attention is markedly compromised. The characteristics of these syndromes suggest that these areas are involved in the control of attention.

3. Most studies of attentional control systems in normal individuals have been carried out via endogenous cuing paradigms on subjects cued as to what to attend to on each trial, which they then voluntarily direct their attention to. These studies have yielded abundant evidence that the orienting of attention to locations or stimuli in the external environment is indeed associated with activity in several specific regions of the dorsal frontal and parietal cortices.

4. In contrast, exogenously induced attention, such as the reorienting of attention to salient or unexpected events, triggers increased activity in cortical regions near the temporoparietal junction and ventral frontal cortex, mainly on the right, which may in turn trigger the involvement of portions of this same dorsal frontoparietal network to implement the attentional orienting itself.

5. Visual search is the process of inspecting a complex visual scene or array for something of particular interest. Such searches have been roughly divided into those that can be performed in parallel across the visual field (detecting an object distinguished by a simple feature), and those that appear to require sequential focused attention on each item (detecting an object with a conjunction of two different features). Theoretical models and some neural studies have suggested that such searches involve stimulus salience maps, possibly located in parietal or parietal-temporal brain regions, along with activity in portions of the frontal and parietal attentional control circuits.

6. These various empirical findings have led to the development of models of attentional control that propose modulation via networks of interacting brain areas. A number of experimental studies testing the interactions between brain areas predicted by these models have provided support for these general ideas.

7. One dominant model holds that in response to both endogenously and exogenously induced attention, the dorsal frontoparietal network, once activated, operates as the attentional orienting control system that sends a biasing signal to the relevant sensory cortices to increase the baseline activity, thus facilitating stimulus processing in those cortices (or other pertinent brain regions). This scheme is consistent with the enhanced sensory activity elicited by attended stimuli, and with the associated improvement in behavioral performance in tasks involving these stimuli.

8. A complementary network of brain regions, known collectively as the default-mode network, is anticorrelated in activation pattern with the dorsal frontoparietal control network. In particular, the default-mode network, which includes

regions in inferior midline frontal cortex and the posterior cingulate cortex, is *deactivated* when subjects are engaged in an attentionally demanding task, and relatively more activated when they are not. The function of this complementary system is not yet clear, but it may play an overarching interactive role with the dorsal frontoparietal network in brain functions related to attentional control.

9. Consideration of attentional control and attentional systems leads to questions about levels of arousal and wakefulness, as well as the highly intriguing but difficult problem of consciousness and its neural basis. Levels of arousal and wakefulness are thought to be controlled by subcortical brainstem regions, particularly those collectively termed the reticular activating system.

10. Studies in both patients and normal subjects have not yet identified a clear neural basis for consciousness in the broader sense of awareness of the world and self. That said, perceptual awareness of sensory stimuli appears to be associated with a modulation of activity in the association sensory cortices, particularly late in processing in a reentrant way, as well as in frontal and parietal cortices that support attention and other higher-level cognitive functions.

Go to the **COMPANION WEBSITE**

sites.sinauer.com/cogneuro2e
for quizzes, animations, flashcards, and other study resources.

Additional Reading

Reviews

CORBETTA, M. AND G. L. SHULMAN (2002) Control of goal-directed and stimulus-driven attention in the brain. *Nat. Rev. Neurosci.* 3: 201–215.

HANNULA, D. E., D. J. SIMONS AND N. J. COHEN (2005) Imaging implicit perception: Promise and pitfalls. *Nat. Rev. Neurosci.* 6: 247–255.

HUSAIN, M. AND P. NACHEV (2007) Space and the parietal cortex. *Trends Cogn. Sci.* 11: 30–36.

MILLER, E. K. AND J. D. COHEN (2001) An integrative theory of prefrontal cortex function. *Annu. Rev. Neurosci.* 24: 167–202.

MOORE, T., K. M. ARMSTRONG AND M. FALLAH (2003) Visuomotor origins of covert spatial attention. *Neuron* 40: 671–683.

POSNER, M. I. AND S. E. PETERSEN (1990) The attention system of the human brain. *Annu. Rev. Neurosci.* 13: 25–42.

REES, G., G. KREIMAN AND C. KOCH (2002) Neural correlates of consciousness in humans. *Nat. Rev. Neurosci.* 3: 261–270.

STERZER, P., A. KLEINSCHMIDT AND G. REES (2009) The neural bases of multistable perception. *Trends Cogn. Sci.* 13: 310–318.

STOERIG, P. AND A. COWEY (1997) Blindsight in man and monkey. *Brain* 120: 535–559.

TONG, F. (2004) Primary visual cortex and visual awareness. *Nat. Rev. Neurosci.* 4: 219–226.

Important Original Papers

ASERINSKY, E. AND N. KLEITMAN (1953) Regularly occurring periods of eye motility, and concomitant phenomena during sleep. *Science* 118: 273–274.

BOYER, J. L., S. HARRISON AND T. RO (2005) Unconscious processing of orientation and color without primary visual cortex. *Proc. Natl. Acad. Sci. USA* 102: 16875–16879.

BRAIN, W. R. (1941) Visual disorientation with special reference to lesions of the right cerebral hemisphere. *Brain* 64: 244–272.

BUSCHMAN, T. J. AND E. K. MILLER (2007) Top-down versus bottom-up control of attention in the prefrontal and posterior parietal cortices. *Science* 315: 1860–1862.

COLBY, C. L., J. R. DUHAMEL AND M. E. GOLDBERG (1996) Visual, presaccadic, and cognitive activation of single neurons in monkey lateral intraparietal area. *J. Neurophysiol.* 76: 641–652.

COOPER, A. A. AND G. W. HUMPHREYS (2000) Coding space within but not between objects: Evidence from Balint's syndrome. *Neuropsychologia* 38: 723–733.

CORBETTA, M., J. M. KINCADE, J. M. OLLINGER, M. P. MCAVOY AND G. L. SHULMAN (2000) Voluntary orienting is dissociated from target detection in human posterior parietal cortex. *Nat. Neurosci.* 3: 292–297.

CORBETTA, M., F. M. MIEZIN, G. L. SHULMAN AND S. E. PETERSEN (1993) A PET study of visuospatial attention. *J. Neurosci.* 13: 602–626.

CORBETTA, M. AND 10 OTHERS (1998) A common network of functional areas for attention and eye movements. *Neuron* 21: 761–773.

FRIEDMAN-HILL, S. R., L. C. ROBERTSON AND A. TREISMAN (1995) Parietal contributions to visual feature binding: Evidence from a patient with bilateral lesions. *Science* 269: 853–855.

GREGORIOU, G. G., S. J. GOTTS, H. ZHOU AND R. DESIMONE (2009) High-frequency, long-range coupling between prefrontal and visual cortex during attention. *Science* 324: 1207–1210.

GRENT-'T-JONG, T. AND M. G. WOLDORFF (2007) Timing and sequence of brain activity in top-down control of visual-spatial attention. *PLoS Biol.* 5: e12.

HOPFINGER, J. B., M. H. BUONOCORE AND G. R. MANGUN (2000) The neural mechanisms of top-down attentional control. *Nat. Neurosci.* 3: 284–291.

KASTNER, S., M. A. PINSK, P. DE WEERD, R. DESIMONE AND L. G. UNGERLEIDER (1999) Increased activity in human visual cortex during directed attention in the absence of visual stimulation. *Neuron* 22: 751–761.

KNIGHT, R. T., S. A. HILLYARD, D. L. WOODS AND H. J. NEVILLE (1981) The effects of frontal cortex lesions on event-related potentials during auditory selective attention. *Electroencephalogr. Clin. Neurophysiol.* 52: 571–582.

LEE, S.-H., R. BLAKE AND D. J. HEEGER (2005) Traveling waves of activity in early visual cortex during binocular rivalry. *Nat. Neurosci.* 8: 22–23.

LIU, T., S. D. SLOTNICK, J. T. SERENCES AND S. YANTIS (2003) Cortical mechanisms of feature-based attentional control. *Cereb. Cortex* 13: 1334–1343.

LUCK, S. J., L. CHELAZZI, S. A. HILLYARD AND R. DESIMONE (1997) Neural mechanisms of spatial selective attention in areas V1, V2, and V4 of macaque visual cortex. *J. Neurophysiol.* 77: 24–42.

MESULAM, M. M. (1981) A cortical network for directed attention and unilateral neglect. *Ann. Neurol.* 10: 309–325.

MOORE, T. AND K. M. ARMSTRONG (2003) Selective gating of visual signals by microstimulation of frontal cortex. *Nature* 421: 370–373.

Moruzzi, G. and H. W. Magoun (1949) Brain stem reticular formation and activation of the EEG. *Electroencephalogr. Clin. Neurophysiol.* 1: 455–473.

O'Connor, D. H., M. M. Fukui, M. A. Piinsk and S. Kastner (2002) Attention modulates responses in the human lateral geniculate nucleus. *Nat. Neurosci.* 5: 1203–1209.

Owen, A. M., M. R. Coleman, M. Boly, M. H. Davis, S. Laureys and J. D. Pickard (2006) Detecting awareness in the vegetative state. *Science* 313: 1402.

Raichle, M. E., A. M. MacLeod, A. Z. Snyder, W. J. Powers, D. A. Gusnard and G. L. Shulman (2001) A default mode of brain function. *Proc. Natl. Acad. Sci. USA* 98: 676–682.

Rihs, T. A., C. M. Michel and G. Thut (2007) Mechanisms of selective inhibition in visual spatial attention are indexed by alpha-band EEG synchronization. *Eur. J. Neurosci.* 25: 603–610.

Serences, J. T., S. Shomstein, A. B. Leber, X. Golay, H. E. Egeth and S. Yantis (2005) Coordination of voluntary and stimulus-driven attentional control in human cortex. *Psychol. Sci.* 16: 114–122.

Sprague, J. M. (1966) Interaction of cortex and superior colliculus in mediation of visually guided behavior in the cat. *Science* 153: 1544–1547.

Steinmetz, M. A. and C. Constantinidis (1995) Neurophysiological evidence for a role of posterior parietal cortex in redirecting visual attention. *Cereb. Cortex* 5: 448–456.

Thompson, K. G., K. L. Biscoe and T. R. Sato (2005) Neuronal basis of covert spatial attention in the frontal eye field. *J. Neurosci.* 25: 9479–9487.

Tong, F., K. Nakayama, J.T. Vaughn and N. Kanwisher (1998) Binocular rivalry and visual awareness in human extrastriate cortex. *Neuron* 21: 753–759.

Treisman, A. and G. Gelade (1980) A feature integration theory of attention. *Cogn. Psychol.* 12: 97–136.

Weissman, D. H., K. C. Roberts, K. M. Visscher and M. G. Woldorff (2006) The neural bases of momentary lapses in attention. *Nat. Neurosci.* 9: 971–978.

Wojciulik, E. and N. Kanwisher (1999) The generality of parietal involvement in visual attention. *Neuron* 23: 747–764.

Woldorff, M. G., C. J. Hazlett, H. M. Fichtenholtz, D. H. Weissman, A. M. Dale and A. W. Song (2004) Functional parcellation of attentional control regions of the brain. *J. Cogn. Neurosci.* 16: 149–165.

Wolfe, J. (1994) Guided search 2.0: A revised model of visual search. *Psychol. Bull. Rev.* 1: 202–238.

Woodman, G. F. and S. J. Luck (1999) Electrophysiological measurement of rapid shifts of attention during visual search. *Nature* 400: 867–869.

Worden, M. S., J. J. Foxe, N. Wang and G. V. Simpson (2000) Anticipatory biasing of visuospatial attention indexed by retinotopically specific alpha-band electroencephalography increases over occipital cortex. *J. Neurosci.* 20: 1–6.

Yantis, S. and 6 others (2002) Transient neural activity in human parietal cortex during spatial attention shifts. *Nat. Neurosci.* 5: 995–1002.

Books

Dennett, D. C. (1991) *Consciousness Explained*. Boston: Little, Brown.

Itti, L., G. Rees and J. K. Tsotsos, eds. (2005) *Neurobiology of Attention*. Amsterdam: Elsevier.

Koch, C. (2012) *Consciousness. The Confessions of a Romantic Reductionist*. Cambridge MA: MIT Press.

Posner, M., ed. (2012) *The Cognitive Neuroscience of Attention*, 2nd Ed. New York: Guilford.

8

Memory: Varieties and Mechanisms

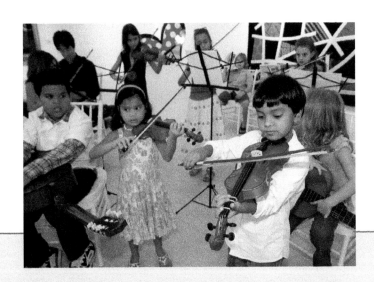

INTRODUCTION

Memory allows us to learn from the past, understand the present, and plan for the future. All cognitive abilities depend on memory to one degree or another. Perception is the result of an interaction between sensory stimuli and stored knowledge about the world. For example, identifying objects depends on accessing preexisting memories about these objects. Attention is also dependent on memory, as past experiences guide the processes of searching for and selecting relevant stimuli in the environment. Our emotional responses are also altered by our memories. In fact, identical stimuli can elicit very different emotional responses in different people, depending on their life experiences. Language depends on concepts and grammatical rules stored in memory. Decision making often requires information that must be retrieved from memory. Finally, our sense of self and our capacity to project ourselves into the future depends on our personal memories.

Memory is not a unitary phenomenon (see Introductory Box). Researchers distinguish between a system that maintains memories for a few seconds or minutes (working memory) and systems that maintain memories for longer periods. The latter include systems that mediate conscious memories for events and facts (declarative memory) and systems that mediate memories that are expressed through task performance (nondeclarative memory). The current chapter begins by introducing some basic concepts and reviewing evidence supporting the distinctions of working memory, declarative memory, and nondeclarative memory. It then focuses on the neural bases of the main forms of nondeclarative memory—namely, priming, skill learning, and conditioning. Finally, the chapter ends by describing cellular mechanisms shared by all memory systems. Declarative memory is the focus of Chapter 9 and working memory is considered together with other executive functions in Chapter 13.

■ INTRODUCTORY BOX **THE CASE OF H.M.**

One of the most consequential discoveries in the history of memory research was serendipitous, resulting from the unexpected effects of a neurosurgical procedure performed in 1953. Patient H.M. (Henry Molaison) was a 27-year-old man who suffered from medically intractable epilepsy that left him unable to work and severely debilitated. With the intent of relieving H.M.'s frequent seizures, neurosurgeon William Scoville removed much of the patient's temporal lobes on both sides, including the amygdala, the entorhinal cortex, and about two-thirds of the hippocampus (Figures A–D). Prior to the surgery, H.M. had been experiencing about 10 minor seizures every day, with a major seizure every few days. Consistent with the assumption that the source of the seizures was in the medial temporal lobes, the surgery was successful in relieving the seizures. Unfortunately, the bilateral removal of these structures had an unforeseen consequence: the surgery left H.M. with a devastating memory deficit.

After the original report of his memory loss, which Scoville and neuropsychologist Brenda Milner published in 1957, more than 100 researchers tested H.M. using a variety of tasks, until his death in 2008. The importance of H.M.'s case comes from the purity of his memory deficit, which showed the major features of amnesia that are often present in other cases, but seldom with the same degree of clarity.

First, although H.M. was severely impaired in memory functions, he had little or no difficulty in other cognitive domains. His sensory and perceptual functions were remarkably preserved. His IQ was normal and even improved a little following surgery, perhaps because of the relief from seizures. Moreover, he had no deficit in executive tasks, including performance on tasks assumed to measure frontal lobe function (see Chapter 13).

Second, H.M.'s memory deficits generalized to all kinds of information and to all sensory modalities. He remembered neither verbal stimuli, such as new names and words, nor nonverbal stimuli, such as faces and spatial layouts. He was unable to remember postsurgery events, regardless of whether the information to be learned or the questions posed were presented visually, auditorily, or in another sensory modality.

Third, although H.M.'s ability to remember new events and facts (declarative memory) was severely impaired, his ability to retain information for brief periods of time (working memory) was intact. For example, when asked to repeat a list of digits (**digit-span task**), he was able to repeat without error about seven to nine digits, which is the normal range. He also had normal working memory for pictorial material.

Finally, and perhaps most important, H.M.'s memory deficits were limited to tasks that require memory of events and facts; his problems did not affect memories expressed through performance, such as motor or cognitive skills. For example, when tracing geometrical figures that could be seen only via a mirror (**mirror drawing task**; Figure E), H.M. showed daily improvements; and these improvements persisted over time,

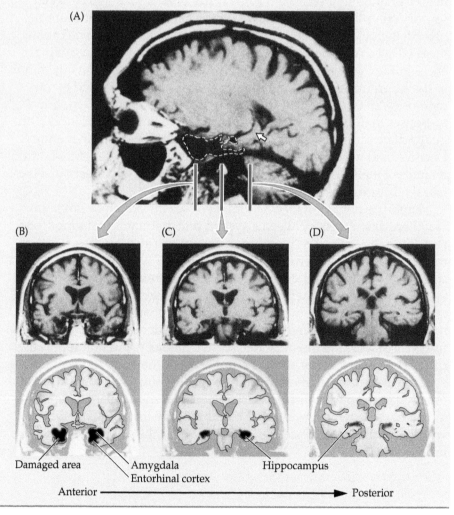

MRI images of H.M.'s brain. (A) The area of H.M.'s anterior temporal lobe destroyed by surgery is indicated by the white dotted line. The intact posterior hippocampus is the banana-shaped object indicated by the white arrow. (This sagittal view shows the right hemisphere; H.M.'s lesions were in fact bilateral.) (B–D) Coronal sections at approximately the levels indicated by the red lines in (A). Image (B) is the most rostral and is at the level of the amygdala. The amygdala and associated cortex are entirely missing. Image (C) is at the level of the rostral hippocampus; again, this structure and the associated cortex have been removed. Image (D) is at the caudal level of the hippocampus; the posterior hippocampus appears intact, although shrunken. The outlines below images (B), (C), and (D) indicate the areas of H.M.'s brain that were destroyed (black shading). (A–D from Corkin et al. 1997.)

■ INTRODUCTORY BOX (continued)

much as in normal subjects (Figure F), even though he did not consciously remember having traced geometrical figures before.

In sum, the case of H.M. made clear for the first time the critical importance of the medial temporal regions in certain types of human memory, stimulating much of the research described in this chapter and the next.

References

CORKIN S, D. G. AMARAL, R. G. GONZALEZ, K. A. JOHNSON AND B. T. HYMAN (1997) H.M.'s medial temporal lobe lesion: Findings from magnetic resonance imaging. *J. Neurosci.* 17: 3964–3979.

MILNER, B., S. CORKIN AND H.-L. TEUBER (1968) Further analysis of the hippocampal amnesic syndrome: A 14-year follow-up study of H.M. *Neuropsychologia* 6: 215–234.

SALAT, D. H. AND 6 OTHERS (2006) Neuroimaging H.M.: A 10-year follow-up examination. *Hippocampus* 16: 936–945.

SCOVILLE, W. B. AND B. MILNER (1957) Loss of recent memory after bilateral hippocampal lesions. *J. Neurol. Neurosurg. Psychiat.* 20: 11–21.

SQUIRE, L. R. (2009) The legacy of patient H.M. for neuroscience. *Neuron* 61: 6–9.

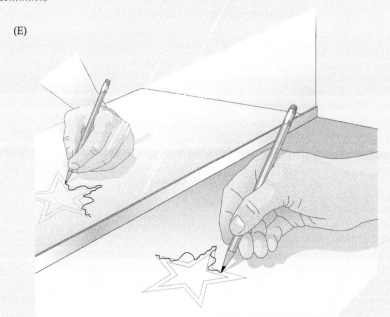

(E)

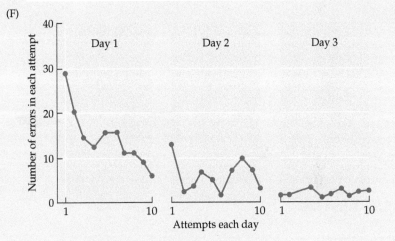

(F)

(E) The mirror drawing task involves tracing geometrical figures seen in a mirror. (F) H.M. shows normal learning in this nondeclarative memory task (errors decrease during the first session), and this learning persists across time (errors start at a lower level the second day). (E,F after Milner et al. 1968.)

Memory Phases, Processes, Systems, and Tasks

Memory is the series of processes whereby the nervous system acquires information from new experiences, retains this information over time, and eventually uses it to guide behavior and plan future actions. This definition points to three basic memory phases shared by all forms of memory: encoding, storage, and retrieval. **Encoding** consists of the processes whereby experiences can alter the nervous system. These alterations, known as *memory traces*, are believed to involve primarily changes in the strength and/or number of synaptic connections between neurons. **Storage** is the retention of memory traces over time. Long-term retention requires cell- and system-level stabilization or *consolidation* processes, which are described in Chapter 9. **Retrieval** is the accessing of stored memory traces, which may lead to a change in behavior and sometimes is associated with the conscious experience of remembering.

Learning—a term closely related to *memory*—is used as a synonym of *encoding* and can also describe gradual changes in behavior as a function of training.

■ BOX 8A INVESTIGATING DECLARATIVE MEMORY IN NON-HUMAN ANIMALS

The most obvious challenge to investigating declarative memory in non-human animals is that they cannot follow verbal instructions or "declare" their memories verbally. However, there are ways of measuring declarative memory in such circumstances.

One such method used in studies on non-human primates is known as a *delayed non-match-to-sample task* (Figure A). A typical trial in this paradigm has three phases. During the *sample phase*, a monkey is shown a single stimulus (e.g., a brown cross) above a well containing a food reward; during the *delay phase*, a door is lowered so the monkey can no longer see the stimulus and reward; and during the *choice phase*, the monkey is presented with the previously rewarded stimulus (the brown cross) along with a new stimulus (e.g., a brown rectangle) that conceals the food reward. This time the animal must select the new (non-matching) stimulus in order to obtain the reward. Using non-match-to-sample tasks, cognitive neuroscientists David Gaffan and Mortimer Mishkin showed that lesions of the medial temporal lobe severely impair memory in monkeys, thus providing the first animal model of the human amnesia syndrome.

Such studies can also be done using rodents—a particularly important advance because the use of rodents allows us to examine the genetic basis of behavior in these animals. The most popular task for measuring declarative memory in rodents is the *Morris water maze*, pioneered by neuroscientist Richard Morris and his group. The animal's task is to swim to a

Testing declarative memory in non-human animals. (A) The delayed non-match-to-sample task. Declarative memory is indexed by the ability to choose the novel stimulus. (B) The Morris water maze. Declarative memory is indexed by the ability to find the hidden platform.

(A)

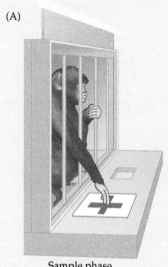
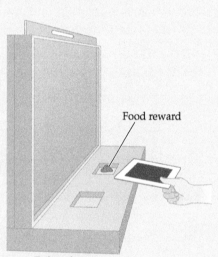
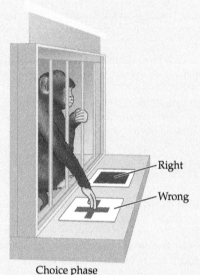

Sample phase   Delay phase   Choice phase

Food reward

Right

Wrong

(B)

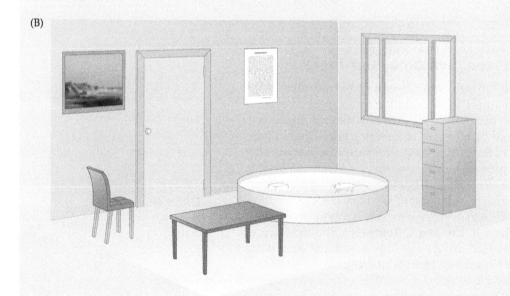
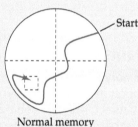
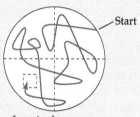

Start

Normal memory

Start

Impaired memory

■ **BOX 8A** *(continued)*

small platform hidden just beneath the surface in a circular tank filled with murky water, which then provides a safe haven (Figure B). Once the animal has learned where to find the platform, the experimenter can assess memory by measuring how long the rat takes to find the platform again, or how much time it spends within the quadrant that contains the platform compared to the other three quadrants of the tank. Given that the murky water

means the animal's view of the tank is the same in all directions, remembered cues from objects in the room (e.g., windows, pictures on the wall) are presumably used to locate the platform.

The Morris water maze measures spatial memory; however, it is also possible to measure nonspatial forms of declarative memory in rodents in paradigms such as the odor association task described in the text and Figure 9.4.

References

D'HOOGE, R. AND P. P. DE DEYN (2001) Applications of the Morris water maze in the study of learning and memory. *Brain Res. Rev.* 36(1): 60–90.

EICHENBAUM, H. AND N. J. COHEN (2001) *From Conditioning to Conscious Recollection: Memory Systems of the Brain.* New York: Oxford University Press.

In this second meaning, the term *learning* refers to the combined effect of all encoding, storage, and retrieval in gradually enhancing the performance of a particular task. For this reason, the second use of *learning* is popular in contexts with multiple learning trials, such as school education, skill learning, and most of the animal memory paradigms.

In addition to memory phases and memory processes, researchers distinguish among different memory systems. Memory systems can be defined as groups of memory processes and associated brain regions that tend to interact to mediate performance over a class of similar memory tasks. This last property illustrates one of the advantages of using psychological constructs (see Chapter 1) such as a memory system: a single construct can account for a whole set of empirical results. The idea that memory systems mediate performance in specific memory tasks does not, however, imply that each memory task measures a single memory system. Although some tasks depend primarily on one memory system, most tasks are sensitive to the contributions of more than one memory system. For this reason, drawing inferences from memory tasks about the operation of memory systems requires converging evidence from several different tasks. For example, the same memory system is assumed to mediate the ability of remembering personally experienced events regardless of whether recall is spoken or written.

The notion of memory systems has a very long history, with some basic ideas going as far back as ancient Greece. As described in the Introductory Box, one of the most important advances in the twentieth century was the report in 1957 of patient H.M., who suffered from amnesia. H.M.'s case showed clearly that memories associated with consciousness depend on medial temporal lobe regions, whereas other types of memory, those expressed through behavior, are independent of these regions. Inspired by the case of H.M., behavioral neuroscientists tried to produce a non-human animal model of his amnesia. Although the role of consciousness cannot be assessed in rodents and monkeys, researchers reasonably assumed that tasks impaired by medial temporal lobe damage measure types of memory similar to those impaired in H.M. (Box 8A).

In parallel with this research, psychologists investigating memory in normal human participants during the 1970s found evidence that retaining information across delays of seconds or minutes (*short-term memory*) involves mechanisms that are fundamentally different from those used for retaining information across delays of hours, days, or weeks (*long-term memory*). The concept of short-term memory, which originally was about simple maintenance of information, was later expanded into the notion of working memory, which includes not only simple maintenance but also operations performed on the information being maintained and mechanisms of attention allocation.

Figure 8.1 **A general taxonomy of memory systems** The working memory (or short-term memory) system maintains information for a few seconds; the long-term memory system maintains information for longer periods. Declarative (explicit) memory is conscious memory for events and facts; nondeclarative (implicit) memory is memory expressed through performance, independently of consciousness.

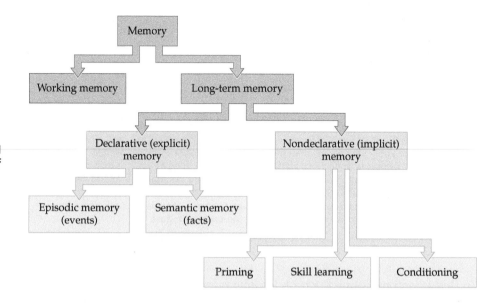

These various developments led to the taxonomy of memory systems illustrated in **Figure 8.1**. **Working memory** mediates the maintenance and manipulation of information online for a few seconds or minutes. In contrast, long-term memory systems mediate the retention of information for longer periods (days, months, decades). Long-term memory systems are typically divided into declarative and nondeclarative types. **Declarative memory** (also known as *explicit memory*) refers to conscious memory for events (*episodic memory*) and facts (*semantic memory*). As noted already, although declarative memory was originally distinguished by having a component of consciousness, researchers have developed tasks that depend on similar brain regions in rodents and monkeys, and that can be used to study declarative memory in non-human animals. **Nondeclarative memory** (also known as *implicit memory*) refers to memories that are expressed through performance independently of consciousness. As described later, there are several different forms of nondeclarative memory. Before considering each memory system (nondeclarative memory in this chapter, declarative memory in the next chapter, and working memory in Chapter 13), it is important to review the evidence supporting these major taxonomic distinctions.

Dissociating Memory Systems

The taxonomy in Figure 8.1 is supported by abundant evidence that the functions of different memory systems can be dissociated by examining the results of brain lesions in human patients and animals, as well as by functional brain imaging and electrophysiology. The next two sections provide some examples from human patients supporting the distinctions between working memory and declarative memory, and between declarative and nondeclarative memory.

Working memory versus declarative memory

The most telling evidence supporting the distinction between working memory and declarative memory has been provided by cases of **amnesia**. This term is typically applied to severe memory loss due to brain damage, but it may also be used to describe our normal lack of memory for events that took place during the first few years of life (**childhood amnesia**) or memory loss due to psychological trauma (psychogenic amnesia). In the case of brain damage, the memory loss may affect information acquired after the damage (**anterograde amnesia**), information acquired before the lesion (**retrograde amnesia**), or both.

Amnesia due to brain lesions most often arises from bilateral damage to the medial temporal lobe. Unilateral damage of these regions usually produces relatively mild memory deficits because the spared medial temporal lobe regions can still support some aspects of memory. But when damage to the medial temporal lobe is bilateral, patients may display severe anterograde amnesia with some degree of retrograde amnesia. The retrograde amnesia typically covers a few years prior to the lesion, as in the case of H.M., but when damage to the medial temporal lobe is extensive, the retrograde amnesia may extend several decades back.

Because of their anterograde amnesia, patients with bilateral damage to the medial temporal lobe cannot form new memories for events. For example, a patient may have a normal conversation with a new doctor, but if the doctor leaves the room, even for a few minutes, the patient may not recognize her when she comes back. The fact that patients with amnesia can maintain a normal conversation implies that working memory is spared, since conversing requires remembering what was said during the last few seconds or minutes.

The finding that people who suffer from amnesia because of damage to the medial temporal lobe are impaired in declarative memory but not in working memory constitutes a *single dissociation*. As explained in Chapter 2, however, single dissociations are not enough to postulate different underlying brain systems. The *double dissociation*, needed to strengthen the case, would require brain-damaged patients who are impaired in working memory but *not* in declarative memory. Such patients have been identified, and their lesions are typically in the left temporoparietal cortex.

One of the most severe cases of working memory deficit resulting from damage to the left temporoparietal cortex is patient K.F. When asked, for example, to repeat back a list of numbers, which normal subjects do correctly up to a maximum of seven or eight digits, K.F. could remember only two digits. Likewise, he could rarely repeat back lists of four words, which is something normal participants can virtually always do (**Figure 8.2A**, left). Yet K.F.'s declarative memory performance was slightly better than normal. In fact, to learn longer lists he needed fewer repetitions than control participants needed, and he remembered the lists for long periods (Figure 8.2A, right). This pattern is opposite the findings in patients with only medial temporal lobe damage (like H.M.), who are impaired in declarative memory but not in working memory (**Figure 8.2B**).

Declarative versus nondeclarative memory

A key feature of medial temporal lobe amnesia is that it impairs declarative memory, as exhibited in tests of recall and recognition but not in nondeclarative memory tasks such as skill learning and priming. For example, H.M. was able to learn to trace geometrical figures projected in a mirror (visuomotor skill) at a normal rate, even though he could not remember the training sessions (see Introductory Box). Conversely, a patient referred to as M.S. showed impaired nondeclarative memory but normal declarative memory. Like H.M., M.S. had surgery to relieve intractable epileptic seizures. However, the brain regions removed

Figure 8.2 Evidence for different anatomical substrates of working and declarative memory (A) Patient K.F. was impaired in immediate word recall, but he needed fewer repetitions than control subjects did to remember word lists for longer periods of time. **(B)** In ontrast, amnesia patients like H.M. tend to show intact working memory but impaired declarative memory. (A after Warrington and Shallice 1969; B after Drachman and Arbit 1966.)

(A) Patient K.F.: Impaired working memory versus preserved declarative memory

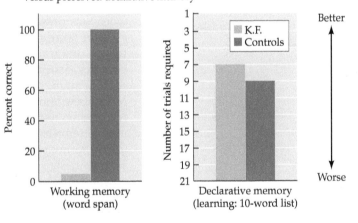

(B) Patient H.M. (amnesic): Preserved working memory versus impaired declarative memory

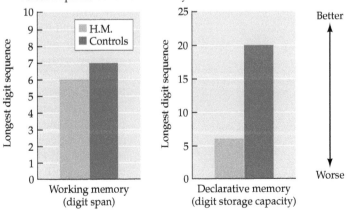

(A)

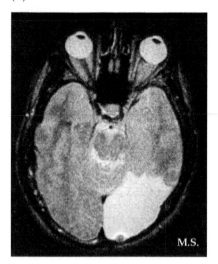

(B) Implicit test

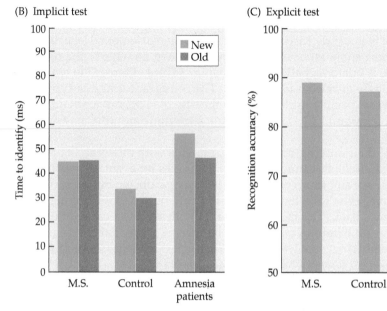

(C) Explicit test

Figure 8.3 Double dissociation of declarative and nondeclarative memory in patient M.S. (A) The surgery performed on M.S. removed the right occipital regions of his brain, including the primary and much of the secondary visual cortex (light area). (B) In an implicit word identification test, M.S. shows impaired priming, whereas amnesia patients show normal priming. (C) In an explicit recognition test, M.S. shows normal performance, but amnesia patients show impaired performance. (After Gabrieli et al. 1995.)

in his case were not the medial temporal lobes but the right occipital regions, including the primary and much of the secondary visual cortex (Figure 8.3A). As a result of the surgery, M.S. became blind in his left visual field. Aside from the vision deficits, he was in good health and showed normal performance on standardized tests of attention, memory, language, perception, and reasoning.

One study compared M.S. to a group of healthy controls and a group of subjects with amnesia using an implicit (nondeclarative) test in which each word was presented for increasing periods until it was identified correctly. Half the words had been seen in a previous session, and half were presented for the first time. As illustrated in Figure 8.3B, control subjects and amnesia patients identified previously seen words after shorter presentations, thus demonstrating *priming*. Despite good word identification performance, however, M.S. showed no priming effect in this task. In contrast, in a declarative (explicit) recognition test, his performance was normal, whereas amnesia patients with medial temporal lobe damage were impaired (Figure 8.3C). Thus, M.S. was impaired in nondeclarative but not in declarative memory, whereas patients with amnesia showed the opposite pattern. M.S.'s priming deficits cannot be attributed to his visual impairment, since he was blind only in the left visual field and, as mentioned, his performance on the (visually mediated) word identification test was normal.

Thus, both of the major distinctions in the taxonomy in Figure 8.1 are supported by clinical cases (for exceptions, see Box 8B). Whereas medial temporal lobe damage tends to impair declarative but not working memory, left temporoparietal damage can disrupt working memory while sparing declarative memory. In addition, medial temporal lobe damage tends to disrupt declarative memory while sparing nondeclarative memory functions, whereas occipital lobe damage may impair nondeclarative memory (tested with visual priming) without altering declarative memory performance.

Finally, note that although some brain regions are differentially involved in working memory (see Chapter 13), declarative memory (see Chapter 9), and nondeclarative memory (see the next section), these functions involve other brain regions that they share. For example, some frontal and parietal regions contribute to both working and declarative memory, as well as to both declarative and

■ BOX 8B MEDIAL TEMPORAL LOBE CONTRIBUTIONS BEYOND DECLARATIVE MEMORY

Although the basic idea that medial temporal lobe regions are critical for declarative memory tasks but not for working memory and nondeclarative memory tasks fits well with most data, there are several exceptions to this general rule.

Regarding working memory, the case of H.M. (see Introductory Box) clearly showed that medial temporal lobe regions are not necessary for maintaining simple familiar stimuli, such as digits, for brief periods of time. However, there are a few reports of patients with medial temporal lobe amnesia who were impaired in complex novel stimuli processed by working memory, such as pictures of unfamiliar objects. In addition, single-cell recordings in monkeys identified medial temporal neurons that showed sustained activity during the delay period of working memory tasks. Moreover, fMRI studies with humans reported medial temporal lobe activation during working memory tasks for a variety of novel visual stimuli.

Turning to nondeclarative memory, we find evidence supporting a role of medial temporal lobe regions in some priming and implicit learning tasks. Although patients with medial temporal lobe amnesia show normal priming for single items,

such as words, some reports claim that they can be impaired in priming for new associations. Furthermore, the implicit memory effect whereby repeated backgrounds enhance visual search was found to be impaired by some forms of medial temporal lobe damage. Likewise, implicit memory effects on eye movements were found to be impaired in patients with medial temporal lobe amnesia and to elicit hippocampal activity in normal participants. Moreover, hippocampal activations were found for old items consciously perceived as new and for subliminally encoded items.

Two main hypotheses have been proposed to explain medial temporal lobe involvement in working memory and nondeclarative memory. One idea, originally proposed by neuroscientists Howard Eichenbaum and Neal Cohen, is that the hippocampus mediates memory for new associations, or *relational memory*, regardless of whether the memories have to be maintained only briefly or are processed outside of consciousness. A related idea is that the medial temporal lobe is critical for processing *flexible memory representations*—those that can be applied in a context different from the one associated with encoding. Although

some authors believe that these two factors are more important for defining medial temporal, and in particular hippocampal, function than consciousness is, most memory researchers believe that consciousness is a major factor and use the memory system taxonomy diagrammed in Figure 8.1.

References

CHUN, M. M. AND E. A. PHELPS (1999) Memory deficits for implicit contextual information in amnesic subjects with hippocampal damage. *Nat. Neurosci.* 2: 844–847.

DEW, I. T. AND R. CABEZA (2011) The porous boundaries between explicit and implicit memory: Behavioral and neural evidence. *Ann. N. Y. Acad. Sci.* 1224: 174–190.

HENKE, K. (2010) A model for memory systems based on processing modes rather than consciousness. *Nat. Rev. Neurosci.* 11: 523–532.

RANGANATH, C. AND R. S. BLUMENFELD (2005) Doubts about double dissociations between short- and long-term memory. *Trends Cogn. Sci.* 9: 374–380.

nondeclarative memory. Moreover, as described later in the chapter, all forms of memory presumably depend on similar cellular and molecular mechanisms.

Nondeclarative Memory

All forms of nondeclarative memory have in common the facts that they are expressed through performance and are independent of conscious awareness. In other words, nondeclarative memory is evidenced by changed behavior, even if the person is unaware that memories from specific past experience are being accessed. Despite these shared properties, the major forms of nondeclarative memory—namely, priming, skill learning, and conditioning (see Figure 8.1)—are very different from each other. **Priming** is a change in the processing of a stimulus due to a previous encounter with the same or a related stimulus, such as completing a word fragment with a previously read word. **Skill learning** is a gradual improvement in performance due to repeated practice, such as mirror drawing in the case of H.M. or riding a bicycle. **Conditioning** consists of simple responses to associations between stimuli, as when a dog salivates at the sound of a can opener associated with food. Thus, whereas priming can result from a single encounter with a stimulus, skill learning requires repeated learning trials. Conditioning also involves multiple learning trials, but typically simpler responses and associations, than skill learning. The sections that follow consider these phenomena in turn.

Priming

Priming is defined as a change in the efficacy of stimulus processing arising from a previous encounter with the same or a related stimulus, in the absence of conscious awareness about the first encounter. In a typical paradigm, participants attend a first session in which they read words, and a second session in which they solve word puzzles seemingly unrelated to the words previously read. For example, they may be asked to complete word fragments (e.g., E_V_L_P_) with the first words that come to mind. Priming is then measured as an increase in the probability of completing word fragments with words presented during the first phase (e.g., the word *envelope*). Critically, this facilitation effect is found even if participants are unaware that they solved the fragments using words previously read in the experiment. In this paradigm, priming is measured as an increase in the probability of generating a particular stimulus, but priming can be measured in many different ways, including increases in processing speed and changes in eye movement patterns.

The requirement that participants be unaware that they are using information from the first session is critical. Participants should complete E_V_L_P_ with *envelope* because this is the first word that comes to mind, not because they tried to recall words from the study list. However, sometimes participants spontaneously realize that some fragments can be completed with words previously seen in the laboratory, and they try retrieve these words to complete the fragments. If this happens, the test is said to be *contaminated by explicit memory strategies*, and its results cannot be considered a valid measure of implicit memory. Several methods have been developed to reduce the chances of explicit memory contamination, such as using shallow or subliminal encoding conditions, or encouraging fast test responses. Such studies may also include priming *and* very similar declarative memory tests; if the two tests show different patterns of results, it is fair to conclude that the priming task was not contaminated.

Figure 8.4 illustrates the major forms of priming. Depending on the relationship between the stimulus that generates the priming effect (the prime) and the stimulus eliciting that effect (the target), priming can be classified as direct or indirect. In **direct priming**, also called *repetition priming*, prime and target stimuli are the same; in **indirect priming** they are different. The most typical form of

Figure 8.4   The major forms of priming (A) This diagram shows the hierarchy of the major types of priming. (B) Here the primes, test cues, and targets are compared for perceptual, conceptual, and semantic priming.

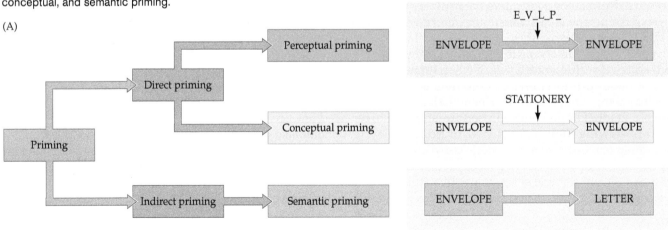

indirect priming is **semantic priming**, in which the prime and the target are semantically related (e.g., *envelope* and *letter*). Depending on the type of cue used in the test, direct priming can be further classified as perceptual or conceptual. In **perceptual priming**, the test cue and the target are perceptually related, as in the aforementioned *word fragment completion test*. In **conceptual priming**, the test cue and the target are semantically or associatively related. For example, in the *category association test*, participants generate words in response to the cue *stationery*, including the target word *envelope*.

Perceptual priming

Abundant evidence suggests that perceptual priming depends on brain systems different from those underlying declarative memory and, in particular, different from those underlying declarative memory for events, called *episodic memory*. In the study whose results are shown in Figure 8.3, patients with medial temporal lobe amnesia were impaired in episodic memory (word recognition) but not in perceptual priming (faster identification of old words). Conversely, patient M.S. with occipital lobe damage was impaired in perceptual priming but not in episodic memory. These results suggest that perceptual priming depends on sensory regions of the cortex, such as visual regions of the occipital lobe.

Consistent with this conclusion, perceptual priming is reduced when the format of the test stimuli changes between encoding and retrieval (called study-test format shifts). For example, perceptual priming in the word fragment completion test is markedly attenuated when items are encoded as pictures rather than as words (e.g., presenting a drawing of an envelope in the encoding phase rather than the word *envelope*). Perceptual priming is reduced not only by study-test shifts in symbols (e.g., from pictures to words) but also by changes in modality (e.g., from auditory to visual presentation), and even by the introduction of more subtle changes (e.g., changing from uppercase to lowercase letters). In general, the greater the perceptual change, the greater the attenuation of perceptual priming. In contrast, performance in episodic memory tests, such as free recall, is not usually disrupted by study-test shifts in stimulus format (**Figure 8.5A**). This is why students readily answer questions in a written exam even if information was originally encoded in an auditory format during a class lecture.

Whereas study-test format shifts affect perceptual priming but not episodic memory, conceptual manipulations tend to produce the opposite effects. For instance, episodic memory is much better for encoding tasks that promote semantic processing (e.g., deciding whether the referent of a word is living or nonliving) than for tasks that promote perceptual processing (e.g., deciding whether the word includes the letter *a*). This effect, known as **levels of processing**, is the reason you think about the meaning of the information that you are reading when studying for an exam rather than paying attention to the font the words are written in. In contrast with episodic memory, perceptual priming is not affected by the levels-of-processing manipulation (**Figure 8.5B**). Taken together with the effects of study-test format shifts (see Figure 8.5A), this finding completes a double dissociation between perceptual priming and episodic memory, and it strongly supports the idea that these two forms of memory depend on different brain systems.

The case of M.S. (see Figure 8.3) and the effects of study-test format shifts (see Figure 8.5A) suggest that perceptual priming depends on sensory cortices. Within these regions, the neural mechanism of perceptual priming is assumed to involve a reduction in neural responses. Single-cell recording studies in monkeys have shown that neurons in visual processing regions show a decreased level of firing when a novel visual stimulus is repeated.

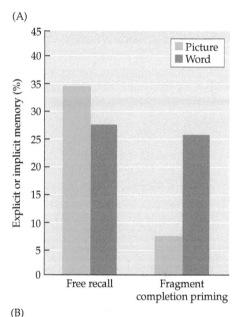

(A)

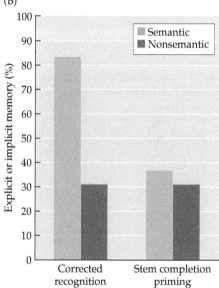

(B)

Figure 8.5 Functional dissociations between episodic memory and perceptual priming (A) Verbal free recall is as good for items studied as words as it is for items studied as pictures, whereas word fragment completion priming is much greater for items studied as words than it is for items studied as pictures. (B) Recognition is better for words encoded under semantic than under nonsemantic study conditions, whereas stem completion priming is similar across these conditions. (A after Weldon and Roediger 1987; B after Graf and Mandler 1984.)

Figure 8.6 Repetition suppression
(A) In this fMRI study of priming, study
and test stimuli were the same object
or different exemplars of the same
object category. (B) The left fusiform
cortex showed significant repetition
suppression in both the same and the
different conditions, whereas the right
fusiform cortex showed it only in the
same condition. (After Koutstaal et al.
2001.)

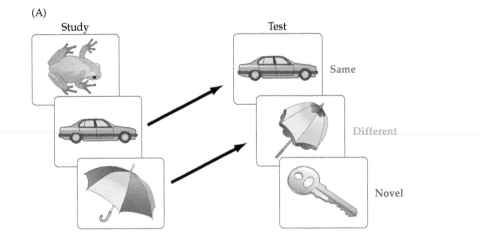

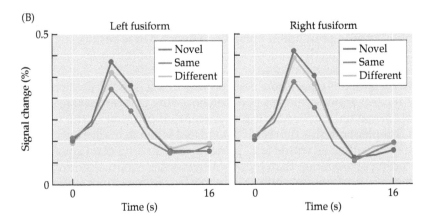

The term **repetition suppression** has been used to describe a similar and presumably related phenomenon observed in functional neuroimaging studies in
which previously encountered (primed) stimuli result in weaker hemodynamic
responses.

For example, one study found that, compared to novel objects, objects
repeated in the identical format elicited reduced activity in bilateral fusiform
regions (Figure 8.6). Interestingly, right and left fusiform regions differed in
their sensitivity to study-test format shifts: presenting different versions of the
same objects eliminated the repetition suppression effect in the right fusiform
gyrus but not in the in the left fusiform gyrus. These results have been interpreted as evidence that, compared to the right fusiform gyrus, the left fusiform
gyrus stores more abstract object representations, which can support priming
across some degree of physical change. However, both left and right fusiform
regions, like occipitotemporal areas, are concerned primarily with perceptual
representations (visual), rather than with the semantic representations that
mediate conceptual priming.

Several theories have been postulated to explain why reduced neural activity (repetition suppression or *neural priming*) leads to enhanced processing of
a stimulus (*behavioral priming*). According to one view, known as **sharpening
theory**, when a stimulus is repeated, neurons that carry critical information
about the stimulus continue to fire vigorously, whereas neurons that are not
essential for processing the stimulus respond less and less, leading to reduced
hemodynamic responses (Figure 8.7). The dropping out of noncritical neurons
is assumed to yield a cortical representation that is both more sparse (fewer

Stimulus   Neurons   PET/fMRI

Repetitions

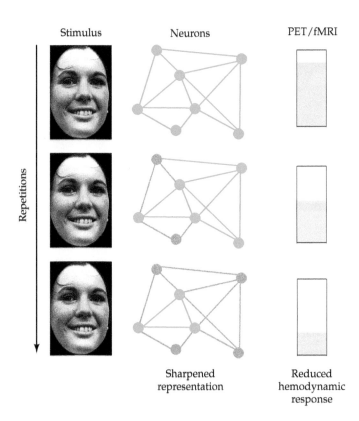

Sharpened representation

Reduced hemodynamic response

Figure 8.7 **Sharpening theory** When a stimulus is repeated, neurons that are not essential for processing the stimulus respond less and less, leading to reduced hemodynamic responses. The sharpened representation is smaller (fewer neurons) and more selective (only critical neurons). (After Henson and Rugg 2003.)

neurons) and more selective (only critical neurons). This sharpened representation could explain behavioral priming effects.

Conceptual priming

Just as perceptual priming reflects prior processing of the perceptual aspects of a stimulus, conceptual priming reflects prior processing of its conceptual aspects. Unlike perceptual priming—but similar to episodic memory—conceptual priming is sensitive to conceptual manipulations but not to perceptual manipulations. Conceptual priming, however, is different from declarative memory. Like perceptual priming—and unlike declarative memory—conceptual priming does not depend on conscious awareness, and it is preserved in amnesia patients with medial temporal lobe damage. Memory performance in these patients is impaired in both perceptual and conceptual memory tests when the tests are explicit, but performance is normal when the tests are implicit. Thus, despite their functional differences, both perceptual and conceptual priming operate independently of the medial temporal lobes.

Given their contrasting properties, perceptual and conceptual priming are likely to depend on different brain regions. Some evidence supporting this idea was provided by research on patients with Alzheimer's disease, who show neural deterioration not only in medial temporal lobe regions but also in lateral temporal and prefrontal cortices. Like patients with amnesia, most patients with Alzheimer's disease are impaired in declarative memory but not in visual perceptual priming. These deficits are consistent with the medial temporal lobe deterioration and relative sparing of the visual cortices. Unlike amnesia patients, however, Alzheimer's patients are impaired in conceptual priming. This deficit suggests that conceptual priming is mediated by brain regions affected in Alzheimer's but not in amnesia, such as lateral temporal and prefrontal cortices.

Figure 8.8 Conceptual priming and the left inferior frontal gyrus The left inferior frontal gyrus showed repetition suppression when the same semantic task was performed during encoding and retrieval (within-task condition) but not when the encoding task was nonsemantic (across-task condition). (After Wagner et al. 2000.)

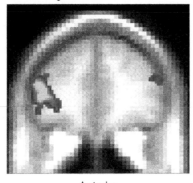

Novel > Repeated

Anterior

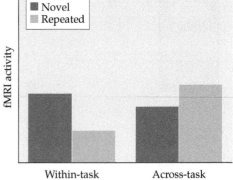

The role of these regions in conceptual priming has been confirmed by functional neuroimaging studies. Within the prefrontal cortex, conceptual priming has been linked to the anterior portion of the left inferior frontal gyrus, an area strongly associated with semantic processing (see Chapter 12). In one fMRI study, for example, participants classified words as either abstract (e.g., *honesty*) or concrete (e.g., *table*) in one task, or as either uppercase or lowercase in a second task. They subsequently repeated the abstract/concrete classification task, which this time included words encountered during the previous abstract/concrete task (*within-task condition*), words encountered during the previous uppercase/lowercase task (*across-task condition*), and novel words. Compared to novel words, the anterior left inferior frontal gyrus showed repetition suppression in the within-task condition but not in the across-task condition (Figure 8.8). This dissociation supports the assumption that the repetition suppression effect in this region reflects the reinstatement of conceptual processes associated with the abstract/concrete task, rather than the recapitulation of perceptual processes associated with just seeing the same words again.

Semantic priming

In both perceptual and conceptual priming, the prime and target stimuli have the same name (e.g., *envelope* in the example in Figure 8.4). In semantic priming, however, the prime and target have different names but are semantically related. In a typical semantic-priming paradigm, participants make simple decisions about each word in a sequence, and response times are faster for words (e.g., *nurse*) that were preceded by semantically related word (e.g., *doctor*) than for words preceded by semantically unrelated words (e.g., *shoe*).

One theoretical account of semantic priming is based on the assumption that semantic memory is organized as a network in which each node corresponds to a concept and each link corresponds to an association between two concepts (Figure 8.9). When a node is accessed it becomes *activated*, or so the argument goes, and activation spreads through

Figure 8.9 Portion of a semantic memory network In this example, activation spreads from the node *doctor* to associated nodes (e.g., *nurse*).

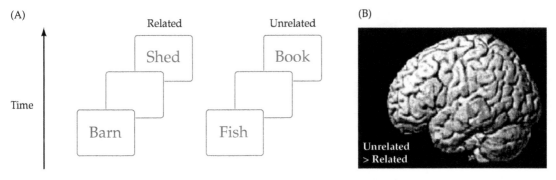

Figure 8.10 Location of neural activation related to semantic priming (A) This functional neuroimaging study of semantic priming compared sequentially presented word pairs that were semantically either related or unrelated. (B) The left anterior temporal cortex showed less activity in the related than in the unrelated condition, thereby linking this region to semantic priming. (After Rossell et al. 2003.)

the network according to the strength of the associations between neurons encoding the concepts. The concept of **spreading activation** has been used to rationalize many semantic memory phenomena, including semantic priming. For example, activation from the node *doctor* spreads to the node *nurse*, so if the word *nurse* is presented before the activation for *doctor* dissipates, this word is processed faster.

In this view, the neural mechanisms of semantic priming should involve brain regions associated with the storage of semantic knowledge, such as left anterior temporal cortical regions. Functional MRI evidence is consistent with this prediction. For example, one study found that when participants were presented with pairs of words, either related or unrelated (**Figure 8.10A**), the only region that showed less activity in the related than in the unrelated condition was the left anterior temporal cortex (**Figure 8.10B**).

The purpose of semantic priming is presumably to facilitate cognitive tasks in everyday life, such as reading with comprehension (see Chapter 12) and problem solving. For example, semantic priming may automatically activate related but not consciously considered ideas when solving a problem, the ideas seeming to simply "pop into our heads" to give an unexpected solution.

Repetition enhancement

Although priming (perceptual, conceptual, or semantic) is usually associated with a reduction in activity (*repetition suppression*), in some conditions it can be associated with the opposite effect: an increase in activity called **repetition enhancement**. According to one theory, whether priming is associated with repetition suppression or enhancement depends on whether the stimuli employed have preexisting memory representations.

Like any form of memory, priming requires a memory trace, which can be defined as an enduring change in the nervous system that stores informational content (as described earlier). For stimuli that have preexisting representations, such as familiar faces, priming could reflect a *modification of stored representations*. But for stimuli without preexisting representations, priming might require the *creation of new representations*. It has been suggested that the former mechanism leads to repetition suppression, whereas the latter leads to enhancement. Support for this theory is not strong, but one fMRI study found a clear dissociation using faces: priming of familiar faces was associated with repetition suppression in the right fusiform gyrus, whereas priming of unfamiliar faces was associated with repetition enhancement (**Figure 8.11**). The repetition suppression effect would reflect access to a sharper representation, whereas repetition enhancement

Figure 8.11 Priming-related decreases and increases in brain activity (A) Familiar and unfamiliar faces were presented twice in this paradigm. (B) The right fusiform gyrus showed repetition suppression (familiar 2 < familiar 1) for the familiar stimuli, but repetition enhancement for the unfamiliar stimuli (unfamiliar 2 > unfamiliar 1). (After Henson et al. 2000.)

(A)

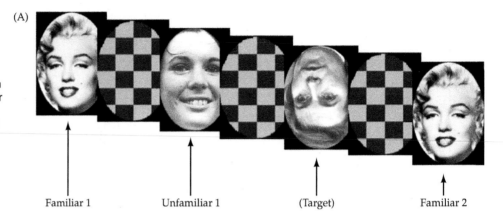

Familiar 1   Unfamiliar 1   (Target)   Familiar 2

(B)

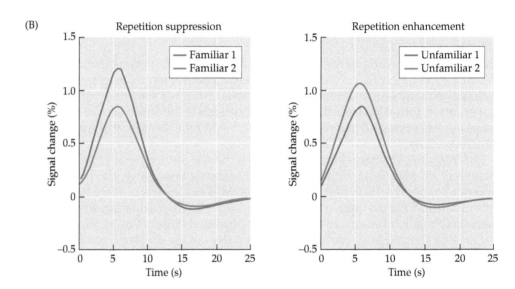

could reflect the retrieval of a new memory representation. The latter idea fits with the fact that episodic retrieval, which is generally assumed to involve the recovery of new memory traces, is associated with increases in brain activity.

In summary, all three priming subtypes (perceptual, conceptual, and semantic) are independent of conscious awareness or the integrity of the medial temporal lobes, depending primarily on different processing in neocortical regions. In functional neuroimaging studies, primed stimuli have been associated with a reduction in neuronal activity known as repetition suppression. Perceptual priming is often associated with repetition suppression in sensory cortex; conceptual priming, with suppression in the anterior left inferior prefrontal cortex; and semantic priming, with suppression in the left anterior temporal cortex. Whereas repetition suppression fits with the idea of modification in a preexisting representation, priming for novel stimuli sometimes yields repetition enhancement, which may reflect the creation of new representations.

Skill Learning

Unlike priming, which can result from a single exposure to a stimulus, *skill learning* refers to gradual changes in behavior due to extensive practice. Skill learning includes learning to play a musical instrument, to ride a bicycle, to throw a baseball, to type on a keyboard, and innumerable other abilities we learn during our lifetimes. Like priming, skill learning is independent of the medial temporal lobes and is preserved in patients with amnesia. Whereas priming depends mainly on the neocortex, skill learning appears to depend more heavily on the interaction between the neocortex and subcortical structures such as the basal ganglia.

Complex skills require fast and accurate responses, efficient processing of sensory stimuli, and the abstraction of stimulus-response patterns. In most real-world skills, these motor, perceptual, and cognitive operations are closely intertwined. For example, playing the piano requires rapid and precise hand and finger movements (*motor operations*) coordinated with quick processing of the score, the keyboard, and the generated sounds (*perceptual operations*), with the aim of fulfilling very specific musical goals (*cognitive operations*). Although motor, perceptual, and cognitive processing progress concurrently, some tasks emphasize one type of operation more than the others. The following sections consider the neural correlates and testing methods of skill learning for tasks that underscore the relevant motor, perceptual, or cognitive operations.

Motor skill learning

We learn innumerable motor skills during life. As babies, we learn to sit, stand, crawl, and walk. As toddlers, we learn to climb stairs, kick a ball, and ride a tricycle. As preschoolers, we learn to hop on one foot, and to bounce, throw, and catch a ball. As school-age children, we learn to skip rope, ride a bicycle, swim, scale fences, use tools, and play a variety of sports. Many children also learn to play a musical instrument. Motor skill learning never ends. As adults, we keep learning new motor skills (e.g., thumb typing on a mobile phone); and as we grow old, we learn to adjust preexisting motor skills to a weaker body. Although a goal of neuroscientists is to understand the neural bases of these various real-world skills, as in other fields the challenge must be made manageable by investigating relatively simple motor learning tasks. These tasks can be roughly divided into two categories: *motor sequence learning tasks*, which focus on the incremental acquisition of movements into a well-executed behavior; and *motor adaptation tasks*, which focus on the process of compensating for environmental changes.

The most thoroughly studied motor sequence learning task is the *serial reaction time (SRT) task*. A typical version of this task involves four screen locations and four spatially mapped response keys (**Figure 8.12A**). On each trial, a stimulus appears in one of the locations and the participant presses the corresponding key. Unbeknownst to the subjects, the order of the stimulus location follows a repeated sequence, typically one that is 10 to 12 units long. The results of such tests show that even when participants are unaware that there is a sequence, the sequence repetition leads to faster reaction times as the

Figure 8.12 Serial reaction time (SRT) task (A) In SRT paradigms, participants press keys corresponding to the locations in which stimuli are presented. (B) When the order of locations follows a repeated sequence, response times become shorter and shorter, even if participants are unaware of the sequence patterns. This improvement in performance reflects implicit learning of the sequence. R, random; S, sequence.

(A)

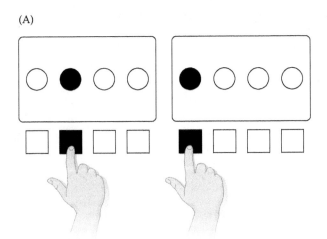

(B)

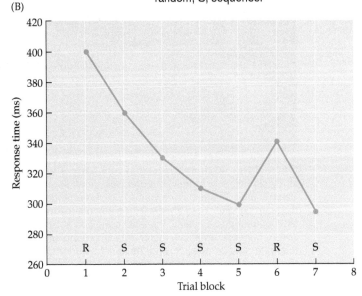

task progresses. Such implicit learning of sequence can be detected by interposing a block of trials in which the order of the stimulus locations is completely random (e.g., trial block 6 in Figure 8.12B); note that reaction times during this block are significantly slower than in neighboring blocks (e.g., trial blocks 5 and 7).

Motor sequence learning tasks such as SRT tasks are preserved in amnesia patients with medial temporal lobe damage but are impaired in patients with basal ganglia disorders, such as the neural degeneration that occurs in Parkinson's or Huntington's diseases (see Chapter 5). Consistent with this evidence, functional neuroimaging of implicit learning in normal subjects shows activation in the basal ganglia. As explained in Chapter 5, the basal ganglia modulate motor and premotor cortices by controlling the starting and stopping of movements. The cerebellum exerts an additional modulatory influence by coordinating movements and correcting errors. Finally, the posterior parietal cortex is involved in processing spatial coordinates for guiding movement (parietal damage may produce *optic ataxia*, a deficit in reaching and saccade accuracy). Thus, it is not surprising that all these regions play an important role in motor skill learning and are frequently activated in functional neuroimaging studies.

Researchers often distinguish two phases of motor sequence learning: an *early learning phase*, when performance improves rapidly within a single training session; and an *advanced learning phase*, when performance improves slowly over multiple practice sessions. The duration of these learning phases depends on the complexity of the task. For example, the early phase may last just a few minutes for a simple four-keystroke sequence, but months for a complex piano piece. Different brain regions are evidently involved in early and advanced learning phases. For example, one study found that during the early learning phase (day 1), motor sequence learning activated the aforementioned motor skill learning network, including motor cortical regions (premotor cortex, pre-supplementary motor area, and supplementary motor area), the basal ganglia (caudate), the cerebellum, and the parietal cortex (Figure 8.13A). The advanced learning phase (day 5) was associated with reduced global activity in most of these regions (Figure 8.13B), possibly reflecting reduced demands for error correction, as well as increased activity in specific subregions of the primary motor cortex and the cerebellum. These increases in activity were correlated with the synchrony of motor responses, confirming their contribution to advanced learning. There is

(A)

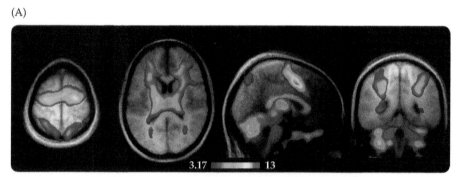

(B)

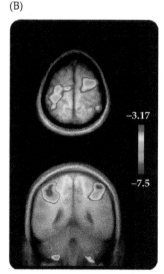

Figure 8.13   Regions associated with early learning of a motor sequence   In this study, participants produced a precisely timed sequence of finger taps in synchrony with visual stimuli. The sequence was a complex arrangement of long and short elements in the learn condition, but always long elements followed by short in the baseline condition. (A) Compared to baseline, the learn condition activated motor cortical regions (premotor cortex, pre-supplementary motor area, and supplementary motor area), the basal ganglia (caudate), the cerebellum, and the parietal cortex during the first session (day 1). (B) Reduced activity during advanced learning (day 5 compared to day 1) was found in primary motor cortex, primary somatosensory cortex, premotor cortex, and the cerebellum. (From Steele and Penhune 2010.)

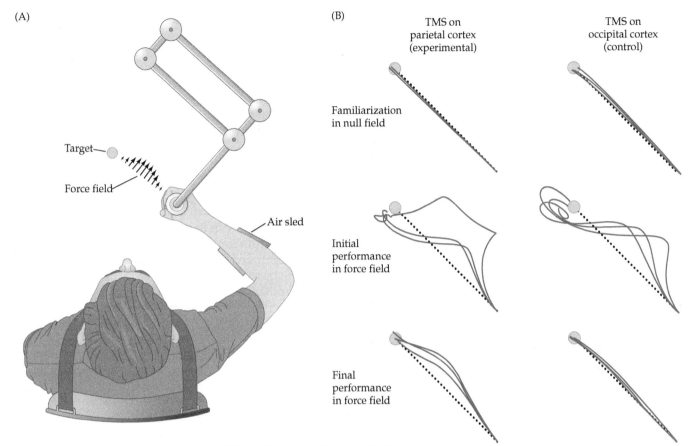

Figure 8.14 Testing motor learning and its basis in paradigms that alter sensory-motor relationships (A) This method of investigating motor learning measures how people learn to adapt their movements to compensate for a force field applied to a handle. (B) TMS interference of the posterior parietal cortex disrupts motor adaptation. (After Della-Maggiore et al. 2004.)

also evidence that the transition from early to advanced phases involves a shift from associative to motor-related regions of the basal ganglia and cerebellum.

Turning to motor adaptation tasks, investigators measure adaptation to externally induced sensory or motor perturbations. In an example of sensory perturbation, subjects wear *prism spectacles* that systematically shift the visual image either horizontally or vertically. In an example of motor perturbation, torque motors are used to create a force field that disturbs the normal movement of a handle (Figure 8.14A). After such manipulations, tracking is initially inaccurate, but it improves rapidly with practice. Functional neuroimaging studies have associated adaptation to novel sensory-motor relationships with activations in the posterior parietal cortex. The causal role of these activations has been confirmed using transcranial magnetic stimulation (TMS). For example, one TMS study found that disrupting parietal function precluded complete adaptation (arm trajectories were never completely straight; Figure 8.14B, left). In contrast, TMS of a control region (occipital cortex) did not produce the same effect (Figure 8.14B, right).

Perceptual skill learning

Perceptual skill learning refers to improvements in processing perceptual stimuli that are identical or similar to stimuli that have been repeatedly encountered. Perceptual skill learning is essential in everyday life. For example, this type of skill learning underlies our ability to understand spoken and written language.

Language comprehension based solely on declarative memory is slow and laborious, as anybody who has tried to learn a foreign language can confirm. However, perceptual skill learning eventually enables us to understand strings of words effortlessly, without the need to consciously retrieve the meanings of individual words or the rules of grammar when we converse.

In language processing, the neural correlates of perceptual skill learning include all the brain regions involved in language comprehension regions, which are reviewed in Chapter 12. Perceptual skill learning plays an equally critical role in processing music (see Chapter 4), and there is some evidence that trained musicians can co-opt language brain regions for the symbolic learning aspects of this task. Perceptual skill learning in the visual domain plays an obvious role in many other circumstances where improved perceptual performance is valued. Radiologists, for example, gradually learn to identify subtle differences in X-ray, CT, MRI, and other medical images. In fact, perceptual learning has been identified as a major factor accounting for better cancer detection accuracy in experienced mammographers compared to less experienced medical residents.

Perceptual skill learning can be studied in the laboratory using simple sensory discrimination tasks. A popular test of this sort is the *mirror reading task*, in which subjects learn to read geometrically altered text (consider also the mirror drawing task discussed earlier). Like many other skill learning tasks, mirror reading is learned normally in patients with medial temporal lobe damage, but impaired in conditions that affect the basal ganglia (see Chapter 5). Functional neuroimaging studies show that, compared to normal reading, mirror reading

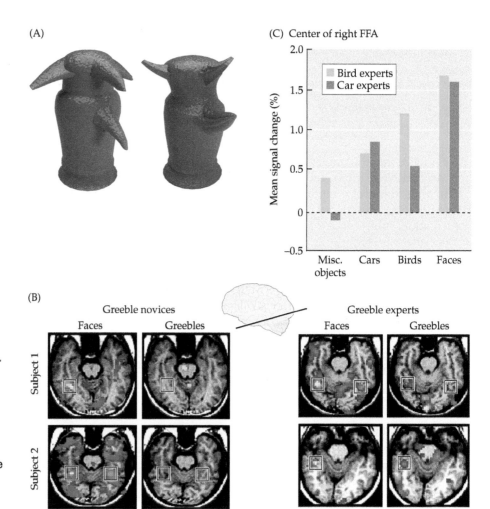

Figure 8.15 Perceptual skill learning (A) Examples of meaningless three-dimensional objects known as Greebles. (B) Expertise in classifying and identifying Greebles is associated with increased activity in the fusiform face area (FFA; boxed areas), suggesting that the FFA is not specific to faces. (C) In car experts, the FFA is more strongly activated by pictures of cars than of birds, whereas in bird experts the opposite pattern is seen. (A courtesy of Isabel Gauthier; B from Gauthier et al. 1999; C after Gauthier et al. 2000.)

elicits activation in occipitotemporal and parietal regions (i.e., in both ventral and dorsal pathways), as well as in the basal ganglia.

Another way to examine perceptual skill learning is to train participants to recognize relatively meaningless three-dimensional objects known as "Greebles" (Figure 8.15A). Cognitive neuroscientists Isabelle Gauthier, Michael Tarr, and collaborators found that expertise in classifying and identifying Greebles is associated with increased activity in the right fusiform region known as the *fusiform face area*, or *FFA* (Figure 8.15B; see also Chapter 3). This observation suggests that, rather than being a face-specific module, the function of the FFA is related to visual expertise. Greebles may activate the FFA because they have some features that resemble faces. However, the FFA of car experts is also more readily activated by pictures of cars than of birds, whereas in bird experts this region is more readily activated by pictures of birds than of cars (Figure 8.15C).

Although motor and perceptual skill learning are described separately in most accounts, acquiring skills typically involves both forms of learning. Moreover, skill learning often involves a shift from perceptual to motor processes. For example, someone learning to drive devotes much visual attention to relevant visual cues and the appropriate motor responses (think of the challenge involved in learning to parallel park). Eventually these stimuli become automatically linked to appropriate motor responses and no longer require conscious mediation. One fMRI study of this shift in perceptual-to-motor learning used a simple task in which participants decided whether a pair of geometrical figures matched. The attentional demands for analyzing feature differences in this task are initially high, but as memory templates for each figure pair are created, visual attention decreases and the role of automatic, learned motor associations increases. Consistent with this result, learning this task is accompanied by a shift from activation in a region associated with visual attention (the intraparietal sulcus; Figure 8.16A) to regions associated with motor processing (the postcentral gyrus; Figure 8.16B).

Cognitive skill learning

Cognitive skill learning refers to problem-solving tasks in which subjects are required to use various cognitive skills to solve a task. An example of this sort of task is probabilistic classification learning, in which participants learn to classify stimuli on the basis of statistical information. In a paradigm called the *weather prediction task*, in each trial participants look at four cards with geometrical shapes that are associated with future weather conditions (Figure 8.17A). Using the

Figure 8.16 Shift of activity from attention to motor-related brain areas during visual learning (A) In each trial, participants decided whether a pair of geometrical figures matched. During early learning, attentional demands for analyzing feature differences elicited greater activity in the intraparietal sulcus, but this activity decreased across sessions (session 1 > sessions 3 and 5). (B) As participants learned to associate each figure pair with a motor response, activity increased in hand areas in motor and sensory cortices (session 5 > sessions 1 and 3). Arrows indicate activations from which the data in the graphs were extracted. (After Pollmann and Maertens 2005.)

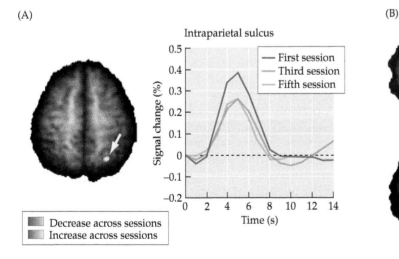

(A)

Intraparietal sulcus

— First session
— Third session
— Fifth session

■ Decrease across sessions
□ Increase across sessions

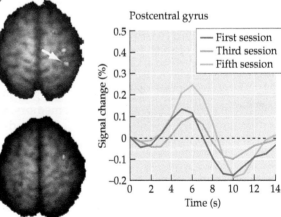

(B)

Postcentral gyrus

— First session
— Third session
— Fifth session

(A)

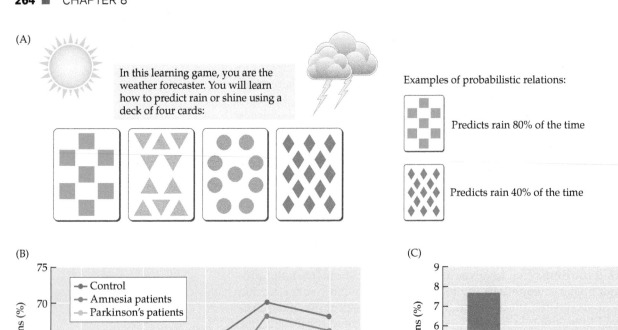

In this learning game, you are the weather forecaster. You will learn how to predict rain or shine using a deck of four cards:

Examples of probabilistic relations:

Predicts rain 80% of the time

Predicts rain 40% of the time

(B)

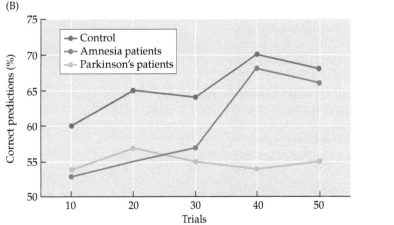

(C)

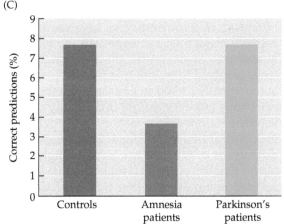

Figure 8.17 Probabilistic classification learning in patients with Parkinson's disease or amnesia (A) The weather prediction task. (B) Subjects with amnesia (medial temporal lobe damage) are slow to learn but eventually reach the same level of performance as controls do; in contrast, the performance of patients with Parkinson's (basal ganglia deficits) never improves. (C) In sharp contrast with probabilistic learning performance, in an episodic memory task (declarative memory) amnesia patients are markedly impaired, whereas Parkinson's patients perform as well as controls. Taken together, the results indicate that the basal ganglia are critical for implicit skill learning but not for episodic memory, whereas the medial temporal lobes are critical for episodic memory but not for implicit skill learning. (After Knowlton et al. 1996.)

cards, the subjects must "forecast" what they think the weather will be. After each decision they are informed whether the prediction was correct. The critical feature of the task is that each of the cards is only probabilistically related to the two possible weather outcomes (e.g., a certain card may be associated with rain only 70 percent of the time); thus, an explicit rule is difficult to infer. Nevertheless, the participants implicitly learn to use the probabilistic information (i.e., they come to associate certain card combinations with an increased probability of rain), and over many trials the accuracy of their predictions slowly improves.

One study found a significant difference in performance in the weather prediction task between amnesia patients who had medial temporal lobe damage, and Parkinson's patients, who had impaired basal ganglia function. Although patients with amnesia improved somewhat more slowly than controls, they eventually learned the task as well as controls did. In contrast, patients with Parkinson's disease never learned the task (**Figure 8.17B**). When these groups of patients were tested in an episodic memory test, the opposite result was found: patients with amnesia were impaired compared to controls, whereas patients with Parkinson's were not (**Figure 8.17C**). Thus, damage of the basal ganglia in Parkinson's patients impaired skill learning but not declarative memory, whereas damage of the medial temporal lobes in amnesia patients impaired declarative memory but not skill learning. These observations are consistent with the idea that episodic memory, as noted earlier, depends on medial temporal lobe structures, whereas cognitive skill learning depends at least to some degree on the integrity of the basal ganglia.

This conclusion about cognitive skill learning is further supported by functional neuroimaging evidence. In one study, normal participants were scanned while they carried out a simplified version of the weather prediction task (**Figure 8.18A**). Consistent with patient studies, the medial temporal lobe was more activated in the paired-association task than in the weather prediction task, whereas the basal ganglia showed the opposite pattern (**Figure 8.18B**). Early trials in this task presumably have a significant episodic memory component that reflects explicit learning of the symbol cards needed to make the

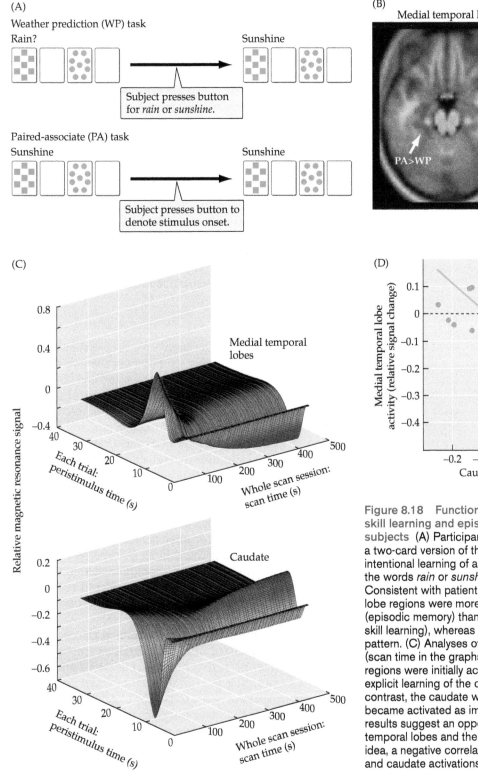

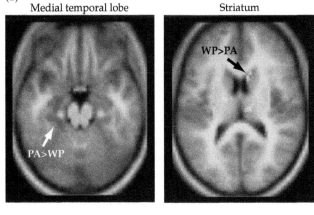

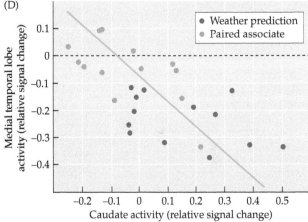

Figure 8.18 **Functional MRI study comparing cognitive skill learning and episodic memory encoding in normal subjects** (A) Participants performed two tasks in the scanner: a two-card version of the weather prediction (WP) task, and intentional learning of associations between pairs of cards and the words *rain* or *sunshine* (paired-associate [PA] task). (B) Consistent with patient data (see Figure 8.17), medial temporal lobe regions were more activated in the paired-associate task (episodic memory) than in the weather prediction task (cognitive skill learning), whereas the basal ganglia showed the opposite pattern. (C) Analyses of activity across weather prediction trials (scan time in the graphs) indicated that medial temporal lobe regions were initially active (first 100 trials), possibly reflecting explicit learning of the cards, but were later deactivated. In contrast, the caudate was originally deactivated and then became activated as implicit learning increased over trials. These results suggest an opposing relationship between the medial temporal lobes and the basal ganglia. (D) Consistent with this idea, a negative correlation was found between medial temporal and caudate activations. (After Poldrack et al. 2001.)

prediction. This interpretation would also explain why patients with amnesia are a bit slower than controls in learning the weather prediction task. Consistent with this idea, the medial temporal lobes are activated during initial trials, but deactivated during most of the learning phase; the basal ganglia (caudate) show the opposite temporal pattern (Figure 8.18C,D). These contrasting temporal patterns suggest an opposing relationship between the medial temporal lobes and the basal ganglia. One possible explanation is a competition between the need for accessible knowledge (medial temporal lobes) versus the need to learn fast, automatic responses in specific situations (basal ganglia).

In sum, there is abundant evidence that skill learning depends on the integrity of the basal ganglia. Patients with basal ganglia disorders, such as Parkinson's and Huntington's diseases, are impaired in motor skill learning tasks, such as the serial reaction time task; in perceptual skill learning tasks, such as mirror reading; and in cognitive skill learning tasks, such as probabilistic classification. In addition to the basal ganglia, however, skill learning involves other brain regions that vary depending on the task. Motor skill learning has been associated with activation of the posterior parietal cortex, supplementary motor area, cingulate cortex, and cerebellum. Perceptual skill learning involves the activation of visual cortices when the learned skills are visually based. Finally, complex cognitive skill learning involves medial temporal regions initially, when the explicit components and rules of the task are being acquired; but these regions are not necessary for subsequent learning of implicit rules, as demonstrated by preserved probabilistic classification learning in amnesia patients. Implicit cognitive learning, like other learned skills, depends on the basal ganglia and the regions of neocortex relevant to the particular cognitive domain.

Conditioning

In addition to priming and skill learning, nondeclarative memory systems include *conditioning*. Conditioning has been intensively studied over the past century, from both psychological and neurobiological perspectives, and can be defined as the generation of a response that is elicited by pairing a neutral stimulus with an appetitive or aversive stimulus that normally elicits the response being studied. There are two broad forms of conditioning: *classical* and *operant*.

In **classical conditioning**, an innate reflex is modified by associating its normal triggering stimulus with an unrelated stimulus that reliably predicts the trigger; the unrelated stimulus eventually will trigger the original response by virtue of this association. This type of conditioning was famously demonstrated by the Russian psychologist Ivan Pavlov's experiments with dogs, carried out early in the twentieth century. The dogs' innate reflex was salivation (the **unconditioned response, or UR**) in response to the sight and/or smell of food (the **unconditioned stimulus, US**). The association was elicited in the animals by repeatedly pairing the sight/smell of food with the sound of a bell (the **conditioned stimulus, CS**). Such conditioning, also called the *conditioned reflex*, was considered established when the CS (the sound of the bell) by itself elicited salivation (the **conditioned response, CR**), even without the presentation of food.

In **operant conditioning**, also known as **instrumental learning**, the probability of a behavioral response is altered by associating the response with a reward (or in some instances a punishment). In psychologist Edward Thorndike's original experiments, carried out in the 1890s, cats learned to escape from a puzzle box by pressing the lever that opened a trap door to get a food reward. Although the cats initially pressed the lever only occasionally—and more or less by chance—the probability of their doing so increased sharply as the animals associated this action with escape and reward. In B. F. Skinner's far more complete and better-known experiments performed a few decades later, pigeons or rats learned to associate pressing a lever with receiving a food pellet in a widely used device that came to be known as a **Skinner box** (see Chapter 1).

In both classical and operant conditioning, it usually takes a number of CS-US training trials for the conditioning to become established—a process called **acquisition**. Furthermore, if the conditioned animal performs the critical response but the US is no longer provided, the conditioned response gradually disappears—a phenomenon called **extinction**. Although the conditioned response is no longer expressed following extinction training, the memory of the CS-US association is stored in the cortex and can be reexpressed upon appropriate retrieval cues (e.g., if the US is reintroduced or the animal reenters the environment in which the conditioned association was initially learned). Such reemergence of conditioned behaviors plagues the clinical treatment of anxiety and addiction, which are believed to be supported in part by conditioning processes, despite the modest success of extinction-based (exposure) therapies. In considering the neural basis of classical conditioning, the paradigms are emotionally neutral. The neural correlates of emotional conditioning are considered with other forms of emotional learning in Chapter 10.

In classical conditioning, it is important to distinguish between delay and trace conditioning. Figure 8.19 illustrates the difference between these two variants of classical conditioning using **eyeblink conditioning** as an example. In this paradigm a puff of air, which elicits a reflexive (automatic) blink, is repeatedly paired with a tone until the tone by itself elicits blinking. The blink reflex is adaptive to the animal in that it causes the membrane protecting the eye to close, shielding the eye from potential toxins or hazards blown in through the airstream. In order for this reflex to be effective, the membrane must close quickly and precisely. In both delay and trace conditioning, the tone (the conditioned stimulus) starts before the air puff (the unconditioned stimulus). The difference is that in **delay conditioning**, the CS is still present when the US starts, and the two terminate at the same time (**Figure 8.19A**); in **trace conditioning**, however, there is a brief time interval between the end of the CS and the start of the US (**Figure 8.19B**). Thus, in trace conditioning the CS must leave some kind of memory trace in the nervous system in order for a CS-US association to be established, whereas this is not the case in delay conditioning. Although the difference between delay and trace conditioning may seem trivial, these different forms of classical conditioning are now known to have different neural correlates.

Eyeblink delay conditioning depends primarily on the cerebellum. For example, patients with cerebellar damage due to different causes (alcohol abuse, disseminated demyelination, tumor removal) failed to acquire eyeblink conditioned responses (**Figure 8.20**). Studies with animals (e.g., rabbits) have shown that within the cerebellum, eyeblink delay conditioning is particularly dependent on the *interpositus nucleus* and the *cerebellar cortex*. In the usual eyeblink conditioning paradigm, both of these structures receive information about the tone (CS) from the auditory system and information about the air puff (US) from the visual and somatic sensory systems. Supporting the critical role of the interpositus nucleus, lesions or transient disruption of this structure lead to deficits in the acquisition and retention of eyeblink delay conditioning. Supporting the role of the cerebellar cortex, mutant mice deficient in

Figure 8.19 Two classical conditioning variants illustrated using an eyeblink paradigm (A) In delay conditioning, the conditioned stimulus (CS) starts before the unconditioned stimulus (US) but is ongoing when the US starts. (B) In trace conditioning, the CS ends before the US starts, leaving a time interval between the two stimuli.

(A) Delay conditioning

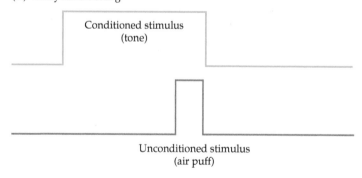

Conditioned stimulus (tone)

Unconditioned stimulus (air puff)

(B) Trace conditioning

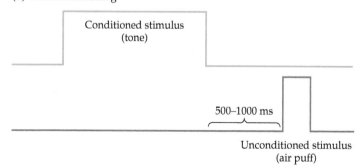

Conditioned stimulus (tone)

500–1000 ms

Unconditioned stimulus (air puff)

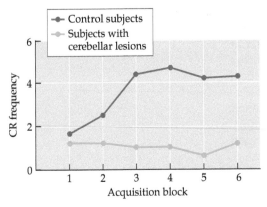

Figure 8.20 Cerebellar damage impairs eyeblink conditioning in humans Mean eyelid conditioned response (CR) frequency in patients with cerebellar lesions and normal control subjects across acquisition blocks. (After Daum et al. 1993.)

Purkinje cells (the output neurons of the cerebellar cortex) are impaired in eyeblink conditioning. As the interpositus nucleus and the cerebellar cortex receive information about the CS and the US, both structures are potentially capable of supporting CS-US associations. Moreover, the deep cerebellar nuclei, including the interpositus nucleus, constitute the final common pathway for output from the cerebellar cortex to other brain regions that control the execution of motor behaviors.

The major difference between the neural correlates of delay and trace conditioning is the role of the hippocampus. Although electrophysiological studies using the eyeblink paradigm in rabbits show the hippocampus to be involved in delay conditioning, damage to the hippocampus does not impair delay conditioning. In contrast, damage to the hippocampus impairs trace conditioning in both experimental animals and human patients.

The finding that trace conditioning depends on the hippocampus creates a problem for the standard taxonomy of memory systems. Is trace conditioning truly a form of nondeclarative memory, then, or is it a form of declarative memory? A possible resolution was provided by a study that investigated delay and trace eyeblink conditioning in amnesia patients with hippocampal damage and in control participants. Immediately after conditioning, participants completed a questionnaire that included a number of questions about their awareness of CS-US contingencies. The results showed that none of the amnesia patients were aware of CS-US contingencies. Nonetheless, all the participants showed delay conditioning (Figure 8.21A). This outcome is consistent with the idea that the delay form of nondeclarative memory is independent of conscious awareness and the hippocampus. In contrast, only the control participants who were aware showed trace conditioning (Figure 8.21B). Thus, trace conditioning depends on awareness of temporal contingencies among stimuli, at least in humans, and is effectively a form of declarative rather than nondeclarative memory.

Turning to operant conditioning, we must distinguish between two main categories of this sort of behavior. Imagine that the route you take when you drive home every evening is characterized by a particular intersection where you always turn right. Turning right because you want to arrive home is a *goal-directed action*; automatically turning right because you always turn right at that

Figure 8.21 Delay and trace eyeblink conditioning in humans Test results for amnesia patients versus controls indicate an underlying difference between delay and trace conditioning. Graphs plot the percentage of differential conditioned eyeblink (CR − CS/CR × 100). (A) All groups showed delay conditioning. (B) Only the control group was aware of the relationship between the tone and the air puff, and only this group showed trace conditioning. These results indicate that trace conditioning depends on the awareness of CS-US contingencies and therefore suggest that trace conditioning is a form of declarative memory. (After Clark and Squire 1998.)

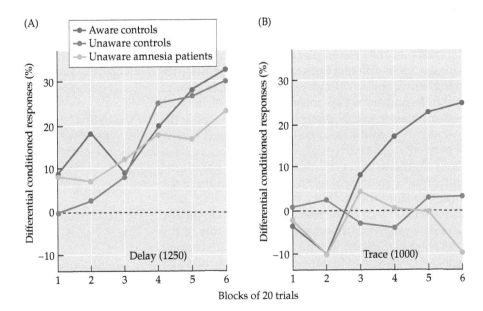

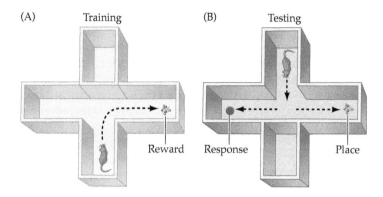

Figure 8.22 Place and response strategies in a cross maze (A) During training, rodents are always placed in the same arm of a maze and reach the food reward by always making the same response (e.g., right turn). (B) On testing, they are placed in a different arm, where they can make either a different response (e.g., left turn) to go to the same place where the reward was previously located (place strategy) or the same response (e.g., right turn) to go to a new arm (response strategy). During testing, only the place arm is baited. (After Yin and Knowlton 2006.)

intersection is a *stimulus-driven habit*. Imagine now that the street where you turn right is blocked and you know that. Avoiding the right turn and using an alternate route indicates that the right turn was goal-directed. But turning right anyway, making an error, is a sign that the action was habitual. In other words, goal-directed actions are sensitive to *action-outcome (A-O) contingencies*, whereas stimulus-driven habits are controlled by *stimulus-response (S-R) associations*.

One way to investigate the distinction between goal-directed actions and stimulus-driven habits uses a paradigm that resembles the driving example. During training, rodents were always placed in the same arm of a maze and had to locate the food reward by always making the same response (right turn in Figure 8.22A). Once they had learned this behavior, they were placed in a different arm (Figure 8.22B), where they could make either a different response to go to a previous reward arm (*place strategy*) or the same response (a right turn) to go to a new arm (*response strategy*). After moderate initial training, most rats used the place strategy (goal-directed), but if the hippocampus was damaged they shifted to a response strategy (habit). After extensive training, rats with intact brains used a response strategy (habit), but if the dorsal striatum (caudate and putamen) was lesioned, they used a place strategy (goal-directed). This double dissociation suggests that goal-directed A-O learning depends on the hippocampus, whereas habitual S-R learning depends on the dorsal striatum.

However, later rodent evidence showed that some regions of the dorsal striatum play an important role in A-O learning. The distinction between A-O and S-R regions of the dorsal striatum corresponds to the distinction between associative and sensory-motor cortico-basal-ganglia loops introduced in Chapter 5 (see Figure 5.21). Some of the evidence is from paradigms in which rodents learn to press one lever for one type of food and another lever for a different type of food. One type of food is then made undesirable (devalued) by producing satiation or taste aversion specific to that food. If behavior is goal-directed, it should decrease in frequency; but if it is habitual, it should continue even if the outcome is undesirable. Studies using this approach have shown that damage to the dorsomedial striatum, which corresponds to the caudate (associative loop), impairs goal-directed A-O learning; whereas damage to the dorsolateral striatum, which corresponds to the putamen (sensory-motor loop), impairs habitual S-R learning. Converging evidence from humans has been found using fMRI.

In sum, conditioning includes classical and operant variants. Classical conditioning is the alteration of an innate reflex, which responds to an unrelated stimulus (CS) that reliably predicts its normal triggering stimulus (US). In delay conditioning, the CS and US overlap; in trace conditioning the CS ends before the US is presented. The most popular nonemotional classical conditioning paradigm is eyeblink conditioning, in which a tone elicits a blink after repeated pairing with an air puff. Delay eyeblink conditioning is critically dependent on the cerebellum. Trace eyeblink conditioning also depends on the hippocampus, but this relationship may reflect contributions of declarative memory. Operant conditioning (instrumental learning) is a change in the probability of a behavioral response associated with a reward (or punishment). Instrumental behaviors include flexible goal-directed actions and inflexible stimulus-driven habits. Whereas goal-directed actions depend more on the dorsomedial striatum (caudate) and the hippocampus, stimulus-driven habits are more dependent on the dorsolateral striatum (putamen).

Cellular Mechanisms of Memory

The preceding sections reviewed the major neural substrates of memory at the *system level*—that is, the extent to which memory depends on gross anatomical structures such as the medial temporal lobes, the cortex, the basal ganglia, and the cerebellum. At the system level the neural substrates of memory are clearly heterogeneous. At the *cellular and molecular levels*, however, *all* the forms of memory seem to depend on changes in neural connectivity and the relative strength of synaptic transmission.

Early in the twentieth century, the German evolutionary biologist Richard Semon coined the term **engram** to refer to the physical and biochemical changes underlying memory storage in the brain. Two related questions about engrams, or **memory traces**, have long fascinated neuroscientists: where are they located in the brain, and how, in neurobiological terms, are they formed?

With respect to the *where* question, an early idea inspired by Pavlovian conditioning was that engrams depend on the integrity of the pathways connecting sensory and motor regions. In the 1920s, American neuroscientist Karl Lashley tested this idea by making cuts in a rat's cortex that would disconnect sensory and motor regions before or after the rats learned to run mazes. Lashley found that the location of the lesions did not matter much, and that only the extent of the tissue destroyed was consequential. This finding is consistent with the idea that an engram consists of a network of neurons with connections distributed over the cortex; thus, only when a large proportion of the network is destroyed is the engram seriously compromised (see the discussion of graceful degradation in Box 8C). This idea does not imply that engrams are randomly distributed. As mentioned already, the modern view is that engrams are defined primarily by the connectivity of the brain regions originally involved in processing the relevant category of information. That is, memory traces for visual information are stored mostly in visual cortices, those for auditory information in auditory cortices, those for motor skills in the motor cortices, and so on.

This general answer to the question of where engrams are located suggests an answer to *how* they are formed. If engrams consist of networks of neurons, then they are formed by a process whereby neurons that once functioned relatively independently begin to work together by virtue of strengthened connections between them. This broad answer was first explicitly proposed in 1949 by Canadian psychologist Donald Hebb, who hypothesized that memories are stored in the brain in the form of networks of neurons that he called *cell assemblies*. Hebb's idea was that through experience (i.e., learning), assemblies gradually become specifically associated with objects, actions, or concepts. To explain how the relevant neurons come to be linked, he proposed that when presynaptic and postsynaptic neurons are simultaneously active (i.e., fire action potentials at the same time), the synaptic connections between them are strengthened. As a result, synaptic associations grow stronger and tend to persist. This mechanism, known today as **Hebbian learning**, is captured in the adage "cells that fire together wire together."

■ BOX 8C CONNECTIONIST MODELS

Unlike sequential processing models, connectionist models assume that information processing occurs in parallel across a large number of distributed units. For this reason, these models are also known as *parallel distributed processing* (*PDP*) *models*. The units, or *nodes*, in connectionist schemes are linked in a network, much as neurons are interconnected in the brain. Thus, connectionist models are also known as *neural network models*.

An example is the model of written-word recognition developed by cognitive scientists James McClelland and his colleague David Rumelhart. Like other connectionist models, it is a network consisting of layers of units. The units of the *input layer* receive information from the environment; in this example, each input unit receives visual information and responds to one particular feature of a written letter (e.g., a horizontal line). The *output layer* consists of units that indicate the outcomes of the processing within the network. Given that this is a model of word recognition, the output units correspond to all the words the model can recognize. Finally, input and output units are connected through one or more *hidden layers*, so called because their units are invisible from the outside. For simplicity, the model in the example here shows only a few letter features, letters, and words.

The network shown responds to only the *first letter* of each word; similar networks would be required to recognize each of the other letters. The connections between units can be excitatory or inhibitory. Some excitatory and inhibitory connections in the figure are obvious. For example, the letter *a* excites the word *able* but inhibits the word *trap* because *able* starts with an *a* but *trap* does not. The inhibitory connections among the units within the same layer ensure that one option will tend to win out over the others. Activation flows not only from input to output layers but also from output to input layers (e.g., the excitatory connection from *able* to the letter *a*).

To see how the model works, consider the sentence "John packed his suitcase and left for a trip." Before such a network reaches the end of the sentence, the node for the word *trip* is activated by semantic associations from the words *suitcase* and *left* (not shown in the figure). This activation facilitates the identification of the letters *t*, *r*, *i*, and *p* and

A connectionist model for written-word recognition. Note that the feature and letter units represent only the first position in each four-letter word. (After McClelland and Rumelhart 1981.)

thus the corresponding feature detectors. At the same time, activation flows in the opposite direction from feature to letter to word detectors in the input layer. A strength of models like this is that they specify how conceptually driven processing (already established in the network) and data-driven processing might interact. Another strength is that they entail a built-in learning mechanism: the modification of connection weights represents stored information that alters the output.

In computer simulations, networks are often "trained" using *supervised learning algorithms* such as *back-propagation*, in which the actual output (e.g., *trap*) is compared to the desired output (e.g., *trip*) and the weights of the connections

from the layers below are modified to reduce subsequent errors. Learning can also be *unsupervised*; for example, the strength of the connection between units may be automatically increased whenever the units are simultaneously active (Hebbian learning, described in the text).

PDP models are attractive in cognitive neuroscience because changing the strength of synaptic connections through individual experience or natural selection is clearly the major way nervous systems store information. The assumption that knowledge is not stored in a single location but is distributed across numerous sites is also consistent with much neu-

(Continued on next page)

■ **BOX 8C** *(continued)*

robiological evidence. Local damage to either the brain or a connectionist model typically degrades performance but doesn't abolish it altogether—a phenomenon called *graceful degradation*.

At the same time, connectionist models have several limitations, including difficulty accounting for rule-based processes in human reasoning; difficulty discerning the strategies being used to solve problems by examining weight patterns of the trained network architecture; and, consequently, difficulty distinguishing among alternative models of the same cognitive process. These caveats notwithstanding, connectionist models have provided cognitive scientists with important insights and a powerful tool.

References

HAYKIN, S. (1998) *Neural Networks: A Comprehensive Foundation*, 2nd Ed. New York: Prentice-Hall.

McCLELLAND, J. L. AND D. E. RUMELHART (1981) An interactive activation model of context effects in letter perception: Part 1. An account of basic findings. *Psychol. Rev.* 88: 375–407.

McCLELLAND, J. L., D. E. RUMELHART AND G. E. HINTON (2002) The appeal of parallel distributed processing. In *Foundations of Cognitive Psychology: Core Reading*, D. J. Levitin (ed.). Cambridge, MA: MIT Press, pp. 57–91.

McCLELLAND, J. L., D. E. RUMELHART AND THE PDP RESEARCH GROUP (1986) *Parallel Distributed Processing: Explorations in the Microstructure of Cognition*. Vol. 2: *Psychological and Biological Models*. Cambridge, MA: MIT Press.

RUMELHART, D. E., J. L. McCLELLAND AND THE PDP RESEARCH GROUP (1986) *Parallel Distributed Processing: Explorations in the Microstructure of Cognition*. Vol. 1: *Foundations*. Cambridge, MA: MIT Press.

Even though they were articulated more than 50 years ago, Hebb's proposals, in essence, remain a plausible basis for understanding memory in cellular terms. Only in the last few decades, however, have neuroscientists begun to understand some of the cellular and molecular mechanisms that allow a strengthening of synaptic connectivity as a result of coincident neuronal activity.

Habituation and sensitization

One of the main difficulties in investigating the cellular bases of memory is the sheer complexity of neuronal circuits and behaviors, particularly in the mammalian brain. One way to simplify this problem is to investigate memory mechanisms in an organism with fewer neurons and a more limited behavioral repertoire. Neuroscientist Eric Kandel and his colleagues pioneered this approach when, beginning in the late 1960s, they carried out studies using the sea slug *Aplysia californica*. The ganglia that make up the nervous system in this animal contain only a few thousand neurons, many of which are large and individually identifiable. Despite the simplicity of its nervous system, the sea slug shows rudimentary learning abilities, which Kandel and his group measured in terms of changes in a simple withdrawal reflex.

A sea slug withdraws its gill when its siphon is lightly touched, presumably as a defensive maneuver, and this simple reflex demonstrates two forms of learning that occur in many animals, including humans: habituation and sensitization. **Habituation** is a reduced response when the same stimulus is repeated over and over; **sensitization** is an increased response to the habituated stimulus when it is paired with an aversive stimulus such as a shock to the animal's tail (**Figure 8.23**). Touching the siphon skin stimulates sensory neurons, which in turn excite interneurons and motor neurons; the excited motor neurons then elicit withdrawal of the gill.

Electrical recordings show that habituation involves a decrease in neurotransmitter release at the synapses between sensory neurons and motor neurons, whereas sensitization involves an increase in neurotransmitter release at these synapses. Whereas the functional changes underlying habituation appear to be confined to the sensory neuron–motor neuron synapse, the tail shock used to elicit sensitization recruits a wider array of sensory neurons, which in turn excite modulatory interneurons that increase neurotransmitter release from the siphon sensory neurons, enhancing gill withdrawal.

Both habituation and sensitization are simple forms of memory. In particular, the modulatory effect of tail shock on the gill withdrawal reflex lasts a matter of minutes, and it can thus be regarded as a model for short-term memory in this system. Moreover, repeated tail shocks over longer periods trigger gene expression, new protein synthesis, and the formation of new synaptic connections, all of which result in enhancement of the gill withdrawal reflex that can last weeks—a model of simple long-term memory.

Long-term potentiation and depression

A second major advance in understanding the cellular mechanisms of memory was accomplished in the early 1970s in studies of hippocampal synaptic transmission carried out by neuroscientists Terje Lømo and Timothy Bliss. As illustrated in Figure 8.24, the researchers stimulated different afferent pathways (e.g., pathways 1 and 2) and recorded responses in a postsynaptic neuron (postsynaptic potentials). They found that when one pathway (e.g., pathway 1) was stimulated with a high-frequency electrical train, the postsynaptic neuron later showed stronger responses to input from the stimulated pathway but not from other pathways (e.g., pathway 2). Because this focal enhancement lasted a long time, they called the phenomenon **long-term potentiation (LTP)**. Although LTP was first localized in the rabbit hippocampus, subsequent research showed that it occurs in many other species and brain regions, including the cortex, the amygdala, the basal ganglia, and the cerebellum. Depending on the locus and stimulation paradigm, LTP can last tens of minutes, hours, or longer.

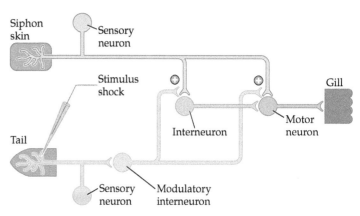

Figure 8.23 Two forms of learning in the sea slug *Aplysia* The simple neuronal circuit in the abdominal ganglion of the sea slug is used in studies of habituation and sensitization. Touching the animal's siphon elicits withdrawal of the gill. When the siphon is repeatedly touched, this response progressively decreases (habituation). Conversely, a shock to the tail enhances the habituated gill withdrawal response (sensitization). (After Squire and Kandel 1999.)

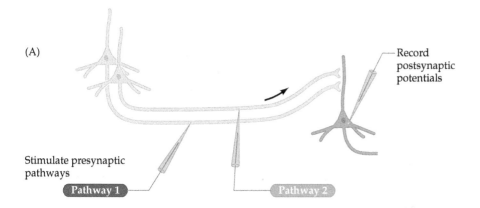

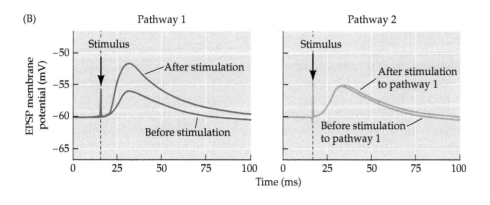

Figure 8.24 Long-term potentiation (LTP) (A) Two pathways in the hippocampus that can be stimulated independently. (B) Following high-frequency stimulation (not shown), the postsynaptic potential elicited by a single stimulus is enhanced, but only for the stimulated pathway. EPSP, excitatory postsynaptic potential. (After Malinow et al. 1989.)

LTP has several properties that advance it as an attractive candidate for one of the major cellular mechanisms of memory. First, LTP can be induced by a single high-frequency train of stimulation—a feature that could explain how some memories can be formed by a single experience. Second, the fact that LTP can last for days or even weeks could explain the persistence of memory over these sorts of time intervals. Third, LTP has a degree of **specificity** that fits well with the specificity of memories. Only those synapses activated during stimulation are enhanced; other synapses—even other synapses on the same neuron—are not affected. Finally, LTP has a property of **associativity** that could underlie memory mechanisms such as Hebbian learning: if a weak and a strong pathway impinging on a target neuron were activated at the same time, then both pathways would tend to become associated via the output of the target cell.

As suggested by the phenomenon of habituation, synaptic *weakening* is equally a part of learning and memory. If synapses continued to increase in strength because of LTP or a similar mechanism, they would eventually reach a point of saturation. It makes sense, therefore, for synaptic potentiation to be counterbalanced by a mechanism of synaptic inhibition. Such a mechanism, known as **long-term depression** (**LTD**), was found in the late 1970s. Whereas LTP occurs with high-frequency stimulation over a brief period, LTD is elicited by low-frequency stimulation over a longer period. LTD can also last several hours and is again specific to activated synapses. As might be expected, LTD can counteract LTP, and vice versa. There is also some evidence that LTD can enhance LTP in neighboring synapses and that it can block the formation of associations that do not follow Hebb's rule.

Linking LTP to memory performance

Although LTP has many of the properties required for memory storage and behavior, it has been studied mainly in vitro. Thus, directly linking LTP and memory performance has been a major research effort in recent years.

One approach has been to seek evidence of **behavioral LTP**—that is, a demonstrated change in synaptic efficacy similar to LTP that follows a natural learning experience. For example, rats raised in an enriched stimulatory environment show enhanced postsynaptic potentials when compared to rats raised in an environment impoverished in stimulation and learning experiences. The enhancement disappears within a few weeks if the enriched rats are placed in the impoverished environment, suggesting that enriched experience is necessary to maintain strong synapses. In addition, changes in synaptic efficacy lasting about 30 minutes have been observed in the rat hippocampus following exploration of a novel environment, which could be indicative of learning and memory storage. There is also evidence that inducing LTP in sensory pathways can enhance synaptic responses to natural sensory stimulation, and that learning experiences can lead to long-term increases in correlated firing among hippocampal neurons that were active during learning (thus showing associativity).

Another approach to linking LTP to naturally occurring learning and memory has been to *prevent* LTP and then determine whether memory is impaired. One way to disrupt LTP is to use "knockout" mice in which a gene for a protein crucial to LTP is eliminated by gene splicing techniques. Neuroscientist Susumu Tonegawa and his colleagues produced a strain of mice that lacked the gene for NMDA receptors in hippocampal region CA1. This receptor protein mediates certain forms of LTP, and indeed the knockout mice showed little or no LTP in the CA1 region of the hippocampus. Mice lacking NMDA receptors were also severely impaired in spatial learning (a property mediated by the hippocampus in rodents), although they were unimpaired in nonspatial learning. Whereas control mice searched for a platform hidden in a water tank only near the location where the platform had been located in previous trials (the *Morris water*

(A) Control

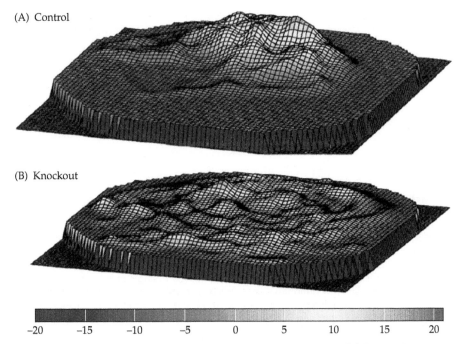

(B) Knockout

−20	−15	−10	−5	0	5	10	15	20

Figure 8.25 Genetic impact on learning the water maze task (A) The landscape shows that control mice focused their search in the trained area, resulting in a high total occupancy peak (yellow) in the old platform position, which they apparently remembered. **(B)** Laboratory mice in which the gene for NMDA receptors was eliminated ("knocked out)" in the hippocampus navigated more or less randomly over the full area of the pool, apparently failing to have learned where the platform should be located. (From Tsien et al. 1996.)

maze; see Box 8A), the NMDA-deficient mice searched widely for the platform, indicating that they had little spatial memory (Figure 8.25).

Efforts to establish behaviorally relevant evidence of LTP involvement have not been limited to the hippocampus or to spatial learning. In the mid-1990s, neuroscientist Joseph LeDoux and collaborators investigated behavioral LTP in the context of auditory fear conditioning, focusing on the pathway connecting the medial geniculate nucleus of the thalamus (a relay station in the auditory sensory pathways; see Chapter 4) to the amygdala. They found that electrical stimulation of this pathway gave rise to LTP in the lateral nucleus of the amygdala, in accord with the fact that synaptic responses in the same nucleus are enhanced by natural auditory stimulation. Although this question is far from settled, there is at least some evidence that LTP is correlated with newly learned behaviors.

Learning-related changes in synaptic morphology

Maintenance of any mechanism of memory that is to last for a long period requires gene expression and the synthesis of new proteins. Among other effects, these changes can, and in some cases do, lead to long-lasting structural alternations in synapses. These morphological changes in neuronal connectivity can be considered the culmination of a process of *synaptic consolidation* discussed in Chapter 9.

For many neurons, learning-related alterations in synaptic morphology appear to involve **dendritic spines**. These are small protrusions from dendritic branches—often mushroom-shaped—that in the neocortex receive excitatory synaptic input from other neurons. Several sorts of morphological changes in dendritic spine structure over periods of a few minutes to hours have been

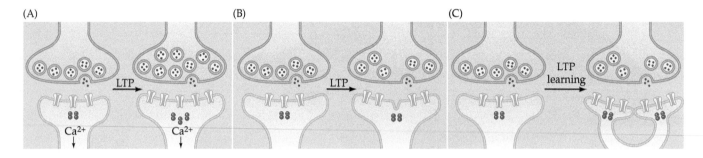

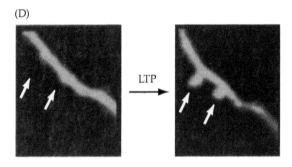

Figure 8.26 Morphological changes in dendritic spines associated with the maintenance of LTP (A) Synapses may increase in number of presynaptic vesicles, postsynaptic receptors, and ribosomes (red circles). (B) Synapses may develop separate synaptic zones divided by a wall or a cleft (perforated synapses) in the spine. (C) A single spine may divide in two. (D) New dendritic spines (white arrows) appear approximately 1 hour after a stimulus that induces LTP. (A–C after Lamprecht and LeDoux 2004; D from Engert and Bonhoeffer 1999.)

observed, some in parallel with the development of LTP and changes in behavior. The simplest changes are in the length and diameter of the "stem" of the mushroom (the spine neck) and/or changes in the size of the mushroom itself (Figure 8.26A). The former changes affect passage of the synaptic signal from the spine to the dendritic shaft, and the latter allow a change in the number of presynaptic terminals in contact with a spine (Figure 8.26B,C). Finally, new spines can emerge from the shaft of the dendrite and others disappear, thereby changing the number of spines and thus synapses in yet another way (Figure 8.26D). All such changes could support memories or their loss by increasing or decreasing synaptic strength over long periods.

In summary, the physical representations of memories (engrams) are assumed to consist of functional and structural changes in synaptic connectivity among neurons that have strengthened or weakened as a result of experience. Long-term maintenance of LTP and other memory mechanisms presumably requires changes in gene expression and the synthesis of new proteins that eventually lead to structural alternations in synaptic morphology and neuronal connectivity. This commonality of mechanisms at the cellular level is quite compatible with functional heterogeneity at the systems level.

Summary

1. The generally accepted taxonomy of memory systems distinguishes three major systems: declarative memory, nondeclarative memory, and working memory. Damage to the medial temporal lobe impairs declarative memory but spares working memory. Other types of lesions can impair working memory without disrupting declarative memory.

2. Nondeclarative memory depends on brain regions other than medial temporal lobes, which vary for different forms of nondeclarative memory: priming, skill learning, and conditioning.

3. Priming is defined as a change in processing of a stimulus due to a previous encounter with the same or a related stimulus in the absence of conscious awareness of the original encounter. The neural correlates of priming include neocortical regions that vary with the type of priming: visual perceptual priming is associated with altered activity in the visual sensory areas in occipitotemporal cortex; conceptual priming, with anterior left inferior prefrontal areas; and semantic priming,

with left anterior temporal areas. In functional neuroimaging studies of priming, these regions typically show a reduction in activity, known as repetition suppression, which may reflect a dropping out of noncritical neurons across repetitions.

4. Skill learning depends on the basal ganglia and is associated with cortical regions that depend on the type of skill learning (motor regions for motor learning, temporal fusiform regions for perceptual learning, and so on).

5. Conditioning is the altered probability of a behavioral response engendered by associating the response with a reward. Eyeblink conditioning has been linked to circuits in the cerebellum. Operant conditioning (instrumental learning) has been associated with the basal ganglia.

6. All varieties of memory appear to depend on the same cellular and molecular mechanisms of neural plasticity. At the cellular level, memories are transiently stored as changes in the efficacy of existing synaptic connections between neurons within particular neuronal assemblies. Longer-lasting memories require more permanent changes in gene expression, protein synthesis, and morphology, including the formation of new synaptic connections.

> Go to the **COMPANION WEBSITE**
>
> sites.sinauer.com/cogneuro2e
> for quizzes, animations, flashcards, and other study resources.

Additional Reading

Reviews

DAYAN, E. AND L. G. COHEN (2011) Neuroplasticity subserving motor skill learning. *Neuron* 72: 443–454.

FOERDE, K. AND D. SHOHAMY (2011) The role of the basal ganglia in learning and memory: Insight from Parkinson's disease. *Neurobiol. Learn. Mem.* 96: 624–636.

GRILL-SPECTOR, K., R. HENSON AND A. MARTIN (2006) Repetition and the brain: Neural models of stimulus-specific effects. *Trends Cogn. Sci.* 10: 14–23.

MILNER, B., L. R. SQUIRE AND E. R. KANDEL (1998) Cognitive neuroscience and the study of memory. *Neuron* 20: 445–468.

NADEL, L. AND O. HARDT (2011) Update on memory systems and processes. *Neuropsychopharmacology* 36: 251–273.

SANES, J. R. AND J. W. LICHTMAN (1999) Can molecules explain long-term potentiation? *Nat. Neurosci.* 7: 597–604.

SQUIRE, L. R., C. E. STARK AND R. E. CLARK (2004) The medial temporal lobe. *Annu. Rev. Neurosci.* 27: 279–306.

YIN, H. H. AND B. J. KNOWLTON (2006) The role of the basal ganglia in habit formation. *Nat. Rev. Neurosci.* 7: 464–476.

Important Original Papers

BUCKNER, R. L., S. E. PETERSEN, J. G. OJEMANN, F. M. MIEZIN, L. R. SQUIRE AND M. E. RAICHLE (1995) Functional anatomical studies of explicit and implicit memory retrieval tasks. *J. Neurosci.* 7: 12–29.

CLARK, R. E. AND L. R. SQUIRE (1998) Classical conditioning and brain systems: The role of awareness. *Science* 280: 77–81.

GABRIELI, J. D. E., D. A. FLEISHMAN, M. M. KEANE, S. L. REMINGER AND F. MORRELL (1995) Double dissociation between memory systems underlying explicit and implicit memory in the human brain. *Psychol. Sci.* 6: 76–82.

GRAF, P., L. R. SQUIRE AND R. MANDLER (1984) The information that amnesic patients do not forget. *J. Exp. Psychol. Learn. Mem. Cogn.* 10: 164–178.

HENSON, R., T. SHALLICE AND R. DOLAN (2000) Neuroimaging evidence for dissociable forms of repetition priming. *Science* 287: 1269–1272.

KNOWLTON, B. J., J. A. MANGELS AND L. R. SQUIRE (1996) A neostriatal habit learning system in humans. *Science* 262: 1747–1749.

MILLER, E. K., L. LI AND R. DESIMONE (1991) A neural mechanism for working and recognition memory in inferior temporal cortex. *Science* 254: 1377–1379.

POLDRACK, R. A. AND 7 OTHERS (2001) Interactive memory systems in the human brain. *Nature* 414: 546–550.

WARRINGTON, E. K. AND L. WEISKRANTZ (1968) New method of testing long-term retention with special reference to amnesic patients. *Nature* 217: 972–974.

YIN, H. H., B. J. KNOWLTON AND B. W. BALLEINE (2004) Lesions of dorsolateral striatum preserve outcome expectancy but disrupt habit formation in instrumental learning. *Eur. J. Neurosci.* 19: 181–189.

Books

FOSTER, J. K. AND M. JELICIC (1999) *Memory: Systems, Process, or Function?* Oxford: Oxford University Press.

EICHENBAUM, H. (2011) *The Cognitive Neuroscience of Memory: An Introduction.* New York: Oxford University Press.

9

Declarative Memory

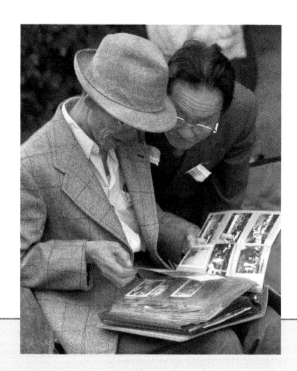

INTRODUCTION

Although nondeclarative forms of memory, such as priming, skill learning, and conditioning, are pervasive in everyday life, declarative memory is what most people mean when they use the term memory—namely, the ability to consciously remember personally experienced events (I parked the car near the exit of the parking lot) and facts shared with others (the name of the actress was so-and-so). Although declarative memory is linked to consciousness, it can be studied in non-human animals (in which consciousness is assumed) by using memory tasks similar to the ones that depend on human declarative memory (for non-human declarative memory tests; see Box 8A).

As noted in Chapter 8, declarative memory is critically dependent on the integrity of the medial temporal lobes. However, this type of memory involves other brain parts as well, including regions of the prefrontal cortex and the posterior parietal cortex. During encoding, memories are assumed to be stored in the medial temporal lobes, as well as in the relevant cortical regions (visual, auditory, and so on), where they are assumed to be made longer lasting by a process called memory consolidation. During retrieval, memory traces in these cortical regions are reactivated, leading to the conscious experience of remembering. Prefrontal and parietal regions are thought to provide the executive and attentional control needed to process and integrate incoming information during encoding, and to select and evaluate memories during retrieval. Although this basic description applies to all forms of declarative memory, there are important differences between declarative memory for events, called episodic memory, and memory for facts, called semantic memory (see Introductory Box). There are also differences between two forms of episodic memory, known as recollection and familiarity.

■ INTRODUCTORY BOX DEVELOPMENTAL AMNESIA

Recall from Chapter 8 that patient H.M. became afflicted with severe amnesia following surgery that removed much of his medial temporal lobes on both sides. After the surgery, H.M. was unable to acquire new declarative memories, including new memories for personally experienced past events (episodic memory) and new memories about facts and language (semantic memory). H.M.'s case left open, however, the question of what happens when medial temporal lobe damage is limited to the hippocampus and spares the surrounding cortices (entorhinal, perirhinal, and para-hippocampal cortices; see Box 9A).

Selective hippocampal damage can occur when the brain is deprived of appropriate oxygen supply (a condition known as hypoxia) because this region has a higher metabolic rate (and thus greater dependence on oxygen) than do most other brain areas. Oxygen deprivation is not uncommon during complications at birth, and depending on the severity of the hypoxia, hippocampal damage can leave children severely impaired as a result of inadequate declarative memory. Surprisingly, however, although these children are impaired in episodic memory, they acquire semantic knowledge relatively normally and are often able to attend mainstream schools.

The first study of such cases reported data for three children who likely suffered hypoxia: Beth, Jon, and Kate. Brain imaging showed hippocampal formations of these children to be smaller than those of normal controls (Figure A). All three suffered from episodic memory deficits, which were noticeable to both the children and their parents, and were confirmed by formal testing. For example, the children were markedly impaired in their ability draw a complex figure from memory (Figure B), as well as in other verbal and nonverbal episodic memory tasks (Figure C). In contrast, as in the case of other patients with medial temporal lobe amnesia, the perceptual abilities

Compared to control subjects, three children with developmental amnesia—Beth, Jon, and Kate—who showed hippocampal atrophy (A) were impaired in visual memory but not visual perception (B). They were also impaired in episodic but not working memory tasks, for both verbal and non-verbal stimuli (C). Remarkably, the three children showed normal reading and comprehension abilities (D). (After Vargha-Khadem et al. 1997.)

(e.g., copying the pattern in Figure B) and working memory abilities (Figure C) of these children were relatively intact.

Another surprising aspect of these cases is that, despite significant hippocampal atrophy and episodic memory impairments, all three children attended mainstream schools and displayed normal levels of speech and language competence, literacy, and factual knowledge (Figure D). In other words, they were impaired in episodic memory but could acquire semantic knowledge at a relatively normal rate.

The dissociation between impaired episodic memory and spared semantic memory has important implications. First, it supports the idea that the hippocampus is specifically associated with episodic memory but not semantic memory. It is not clear which brain region supports semantic learning in Beth, Jon, and Kate or the rest of us, but the implication is that semantic memory is mediated by the medial temporal lobe cortices (i.e., the perirhinal, entorhinal, and parahippocampal cortices; see Box 9A).

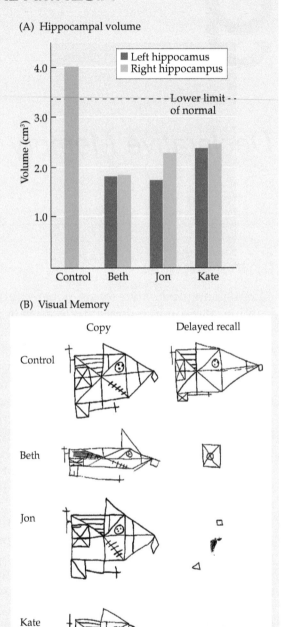

(A) Hippocampal volume

(B) Visual Memory

This chapter first introduces some basic concepts and assumptions about the taxonomy of declarative memory, and the neural mechanisms underlying encoding, storage, and retrieval. The second section focuses on the nature of medial temporal lobe representations, distinguishing the role of the hippocampus and other medial temporal lobe structures. The following sections focus on the organization and access of semantic and episodic memory traces stored in the cortex, and contributions of the prefrontal and parietal cortices during

■ INTRODUCTORY BOX (continued)

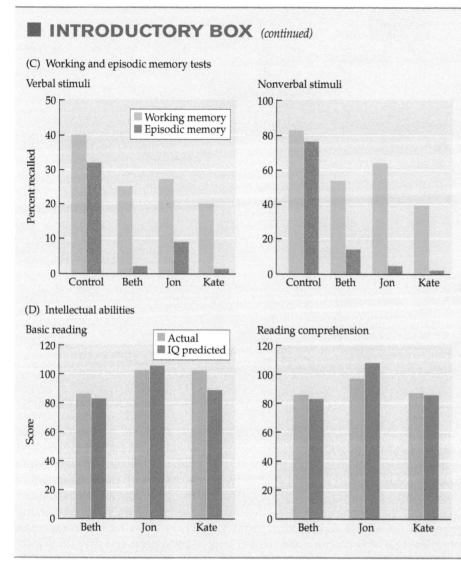

(C) Working and episodic memory tests

Verbal stimuli

Nonverbal stimuli

(D) Intellectual abilities

Basic reading

Reading comprehension

This dissociation also has implications for theories of memory development. According to one view, semantic memory develops after episodic memory because general concepts (e.g., the idea of a "dog") are assumed to be abstracted from individual experiences (e.g., encountering specific dogs). An alternative view, however, is that episodic memory develops after semantic memory, since understanding the meaning of an event (what happened) is a requirement for associating core content to contextual details of the event (where, when, and how it happened). The finding that Beth, Jon, and Kate could accumulate a wealth of semantic knowledge despite pronounced episodic memory deficits is consistent with the second view.

References

DE HAAN, M., M. MISHKIN, T. BALDEWEG AND F. VARGHA-KHADEM (2006) Human memory development and its dysfunction after early hippocampal injury. *Trends Neurosci.* 29: 374–381.

SQUIRE, L. R. AND S. ZOLA (1998) Episodic memory, semantic memory, and amnesia. *Hippocampus* 8: 205–211.

VARGHA-KHADEM, F., D. G. GADIAN, K. E. WATKINS, A. CONNELLY, W. VAN PAESSCHEN AND M. MISHKIN (1997) Differential effects of early hippocampal pathology on episodic and semantic memory. *Science* 277: 376–380.

encoding and retrieval. Finally, the last section describes what is known about memory consolidation.

Basic Concepts and Assumptions

This section introduces a few basic terms and hypotheses. One set of terms refer to the different forms of declarative memory, and another, to the processes describing how declarative memory operates. The section ends with a simple theory of how these declarative memory processes are mediated by the brain and basic findings supporting the theory.

A taxonomy of declarative memory

Chapter 8 introduced basic distinctions of working memory, declarative memory, and nondeclarative memory. Here we focus on different types of declarative memory (yellow boxes in **Figure 9.1**). Each type is defined by conscious memory for events versus facts, and the qualities associated with those events and facts. Memory for events is known as **episodic memory**, and memory for facts is known as **semantic memory**—a distinction introduced by psychologist Endel

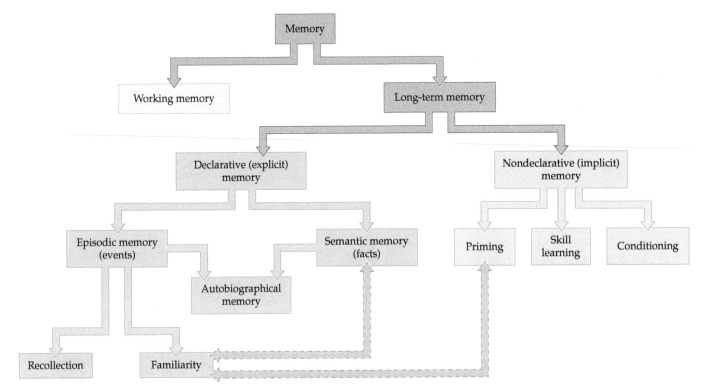

Figure 9.1 **The memory system taxonomy and forms of declarative memory** The main branches of the memory system are working memory, declarative memory, and nondeclarative memory. Declarative memory can be subdivided into episodic memory (conscious memory for events) and semantic memory (conscious memory for facts). Both episodic and semantic memory contribute to people's memories of their own lives, or autobiographical memory. Episodic memory can be further subdivided into recollection and familiarity. Although familiarity is usually classified as a form of episodic memory, its mechanisms are also related to those of semantic memory and priming.

Tulving in the early 1970s. The term *episodic memory* thus refers to memories of events that an individual has experienced personally in a specific place and at a particular time (i.e., from an *episode*). In contrast, *semantic memory* refers to knowledge about the world that individuals share with other members of their culture, including the knowledge of a native language and facts learned in school. For example, remembering listening to reggae music in your living room last Sunday is an episodic memory, whereas knowing that reggae is a popular style of Jamaican music characterized by syncopated rhythm is a semantic memory.

In the laboratory, episodic memory is sometimes defined as consisting of memories encoded during the experiment, such as a list of words presented on a computer; semantic memory, on the other hand, is defined as information that the participants had encoded before the experiment started, such as knowing that a dog is a mammal. In life, episodic and semantic memories interact and to some degree overlap. In fact, memory for the events of our own lives, called **autobiographical memory**, is a complex mixture of episodic and semantic memories (see Figure 9.1). For example, the semantic knowledge that the river Seine runs through Paris, that the Louvre is a famous museum in that city, and that long lines are common at famous museums may affect our reconstruction of autobiographical memories of a particular day actually spent in Paris. Conversely, semantic memories can also be associated with episodic memories of the learning events (e.g., the day in French class when Paris was the topic of discussion).

Episodic memory is typically subdivided into two additional categories: *recollection* and *familiarity*. **Recollection** refers to memories of a past event that include specific associations and contextual details; **familiarity** refers to the sense that we experienced an event at some point in the past, even though no specific associations or contextual details come to mind. An example of familiarity without recollection is seeing a person's face and knowing that you have seen that person before, but being unable to remember any specific previous encounter or information about the person, such as the person's name. The classification of familiarity as a form of episodic memory is a topic of some debate because familiarity involves conscious memory for events, but its neural mechanisms are related to those underlying semantic memory and priming (dashed arrows in Figure 9.1).

A simple neurological model of encoding, storage, and retrieval

As illustrated by the case of H.M. described in Chapter 8, damage to the medial temporal lobe impairs declarative memory but spares nondeclarative forms of memory, such as priming and skill learning. A generally accepted explanation of why medial temporal lobe regions are critical for declarative memory is that they store pointers to the locations of memory traces that were stored in the cortex during their formation. To pursue this explanation, which provides an organizing principle for this chapter, it is useful to start with a very simple model of how different brain regions contribute to the encoding, storage, and retrieval phases introduced in Chapter 8. The model in Figure 9.2 is described here using episodic memory as an example, but it also applies to semantic memory.

During the *encoding phase* (Figure 9.2A), different aspects of an event are thought to be stored in the same regions that are involved in perceiving the event. For example, memory traces from a birthday party would include memories about the color of the balloons stored in visual cortex, memories about the music stored in auditory cortex, memories about dancing stored in motor cortex, and so forth (for simplicity, Figure 9.2A shows only auditory and visual memory traces). As noted in Chapter 8, memory traces consist of alterations in the synapses. For example, encoding a memory about a red balloon can be assumed to involve strengthened synapses between groups of neurons coding for "red" and for "balloon." However, remembering a complex event, such as a birthday party, is much more than remembering simple perceptual associations; it requires simultaneous access to many different aspects of an event, including not only *what* happened but also *where*, *when*, and *how* it happened.

According to the model, simultaneous access to all these traces can be accomplished because the hippocampus stores a summary representation of the whole event with pointers to the locations of the traces distributed over the cortex. This hippocampal representation is sometimes called an *index*, emphasizing the idea that the representation is not the main information about the event, but a pointer to where the main information can be found and accessed, much like the index in this book. In sum, in the encoding of declarative memory, two types of representations are created: distributed cortical traces and hippocampal indices.

Figure 9.2 A simple model of episodic memory encoding, storage, and retrieval (A) During encoding, each aspect of an event is stored in the cortical area involved in processing (perceiving) this aspect of the event (visual information is stored in visual cortex, auditory information in auditory cortex, and so on). The hippocampus is assumed to store a summary representation, or *index*, pointing to the locations of memory distributed over the cortex. (B) During storage, the traces for some memories are stabilized—a process known as consolidation. (C) During retrieval, a retrieval cue may access the hippocampal index, which leads to simultaneous access of the various cortical traces and the experience of remembering the original event. HC, hippocampus; PFC, prefrontal cortex; PPC, posterior parietal cortex.

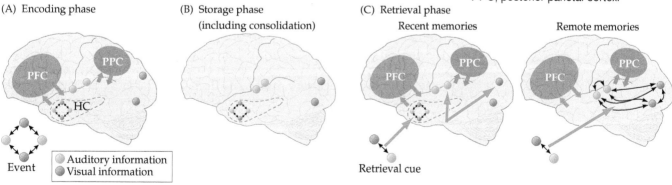

(A) Encoding phase

(B) Storage phase (including consolidation)

(C) Retrieval phase — Recent memories — Remote memories

PPC PFC HC Event Auditory information Visual information Retrieval cue

Time

During the *storage phase* (Figure 9.2B), some memory traces are strengthened and become long lasting, whereas other memories are presumably lost. The strengthening process is known as **consolidation** and is specifically considered at the end of the chapter. The assumption that some memories are lost during storage is difficult or impossible to prove in complex organisms because the fact that a particular memory cannot be retrieved does not imply that the memory does not exist; the memory may be *available* but not *accessible*. However, in animal models in which learning can be linked to synaptic changes, alterations in synaptic form and function reverse over time in parallel with behavioral measures of forgetting, suggesting that some memories do become lost.

The *retrieval phase* (Figure 9.2C) is usually triggered by a **retrieval cue**, typically a piece of information associated with a particular aspect of the original event. Retrieval cues may be external or internal, and the retrieval process may be involuntary or voluntary. For example, seeing a person at work (external cue) who was at a recent party may spontaneously remind you of the party (involuntary retrieval). Alternatively, you can intentionally try to remember the party (voluntary retrieval) by generating an image of the house where the party was held or of the host (internal cue). In episodic memory tests in the lab, the cues are typically external (e.g., the word *house* provided by the experimenter), and retrieval is usually voluntary (e.g., trying to recall the word that was paired with *house*).

In the case of recent memories, access to cortical traces is assumed to be mediated by the hippocampus: the retrieval cue accesses the hippocampal index, which leads to access of the distributed cortical memory traces, and in turn to the experience of remembering the original event. In the case of remote memories, however, because direct associations have been created among distributed cortical traces (a process explained in the discussion of consolidation at the end of the chapter), these traces can be accessed directly by retrieval cues, bypassing the hippocampus.

So far, we have considered only the roles of the medial temporal lobe and modality-specific cortical regions. What about other brain regions, including the prefrontal and posterior parietal regions mentioned earlier (see Figure 9.2)? Prefrontal regions mediate both semantic/linguistic processes (see Chapter 12) and executive functions (see Chapter 13) that directly contribute to encoding and retrieval. During encoding, these processes are thought to help link incoming stimuli with preexisting knowledge and organize them into meaningful units that can be more easily remembered. During retrieval, the prefrontal regions help guide the memory search, evaluate the information recovered, and underlie decisions about its validity. Posterior parietal regions support attentional control processes (see Chapter 7), which are critical for selecting information during encoding and for guiding the memory search during retrieval. Prefrontal and posterior parietal regions are less critical during storage, but they may play a role during consolidation.

Using the model to explain the effects of brain damage

The general model can account well for three features of declarative memory loss following brain damage. First, it can explain well why small lesions in the cortex tend to produce very mild or no declarative memory deficits, whereas bilateral lesions of the same size in the medial temporal lobes can produce severe amnesia. Since the memory traces for one event are distributed over the cortex, a single lesion is unlikely to destroy associated memory traces (recall Karl Lashley's experiments and the idea of *graceful degradation* in connectionist models described in Box 8C). In contrast, the medial temporal lobes store the locations of most cortical memory traces within a small region, and hence, damage to this small region can block access to a vast number of cortical memory traces.

To use a simple metaphor, imagine a large, multifloor library with a single computer in the basement containing the records that show the locations of all books in the library. Whereas a small fire in one of the floors could damage a fraction of the books, a similar fire in the basement could destroy the computer and prevent access to all books stored in the library (a situation analogous to *retrograde amnesia*). The books are still there, but one cannot find them without the computer records. Without the computer, it is also impossible to log the locations of new books received after the computer damage. These new books may be accessible immediately after delivery while they are still at the receiving counter (which would be analogous to working memory), but not after being shelved somewhere in the library if no record of their storage location is kept (a situation analogous to *anterograde amnesia*).

Second, the model can explain why cortical damage can produce selective memory loss, whereas memory loss following medial temporal lobe damage is global, affecting all modalities and types of stimuli. For example, some forms of cortical damage can impair knowledge for living things without disrupting knowledge for nonliving things, or vice versa (see the discussion of storage later in the chapter). In contrast, patients with medial temporal lobe amnesia like H.M. are typically impaired in remembering all kinds of knowledge and events, regardless of their semantic category or modality. According to the model, cortical memory traces are organized by modality and can also be organized by category, but medial temporal lobe regions like the hippocampus store the indices for all kinds of memory traces. Returning to the library metaphor, whereas damage in one floor may be selective to one type of book (e.g., poetry books), damage to the basement computer will affect the records for all types of books.

Finally, the model can explain why medial temporal lobe damage tends to produce anterograde amnesia together with retrograde amnesia for recent events (e.g., a few years before the lesion) but usually spares memory for remote events (e.g., from childhood). According to the model, the cortical traces for recent memories are disconnected from each other; hence, they can be accessed together only via the indices stored in the hippocampus. However, as memories are repeatedly retrieved, their cortical traces become directly associated with each other, so they can be accessed together independently of the hippocampus. This process, known as *system consolidation*, is explained at the end of the chapter. Again using the library metaphor, imagine that each time you gather the set of "books" associated with one event (e.g., the balloon, music, and dancing "books" for a particular birthday party), you place Post-it notes on some books indicating the location of some of the other books in the set. After doing this many times, finding one or a few books in the set is enough to find all the other books in the set, even if the basement computer is not available.

The remainder of the chapter focuses on different aspects of the model depicted in Figure 9.2, including (1) the nature of medial temporal lobe representations, (2) the cortical regions that store semantic and episodic memory traces, (3) the contributions of prefrontal regions during encoding and retrieval, (4) the role of parietal regions during encoding and retrieval, and (5) consolidation processes during the storage phase.

The Nature of Medial Temporal Lobe Representations

Given the dramatic effects of medial temporal lobe damage in human and non-human animals, there is no doubt that these regions play a fundamental role in episodic memory. However, the specific contributions of different medial temporal lobe subregions to declarative memory are topics of much debate. The following sections consider theories of hippocampal function, and theories about the function of various medial temporal subregions described in Box 9A.

■ BOX 9A ORGANIZATION OF THE MEDIAL TEMPORAL LOBE MEMORY SYSTEM

The medial temporal lobe memory system consists of the hippocampus and the surrounding rhinal cortex and parahippocampal cortex (Figure A). The amygdala is located in the anterior part of the medial temporal lobe; although it modulates declarative memory processing, the amygdala is not considered a memory region per se.

The main output of the hippocampus is the *fornix*, a tract that connects the hip-pocampus to the mammillary bodies, and the mammillary bodies in turn project to the anterior nucleus of the thalamus. The rhinal cortex consists of the entorhinal cortex medially, and the perirhinal cortex laterally (Figure B). Taken together, the entorhinal, perirhinal, and parahippocampal cortices constitute the parahippocampal gyrus. (The *parahippocampal gyrus* should not be confused with the *parahippocampal cortex*, which is only the poste-rior half of the gyrus.) The perirhinal and parahippocampal cortices receive inputs from unimodal and polymodal associa-tion areas in frontal, parietal, temporal, and cingulate cortices (Figure C). In humans and other primates, the perirhinal and parahippocampal cortices project

(A) Medial temporal lobe regions within the brain. (B) Three-dimensional view of the subregions of the medial temporal lobe. (C) Neural connections among medial tem-poral lobe regions, as well as between these regions and the rest of the brain. (A–C after Lavenex and Amaral 2000.)

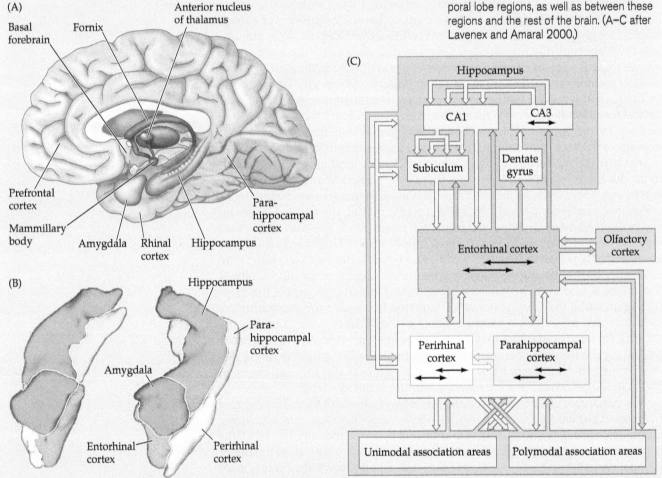

Theories of hippocampal memory function

According to the **cognitive map theory** proposed by neuroscientists John O'Keefe and Lynn Nadel, the main role of the hippocampus is to mediate memory for spatial relations among objects in the environment. The strongest evidence for this theory is the existence of place cells in the rodent hippocampus. These neurons become active only when the animal is in a particular spatial location

■ **BOX 9A** *(continued)*

to the entorhinal cortex, which provides the predominant cortical input to the hippocampus.

Of these regions in the medial temporal lobe, the one that has received the most attention is the hippocampus (which gets its name derived from its seahorse-like shape). The hippocampus is not a homogeneous structure but consists of several interconnected subregions, including the *dentate gyrus*, the *cornus Ammon* (Latin for "horn of Ammon," and often referred to by its abbreviation,

"CA"), and the *subiculum* (Figure D). Input from the entorhinal cortex reaches all three hippocampal subregions. In addition, several internal "loops" connect the dentate gyrus to the CA3 and CA1 regions, to the subiculum, and then back to entorhinal cortex (Figure E).

Thus, the organization of the medial temporal lobe can be thought of as a hierarchical sequence in which information is processed through perirhinal, parahippocampal, and entorhinal cortices, finally reaching the hippocampus. It is clear,

however, that the cortices of the parahippocampal gyrus do not simply funnel information to the hippocampus. On the contrary, each of these cortices consists of several subregions that are densely associated by reciprocal connections and clearly carry out extensive processing in their own right. Moreover, these different cortices are linked to each other by rich intrinsic connections, and hence they collaborate in processing incoming information before it reaches the hippocampus.

References

AMARAL, D. G. (1999) Introduction: What is where in the medial temporal lobe? *Hippocampus* 9: 1–6.

LAVENEX, P. AND D. G. AMARAL (2000) Hippocampal-neocortical interaction: A hierarchy of associativity. *Hippocampus* 10: 420–430.

(D) Nissl-stained coronal section of the hippocampus. The 4-millimeter squares (the typical spatial resolution of fMRI studies) illustrate the difficulty of distinguishing medial temporal lobe subregions using functional neuroimaging. *, collateral sulcus; ab, angular bundle; cf, choroidal fissure; DG, dentate gyrus; EC, entorhinal cortex; FG, fusiform gyrus; hf, hippocampal fissure; PRC, perirhinal cortex; PaS, parasubiculum; PrS, presubiculum; S, subiculum; V, ventricle. (E) Connections within subregions of the hippocampus, including the entorhinal-dentate-CA-subiculum-entorhinal loop. (D from Amaral 1999.)

(D)

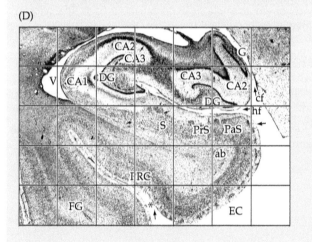

(E)

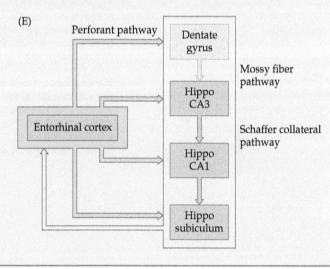

in its local environment (Figure 9.3A). Place cells also have been identified in the human hippocampus. For example, one study had epileptic patients with implanted electrodes play a "taxi driver" computer game in which they had to drive passengers to target locations in a virtual town (Figure 9.3B). As in rats, some neurons of the hippocampus were active only when the "taxi" passed through specific locations of the simulated town.

According to the **relational memory theory** put forward by neuroscientists Howard Eichenbaum and Neal Cohen, the hippocampus mediates memory for new associations in general. Consistent with this idea, the hippocampus is critical for remembering nonspatial associations in rodents, such as new associations between odors. In the *odor association task*, for example, treats such as Froot Loops cereal are hidden in cups of differently odorized sand (Figure 9.4A). Rats are trained to prefer Odor A over Odor B, Odor B over Odor C, Odor

(A)

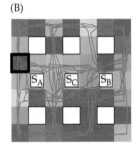
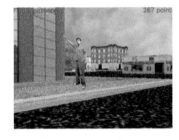
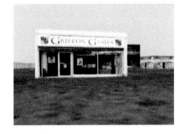
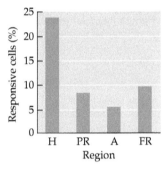

(B)

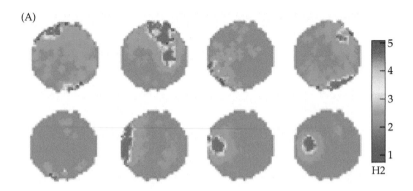

Figure 9.3 Place cells in the hippocampus (A) In the rat, place cells fire when the animal is in a specific spatial location–for example, in an open circular cage. The color code here shows the firing pattern of eight different place cells, with red indicating intense activity. Note that each cell being recorded from is active only when the rat is in a particular position in its environment (shown here, from above, as the circular arena the animal is exploring). The color scale shows the cell firing rate in hertz. (B) A neuron in the human hippocampus was active only when the subject was in a specific location (red square) of a virtual town (red lines indicate the trajectory of the "taxi"). Lettered squares are store locations, and blank white squares are nontarget buildings. The graph on the right shows that although most place cells in humans were found in the hippocampus (H), some were also found in the parahippocampal region (PR), the amygdala (A), and the frontal lobes (FR). (B from Ekstrom et al. 2003.)

(A)

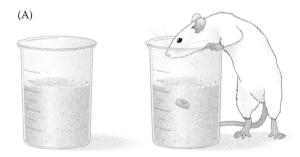

(B)

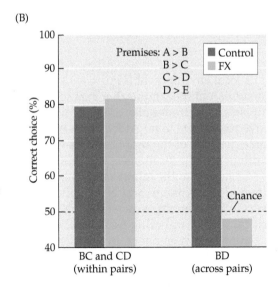

Figure 9.4 Relational memory for odor associations and transitive inference in rodents (A) In this paradigm, declarative memory is indexed by a rat's ability to choose cups associated with a series of odors that have been differentially rewarded. (B) Rats with fornix (FX) lesions that disrupt hippocampal output can remember their choices within individual odor pairs (B > C and C > D), but they fail to show memories for relationships across pairs (B > D). (After Dusek and Eichenbaum 1997.)

Figure 9.5 Amnesia patient K.C. (A) K.C.'s ability to play chess and to remember general knowledge of the world (semantic memory) was not affected by his brain lesions. (B) Sagittal MRI slice showing K.C.'s bilateral hippocampal and parahippocampal damage. (A from Tulving 2002; B from Rosenbaum et al. 2000.)

(A)
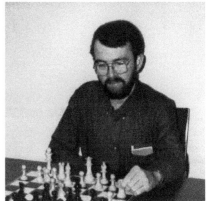

(B)
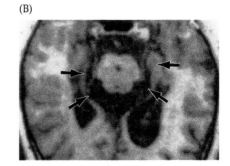

C over Odor D, and so on. Rats with fornix lesions, which disrupt the output of the hippocampus, can remember trained pairs, such as B is better than C and C is better than D, but they cannot infer relationships across pairs, such as B is better than D (*transitive inference*; Figure 9.4B).

The **episodic memory theory**, promoted by Endel Tulving, Morris Moscovitch, and other researchers, postulates that the hippocampus is critical for episodic memory but not for semantic memory. Consistent with this view, selective hippocampal damage tends to impair episodic more than semantic memory. As mentioned in the Introductory Box, children with hypoxia-related hippocampal damage are severely impaired in episodic memory but can acquire new vocabulary and knowledge.

Another example is the amnesia patient K.C. (Figure 9.5A), who suffered a motorcycle accident in which he sustained damage to several brain regions, including the hippocampus (Figure 9.5B). As with patient H.M., K.C.'s intellectual abilities were well preserved: he is able to read, write, and play chess at much the same level as before his accident. However, he cannot remember events that happened before or after the accident (i.e., he has both anterograde and retrograde amnesia). By contrast, his memory for semantic information acquired before the accident is intact. He has a good vocabulary, and his knowledge of subjects such as mathematics, history, and geography is similar to that of others with comparable education. He has difficulty forming new semantic memories but can learn simple semantic associations with many repetitions. Thus, medial temporal lobe damage can, in at least some cases, impair episodic memory while sparing retrograde semantic memory.

Moreover, whereas hippocampal lesions impair episodic more than semantic memory, damage to cortical regions in the anterior temporal lobe tends to disrupt semantic more than episodic memory. The latter pattern is displayed by patients with the progressive disorder known as **semantic dementia**. Semantic dementia is a variant of frontotemporal dementia, which typically starts with word-finding deficits (*anomia*) and progresses into a severe loss of knowledge and language. For example, patient A.M., who displayed the left anterior temporal atrophy typical for this disorder (Figure 9.6A), was severely impaired in nonverbal semantic knowledge tests (e.g., deciding whether a pyramid shape fits better with palm trees or with pine trees; Figure 9.6B), but performed

Figure 9.6 Semantic dementia (A) Coronal-section MRI of A.M., a patient with semantic dementia, showing severe left-lateralized atrophy of the anterior temporal cortex, including the parahippocampal, fusiform, and inferior temporal gyri. The left hippocampus is only mildly atrophied. (B) Subjects suffering from semantic dementia perform poorly on tests of semantic knowledge such as the "pyramid and palm trees" test. Here participants are asked to indicate which of the bottom two images fits better with the top image. (A from Hodges and Graham 2001.)

(A)
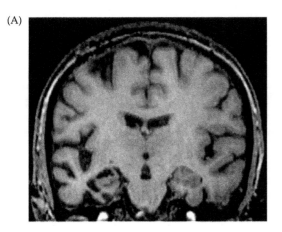

(B)
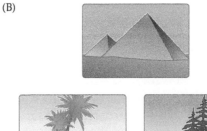
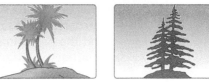

(A) Left hippocampus

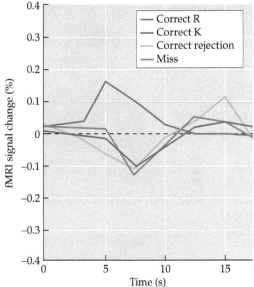

(B)

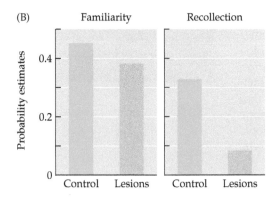

Figure 9.7 **Evidence for a greater hippocampal role in recollection than in familiarity** (A) In this fMRI study, the hippocampus showed greater activity for recognition responses based on recollection ("remember," or R, responses) than for those based on familiarity ("know," or K, responses). (B) Compared to controls, rats with selective hippocampal lesions are impaired in recollection but not in familiarity. (A after Eldridge et al. 2000; B after Fortin et al. 2004.)

normally on nonverbal episodic memory tasks (e.g., delayed recall of the complex figure in the Introductory Box). Thus, the combined results of amnesia and semantic dementia cases suggest that the hippocampus is more critical for episodic than semantic memory, whereas left anterior temporal cortex is more critical for semantic than episodic memory.

Evidence regarding hippocampal function can be consistent with more than one theory. For example, evidence that the hippocampus is associated with recollection rather than familiarity fits well with both relational memory and episodic memory theories because recollection requires relational memory and is also the prototypical form of episodic memory. Several methods have been used to distinguish recollection from familiarity. In one method, participants are asked to use introspection to distinguish between recognition trials that elicit memory for contextual details ("remember," or R, responses) and trials in which the item is recognized but no contextual details come to mind ("know," or K, responses).

Consistent with both the relational and episodic memory theories, fMRI studies have shown that "remember" responses tend to elicit greater hippocampal activity than "know" responses (Figure 9.7A). Recollection and familiarity measures can also be estimated from the proportion of correct and incorrect responses. A study that used this method to assess memory for odors in rats found that selective hippocampal lesions impaired recollection estimates but not familiarity estimates (Figure 9.7B). Thus, converging lines of evidence from humans and animals link the hippocampus to recollection rather than familiarity, supporting a role for this structure in both relational memory and episodic memory.

Differences between medial temporal lobe subregions

An issue of obvious importance is how hippocampal memory functions are related to the functions of surrounding medial temporal structures, such as the perirhinal and parahippocampal cortices described in Box 9A. Several ideas about functional differences between the hippocampus and medial temporal cortices have been proposed.

According to a *two-process theory*, the hippocampus processes information relatively slowly and is relational and spatial, whereas the perirhinal cortex processes information more rapidly and is item-based. In this conception, neurons in the hippocampus signal information about spatial positions or associations between items (i.e., recollection), whereas neurons in the perirhinal cortex signal information about the novelty of individual items (i.e., differences in familiarity). Consistent with the latter hypothesis, single-cell recordings in experimental animals have shown that perirhinal neurons do indeed show a stronger response when an item is first presented than when the same item is shown again (Figure 9.8A).

Functional neuroimaging studies have also suggested that the hippocampus and the perirhinal cortex make different contributions to recollection and familiarity. For example, the hippocampus shows a sharp increase in

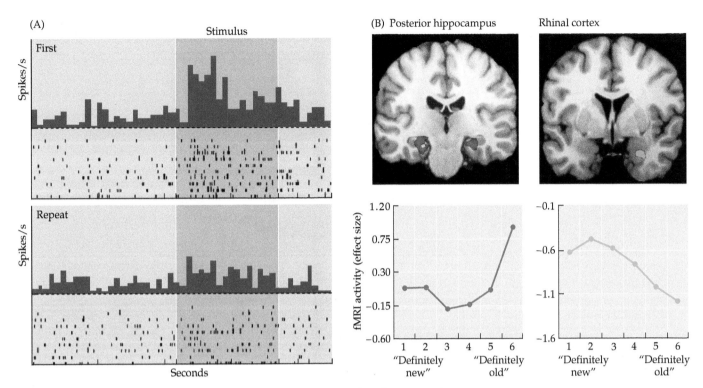

Figure 9.8 Evidence of functional differences between the perirhinal cortex and the hippocampus (A) Neurons in the perirhinal cortex show a strong response when an item is first presented (top panel) but not when the item is repeated (bottom panel). (B) Functional MRIs show that activity in the hippocampus increases sharply for items recognized as "definitely old," whereas activity in rhinal cortex decreases gradually as items become more familiar. (A after Xiang and Brown 1998; B after Daselaar et al. 2006.)

activity when participants are sure they have encountered an item before (i.e., giving a "definitely old" response on test), consistent with its putative role in recollection. Activity in perirhinal cortex, by contrast, decreases gradually as items are regarded as more and more familiar, consistent with a greater role in familiarity than in recollection (Figure 9.8B). It is unclear, however, whether the decrease in perirhinal activity measured with fMRI reflects the reduction in firing rate measured with single-cell recording studies seen in Figure 9.8A. It is also uncertain how familiarity-related perirhinal reductions pertain to the repetition suppression mechanisms assumed to mediate priming. Several authors have suggested that familiarity could be linked to nondeclarative memory phenomena, such as conceptual priming.

More recently, several researchers have proposed *three-process theories* that include not only the hippocampus and the perirhinal cortex, but also the parahippocampal cortex. According to one of these theories, the perirhinal cortex is concerned with *memory for objects*, the parahippocampal cortex is involved in *memory for spatial layouts*, and the hippocampus integrates the two types of information and hence is involved in *domain-general relational memory* (Figure 9.9). Three-process theories have several strengths. They account for evidence linking the perirhinal cortex to familiarity and the hippocampus to recollection. In addition, the distinction between perirhinal and parahippocampal functions fits well with anatomical connectivity, lesion, and functional neuroimaging evidence. The perirhinal cortex receives most of its visual input from the ventral ("what") pathway, and the parahippocampal cortex receives most of its

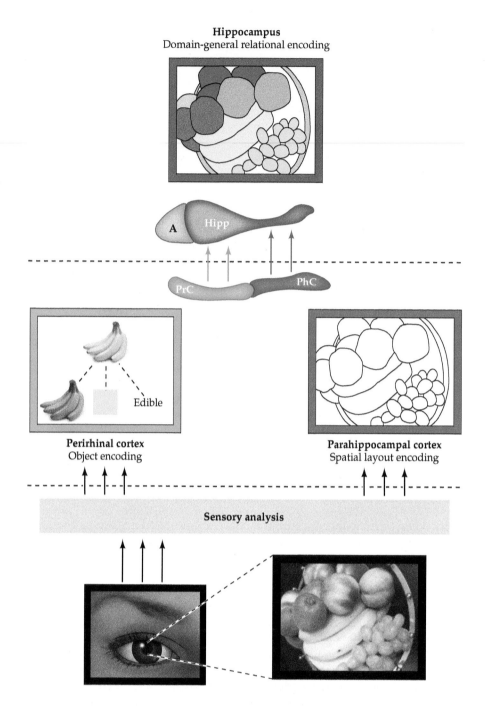

Figure 9.9 A three-process theory of medial temporal lobe functions The perirhinal cortex (PrC) is concerned with memory for objects; the parahippocampal cortex (PhC), with memory for spatial layouts; and the hippocampus (Hipp), with domain-general relational memory. A, amygdala. (After Davachi 2006.)

visual input from the dorsal ("where") pathway (see Chapter 3). In monkeys, perirhinal lesions tend to impair object memory rather than spatial memory, whereas parahippocampal lesions yield the opposite pattern. It is worth noting, however, that in humans the parahippocampal cortex appears to play a more general role in context memory and is not limited to spatial memory.

In sum, all the major theories of hippocampal function—the cognitive map, relational memory, and episodic memory theories—are supported by substantial evidence. One possibility is that all of these theories are correct in some measure and could be integrated. For example, it has been suggested that spatial memory functions are more pronounced in the right hippocampus, whereas general relational functions are more the province of the left hippocampus. Moreover, the relational memory and episodic memory theories are already closely related, and as noted earlier, both views are consistent with evidence linking the hippocampus to recollection. Recent three-process theories are promising and may eventually provide a more integrative theory for the various medial temporal lobe regions.

Cortical Regions Storing Semantic and Episodic Memory Representations

As noted earlier in the description of the general model of memory in Figure 9.2, in episodic memory it is generally assumed that different aspects of an event (visual, auditory, etc.) are stored within the cortical regions specialized in processing each type of information (visual cortex, auditory cortex, etc.). A similar assumption is made in semantic memory regarding the storage of conceptual knowledge. Although cortical storage mechanisms are probably shared, studies of semantic and episodic memory have typically emphasized different aspects of these shared mechanisms.

Since studies of semantic memory generally focus on knowledge acquired before the experiment (e.g., knowing that dogs are mammals), they do not usually investigate the encoding phase. By contrast, studies of episodic memory generally focus on memories formed in the laboratory, and they tend to investigate both encoding and retrieval phases. Partly because of this difference, semantic memory studies tend to focus on differences between cortical storage for different types of knowledge (e.g., animals versus tools), whereas episodic memory studies tend to focus on whether cortical regions engaged during encoding are recruited again during retrieval. In other words, semantic memory studies tend to focus on memory *organization*, whereas episodic memory studies tend to focus on memory *reactivation*.

The organization of semantic knowledge in the cortex

There are two main theories of how semantic knowledge is organized in the cortex: sensory/functional theory and domain-specific theory. According to the **sensory/functional theory**, advanced by neuropsychologists Elizabeth Warrington, Tim Shallice and other researchers, conceptual knowledge is organized by the sensory (form, color, etc.) and functional (motions, actions, etc.) properties of real objects. For example, the concept of "ice cream" would be distributed over visual regions that process associated colors (e.g., red, brown) and shapes (e.g., cone); the gustatory regions that process associated tastes (e.g., strawberry, chocolate); and the somatosensory/motor regions that process associated actions (e.g., licking, cone holding). According to the **domain-specific theory**, proposed by neuropsychologist Alfonso Caramazza and collaborators, concepts in the brain are organized by semantic categories rather than properties. This idea does not apply to all semantic categories, but only to those assumed to have special significance for well-being. These include animals, fruits/vegetables, conspecifics, and nonliving things that would have been important during evolution.

The sensory/functional theory, which is an instance of *embodied cognition*, is supported by abundant functional neuroimaging evidence that processing

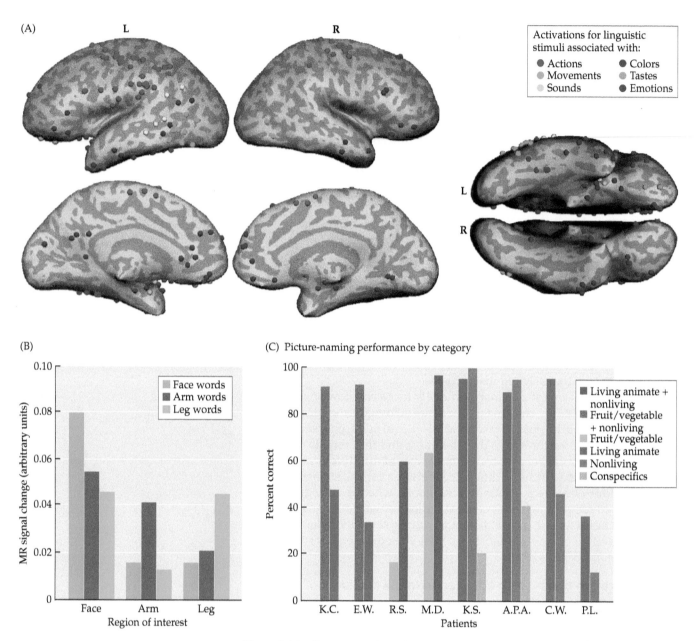

Figure 9.10 Representation of semantic knowledge in the brain (A) Locations of activation, as indicated by functional neuroimaging studies that used linguistic materials (words, phrases, or sentences) to assess modality-specific knowledge representation. (B) Brain activity elicited by words associated with motor actions made with the face (e.g., *lick*), the arm (e.g., *pick*), or the leg (e.g., *kick*) in regions of interest within primary motor cortex. The regions of interest were identified with a localizer scan in which participants moved their tongue, hands, or feet. (C) Examples of patients with domain-specific semantic deficits. Some patients are disproportionately impaired in knowledge about living things compared to nonliving things; others have greater deficits with nonliving things or conspecifics. (A from Binder and Desai 2011; B after Hauk et al. 2004; C after Mahon and Caramazza 2011.)

linguistic stimuli activates brain regions associated with their corresponding sensory and functional properties. For example, words such as *trumpet* activate auditory cortex, words such as *jump* activate motor cortex, words such as *chocolate* activate gustatory cortex, and so on (Figure 9.10A). Importantly, these effects can be found not only during tasks that require intentional retrieval of the objects' properties, which could elicit visual imagery and top-down attentional modulation of sensory and motor cortices, but also during passive reading tasks. For example, passively reading words like *lick*, *pick*, and *kick* activates, respectively, tongue, finger, and feet areas of primary motor cortex (Figure 9.10B). These results suggest that the activation of property-related cortices mediates language comprehension. Evidence that these activations are not epiphenomenal includes, for example, the finding that motor disorders (such as Parkinson's disease) and TMS-based disruption of motor cortex can produce selective deficits in the comprehension of action verbs.

The domain-specific theory is supported primarily by evidence from brain-damaged patients who show disproportionate and even selective impairments for one semantic category compared to others. Over 100 cases of these category-specific semantic deficits have been reported. Most of them show impaired knowledge for living things compared to nonliving things, but the converse pattern and other selective deficits have also been observed (see examples in Figure 9.10C). Although the location of the damage in these conditions is variable and somewhat controversial, animate knowledge deficits are often associated with lesions of the temporal cortex, and deficits in inanimate knowledge, with frontoparietal damage.

Supporters of the sensory/functional theory have explained the living-nonliving dissociation by arguing that the ability to identify living things depends more on sensory knowledge (stored in temporal cortices), whereas the ability to identify nonliving things depends more on functional knowledge (stored in frontoparietal cortices). However, this argument cannot easily explain why the affected category (e.g., tools) is sometimes impaired in both sensory and functional knowledge (e.g., both the shape and the actions associated with a hammer), and why semantic deficits for living things may occur without sensory deficits. In addition, some functional neuroimaging evidence fits better with the domain-specific theory than with the sensory/functional theory. Thus, both theories are partly correct, and they need to be integrated into a more general theory.

Sensory/functional and domain-specific theories are concerned primarily with the representation of relatively concrete semantic knowledge, such as the properties of objects. But are there also regions that store abstract semantic knowledge, like the one required for generalizing and reasoning? For example, if the knowledge about "ice cream" is stored in the brain regions that process sweetness and licking, and the knowledge about "potato chips" is stored in the regions that process saltiness and chewing, where are concepts like "snack" or "carbohydrate" stored? According to a distributed-only view, there are no specialized regions for abstract concepts; these concepts are represented by the same distributed network that mediates concrete sensory/functional features (Figure 9.11A). According to the distributed-plus-hub view, by contrast, in addition to direct connections among sensory/functional regions, there is a single "hub" in anterior temporal cortex that stores abstract, amodal representations for all semantic categories (Figure 9.11B).

The distributed-plus-hub view fits with anatomical evidence that the anterior temporal lobe is connected to sensory and motor cortices, and is considered a locus of the caudal-to-rostral convergence of information along the temporal lobes. The anterior temporal lobe is also proximal to the amygdala and the orbitofrontal cortex, which could help link semantic knowledge to emotion and reward. Moreover, the anterior temporal lobe is immediately adjacent to medial temporal regions that mediate rapid learning of new episodic information, such as the hippocampus, which could provide the seeds for the acquisition of new conceptual knowledge.

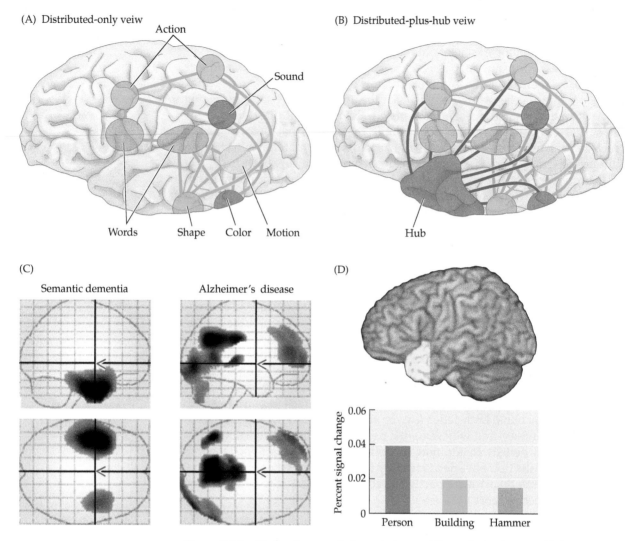

Figure 9.11 Abstract semantic knowledge and the anterior temporal lobes
(A) According to a *distributed-only* view, abstract semantic knowledge is mediated by the same distributed network that mediates concrete knowledge. (B) According to the *distributed-plus-hub* view, abstract semantic knowledge is supported by an amodal "hub" in the anterior temporal lobes. (C) The brain areas showing reduced metabolism in semantic dementia are primarily the anterior temporal lobes (left panel), whereas in Alzheimer's disease they are primarily the posterior midline and temporoparietal regions (right panel). (D) In this fMRI study, participants learned facts about specific people (e.g., Alex works as an insurance agent), specific buildings (e.g., the Newport Building is used for voter registration), and specific hammers (e.g., the Brooks hammer is used to shatter window glass). Activity in anterior temporal regions (both left and right, but only left is shown) was significantly greater for person facts than for building or hammer facts. (A–C after Patterson et al. 2007; D after Simmons et al. 2010.)

The strongest evidence for the idea that the anterior temporal lobe is a semantic hub is provided by semantic dementia cases. As noted earlier, this variant of frontotemporal dementia is associated with atrophy of the anterior temporal lobes and with global semantic knowledge loss. Neuroimaging studies have confirmed that, unlike forms of dementia involving more widespread damage such as Alzheimer's disease, semantic dementia is associated primarily with anterior temporal lobe dysfunction (Figure 9.11C). Semantic dementia impairs all kinds of knowledge, regardless of the modality of reception and expression. A semantic dementia patient who cannot name an object as a "telephone" when shown a photo of one will also fail to identify its sound or to draw a picture of it. The global nature of this semantic deficit is consistent with the idea of an amodal, domain-general representational hub in the anterior temporal lobe.

However, the idea that the anterior temporal lobe is a semantic hub has not received strong support from functional neuroimaging studies. In fact, left inferior frontal, posterior temporal, and temporoparietal activations are more frequent in these studies than are anterior temporal activations. It has been suggested that the scarcity of anterior temporal lobe activation in fMRI studies reflects a poor signal-to-noise ratio in this region that is due to the proximity to air-filled sinuses. However, this explanation cannot explain why the fMRI activations found in this area are often associated with social conceptual knowledge, such as processing famous faces, rather than with knowledge in general. Hub supporters argue that the social tasks are more sensitive because they require more specific identification (e.g., recognizing a particular famous person). Yet a recent fMRI study that compared learning facts about specific people, specific buildings, and specific hammers found greater anterior temporal activity for people compared to the other two categories (Figure 9.11D). In sum, although the idea that the anterior temporal lobe is an abstract knowledge hub fits well with anatomical and lesion evidence, functional neuroimaging evidence has often linked the anterior temporal lobes more to social knowledge than to knowledge in general.

The reactivation of cortical regions for recent episodic memories

According to the memory model described at the beginning of the chapter, retrieval of recent episodic memories requires access to hippocampal indices, which in turn lead to the reactivation of cortical memory traces. Let's consider the latter first. Relevant evidence for this process has been provided by single-cell recording studies in non-human animals and by functional neuroimaging studies in humans.

As an example of single-cell recording evidence, one study trained monkeys until they could remember associations between pairs of pictures (e.g., between pictures 12 and 12' in Figure 9.12A). At test, one of the pictures was presented during the cue period, and after a delay, monkeys had to choose the associated picture. Many neurons in anterior temporal cortex showed a firing pattern consistent with reactivation. For example, a neuron that fired selectively to picture 12 when this picture was presented during the cue period (Figure 9.12B) also fired when picture 12' was the cue, but in this case the firing occurred later, during the delay period (Figure 9.12C), consistent with the retrieval of picture 12' before the choice period. This type of neuron, which the authors called "pair-recall neurons," could be the neurons whose synapses stored the associations between the pictures.

At a coarser level, functional neuroimaging studies can detect cortical reactivation in humans. In a typical paradigm (Figure 9.13A), participants study cues (e.g., words) in two different contexts (e.g., words paired with associated pictures or with associated sounds). At test, the cues are presented without their contexts (e.g., words alone) while participants make old-versus-new recognition or context memory decisions. The presence of encoding-related reactivations is demonstrated by retrieval activity in brain regions associated with the study contexts (e.g., visual cortex versus auditory cortex), even though these contexts were not presented during retrieval. Since context-related activity cannot be attributed to the test cues, it can be reasonably inferred as resulting from reactivation of the encoding context. Reactivation has been demonstrated for a variety of sensory contexts besides visual and auditory modalities. For example, objects encoded with odors reactivate piriform cortex during retrieval, and objects encoded with emotional pictures reactivate the amygdala during retrieval.

(A)

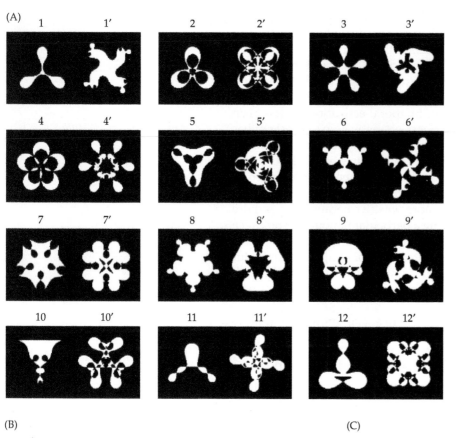

(B)

(C)

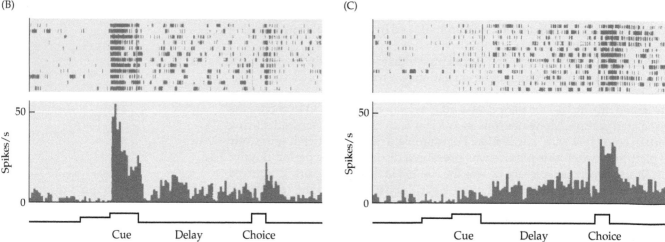

Figure 9.12 **Reactivation of visually paired associates in monkeys' inferior temporal cortex** (A) Monkeys were extensively trained until they learn to associate the two visual patterns in each pair. (B,C) At test, monkeys were presented with one member of a pair (e.g., 12) and after a delay they had to distinguish between the other member of the pair (e.g., 12′) and a distracter pattern (e.g., 11′). "Pair-recall" neurons responded more strongly to one picture (e.g., picture 12) during the cue period (B), as well as to its associated picture (e.g., picture 12′) during the delay period (C), suggesting that they store the memory for the newly learned association. (After Sakai and Miyashita 1991.)

Although these examples are all about the reactivation of sensory contexts, memory theories also predict reactivation of the encoding operations or strategies. In fact, the fundamental memory principle known as **transfer-appropriate processing** postulates that memory success is a function of the overlap between encoding and retrieval operations. A classic behavioral study supporting this idea found that when participants learned words by focusing either on semantics (e.g., Is *brain* a part of the body?) or on phonology (e.g., Does *brain* rhyme with *train*?), the semantic encoding task yielded better performance in a typical retrieval test emphasizing word meaning (e.g., Did you read the word *brain*?), whereas the phonology encoding task yielded better performance in a retrieval test emphasizing word sound (e.g., Did you read a word that rhymes with *train*?). In other words, whether a particular encoding task yields

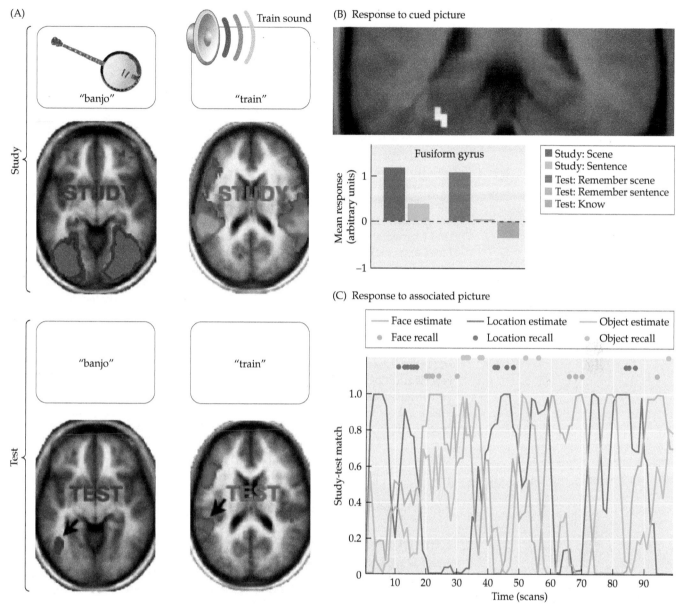

Figure 9.13 **Detecting reactivation during episodic memory retrieval in humans** (A) A typical paradigm for measuring reactivation activity. Participants study words paired with pictures or paired with sounds, and at test, the words are presented alone while participants make old-versus-new recognition or context memory decisions. Since the words are presented alone, differences in retrieval activity as a function of encoding context are interpreted as reactivation. (B) A fusiform gyrus region showed greater activity for scene than for sentence encoding tasks, and the same region was reactivated during retrieval, particularly for "remember" responses. (C) Multivoxel pattern analysis (MVPA) classifiers trained in distinguishing distributed activation patterns for faces, locations, and objects showed reactivation of these patterns before items in the corresponding categories were recalled. (A after Danker and Anderson 2010, with brain images from Wheeler et al. 2000; B after Johnson and Rugg 2007; C after Polyn et al. 2006.)

good memory performance depends on how well the cognitive operations recruited by the encoding task match the operations engaged by the test.

The concept of transfer-appropriate processing suggests that retrieval reactivations may reflect not only sensory aspects of the encoding context, but also the specific strategies used to encode the stimuli. Consistent with this idea, functional neuroimaging studies have identified retrieval reactivations that reflect the use of motor or visual imagery during encoding. As an example of motor imagery, one study found that when participants learned action phrases such as "roll the ball," retrieval activations were stronger in motor and somatosensory cortices if, rather than covertly rehearsing the phrase, they imagined themselves performing the action. As an example of visual imagery reactivations, one study had participants encode each word either by imagining the referent object in a visual scene or by generating a sentence including the word. In the test phase, only words were presented, and participants made "remember" (recollection), "know" (familiarity), or "new" responses. As illustrated in Figure 9.13B, the same fusiform region that showed greater activity for scene imagery than for sentence generation during encoding also showed greater activity for words encoded in the scene than for words encoded in the sentence task, even though the test stimuli were identical. This effect was greater for "remember" than for "know" responses, suggesting that the reactivation of encoding details contributes to the experience of recollection.

Whereas the foregoing reactivations were detected in the overall *amount* of activity within a certain brain region, the recapitulation of encoding contexts or operations can also be observed in the *distributed pattern* of retrieval activations. The reactivation of distributed activation patterns has been investigated using *multivoxel pattern analysis* (*MVPA*; see Chapter 2). For example, a study that trained an MVPA classifier to distinguish among activation patterns for faces (e.g., Jack Nicholson), locations (e.g., the Taj Mahal), and objects (e.g., a tree) identified the reactivation of these distributed patterns during retrieval just before participants recalled the names of faces, locations, or objects (Figure 9.13C). In other words, distributed activation patterns predicted the types of stimuli participants were about to recall. MVPA studies have also been applied to item recognition and source memory tasks.

In addition to involving the reactivation of cortical memory traces, the model in Figure 9.2 assumes that for nonconsolidated memories, retrieval entails the reactivation of hippocampal indices. Hippocampal reactivation has also been investigated using MVPA. In one study, for example, participants repeatedly viewed short video clips of three distinct everyday events (e.g., taking a drink from a disposable coffee cup and throwing the cup into a trash can). Then, while in the MRI scanner, they recalled the movie clips with their eyes closed. MVPA classifiers were trained on half of the imaging data during recall and were then applied to the other half. Using only activation patterns within the hippocampus, the classifiers were able to successfully identify the particular video clip being recalled by individual participants.

Contributions of the Prefrontal Cortex to Encoding and Retrieval

Evidence for the role of prefrontal regions during memory encoding and retrieval phases comes from both neuroimaging and patient studies. Functional neuroimaging has the advantage of providing independent measures of brain activity during encoding and retrieval. In contrast, evidence from brain-damaged patients cannot easily distinguish between these two memory phases; when damage of a certain brain region, such as the prefrontal cortex, impairs memory performance, it is unclear whether this impairment reflects an encoding deficit, a retrieval deficit, or both. On the other hand, patient studies provide information about whether a certain region is actually necessary for memory performance.

Functional neuroimaging of episodic encoding

A powerful way to isolate the neural correlates of episodic encoding is the *subsequent memory paradigm*. This method, described in Box 9B, involves comparing encoding-phase activity for items that are remembered versus those forgotten in a subsequent memory test. As Figure 9.14A illustrates, the left inferior frontal gyrus tends to show greater encoding activity for words that are subsequently remembered than for words forgotten. These differences in activity, known as

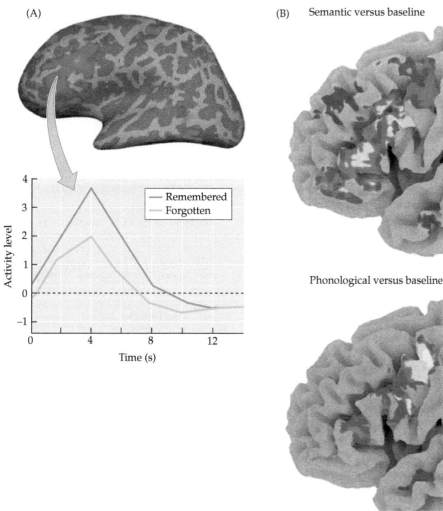

(A)

(B) Semantic versus baseline

Phonological versus baseline

Figure 9.14 Subsequent memory effects and semantic processing in the left inferior frontal gyrus (A) Greater encoding activity is seen in the left inferior frontal gyrus for words that were subsequently remembered than for words subsequently forgotten. This difference is known as a subsequent memory effect (SME). (B) Evidence that the anterior part of the left inferior frontal gyrus is associated with semantic processing. This region was activated when participants attended to meaningful associations among semantically related words (e.g., *tiger*, *circus*, *jungle*) but not when they attended to sound associations between phonologically related words (e.g., *skill*, *fill*, *hill*). (A after Paller and Wagner 2002; B from McDermott et al. 2003.)

subsequent memory effects (SMEs), are also typically found in medial temporal lobe and dorsal parietal lobe regions. In general, SMEs in the inferior frontal gyrus tended to occur in the left hemisphere for verbal stimuli and bilaterally for visual stimuli.

The results of language studies suggest that SMEs in the anterior part of the left inferior frontal gyrus are likely to reflect enhanced semantic processing, whereas SMEs in the posterior part are more likely to reflect phonological processing. The posterior part includes the region known as *Broca's area*, and damage to this region is associated with a deficiency called production aphasia (see Chapter 12). The dissociation between semantic and phonological processing in anterior compared to posterior parts of the left inferior frontal gyrus has been confirmed by several fMRI studies (Figure 9.14B).

■ BOX 9B FUNCTIONAL NEUROIMAGING METHODS TO STUDY EPISODIC MEMORY

As described in Chapter 2, functional neuroimaging provides a powerful method to investigate the neural correlates of cognitive functions. With respect to episodic memory, these methods are especially useful in that they can distinguish between encoding and retrieval. In studies of brain-damaged patients who are impaired in episodic memory, it is difficult or impossible to know whether the impairment reflects encoding deficits, retrieval deficits, or both. Functional neuroimaging studies of normal subjects, however, have identified differences in the involvement of several brain regions in encoding versus retrieval.

In working to isolate activity specifically associated with successful encoding or retrieval operations, the event-related potential (ERP) designs described in Chapter 2 are well suited to this purpose because they allow a direct comparison between successful and unsuccessful trials during encoding and/or retrieval. When applied to encoding, this method is known as the *subsequent memory paradigm* and involves four steps (Figure A).

In Step 1, participants study a series of items (*a,b,c…*) while their brain activity is recorded. Step 2 requires that they perform encoding trials, remembering some of the studied items and forgetting

others. On the basis of retrieval performance, in Step 3 the encoding trials are coded as subsequently remembered or subsequently forgotten; activity during these two types of encoding trials is compared in Step 4. Greater activity for subsequently remembered than for forgotten trials, assumed to reflect successful encoding processes, is known as *subsequent memory effects (SMEs)*.

The subsequent memory paradigm has been used in ERP studies since the early 1980s by cognitive neuroscientist Kenneth Paller and other researchers. In ERP studies, SMEs tend to be seen over frontoparietal scalp regions. Although

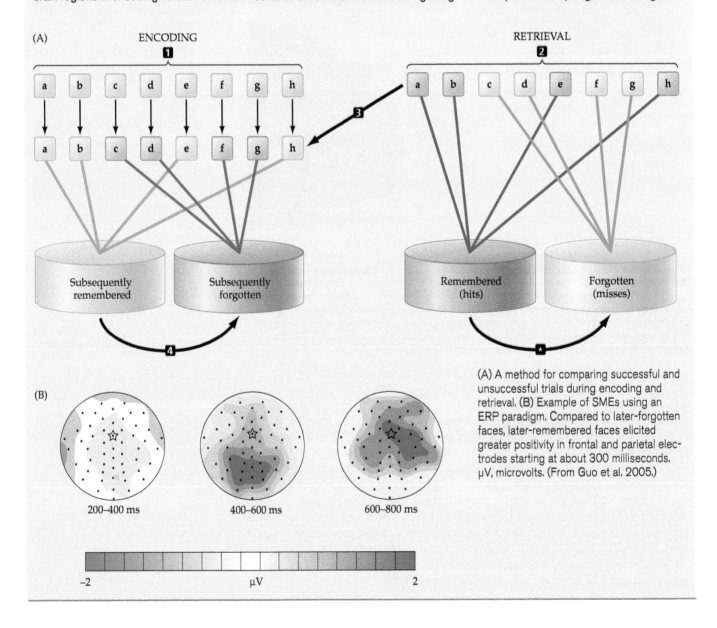

(A) A method for comparing successful and unsuccessful trials during encoding and retrieval. (B) Example of SMEs using an ERP paradigm. Compared to later-forgotten faces, later-remembered faces elicited greater positivity in frontal and parietal electrodes starting at about 300 milliseconds. μV, microvolts. (From Guo et al. 2005.)

200–400 ms   400–600 ms   600–800 ms

−2   μV   2

■ **BOX 9B** *(continued)*

the neural generators of scalp ERPs are uncertain, this method has the advantage of providing fine temporal resolution. As an example, Figure B, which shows that ERPs for later-remembered and forgotten faces start to diverge around 300 milliseconds after stimulus onset—a distinction that persists until about 800 milliseconds. This time window provides a useful limit on speculation about the cognitive processes supporting successful face encoding.

As illustrated by the right-hand panel in Figure A, successful versus unsuccessful trials (i.e., hits versus misses) can also be compared during retrieval. An alternative approach to isolating activ-ity associated with retrieval success is to compare hits to correct rejections of new items. An important advantage of the hit-versus-miss contrast is that the same sets of items are compared as in the subsequent memory paradigm (e.g., *a,b,e,h* versus *c,d,f,g* in Figure A). An advantage of the hit-versus-correct-rejection comparison is that it is based on correct responses, and hence not contaminated with error production and detection processes. A problem of using correct rejections as the baseline, however, is that new items elicit novelty detection processes that may contaminate retrieval-related activations.

References

BUCKNER, R. L. AND M. E. WHEELER (2001) The cognitive neuroscience of remembering. *Nat. Rev. Neurosci.* 2: 624–634.

GUO, C., J. L. VOSS AND K. A. PALLER (2005) Electrophysiological correlates of forming memories for faces, names, and face–name associations. *Brain Res. Cogn. Brain Res.* 22: 153–164.

PALLER, K. A. AND A. D. WAGNER (2002) Observing the transformation of experience into memory. *Trends Cogn. Sci.* 6: 93–102.

SMEs are usually found in the *inferior* frontal gyrus (ventrolateral prefrontal cortex; Figure 9.15A), but rarely in the *middle* frontal gyrus (dorsolateral prefrontal cortex). This pattern may reflect the simple nature of the stimuli commonly used in SME studies (e.g., unrelated words), which do not typically require the organizing functions attributed to dorsolateral prefrontal regions (see Chapter 13). To investigate this idea, participants can be scanned while they are reordering or rehearsing words in working memory. The participants are later tested outside the scanner for memory of the learned words. The left dorsolateral prefrontal region in this study showed a significant SME (Figure 9.15B), but only for the reorder condition (Figure 9.15C). This finding suggests that the dorsolateral prefrontal region contributes to successful episodic encoding through its role in organizing or manipulating information within working memory.

Functional neuroimaging of episodic retrieval

Consider trying to remember what you had for breakfast the day before yesterday. Your train of thought might go something like this:

> Hmm … the day before yesterday I had a class in the morning and I didn't have much time for breakfast. I had something in the kitchen. I made coffee, which I always have in the morning, and I probably made some eggs … No, I didn't have eggs because I was in a hurry … Now, I remember! I grabbed a slice of bread and ate it while walking out of the apartment.

This example illustrates typical components of episodic memory retrieval. A **retrieval cue** (the question about breakfast) triggers a **memory search** that narrows the focus to a particular time and place (the day before yesterday, in the kitchen), which leads to the **recovery** of increasingly specific stored memory traces (grabbing a slice of bread, eating it while walking). Descriptively at least, the information recovered is evaluated by a **monitoring** process that can reject inappropriate memories (e.g., eggs), leading to further refinement. While these different processes are taking place, a hypothetical mental state known as **retrieval mode** is assumed to keep continuous attentional focus on the past

(A)

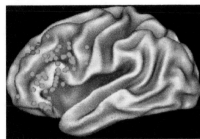

(B)

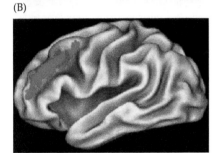

(C)

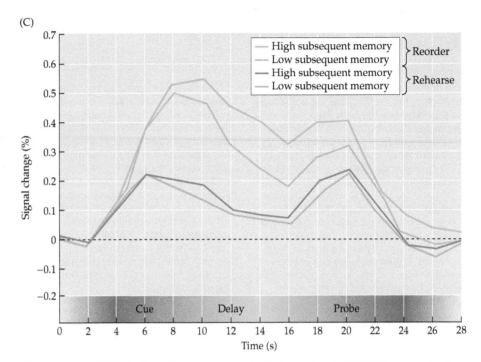

Figure 9.15 **SMEs in the inferior versus middle frontal gyri** (A) SMEs are typically found in the left inferior frontal gyrus (green dots) but rarely in the middle frontal gyrus (red dots). (B) However, when the encoding task requires organizing information within working memory, the middle frontal gyrus (shown in red) shows a robust SME. (C) This region showed a significant SME during the delay period of a working memory task when participants reordered words during this period but not when they just rehearsed them. (After Blumenfeld and Ranganath 2006.)

events in question. All these processes tend to operate very fast, and we are usually unaware of their operations. In the laboratory, however, the cognitive and neural mechanisms of these processes can be investigated by measuring the effects of experimental variables on various episodic memory tests.

Episodic memory tests include item recognition, recall, and source memory tests. In a typical **item recognition test**, participants are presented with items (e.g., words) previously encountered in the laboratory (old) intermixed with items never encountered in the context of the laboratory (new), and they are asked to classify each item as either "old" or "new". Correct responses include responding "old" to an old item (**hit**) and responding "new" to a new item (**correct rejection**); incorrect responses include responding "old" to a new item (**false alarm**) and responding "new" to an old item (**miss**; Table 9.1).

In a **recall test**, the target information is not provided by the experimenter and must be generated by the participant in response to contextual information, which is broad in a *free-recall test* ("Recall the words you read at the beginning of the experiment") or item-specific in a *cued-recall test* ("Recall the word that was paired with the word *house*").

In a **source** (or **context**) **memory test**, participants are provided with items and must retrieve the spatial, sensory, or semantic context associated with the item during encoding (e.g., "Was the word *house* presented on the left or the right side of the screen?").

One variable often measured or manipulated by functional neuroimaging researchers is the amount of information successfully retrieved. Since this amount is assumed

TABLE 9.1 Four Recognition Memory Outcomes

	RESPONSE	
ITEM CLASSIFICATION	"OLD"	"NEW"
Old	Hit	Miss
New	False alarm	Correct rejection

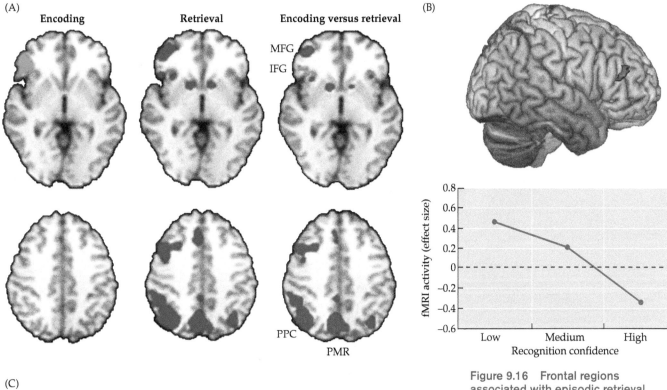

Figure 9.16 Frontal regions associated with episodic retrieval processes (A) Meta-analysis showing brain regions frequently activated during successful encoding (SMEs) and retrieval (hits minus correct rejections). Whereas the left inferior frontal gyrus (IFG) is more frequently activated during encoding, the left middle frontal gyrus (MFG) and the posterior parietal cortex (PPC) are more frequently activated during retrieval. PMR, posterior midline region. (B) This study showed right dorsolateral prefrontal activity to be greater for low-confidence than for high-confidence recognition responses, possibly reflecting monitoring. (C) The right frontopolar cortex showed sustained activity during an episodic retrieval task, possibly reflecting retrieval mode. Dashed lines indicate average activity and show differences during the block (gray bars) but not during the interblock intervals. (A from Spaniol et al. 2009; B after Fleck et al. 2006; C after Velanova et al. 2003.)

to be greater for hits than for correct rejections, regions showing greater activity for hits than for correct rejections are presumed to be involved in recovering memories and/or holding recovered information within working memory. These regions typically include left inferior and left middle frontal gyri, as well as the posterior parietal and posterior midline regions considered in the next section (Figure 9.16A). These regions are also associated with successful retrieval during source memory tasks. Activations in the left middle frontal gyrus tend to be more frequent during retrieval than during encoding, possibly reflecting greater demands of working memory manipulation during memory search. Conversely, activations in the anterior left inferior frontal gyrus tend to be more pronounced during encoding than during retrieval, possibly reflecting greater semantic processing contributions during encoding.

Another variable often measured in functional neuroimaging studies of episodic retrieval is confidence. In general, "old" responses made with high confidence are assumed to involve greater information recovery than those made with low confidence. Conversely, monitoring processes are assumed to be more demanding for low-confidence than for high-confidence responses. Using this logic, fMRI studies have linked monitoring processes to activity in right dorsolateral prefrontal cortex, which tends to show greater activity for low-confidence than for high-confidence recognition decisions (Figure 9.16B). It is worth mentioning, however, that the same region also shows greater activity for low-confidence than for high-confidence perceptual decisions, suggesting that this region mediates monitoring processes that are shared by episodic retrieval and other cognitive functions.

Finally, retrieval processes also differ in their temporal characteristics. In a typical episodic retrieval test that includes several items from the same past event (e.g., a study list), memory recovery and monitoring processes are assumed to vary from trial to trial, and to dissipate during the intertrial interval. Retrieval mode, however, is assumed be sustained throughout the task, including the interval between the trials. One way of distinguishing sustained from transient activations is to use the hybrid block/event-related designs described in Chapter 2. For example, a hybrid fMRI study found that the right anterior prefrontal cortex showed sustained activity during episodic retrieval (Figure 9.16C), thereby linking this region to retrieval mode, rather than to more transient event-related processes.

Effects of frontal lobe lesions

Whereas medial temporal lobe lesions are associated with a devastating amnesia syndrome, frontal lobe lesions typically cause only mild declarative memory deficits, and only in certain tasks. In general, the effects of frontal damage on declarative memory appear to be a function of the strategic demands of the task. Recall and source memory tests, which depend more on strategic control processes, tend to be more affected by frontal lesions than recognition memory tests are. For example, in one study patients with frontal lobe damage, age-matched controls, and younger controls were presented a series of facts that previous testing indicated they had not known prior to the study. After a delay, participants performed recognition and source memory tests for the facts. In the source memory test, they had to indicate whether they had learned the fact during the experiment or had known it all along (the latter being an "incorrect" answer). Although the three groups performed at about the same level in recognition, frontally damaged patients made many more errors in identifying the source of the memories than did the two control groups (Figure 9.17A).

Source memory deficits in frontal lobe patients may reflect impairments in encoding processes, such as semantic processing and working memory manipulation, and/or impairments in retrieval processes, such as organizing the memory search and monitoring retrieved information. Functional neuro-imaging evidence can be used to predict which processes will be more affected depending on the location of the lesion. For example, given that fMRI studies have linked monitoring processes to the right dorsolateral prefrontal cortex (see Figure 9.16B), damage to this region should lead to a monitoring failure. Consistent with this idea, cognitive neuroscientist Daniel Schacter and colleagues reported a patient (B.G.) with a large right dorsolateral prefrontal lesion who showed a severe deficit in rejecting new items. As illustrated in Figure 9.17B, B.G. produced an abnormally high proportion of "old" responses to nonstudied items (false alarms), many of which he classified as remembered rather than known. Control participants very rarely classify false alarms as remembered. This sort of impairment suggests a monitoring deficit.

Although dorsolateral prefrontal lesions may lead to increased false alarms in laboratory memory tasks, they are not typically associated with false memories for complex autobiographical events, or **confabulations**. Patients suffering from confabulation report personal events that never happened. Confabulations may be *spontaneous*, generated by the patient without any apparent prompting; or *provoked*, generated in response to direct questions. Sometimes confabulations

(A)

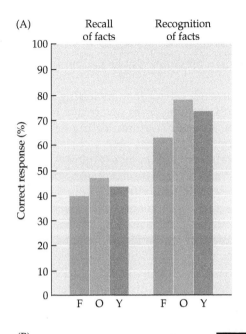

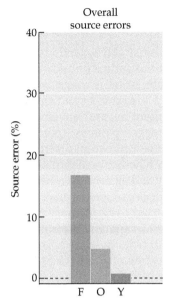

Figure 9.17 Recall, recognition, and source memory in patients with frontal lobe damage (A) Patients with frontal lobe damage (F) were compared with age-matched controls (O) and with younger control subjects (Y). Performance on recognition memory was similar across all three groups, but source memory was significantly impaired in patients with frontal lobe damage. (B) Patient B.G., who has a large lesion of the right dorsolateral prefrontal cortex, is impaired in memory monitoring. He showed a very high false-alarm rate for nonstudied words, many of which he classified as remembered rather than known. (C) Overlapping lesions in a group of confabulating patients. The colors represent the number of patients with lesions that overlap, ranging from one patient (purple) to all patients (red). (A after Janowsky et al. 1989; B after Schacter et al. 1996; C from Gilboa et al. 2006.)

(B)

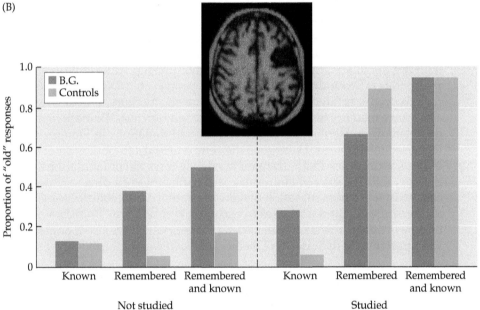

(C)

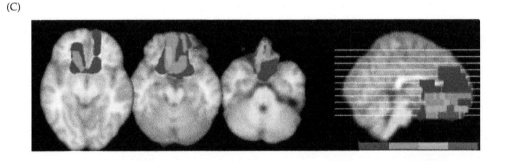

involve misplacing an event in time and/or place, such as the case of a patient who remembered an imaginary trip abroad to visit a relative when the meeting with the relative actually occurred while the patient was in the hospital. Other times confabulations can be fantastic, such as the case of a patient who claimed that his father had been abducted by aliens over the weekend. This bizarre confabulation was apparently a blend of two different memories: (1) the father missed his usual weekend visit, and (2) in a previous visit he had brought toy aliens for the patient's children.

Confabulation is a sign found in numerous disorders, including schizophrenia, Korsakoff's syndrome (dementia arising from severe alcoholism), other dementias, and aneurysms of the anterior communicating artery. In brain-damaged patients, spontaneous confabulation has been associated with lesions in ventromedial prefrontal and orbitofrontal regions (Figure 9.17C). It is unclear whether confabulations reflect difficulty in discriminating between internally and externally generated representations, confusion about temporal order, deficits in strategic retrieval processes, or a combination of these problems.

In sum, episodic memory encoding and retrieval have been associated with activations in specific prefrontal regions and with patients that have frontal damage deficits in some episodic retrieval tests. During episodic encoding, subsequent memory effects (SMEs) are typically found in the left inferior frontal gyrus for verbal stimuli and bilaterally for pictorial stimuli. The anterior part of the left inferior frontal gyrus has been associated with semantic processing; the posterior part, with phonological processing. Dorsolateral prefrontal regions may also show SMEs when stimuli are more complex and require organization of the information in working memory to facilitate subsequent memory retrieval. Episodic retrieval involves a variety of processes, including memory search, monitoring, and retrieval. Successful memory recovery has been associated with left dorsolateral prefrontal regions; monitoring, with right dorsolateral prefrontal cortex; and retrieval, with frontopolar cortex. Damage to prefrontal regions produces larger impairments on strategic memory tests, such as recall and source memory tests, than on simple recognition tests. Damage to the right dorsolateral prefrontal cortex has been linked to deficits in monitoring and increased false alarms. Damage to the ventromedial and orbitofrontal regions may sometimes lead to a dramatic tendency toward confabulations. Taken together with functional neuroimaging results, these findings are generally consistent with the assumption that the prefrontal cortex contributes semantic and executive control processes to encoding and retrieval. Prefrontal regions operate in tight connection with parietal regions, which are also thought to play an important role in declarative memory, as reviewed in the following section.

Contributions of the Posterior Parietal Cortex to Encoding and Retrieval

Although the parietal cortex is not a region traditionally associated with memory, recent evidence suggests it plays an important role in declarative memory, both during retrieval and during encoding.

The role of posterior parietal cortex during retrieval

The role of posterior parietal cortex during episodic memory retrieval was first detected by ERP studies of recognition, which consistently showed a parietal positivity that is greater for hits than for correct rejections at about 400 to 800 milliseconds after the stimulus (Box 9C). Event-related fMRI studies later confirmed the parietal origin of these effects and showed that activation patterns differ for dorsal and ventral parietal cortex (the anatomy is illustrated in Figure 9.18). As Figure 9.19A shows, activations associated with familiarity and low-confidence recognition are more frequent in dorsal parietal cortex, whereas activations associated with recollection and high-confidence recognition trials are more frequent in ventral parietal cortex.

Figure 9.18 Gross anatomy of posterior parietal cortex Posterior parietal cortex (PPC) consists of the parietal regions posterior to the somatosensory cortex and can be divided into dorsal and ventral components. Dorsal PPC includes the intraparietal sulcus (IPS) and the superior parietal lobule, which extends medially into the precuneus region. Ventral parietal cortex consists of the angular gyrus and the supramarginal gyrus, which includes the area known as the temporoparietal junction (TPJ).

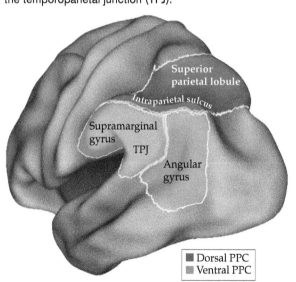

Superior parietal lobule
Intraparietal sulcus
Supramarginal gyrus
TPJ
Angular gyrus

■ Dorsal PPC
■ Ventral PPC

■ BOX 9C ERP STUDIES OF EPISODIC RETRIEVAL

Studies of episodic memory retrieval using event-related potentials have identified three consistent differences between recalling old and new items. First, about 300 to 500 milliseconds after a stimulus is presented, new items tend to elicit greater negative voltage over midfrontal regions than do old items. This *frontal negativity* (*FN*) *effect* has been called the FN400 effect to distinguish it from the central parietal N400 effect typically associated with semantic processing. The FN400 effect responds similarly to studied items and to new items that appear familiar, and to both deeply and shallowly encoded items (Figure A). Because of these and other findings, the FN400 effect has been attributed to familiarity.

Second, 400 to 800 milliseconds after the stimulus, old items tend to elicit more positive voltage over parietal electrodes than new items do. This effect is typically left-lateralized for verbal materials, and it is known as the **left parietal effect**. This phenomenon tends to be more pronounced when higher (more complex) levels of recollection are required. For example, the effect tends to be greater for deeply encoded items than for shallowly encoded items (Figure B); for words judged as "remembered" rather than "known"; and for words accompanied by successful rather than unsuccessful source retrieval. The source of the left parietal effect is most likely the left posterior parietal region, since it is typically activated during PET and fMRI studies of episodic retrieval and is strongly associated with retrieval success.

Finally, at 600 to 1200 milliseconds poststimulus, old items sometimes elicit a more positive response over right frontal regions than do new items; this is known as the **right frontal effect**. The right fron-

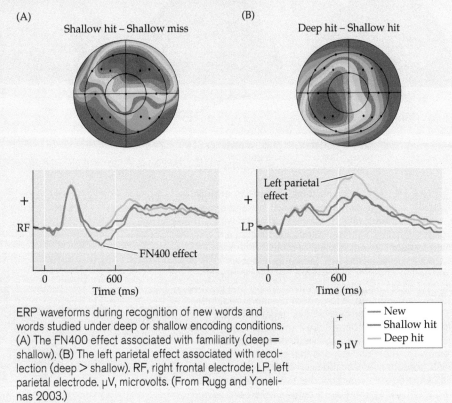

ERP waveforms during recognition of new words and words studied under deep or shallow encoding conditions. (A) The FN400 effect associated with familiarity (deep = shallow). (B) The left parietal effect associated with recollection (deep > shallow). RF, right frontal electrode; LP, left parietal electrode. μV, microvolts. (From Rugg and Yonelinas 2003.)

tal effect is usually apparent during tasks that entail demanding source memory decisions and is assumed to reflect postretrieval operations. This idea fits the extended time course of the right frontal effect, and it is consistent with functional neuroimaging and lesion evidence linking the right prefrontal cortex to monitoring.

References

CURRAN, T., K. L. TEPE AND C. PIATT (2006) ERP explorations of dual processes in recognition memory. In *Binding in Human Memory: A Neurocognitive Approach*, H. D. Zimmer, A. Mecklinger and U. Lindenberger (eds.). Oxford: Oxford University Press, pp. 467–492.

RUGG, M. D. (2004) Retrieval processing in human memory: Electrophysiological and fMRI evidence. In *The Cognitive Neurosciences*, 3rd Ed., M. S. Gazzaniga (ed.). Cambridge, MA: MIT Press, pp. 727–737.

RUGG, M. D. AND A. P. YONELINAS (2003) Human recognition memory: A cognitive neuroscience perspective. *Trends Cogn. Sci.* 7: 313–319.

To explain this dissociation, one theory, known as the *attention to memory* (*AtoM*) *model* and proposed by cognitive neuroscientists Roberto Cabeza, Elisa Ciaramelli, and Morris Moscovitch, extends the distinction between ventral and dorsal attention systems (see Chapter 7) to memory. This theory postulates that the dorsal parietal cortex mediates top-down attention processes, which are required by demanding memory search and monitoring operations, whereas ventral parietal cortex mediates bottom-up attention processes, which are captured by salient memories or retrieval cues. The AtoM theory explains dorsal parietal activations for familiarity and low-confidence recognition trials, which involve greater memory search and monitoring; and ventral parietal activations for recollection and high-confidence recognition trials, which involve the

(A) Retrieval　　　　　　　　　　　　　　　　(B) Encoding

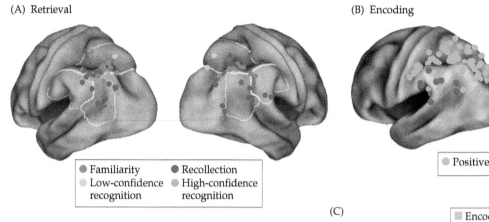

● Familiarity　　　● Recollection
○ Low-confidence　● High-confidence
　recognition　　　　　recognition

● Positive SME　　● Negative SME

Figure 9.19 Posterior parietal activations during episodic retrieval and encoding (A) Meta-analysis showing that retrieval activations associated with recollection and high-confidence recognition are more frequent in ventral parietal cortex, whereas activations associated with familiarity and low-confidence recognition are more frequent in dorsal parietal cortex. (B) Meta-analysis showing that positive SMEs (remembered > forgotten) are more frequent in dorsal parietal cortex, whereas negative SMEs (forgotten > remembered) are more frequent in ventral parietal cortex. (C) Across five different studies, the same ventral parietal regions that showed a negative SME (forgotten > remembered) during encoding also showed success-related activity (remembered > forgotten) during retrieval—a pattern called *encoding-retrieval flip*. (A after Cabeza et al. 2008; B after Uncapher and Wagner 2009; C after Daselaar et al. 2009.)

(C)

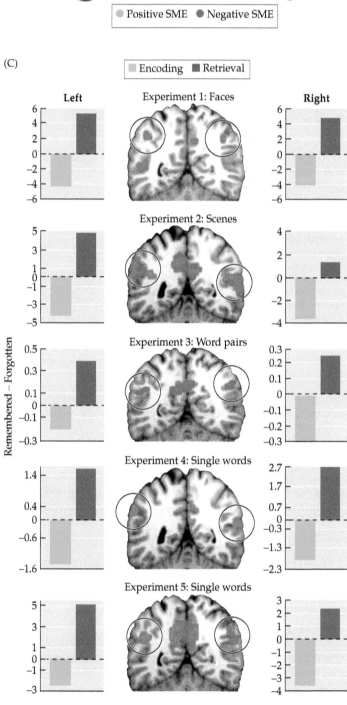

□ Encoding　■ Retrieval

recovery of salient episodic details. An alternative theory of ventral parietal cortex function, known as the *episodic buffer hypothesis*, proposes that this region mediates the maintenance of recovered multisensory episodic memories within working memory.

Thorough neuropsychological assessment of patients with ventral parietal lesions revealed subtle memory deficits. One study found that when these patients were asked to describe autobiographical memories, they produced fewer episodic details than did controls. However, when specific questions about these details were posed, the patients were able to generate the missing details. This finding suggests that the episodic details were available but not spontaneously attended. Likewise, another study found that in the "remember"/"know" paradigm, ventral parietal patients produced fewer "remember" responses; but when tested in a source memory task in which episodic details were specifically tested, they performed as well as controls did. Again, episodic details apparently were available but were not spontaneously attended. The finding that ventral parietal lesions impair not memory retrieval per se, but only the ability to spontaneously attend to the retrieval output, fits well with the AtoM model. However, an important challenge for any theory of parietal contributions to declarative memory is to explain not only retrieval findings but also encoding findings.

The role of posterior parietal cortex during encoding

As during retrieval, dorsal and ventral parietal regions show very different activation patterns during encoding. In fact, the dorsal-ventral dissociation is even more dramatic during encoding (**Figure 9.19B**); whereas dorsal parietal regions show greater activity for subsequently remembered than for forgotten trials (positive SMEs), ventral parietal regions show the reverse effect: greater activity for subsequently forgotten than remembered items (negative SMEs). Thus, the same ventral parietal regions that are associated with retrieval success (recollection, high-confidence recognition) are associated with encoding failure (subsequent forgetting). A study that compared activity for remembered versus forgotten trials during encoding and during retrieval in five experiments using different stimuli confirmed that the same ventral parietal regions that showed negative SMEs during encoding (subsequently forgotten greater than subsequently remembered) also showed success effects during retrieval (remembered more than forgotten; **Figure 9.19C**).

A possible explanation of this "encoding-retrieval flip" is provided by the attention to memory model's assumption that the ventral parietal cortex mediates bottom-up attention. During retrieval, bottom-up attention is associated with memory success because it reflects the capture of attention by recovered memories. During encoding, by contrast, information to be learned is the focus of top-down attention, and bottom-up attention is more likely to reflect attention shifts to unrelated environmental stimuli or spontaneous thoughts, away from the items that are meant to be encoded. For this reason, bottom-up attention during encoding is more likely to reflect distraction and to be associated with encoding failure. These ideas, however, remain highly speculative.

In sum, posterior parietal regions play a role in episodic memory retrieval and encoding. During retrieval, dorsal parietal cortex is associated with familiarity and low-confidence recognition, whereas ventral parietal cortex is associated with recollection and high-confidence recognition. One possible explanation of this pattern is that, similar to what happens during perception, dorsal parietal cortex is involved in top-down attention and ventral parietal cortex is involved in bottom-up attention. Consistent with a role in bottom-up attention, damage to ventral parietal cortex impairs not the ability to retrieve episodic details, but only the ability to spontaneously report these details. During encoding, dorsal parietal regions are associated with encoding success (positive SME), whereas ventral parietal regions are associated with encoding failure (negative SME). Thus, ventral parietal regions are associated with retrieval success and with encoding failure. The reasons for this encoding-retrieval flip are still unknown.

Memory Consolidation

The term *consolidation* (from the Latin for "to make firm") refers to the progressive stabilization of long-term memory that follows the initial encoding of memory traces. The discussion that follows distinguishes between synaptic and system consolidation, describes theories of system consolidation, considers the roles of the hippocampus and the cortex as complementary learning systems, and reviews evidence of consolidation during sleep.

Synaptic versus system consolidation

Consolidation occurs at both cellular and system levels, known respectively as *synaptic consolidation* and *system consolidation*. **Synaptic consolidation** is accomplished within a few minutes to hours after encoding. It involves changes in gene expression, protein synthesis, and other mechanisms of synaptic plasticity that allow the persistence of memory traces at the cellular level (see Chapter 8). In vertebrate animal models, synaptic consolidation occurs in regions of the brain pertinent to long-term memory storage. One way of disrupting synaptic consolidation is to administer *protein synthesis inhibitors*. These drugs block long-term synaptic changes but do not impair the perceptual and motor processes required for task performance. In Figure 9.20A, for example, protein-synthesis inhibitors disrupted nondeclarative memory when administered during the first hour after training but not thereafter, indicating that synaptic consolidation was completed within this time. Similar synaptic consolidation processes presumably apply to all memory systems.

In contrast, the phrase **system consolidation** has been applied to changes in neural connectivity that can take days, months, or even years, and it involves a change in the brain regions supporting certain types of memory. System consolidation is said to occur when a particular brain region that was necessary for post-encoding memory performance is no longer required, or when it can be demonstrated that another brain region is now needed to preserve the memory. Although system consolidation involves changes at cellular and molecular levels, the term emphasizes a description at the system level—namely, a change in relative contributions of different brain regions. System consolidation applies to both declarative and nondeclarative memory and can be observed even in invertebrates, but typically the term is used to describe changes in the role of the medial temporal lobe regions in declarative memory.

Figure 9.20 Synaptic and system consolidation show different time courses (A) Synaptic consolidation was demonstrated in this example by administering a protein synthesis inhibitor to goldfish at different times following learning. Sensitivity to the drug lasted about an hour. (B) System consolidation was demonstrated here by damaging the hippocampus of rats at different times following contextual fear conditioning. Sensitivity to the lesion lasts about a month. (After Dudai 2004; data in A from Agranoff et al. 1966; data in B from Kim and Fanselow 1992.)

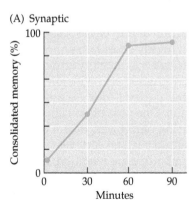
(A) Synaptic

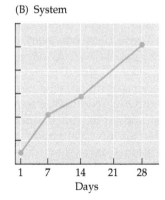
(B) System

System consolidation was first described in 1982 by the French psychologist Théodule-Armand Ribot, who noted that memory loss following brain damage affects recent memories to a greater extent than remote memories; this temporal gradient became known as *Ribot's law*. Indeed, the medial temporal lobe amnesia displayed by H.M. and similar patients shows such a temporal gradient. Studies on human patients are limited, however, because the locations of the lesions cannot be controlled and the assessment of memory must rely on retrospective measures, such as memory for news events and the like. By contrast, in animal studies it is possible to selectively damage a region that is assumed to be critical for system consolidation at different times after encoding. For example, hippocampal lesions in rats impaired declarative memory during the first month after encoding but not thereafter (Figure 9.20B). Although in this example system consolidation occurred within a month, temporal gradients in amnesia patients suggest that some forms of system consolidation in humans may take years.

Theories of system consolidation in declarative memory

There are two main theories of system consolidation: standard consolidation theory and multiple-trace theory. The **standard consolidation theory** was introduced earlier, in the description of the basic neurological memory model in Figure 9.2. As previously noted, the standard assumption is that in the case of recent events, the various cortical memories for one event (e.g., the color of the balloons, the sound of the music, and action of dancing at a birthday party) are disconnected from each other, and hence they can be reactivated together only via the indices stored in the hippocampus (see retrieval of recent memory in Figure 9.2C). In the case of remote memories, by contrast, repeated reactivation of the cortical traces in the time since the original forming of the memory presumably leads to the establishment of direct connections between the distributed cortical traces. As a result, cortical traces for remote memories can be reactivated as a unit, independently of the medial temporal lobes (see retrieval of remote memory in Figure 9.2C).

This point is further illustrated in Figure 9.21: before consolidation, the connections between the hippocampus and cortical units are essential for reactivation; after consolidation, direct connections are established among the cortical units, and the cortical-hippocampal connections become less critical for retrieval. This hypothetical consolidation process is sometimes described as a "transfer" of memories from the hippocampus to the cortex, but, as illustrated in Figure 9.21, memories are not really transferred; what is transferred, or expanded, is the ability to enact the reactivation process.

In 1997, Lynn Nadel and Morris Moscovitch pointed out problems with this standard consolidation theory. One problem they noted is that in some patients

Figure 9.21 The standard model of declarative system consolidation As time passes and memories are repeatedly reactivated, direct associations are formed among cortical units, and the connections with the hippocampus become less critical for retrieving the memory. (After Frankland and Bontempi 2005.)

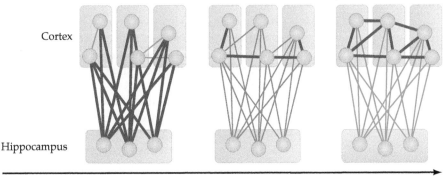

Cortex

— Necessary connection
— Unnecessary connection

Hippocampus

Time

with medial temporal lobe amnesia, retrograde amnesia for autobiographical (episodic) memory information can be quite extensive, occasionally spanning almost the entire life of the individual. If interpreted according to standard consolidation theory, this observation would suggest that the consolidation process may take more than 40 years—as long as the average human life span throughout much of history.

To explain this and other phenomena, Nadel and Moscovitch proposed an alternative model, called the **multiple-trace theory**, in which episodic memories, consolidated or otherwise, always depend on the hippocampus. In this account, the temporal gradient found in some amnesia patients is due not to transfer to the cortex, but to the *number* of memory traces for an event stored in the hippocampus. A central idea of the multiple-trace theory is that each time a memory is reactivated, a new memory trace for the memory is stored in the hippocampus. As a result, remote events are encoded by multiple hippocampal traces and become more resistant to partial hippocampal damage. Thus, partial damage of the hippocampus would yield a temporally graded amnesia, similar to the one predicted by standard consolidation theory. However, the multiple-trace theory further predicts that when hippocampal damage is complete, retrieval of both recent and remote memories should be equally affected, and hence, the retrograde amnesia should be complete (flat) rather than temporally graded. As for semantic memories, the theory postulates that they are gradually extracted from repeated episodes and are stored in the cortex independently of the hippocampus. At present, there is evidence for both the standard and multiple-trace theories, and their respective strengths and weaknesses are the topic of much debate.

Consolidation, reactivation, and sleep

A number of studies in recent years have made the case that consolidation is promoted by memory reactivation during memory retrieval (discussed earlier) and, more surprisingly, during sleep. The idea that memories are also reactivated, or *replayed*, during sleep was suggested by behavioral evidence indicating that sleeping soon after learning attenuates forgetting and enhances resistance to inference. Electroencephalographic (EEG) studies suggested that rapid-eye-movement (REM) sleep is more important for nondeclarative memory consolidation, whereas slow-wave sleep is more important for declarative memory consolidation.

For example, one study implanted electrodes in the hippocampus and visual cortex of rats, and measured neuronal firing in these brain regions while the rats ran in a figure-eight maze, as well as during periods of slow-wave sleep before and after maze running. Localized firing fields were found not only in hippocampal place cells but also in visual cortex. The cells that fired in specific locations could be ordered in a sequence (e.g., sequence 01234567 in Figure 9.22A). The most striking finding was that in both the hippocampus and the visual cortex, the firing sequences found during maze running were replayed during subsequent slow-wave sleep. Moreover, replay events in the hippocampus and visual cortex were coordinated, suggesting simultaneous reactivation in the two regions. This simultaneous hippocampal-cortical reactivation was proposed to gradually strengthen cortical-cortical synapses, leading to memory consolidation.

Although this evidence is intriguing, to establish a causal link between sleep replay and memory enhancement, it is important to directly manipulate sleep replay. To investigate this idea, researchers presented stimuli during sleep that are associated with the learning experience and can promote replay. In one such study, participants learned object-location associations while a specific odor (the scent of roses) was present in the room. Presenting the same smells

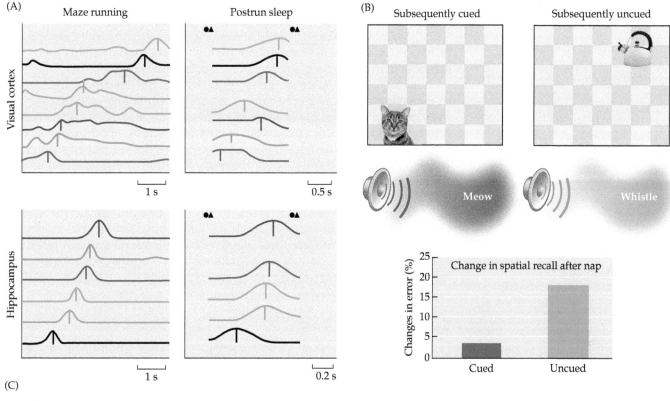

Figure 9.22 Consolidation-related changes during sleep and rest (A) Average firing rate of hippocampal and visual cortex cells while rats were running through a figure eight–shaped maze, and later while they were sleeping after the run. Each line corresponds to one cell. In both regions, firing sequences identified during maze running were replayed during slow-wave sleep, and firing in the two regions was coordinated during sleep consistent with memory reactivation. (B) In this behavioral and ERP study, participants learned object-spatial associations while listening to sounds associated with each object. During a nap after learning, the sounds for half of the objects were presented during slow-wave sleep. Spatial memory after the nap improved for cued objects but not for uncued objects. (C) Functional connectivity between the FFA and LOC regions measured during rest was enhanced after participants learned a series of object-face associations but not scene-face associations. (A after Ji and Wilson 2007; B after Rudoy et al. 2009; C after Tambini et al. 2010.)

again during slow-wave sleep increased hippocampal activity and improved memory for object locations the next day. In another study (Figure 9.22B), participants learned associations between objects and spatial locations (e.g., cat near the bottom left) while listening to a sound associated with each object. During a nap after learning, the sound for half of the objects was presented during slow-wave sleep. Spatial memory after the nap improved for cued but not uncued objects.

While most studies of consolidation-related reactivation have focused on sleep, consolidation presumably happens during rest while awake too. For example, a recent fMRI study found that functional connectivity among relevant cortical regions was greater during a rest period after learning than during a rest period before learning. More specifically, functional connectivity between regions associated with processing objects (lateral occipital complex, LOC) and faces (fusiform face area, FFA; see Chapter 3) was enhanced after learning object-face associations but not after learning scene-face associations (Figure 9.22C). Moreover, learning object-face associations also enhanced connectivity between LOC and the hippocampus, and this increase in connectivity predicted subsequent memory for the object-face associations.

In short, consolidation occurs at both cellular and system levels. Synaptic consolidation involves changes in synaptic morphology and takes a few minutes or hours. System consolidation (which must also depend on synaptic connectivity) involves reorganization in the brain regions supporting long-term memories and may take days, months, or even years. According to the standard theory of declarative system consolidation, recent memories depend on the medial temporal lobes, but, through repeated reactivation, direct associative connections are created among cortical traces, and memories can be accessed independently of the medial temporal lobes. This idea can explain the temporally graded retrograde amnesia in patients with medial temporal lobe damage. According to multiple-trace theory, however, the temporal gradient reflects a greater number of hippocampal traces for remote memories. But both theories agree that consolidation involves memory reactivation, which happens not only during intentional retrieval, but also during sleep and rest.

Summary

1. Declarative memory is conscious memory for events (episodic memory) and facts (semantic memory). Episodic memory may involve remembering contextual details (recollection) or merely having vague feelings of knowing (familiarity).

2. According to the most popular model of declarative memory, during encoding, memory traces are stored in the cortical regions that process each type of information; at the same time, the hippocampus stores indices pointing to these cortical locations. During this period of storage, some memories are strengthened (by consolidation) while others are lost. During retrieval, activation of hippocampal index representations leads to the reactivation of cortical traces. Damage to the hippocampus prevents access to cortical memory traces, producing memory loss (amnesia). Importantly, the hippocampus is no longer needed after memories have been consolidated, explaining why amnesia patients like H.M. can often remember remote memories. Prefrontal and parietal regions are assumed to mediate control processes during both encoding and retrieval.

3. Hippocampal memory representations have been described as spatial, relational, or episodic. Developmental and adult amnesia cases suggest that the hippocampus is more critical for episodic than for semantic memory. Conversely, semantic dementia cases indicate that the anterior temporal lobe is more critical for semantic than for episodic memory. The hippocampus has also been more strongly linked to recollection than to familiarity.

4. According to a three-process model, the perirhinal cortex is concerned with memory for objects; the parahippocampal cortex, with memory for spatial layouts; and the hippocampus, with domain-general relational memory.

5. The organization of semantic knowledge may reflect the sensory and functional properties of objects and/or semantic categories. Semantic dementia cases suggest that the anterior temporal lobes could be an amodal semantic "hub," with some links to social knowledge.

6. Functional neuroimaging studies and single-unit recordings show that regions activated during encoding tend to be reactivated during retrieval. Consistent with transfer-appropriate processing, this reactivation varies with specific encoding strategies.

7. The left inferior frontal gyrus has been associated with successful episodic encoding, possibly because of its role in semantic processing. The left middle frontal gyrus has been associated with organizing information during encoding and during retrieval. The right dorsolateral prefrontal cortex has been linked to monitoring processes; and the frontopolar cortex, to retrieval mode.

8. Posterior lateral parietal regions are often activated in episodic retrieval. Dorsal parietal activations have been linked to top-down attention; and ventral parietal

activations, to bottom-up attention. During encoding, ventral parietal activations are associated with subsequent forgetting.

9. Encoding is not completed immediately, but requires a process of synaptic consolidation, involving gene expression, protein synthesis, and synaptic plasticity.

10. System consolidation is the formation of direct connections among cortical traces, which allows these traces to be accessed independently of the hippocampus and could explain why remote memories are often spared by hippocampal damage. According to a multiple-trace theory, the sparing of remote memories reflects the creation of new hippocampal traces each time a memory is reactivated.

11. Consolidation is promoted by memory reactivation, whether by intentional practice, during slow-wave sleep, or at rest.

Go to the **COMPANION WEBSITE**

sites.sinauer.com/cogneuro2e
for quizzes, animations, flashcards,
and other study resources.

Additional Reading

Reviews

BROWN, M. W. AND J. P. AGGLETON (2001) Recognition memory: What are the roles of the perirhinal cortex and hippocampus? *Nat. Rev. Neurosci.* 2: 51–61.

CABEZA, R., E. CIARAMELLI, I. R. OLSON AND M. MOSCOVITCH (2008) The parietal cortex and episodic memory: An attentional account. *Nat. Rev. Neurosci.* 9: 613–625.

DANKER, J. F. AND J. R. ANDERSON (2010) The ghosts of brain states past: Remembering reactivates the brain regions engaged during encoding. *Psychol. Bull.* 136: 87–102.

DAVACHI, L. (2006) Item, context and relational episodic encoding in humans. *Curr. Opin. Neurobiol.* 16: 693–700.

DUDAI, Y. (2004) The neurobiology of consolidations, or, how stable is the engram? *Annu. Rev. Psychol.* 55: 51–86.

EICHENBAUM, H., A. R. YONELINAS AND C. RANGANATH (2007) The medial temporal lobe and recognition memory. *Annu. Rev. Neurosci.* 30: 123–152.

LAMPRECHT, R. AND J. LEDOUX (2004) Structural plasticity and memory. *Nat. Rev. Neurosci.* 5: 45–54.

MARTIN, A. (2007) The representation of object concepts in the brain. *Annu. Rev. Psychol.* 58: 25–45.

NADEL, L. AND M. MOSCOVITCH (1997) Memory consolidation, retrograde amnesia and the hippocampal complex. *Curr. Opin. Neurobiol.* 7: 217–227.

PATTERSON, K., P. J. NESTOR AND T. T. ROGERS (2007) Where do you know what you know? The representation of semantic knowledge in the human brain. *Nat. Rev. Neurosci.* 8: 976–987.

SQUIRE, L. R., C. E. STARK AND R. E. CLARK (2004) The medial temporal lobe. *Annu. Rev. Neurosci.* 27: 279–306.

Important Original Papers

BERRYHILL, M. E., L. PHUONG, L. PICASSO, R. CABEZA AND I. R. OLSON (2007) Parietal lobe and episodic memory: Bilateral damage causes impaired free recall of autobiographical memory. *J. Neurosci.* 27: 14415–14423.

BUCKNER, R. L., S. E. PETERSEN, J. G. OJEMANN, F. M. MIEZIN, L. R. SQUIRE AND M. E. RAICHLE (1995) Functional anatomical studies of explicit and implicit memory retrieval tasks. *J. Neurosci.* 15: 12–29.

DAVIDSON, P. S. R. AND 8 OTHERS (2008) Does lateral parietal cortex support episodic memory? Evidence from focal lesion patients. *Neuropsychologia* 46: 1743–1755.

JI, D. Y. AND M. A. WILSON (2007) Coordinated memory replay in the visual cortex and hippocampus during sleep. *Nat. Neurosci.* 10: 100–107.

MOSCOVITCH, M. AND B. MELO (1997) Strategic retrieval and the frontal lobes: Evidence from confabulation and amnesia. *Neuropsychologia* 35: 1017–1034.

POLYN, S. M., V. S. NATU, J. D. COHEN AND K. A. NORMAN (2005) Category-specific cortical activity precedes retrieval during memory search. *Science* 310: 1963–1966.

RASCH, B., C. BUECHEL, S. GAIS AND J. BORN (2007) Odor cues during slow-wave sleep prompt declarative memory consolidation. *Science* 315: 1426–1429.

RUDOY, J. D., J. L. VOSS, C. E. WESTERBERG AND K. A. PALLER (2009) Strengthening individual memories by reactivating them during sleep. *Science* 326: 1079.

SAKAI, K. AND Y. MIYASHITA (1991) Neural organization for the long-term memory of paired associates. *Nature* 354: 152–155.

WAGNER, A. D. AND 7 OTHERS (1998) Building memories: Remembering and forgetting of verbal experiences as predicted by brain activity. *Science* 281: 1188–1191.

Books

BADDELEY, A., M. A. CONWAY AND J. P. AGGLETON, EDS. (2002) *Episodic Memory: New Directions in Research.* Oxford: Oxford University Press.

EICHENBAUM, H. AND N. J. COHEN (2004) *From Conditioning to Conscious Recollection: Memory Systems of the Brain.* New York: Oxford University Press.

TULVING, E. (1983) *Elements of Episodic Memory.* Oxford: Oxford University Press.

SQUIRE, L. R. AND E. R. KANDEL (1999) *Memory: From Mind to Molecules.* New York: Holt.

10

Emotion

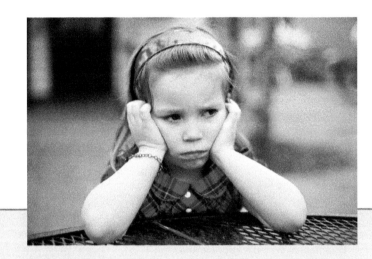

INTRODUCTION

The discussion of cognitive functions so far has avoided the question of how behavior is shaped by an individual's emotions and social context. In fact, the social and emotional aspects of brain function are central factors in mobilizing bodily resources appropriate to adjusting to particular circumstances, to evaluating goals, to setting priorities for action, and to meshing one's own behavior appropriately with that of others. Although neuroscience has sometimes neglected these complex influences on what we think and do in favor of issues that can be more readily understood in reductionist terms, it has become increasingly clear that emotional and social influences are amenable to the same conceptual and methodological approaches that have been used successfully to study other cognitive functions, albeit with some additional ethical constraints (see Introductory Box).

The term **affective neuroscience** broadly refers to the subfield within cognitive neuroscience that is concerned with understanding emotional aspects of brain function. Accordingly, this chapter and the next review the history, phenomenology, and neural substrates of emotional and social processes and their interactions with other cognitive functions. Historically, studies of emotion were often framed in a psychosomatic tradition that attempted to understand how bodily reactions are linked to brain function. This work led to the *limbic system theory of emotion* in the mid-twentieth century, which emphasized visceral (autonomic) functions associated with brain regions surrounding the medial forebrain. Although investigators have long since recognized that a broader perspective is required to bring together the many neural systems involved, at present there is no agreed-upon neurobiological account of how the brain and body interact to generate integrated emotional states. Despite the absence of a unified theory of emotion and social behavior, many recent advances have been made, particularly in understanding how emotions influence other cognitive functions, such as attention, memory, and executive control, and these topics remain very much in the forefront of cognitive neuroscience research.

■ INTRODUCTORY BOX   THE NEUROSCIENCE AND NEUROETHICS OF POSTTRAUMATIC STRESS DISORDER

For months after the attack, I couldn't close my eyes without envisioning the face of my attacker. I suffered horrific flashbacks and nightmares. For four years after the attack I was unable to sleep alone in my house. I obsessively checked windows, doors, and locks ... I lost all ability to concentrate or even complete simple tasks. Normally social, I stopped trying to make friends or get involved in my community.

P. K. PHILIPS, http://www.adaa.org/ living-with-anxiety/personal-stories

The condition described in the vivid personal example above is known as **posttraumatic stress disorder (PTSD)**. PTSD emerges following exposure to a traumatic stressor—such as rape, robbery, or combat—that elicits feelings of fear, horror, or helplessness in response to bodily injury or threat of death to oneself or another person. Community-based studies in the United States estimate that 50 percent of people will have a traumatic experience during their lifetime, although only about 5 percent of men and 9 percent of women will develop PTSD as a result. Symptoms include persistently reexperiencing the traumatic event, avoiding reminders of the event, numbed responsiveness, and heightened arousal. PTSD is often accompanied by depression and substance abuse, each of which complicates treatment and recovery. While cognitive-behavioral therapies and antianxiety and antidepressant medications often help, there is no cure for this debilitating condition and its chronic stress, which can persist for decades.

Some of the structural abnormalities associated with PTSD are reductions in hippocampal and amygdala volume (Figure A) and altered dendritic remodeling in these structures. Hippocampal atrophy has been linked to declarative memory deficits and PTSD symptom severity, and functional impairments in the amygdala are associated with hyperarousal symptoms and exaggerated responses to threats. Problems with fear reduction are further exacerbated by hyporesponsiveness in the rostral anterior cingulate and ventromedial prefrontal cortex (vmPFC), which provide inhibitory control over neurons in the amygdala (Figure B). Treatment with serotonin reuptake inhibitors

(A)

Legend:
- Subjects with both abuse and PTSD
- Subjects with abuse but not PTSD
- Subjects with neither abuse nor PTSD

Hippocampal volume (mm³): y-axis from 600 to 1300, x-axis Left hippocampus, Right hippocampus

(B)

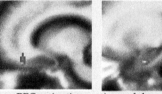

SCR magnitude graph: y-axis −0.1 to 0.3, legend CS+ CS−, x-axis PTSD, Control

PTSD vs. Control
CS+ > CS− (late extinction learning)

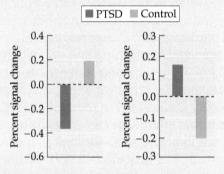

vmPFC activation   Amygdala activation

PTSD   Control

Percent signal change graphs

Brain abnormalities associated with PTSD. (A) The volume of the hippocampus is reduced in adult patients with PTSD and childhood abuse, compared both to abused individuals who never developed PTSD and to healthy individuals. Estimates of the magnitude of the hippocampal atrophy vary across studies, ranging from 2 to 12 percent. (B) Compared to trauma-exposed control subjects, PTSD patients have a difficult time extinguishing fear responses to cues that previously predicted a threat. During fear conditioning, one cue (CS+) predicted delivery of a mild shock, whereas another cue (CS−) did not. Participants then underwent an extinction procedure in which the shock was removed and the CS+ was now "safe." Even though the cue no longer predicted a shock, the PTSD patients continued to show greater skin conductance responses (SCRs)—a measure of sympathetic arousal—and greater amygdala activity to the CS+ during the extinction test. In addition, they failed to engage the ventromedial prefrontal cortex (vmPFC) during the extinction test. This functional activity pattern is indicative of persistent hyperreactivity to threats and difficulty engaging executive control processes to suppress acquired fears when they are not appropriate to express. (A after Bremner et al. 2003; B after Milad et al. 2009.)

such as Prozac may partially reverse hippocampal volume differences and alleviate anxiety symptoms, although no single treatment cures the myriad behavioral problems of this complex and debilitating disorder. Currently, a major focus of research is to determine whether the brain alterations lead to PTSD or are a consequence of dealing with the chronic stress associated with the syndrome. Some twin studies suggest that reduced hippocampal volume and fear extinction abilities may predispose individuals to

developing PTSD after experiencing a traumatic event.

Researchers and clinicians interested in PTSD face many challenges. Since it is generally considered unethical to induce physical or psychological trauma in the laboratory, the topic is difficult to approach experimentally. For instance, is it ethical to have PTSD patients relive their painful past experiences for the purpose of studying these extreme emotions in the laboratory? As new treatments develop, additional dilemmas have emerged. If

■ **INTRODUCTORY BOX** *(continued)*

a pharmacological agent selectively blocks emotional memories, should it be administered to all rape victims? If a genetic variant of a molecular marker is discovered to be a risk factor for developing PTSD, should military recruits be screened for it? Is it ethical to expose research animals to chronic stress to investigate its neurobiological mechanisms?

Questions like these raise ethical concerns not only for PTSD patients but for emotion research generally. A primary goal of such research is to improve the human condition and alleviate the suffering of patients afflicted with affective disorders. On the one hand, it is incumbent on researchers to study emotional phenomena that mimic or elicit the emotions associated with the disorder of interest. On the other hand, if emotions are evoked only weakly in the laboratory, the

mechanisms uncovered may bear little resemblance to those that operate in the real world, but evoking stronger emotions may cause harm to a study volunteer. As with all other scientific research, a balance must be struck between the risks posed to an individual participant and the ultimate benefit to society.

References

BREMNER, J. D. (2006) Traumatic stress: Effects on the brain. *Dialogues Clin. Neurosci.* 8: 445–461.

BREMNER, J. D. AND 13 OTHERS (2003) MRI and PET study of deficits in hippocampal structure and function in women with childhood sexual abuse and posttraumatic stress disorder. *Am. J. Psychiatry* 160: 924–932.

CANLI, T. AND Z. AMIN (2002) Neuroimaging of emotion and personality: Scientific evidence and ethical considerations. *Brain Cogn.* 50: 414–431.

GLANNON, W. (2006) Neuroethics. *Bioethics* 20: 37–52.

KESSLER, R. C., A. SONNEGA, E. BROMET, M. HUGHES AND C. B. NELSON (1995) Posttraumatic stress disorder in the National Comorbidity Survey. *Arch. Gen. Psychiatry* 52: 948–960.

MILAD, M. R. AND 9 OTHERS (2009) Neurobiological basis of failure to recall extinction memory in posttraumatic stress disorder. *Biol. Psychiatry* 66: 1075–1082.

SHIN, L. M. AND I. LIBERZON (2010) The neurocircuitry of fear, stress, and anxiety. *Neuropsychopharmacology* 35: 169–191.

What Is Emotion?

In everyday use, the word **emotion** typically refers to conscious feelings, like love, jealousy, contempt, anger, and despair. Because consciousness itself defies clear neurobiological explanation (see Chapter 7), defining emotions solely in terms of these subjective feeling states is problematic for scientific study. Among other difficulties, a definition in these terms implies that organisms with less self-awareness do not experience or use emotions the way humans do. Yet, as Charles Darwin noted in the late nineteenth century, many non-human animal species produce affective displays during predator-prey interactions, sex and mating, and maternal care of the young that are similar to those observed in humans (see Chapter 15). As a consequence of this broader view, researchers today conceptualize emotion as a composite of *feelings, expressive behavior,* and *physiological changes* (Figure 10.1).

In functional terms, emotions are considered dispositions toward behaviors that help an organism deal with biologically significant events. To illustrate, an emotion like fear at the sight of a predator engages defensive behavior that prepares the organism to fight or to flee, redistributing blood flow from internal organs to peripheral muscles, releasing stress hormones, increasing sensory vigilance, facilitating reflexes, and altering breathing, heart rate, and blood pressure. Learning from such experiences helps one flexibly alter behavior to yield beneficial outcomes in similar circumstances in the future. In some individuals, however, such learned associations may also contribute to the development of phobias and other affective disorders (see Introductory Box). By focusing on how specific emotional circumstances elicit changes in behavior and physiology (rather than on conscious experiences of internal states that constitute feelings), scientific models of emotion in health and disease have become easier to describe at the neural level.

In sum, emotions are sets of physiological responses, action tendencies, and subjective feelings that adaptively engage humans and other animals to react to events of biological and/or individual significance. This perspective has

Figure 10.1 **The components of emotions** Emotions can be broken down into three components, each of which can be studied independently: behavioral action (a motor output, such as social approach); conscious experience (a subjective feeling, such as love); and physiological expression (autonomic activity, such as increased heart rate). For healthy emotions, these components are generally integrated into a coherent pattern that defines a particular emotion and leads to the facilitation of biologically useful responses. In various forms of psychopathology, however, these normal patterns are discordant. For example, patients who suffer from schizophrenia often show increased autonomic arousal despite reduced motor output.

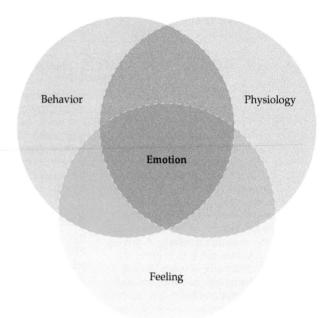

several corollaries. First, emotions are typically triggered by conditions and events in the local environment, although thoughts or memories of more remote experiences can also trigger emotions. Second, emotions include behavioral and physiological changes that may not be accessible to conscious awareness but are nonetheless amenable to investigation. Third, emotions facilitate social interactions that are beneficial to survival and propagation of the species. By investigating emotional reactions in individuals, across cultures and species, it is possible to determine the neurophysiological signatures of specific emotions, their interactions with cognitive processes, and, in humans, their relation to self-reported feelings.

Psychological Classification of Emotions

Theories about how emotions are organized and related to one another have evolved greatly over the years. This section describes the major psychological perspectives on these questions; the following section indicates how these ideas have been informed and refined as newer methods have examined and clarified the neural bases of emotional behavior.

Categorical theories

Categorical theories regard each emotion as a discrete, independent entity and typically distinguish a small set of basic emotions from a larger pool of complex emotions. **Basic emotions** are taken to be innate, pan-cultural, evolutionarily old, shared with other species, and expressed by particular physiological patterns and facial configurations. In contrast, **complex emotions** are learned, socially and culturally shaped, evolutionarily new, most evident in humans, and typically expressed by combinations of the response patterns that characterize basic emotions. Complex emotions tend to be influenced by language usage and emerge later in development. Researchers interested in distinguishing and classifying basic and complex emotions use techniques that monitor physiological responses, as well as techniques for coding and analyzing facial or vocal expressions. Because basic emotions can be studied readily in nonhuman animals, the biology of these emotions has been well characterized.

Nonetheless, researchers still debate which emotions are basic. Although different taxonomies posit between four and nine basic emotions, most include

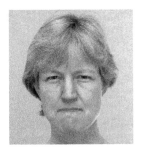

Anger

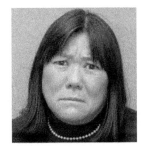

Sadness

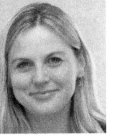

Happiness

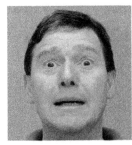

Fear

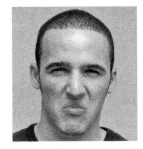

Disgust

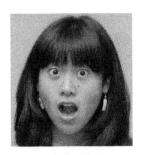

Surprise

Figure 10.2 Categorical theories of emotion Posed facial expressions are taken to exemplify discrete emotion categories. Emotions typically classified as *basic* are depicted here and include (from left to right and top to bottom) anger, sadness, happiness, fear, disgust, and surprise. Note that most of the basic emotions are unpleasant in valence.

a similar core set: anger, sadness (distress), happiness (joy), fear, disgust, and surprise (Figure 10.2). But even basic emotions like disgust take on nuanced forms and expanded functions in humans. For instance, moral disgust is elicited by acts that violate an individual's innocence or integrity, such as rape, and it manifests itself in a facial expression that emphasizes a curled upper lip. Physical disgust, in contrast, is evoked by bad tastes or odors and accompanied by a different aspect of facial expression, a "wrinkled" nose.

As one might expect, not only are complex emotions more difficult to categorize than basic emotions; they are also more difficult to study. The external features of expression for more complex emotions are more subtle, occur in more varied contexts, and have more prominent cross-cultural differences. Take the emotion pride as an example. Pride is elicited when a person takes credit for a personal accomplishment that boosts self-esteem, such as winning a marathon or a chess tournament. This response is often expressed by a modest smile combined with erect postural gestures of dominance (shoulders back, chin up, arms raised). This body profile, which is harder to quantify than facial expression alone, tends to distinguish pride from other positive emotions. There are also wide variations in the circumstances and frequency with which pride is expressed in social settings, because of cultural value systems. For instance, some East Asian cultures promote an expanded concept of self that includes relatives or the larger community. In these cultures, expressions of pride arising from one's own accomplishments may be viewed negatively and are often curtailed.

Dimensional theories

In contrast to categorical theories, dimensional theories consider each emotion a point within a complex space that includes two or more continuous dimensions. Most researchers consider **arousal** (the physiological and/or subjective intensity of the emotion) and **valence** (its relative pleasantness) to be critical dimensions, and they use techniques that enable analyses on ordinal scales. For instance, subjects might be asked to rate movie clips that vary in emotional content on a 9-point valence scale ranging from "very unpleasant" to "very pleasant."

Two models of this sort have been proposed. One way to represent emotions dimensionally is to use **vector models**. Vector models tend to order emotions

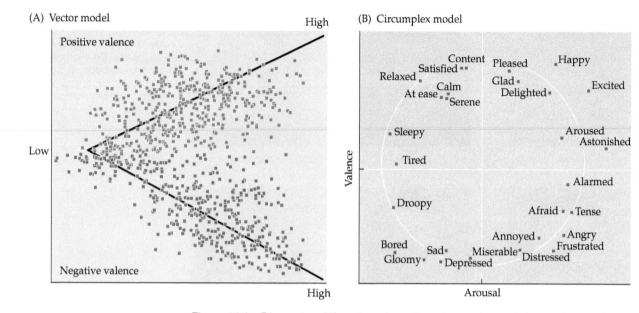

(A) Vector model

Positive valence

High

Low

Negative valence

High

(B) Circumplex model

Content
Relaxed Satisfied Pleased Happy
Calm Glad Excited
At ease Serene Delighted
Sleepy Aroused
Astonished
Tired
Alarmed
Droopy Afraid Tense
Annoyed Angry
Bored Frustrated
Gloomy Sad Miserable Distressed
Depressed

Valence

Arousal

Figure 10.3 Dimensional theories of emotion: the vector and circumplex models (A) Vector models are supported by studies in which participants rate pictures on ordinal scales of arousal and valence. The ratings are then plotted on two coterminating axes that reflect unipolar dimensions of positive and negative valence. Plotting the mean ratings given to hundreds of pictures by a large number of individuals results in a boomerang shape in which the most arousing stimuli of each valence are plotted the farthest away from the neutral endpoint that joins the two axes. Individual pictures that are rated similarly cluster together on the boomerang. (B) Circumplex models are supported by studies in which participants rate words on ordinal scales of arousal and valence. The ratings are then plotted on orthogonal axes of arousal (activation) and valence (pleasantness) that intersect in the middle of the scales. Words that represent similar emotions cluster together along the circumference of the circle. (A after Lang et al. 1993; B after Russell 1980.)

along axes of positive and negative valence that are oriented at 90 degrees and meet at a common neutral endpoint, forming a boomerang shape when plotted on a graph (Figure 10.3A). In these models, arousal is represented by the distance from the neutral endpoint along each arm of the boomerang and is functionally equivalent to increases in valence. Alternatively, the motivational concepts of approach (activation) and avoidance (inhibition) can be used as the axes. Vector models have been supported by experimental studies that ask participants to rate the emotional properties of pictures, sounds, and memories.

In contrast to vector models, **circumplex models** order emotions around the circumference of a circle centered at the intersection of two orthogonal axes, of arousal and valence (Figure 10.3B). Emotions that cluster together in the resulting graph are taken to be similar in their dimensional features. Studies that ask participants to rate the emotional properties of words, facial expressions, and music tend to support the validity of this class of models. Such models are also tested with psychophysiological measures that index arousal and valence (Box 10A).

Either circumplex or vector models can represent individual emotions. However, the genesis of individual emotions is accounted for simply by their position along valence-arousal or approach-avoidance axes. As a result, dimensional theorists do not look for discrete neural systems underlying each emotion; instead they argue that seeking the neural correlates of the dimensional axes and their impact on cognition and behavior will be more fruitful.

TABLE 10.1 Component Process Theories of Emotion[a]

APPRAISAL CRITERIA	JOY	ANGER	FEAR	SADNESS
Novelty[b]	High	High	High	Low
Pleasantness	High	Open	Low	Open
Goal significance				
Outcome certainty	High	Very high	High	Very high
Conduciveness	Conducive	Obstructive	Obstructive	Obstructive
Urgency	Low	High	Very high	Low
Coping potential				
Agency	Self/other	Other	Other	Open
Control	High	High	Open	Very low
Power	High	High	Very low	Very low
Adjustment	High	High	Low	Medium

Source: ELLSWORTH, P. AND K. R. SCHERER (2003) Appraisal processes in emotion. In *Handbook of Affective Sciences*, R. J. Davison, K. R. Scherer and H. H. Goldsmith (eds.). New York: Oxford University Press, pp. 572–595.

[a]Component process theories maintain that emotions arise from combinations of specific appraisals of an emotion-eliciting situation.

[b]Both joy and anger can be elicited by novel situations. However, situations that induce anger tend to be obstructive to obtaining one's goals and are accompanied by a high sense of urgency to act, whereas those that induce joy tend to be conducive to one's goals and have a low sense of urgency. Different emotions resemble each other to the extent that they share some of these component cognitive processes.

Component process theories

Rather than viewing emotions as fixed states, component process theories attempt to capture the fluid nature of emotions, which require flexible interactions of multiple component processes. These theories emphasize processes that are involved in cognitively appraising the emotional meaning of events, as well as the link between the appraisal outcome and a behavioral and physiological response. In this view, emotions are related according to the similarity of the appraisal processes engaged.

Some investigators argue that important appraisals include the sense of urgency for action in response to the elicitor, how well a person can cope with the presence of the elicitor, and whether the elicitor facilitates or impedes progress toward a goal (Table 10.1). In this view, emotions are organized in the brain according to their overlap in recruiting specific appraisal mechanisms, which may vary across individuals, depending on social context and cultural influences. Because of their complexity, component process models have not been extensively tested with neuroscientific methods.

Early Neurobiological Theories of Emotion

Neurobiological research has not yet provided a compelling answer to the question of which, if any, of the psychological theories posited thus far provides the best account of how emotions are generated. In general, the search for neural substrates of emotion has been guided by breaking down the concept of emotion into different information-processing stages. In particular, three stages have been broadly characterized: (1) the *evaluation* of sensory input; (2) the conscious *experience* of a feeling state; and (3) the *expression* of behavioral and physiological responses. Neurobiological accounts have differed in how these stages are related to one another conceptually, anatomically, and temporally.

■ BOX 10A PSYCHOPHYSIOLOGY AND THE BRAIN-BODY LINK

Psychophysiology is a discipline that relates psychological constructs, such as emotion, to measurable changes in the body. This field broadly covers both central and peripheral neural measures, as well as musculoskeletal, endocrine, and immune system responses. In emotion research, characterizing changes in body function is important for verifying and quantifying emotional reactions, especially when self-report of emotion may not be reliable or even possible (as in non-human animals or preverbal infants).

As described in the text, early emotion theorists noted a strong link between emotions and changes in the state of the body's internal organs (viscera), as anyone who has experienced the "butterflies" of a first date or the "pangs" of regret can attest. The viscera are regulated by the autonomic nervous system, which affects a vast array of bodily changes, including cardiac, respiratory, digestive, and reproductive functions. The autonomic nervous system comprises a sympathetic division and a parasympathetic division, which are independent and complementary subsystems (Figure A). The *sympathetic division* is concerned mainly with functions related to fight-or-flight behaviors, and these responses are effected by a series of ganglionic relays along the vertebral column that innervate the target organs. By contrast, the *parasympathetic division* regulates rest-and-digest functions under more peaceful circumstances; the ganglia that regulate these functions are generally in or near the organs themselves.

Finally, the gut is innervated by neurons that reside in a large number of ganglia referred to collectively as the *enteric nervous system*. The enteric system is for the most part locally regulated, permitting relatively independent activity of digestive functions. The balance between these systems is important for maintaining homeostasis and meeting the body's essential metabolic and physiological needs. The autonomic motor neurons in the spinal cord and brainstem are under descending control of neurons in the hypothalamus, which in turn, is regulated by limbic and prefrontal structures. The viscera send feedback to the brain via afferent projections of the vagus, glossopharyngeal, oculomotor, and facial nerves to brainstem nuclei.

Two peripheral psychophysiological indices that have been particularly useful for distinguishing emotions along the dimensions of arousal and valence are *skin conductance* and *startle responses* (see the text for a discussion of dimensional theories of emotion). The skin conductance response (SCR) is an autonomic index of electrodermal activity taken from electrodes placed over the palmar surface of the hands and feet. At these locations, eccrine sweat glands are highly concentrated, about 900 glands per square centimeter (glands of another class—the apocrine glands—are located in the armpit and pubic regions). Activity of the sweat glands during emotional arousal, as is commonly experienced during public speaking, increases the electrical conductance of the skin surface. Eccrine sweat gland activity as a result of arousal is mediated solely by the sympathetic nervous system; thus, skin conductance is a good measure of the sympathetic response to arousing circumstances, and by the same token a good indicator of the arousal levels associated with specific emotions.

Several different aspects of the skin conductance can be assessed. The average skin conductance level over time is a measure of the basal (tonic) level of arousal. Spontaneous fluctuations in the baseline level are taken as measures of anxiety or contextual fear because they occur in the absence of a particular sensory stimulus. Finally, phasic SCRs are amplitude modulations that have a characteristic time course and profile time-locked to the onset of a sensory stimulus (Figure B). The fact that the temporal profile of this response is similar to that of the hemodynamic response measured with fMRI conveniently facilitates the design of studies that combine the two techniques.

Because fear and anxiety are linked to high arousal states, the SCR is a good measure of these emotions, and it is widely used in "lie detector" (polygraph) tests in criminal cases. However, skin conductance is modulated by other factors, such as sexual arousal, as well as attentional orienting responses to novel stimuli, complicating the interpretation of polygraph tests. Skin conductance has also been used to identify stimulus-evoked arousal responses that arise unconsciously. For instance, patients with prosopagnosia (see Chapter 3) often show SCRs when viewing pictures of family members, despite being unable to consciously recognize the individuals by sight alone.

The **startle response** is a protective musculoskeletal reflex elicited by intense and unexpected sensory stimuli (e.g., a flash of light or a loud noise). Such stimuli interrupt ongoing thoughts and behavior to evaluate the location and significance of sensory input. The startle response is mediated by subcortical neural circuitry that includes the brainstem reticular formation, which plays a key role in arousal and interfaces with sensory and motor functions. This complex set of nuclei is modulated by descending corticolimbic projections, including projections from the amygdala.

A component of the startle response that is readily measured in both humans and experimental animals is the eyeblink reflex, which helps protect the eye from unexpected noxious stimuli. Eyeblink startle is measured either by electromyographic recordings of activity in the orbicularis oculi muscle or by infrared monitoring of eyelid closure (Figure C). Several measures can be extracted from such recordings, including the probability of blinking in response to a stimulus, the magnitude of the blink, and its latency after the stimulus.

Startle responses are influenced by attention; for instance, when we attend to visual stimuli, startle responses to an auditory stimulus are attenuated, and vice versa. Thus, startle can be used to determine the relative allocation of sensory or other processing resources to a particular aspect of the environment. This attentional influence is further modulated by emotion. In circumstances that generate fear (e.g., walking down a dark alley at night), startle responses are potentiated: a sudden noise or touch will elicit a larger startle response than in the circumstance of walking down a well-populated street during the day. Fear-potentiated startle has been particularly beneficial in the development of animal models of anxiety

Emotional states induce changes in autonomic and musculoskeletal activity. (A) Overall scheme of the autonomic nervous system. Note that the sympathetic branch contains a paravertebral column alongside the spinal cord that coordinates activity among the target organs. The innervation of target organs is typically cholinergic (stimulated by acetylcholine) from the parasympathetic division and noradrenergic (stimulated by norepinephrine) from the sympathetic division. These divisions generally elicit complementary changes in the viscera.

■ BOX 10A (continued)

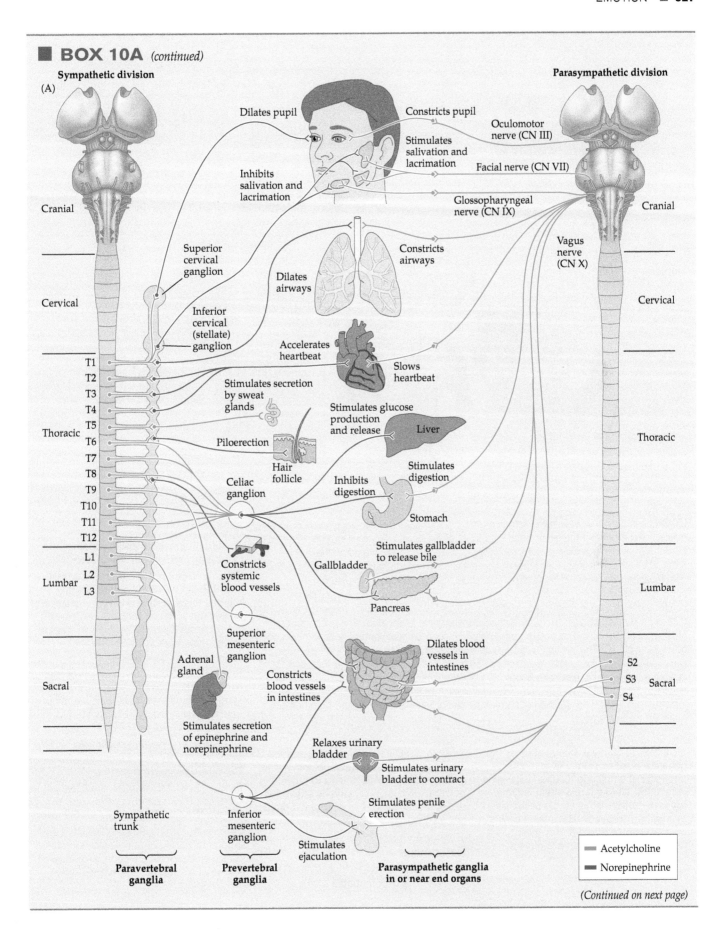

Sympathetic division

(A)

Cranial

Cervical

T1
T2
T3
T4
T5
T6
T7
T8
T9
T10
T11
T12

Thoracic

L1
L2
L3

Lumbar

Sacral

Dilates pupil

Inhibits
salivation and
lacrimation

Superior
cervical
ganglion

Inferior
cervical
(stellate)
ganglion

Dilates
airways

Accelerates
heartbeat

Stimulates secretion
by sweat
glands

Piloerection

Celiac
ganglion

Hair
follicle

Inhibits
digestion

Constricts
systemic
blood vessels

Superior
mesenteric
ganglion

Adrenal
gland

Constricts
blood vessels
in intestines

Stimulates secretion
of epinephrine and
norepinephrine

Sympathetic
trunk

Inferior
mesenteric
ganglion

Stimulates
ejaculation

**Paravertebral
ganglia**

**Prevertebral
ganglia**

Parasympathetic division

Constricts pupil

Stimulates
salivation and
lacrimation

Oculomotor
nerve (CN III)

Facial nerve (CN VII)

Glossopharyngeal
nerve (CN IX)

Vagus
nerve
(CN X)

Cranial

Cervical

Constricts
airways

Slows
heartbeat

Stimulates glucose
production and release

Liver

Stimulates
digestion

Stomach

Stimulates gallbladder
to release bile

Gallbladder

Pancreas

Dilates blood
vessels in
intestines

Relaxes urinary
bladder

Stimulates urinary
bladder to contract

Stimulates penile
erection

**Parasympathetic ganglia
in or near end organs**

Thoracic

Lumbar

S2
S3
S4

Sacral

Acetylcholine
Norepinephrine

(Continued on next page)

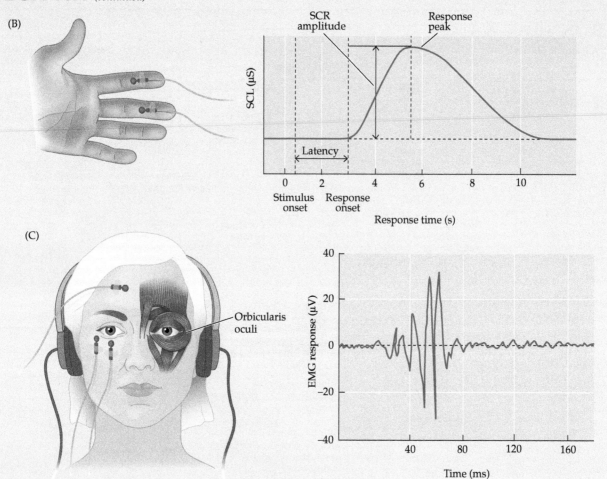

(B) Skin conductance reflects the activity of sweat glands. Skin conductance level (SCL) is typically recorded from the second and third digits of the hand, although it can be recorded from the palm or the bottom of the foot as well. The eccrine sweat glands on these body parts receive no parasympathetic innervation, making skin conductance an attractive dependent measure of sympathetic activation. If the task requires a motor response from the hand, to avoid movement artifacts the nondominant hand is used for recording. The skin conductance change in response to a stimulus (i.e., the skin conductance response, or SCR), measured in microsiemens (μS), has a characteristic onset latency (usually 1–2 seconds after stimulus onset) and peak latency (usually 1–4 seconds later) before decaying back to baseline levels. (C) The startle response is an example of a musculoskeletal reflex. The eyeblink component of the startle response can be measured by electrodes over the orbicularis oculi muscle (a ground electrode is typically placed on the forehead). Unlike the SCR, the electromyographic (EMG) response, measured in microvolts (μV), has a rapid onset (<50 milliseconds) and a brief duration (<100 milliseconds), and it is more sensitive to emotional valence than to arousal.

disorders. In contrast, circumstances that generate positive emotions or moods reduce startle amplitude relative to baseline conditions, although this effect is generally less robust than is startle potentiation by negative emotions. Because it can be modulated upward or downward as a function of valence, startle is more sensitive to this dimension of emotion than is skin conductance.

Thus, psychophysiological measures such as the skin conductance and startle responses can be combined to provide powerful physiological indices of two fundamental dimensions of emotion: arousal and valence.

References

AMELI, R., C. IP AND C. GRILLON (2001) Contextual fear-potentiated startle conditioning in humans: Replication and extension. *Psychophysiology* 38: 383–390.

CRITCHLEY, H. D., R. ELLIOTT, C. J. MATHIAS AND R. J. DOLAN (2000) Neural activity relating to generation and representation of galvanic skin conductance responses: A functional magnetic resonance imaging study. *J. Neurosci.* 20: 3033–3040.

DAVIS, M., J. M. HITCHCOCK AND J. B. ROSEN (1991) Neural mechanisms of fear conditioning measured with the acoustic startle reflex. In *Neurobiology of Learning, Emotion, and Affect*, J. I. Madden (ed.). New York: Raven, pp. 67–96.

HUGDAHL, K. (1995) *Psychophysiology: The Mind-Body Perspective.* Cambridge, MA: Harvard University Press.

LANG, P. J., M. M. BRADLEY AND B. N. CUTHBERT (1990) Emotion, attention, and the startle reflex. *Psychol. Rev.* 97: 377–395.

ÖHMAN, A. AND J. J. SOARES (1993) On the automatic nature of phobic fear: Conditioned electrodermal responses to masked fear-relevant stimuli. *J. Abnorm. Psychol.* 92: 121–132.

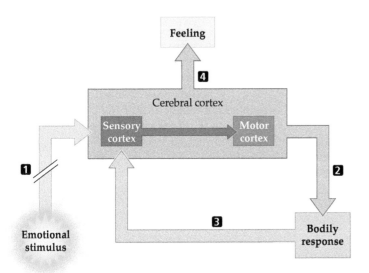

Figure 10.4 The James-Lange feedback theory of emotion An eliciting stimulus (1) directly causes a bodily reaction (2), which feeds back into the brain (3) to generate an emotional feeling (4). According to this theory, no specialized brain region for processing emotion exists, and bodily reactions and feelings have a one-to-one correspondence.

The James-Lange feedback theory

The late-nineteenth-century psychologist William James posed the following question about emotion: "Do we run from a bear because we are afraid, or are we afraid because we run?" Although most of us would submit that the act of running from a bear is initiated by a fearful feeling, James took the opposite stance. He believed that the act of running itself (combined with increased sweating, rapid breathing, increased heart rate, and other physiological manifestations) generated the fear. Thus, from James's perspective, the experience of an emotion depended on a prior set of changes in the body that fed back to the brain (Figure 10.4).

This theory rests on two assumptions: first, that a deterministic relationship exists between bodily reactions and emotions; and second, that no emotions are felt in the absence of bodily reactions, since those reactions are causal. James did allow for individual differences in emotion and acknowledged that situational context might alter the response profile. Nevertheless, in this view the physiological pattern for each emotion must be reasonably consistent among individuals.

The Danish physiologist Carl Lange also proposed a feedback theory of emotion in the late nineteenth century. Although James accommodated other bodily feedback signals, such as those arising from the facial musculature (as emphasized by his contemporary Duchenne; see Box 5B), Lange postulated that cardiac function was most relevant for emotion. Not surprisingly, Lange was less concerned about explaining conscious awareness of emotion, since, unlike James, he was a physiologist. Despite the two men's differences in theoretical orientation, these early feedback ideas of emotion are now referred to as the **James-Lange feedback theory.**

Although James did not postulate dedicated neural structures for emotional processing, Lange felt that brainstem nuclei that control cardiac function were important. Lange also believed that specific feelings emerged directly from the pattern of somatic feedback to diffuse cortical sites in the brain. In any event, the James-Lange theory highlighted the relationship between brain activity and physiological reactions—an idea that was further developed in the early twentieth century as a wealth of information was uncovered about the functions and anatomy of the autonomic nervous system.

The Cannon-Bard diencephalic theory

In the 1920s, physiologist Walter Cannon and his student Philip Bard challenged the James-Lange theory. Cannon and Bard argued that responses of

No sham rage

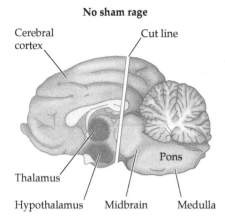

Sham rage remains

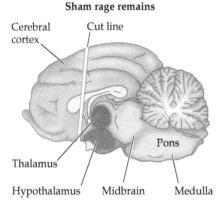

Figure 10.5 Emotions in decorticate animals Transection experiments show that decorticate animals can express an integrated emotional reaction such as sham rage, but only if the neural pathways are interrupted above the level of the diencephalon (hypothalamus and thalamus). Cuts below the diencephalon disconnect the forebrain from the rest of the body and preclude centrally generated autonomic and motor control.

the autonomic nervous system (see Box 10A) were too undifferentiated to yield the variety of emotional states that we experience. For example, flushing of the skin increases during embarrassment, anger, and sexual arousal. Therefore, the presence of a specific peripheral response could not uniquely determine which emotion would be felt. They also pointed out that neurohormonal feedback from the body's endocrine organs to the brain would take too long to account for the abrupt onset of emotions (although direct neural feedback from the facial musculature potentially could). Finally, they showed that hormonal feedback was insufficient to generate emotions; systemic injection of hormones such as norepinephrine (which stimulates a variety of sympathetic responses associated with emotions such as fear and anger) does not consistently result in a particular emotional state. Cannon and Bard instead suggested that the autonomic nervous system coordinates the body's general fight-or-flight response, which mobilizes the body's resources in preparation for appropriate action in an emotionally arousing situation.

Cannon and Bard went on to investigate the effects of surgically disconnecting the cerebral cortex from the brainstem and other subcortical nuclei in experimental animals (Figure 10.5). They found that decorticate animals could exhibit integrated emotional reactions, such as defensive behavior, only if the transection occurred above the level of the diencephalon (**hypothalamus** and **thalamus**). These findings were bolstered by the studies of Walter Hess, a contemporary of Cannon and Bard who showed further that electrical stimulation of the hypothalamus elicits emotional reactions in the cat, including **sham rage**, in which hissing, growling, and attack behaviors are directed randomly toward innocuous targets.

Cannon and Bard therefore proposed that when an emotional stimulus was processed by the diencephalon, it was directed simultaneously to the neocortex for the generation of emotional feelings, and to the rest of the body for the expression of emotional reactions (Figure 10.6). This idea is known as the **Cannon-Bard theory** (or *diencephalic theory*) of emotion, and it represents one of the first parallel-processing models of brain function—a theme in brain organization that appears in many contexts in cognitive neuroscience. The theory's focus on the hypothalamus emphasizes the key relationship between emotional information processing in the brain and the activity of the autonomic

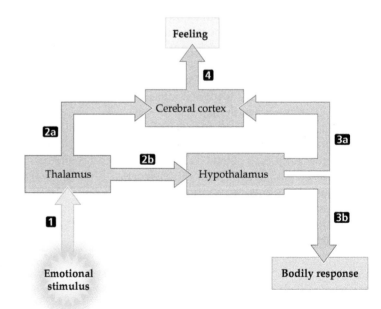

Figure 10.6 The Cannon-Bard theory of emotion Input from emotion-provoking stimuli (1) is directed in parallel from the thalamus to the cortex directly (2a) or indirectly (2b, 3a) for the generation of feelings (4), and from the thalamus to the hypothalamus (2b) for bodily expression (3b).

nervous system. It also paved the way for more elaborate parallel-processing models of emotion. Although the Cannon-Bard and James-Lange theories differ in orientation, both ideas postulate an important role for the body in generating emotions, and both argue that conscious emotional states are processed in the neocortex.

The Papez circuit and Klüver-Bucy syndrome

Working in the late 1930s, neuroanatomist James Papez described a circuit for emotion in the medial walls of the forebrain. These brain regions, which the French neuroanatomist Paul Broca had earlier called "la grande lobe limbique" (the Latin word *limbus* means "rim" or "border"), are evolutionarily older than the neocortex. Structures contained within Papez's circuit straddle the diencephalon and forebrain and include the anterior thalamus, hypothalamus, hippocampus, and cingulate gyrus. Papez's rationale in identifying this circuit was based on brain structures directly connected with the hypothalamus, the locus most central to the Cannon-Bard theory (Figure 10.7).

About the same time that Papez was carrying out this anatomical research, psychologist Heinrich Klüver and neurosurgeon Paul Bucy serendipitously discovered the emotional consequences of removing the temporal lobes in the rhesus monkey. They made the following remarkable observations:

> The animal does not exhibit the reactions generally associated with anger and fear. It approaches humans and animals, animate as well as inanimate objects, without hesitation, and although there are no motor deficits, tends to examine them by mouth rather than by use of the hands … Various tests do not show any impairment in visual acuity or in the ability to localize visually the position of objects in space. However, the monkey seems to be unable to recognize objects by the

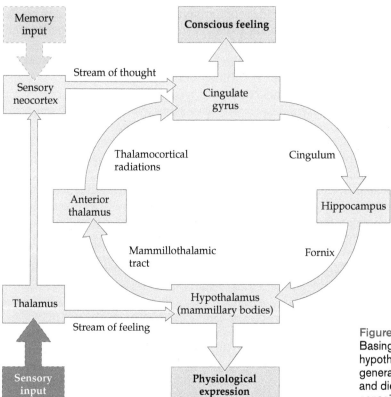

Figure 10.7 The Papez circuit for emotional processing Basing his work on known anatomical projections to the hypothalamus, Papez described a fundamental circuit for generating emotions involving portions of the limbic forebrain and diencephalon. The cingulate gyrus was assumed to signal conscious emotional feelings.

sense of sight. The hungry animal, if confronted with a variety of objects, will, for example, indiscriminately pick up a comb, a bakelite knob, a sunflower seed, a screw, a stick, a piece of apple, a live snake, a piece of banana, and a live rat. Each object is transferred to the mouth and then discarded if not edible.

H. KLÜVER AND P. BUCY 1939

These observations led to the description of a new syndrome, and its extension to human patients, that included loss of fear, visual agnosia, hyperorality, altered food preferences, hypersexuality, and increased exploratory behaviors. This constellation of behavioral changes is now known as **Klüver-Bucy syndrome**. The major hallmark of this disorder is the inability to evaluate the emotional and motivational significance of objects in the environment, particularly by the sense of sight. Because the brain ablation in the affected monkeys included the hippocampus (the only component of the Papez circuit that resides in the temporal lobe), damage to this structure was hypothesized to underlie the behavioral deficits.

Subsequent studies showed this speculation to be incorrect, primarily because selective damage to the hippocampus in monkeys yielded few signs of Klüver-Bucy syndrome. Instead, disconnection of the frontal lobe and other areas from the amygdala, which resides just anterior to the hippocampus in the medial temporal lobe, is critical for producing aspects of the syndrome. Regardless, Klüver and Bucy's dramatic behavioral descriptions, combined with Papez's neuroanatomical circuit, provided the backdrop for the further refinement of emotion theory that dominated the rest of the twentieth century—namely, the **limbic system theory**.

The limbic system theory and its challenges

As a clinician in the tradition of psychosomatic medicine, Paul MacLean, working in the 1940s through the 1970s, offered a compelling neurobiological account of emotion that integrated the ideas of Cannon and Bard, Klüver and Bucy, Papez, and even Freud. MacLean argued that evolutionarily older (three-layered) cortex in the medial wall of the forebrain (as well as the underlying subcortical structures) played a general role in body functions related to survival. He renamed what had been called the rhinencephalon (or "smell brain," because of its prominent olfactory connections) the "visceral brain." The visceral brain included structures in the Papez circuit, Broca's limbic lobe (including pyriform, rhinal, subcallosal, and parasplenial cortices), and subcortical nuclei like the septum and portions of the basal ganglia (**Figure 10.8A**). Later, MacLean added the amygdala and orbitofrontal cortex to the visceral brain and called this set of structures the *limbic system*. The centerpiece of the limbic system concept is the **hippocampus**, which contains an orderly array of pyramidal neurons that MacLean thought of as a "keyboard" upon which the emotions played. In this conceptualization, the hippocampus was the seat of emotional feelings and the integrator of emotional reactions.

Despite the continued prominence of this theory, it has come under increasing scrutiny in recent years. One problem with the limbic system concept is that there are no independent anatomical criteria for defining the regions within the system and those without. Although the limbic system theory grew out of Papez's circuit model of hypothalamic connectivity, many brainstem nuclei that are connected directly to the hypothalamus were not included. Similarly, on functional grounds, many brainstem nuclei are directly involved in autonomic regulation but are curiously absent from the visceral-brain concept.

In short, MacLean's collection of brain areas does not have the same degree of functional or structural coherence as do other brain systems (e.g., the sensory

(A)

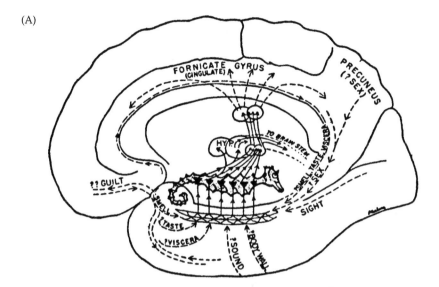

Figure 10.8 **Components of the limbic forebrain and their connections** (A) MacLean's original 1949 drawing of the visceral brain is reproduced here. In MacLean's interpretation, the cornerstone of this system was the hippocampus ("seahorse") and its connections to the hypothalamus. (B) More contemporary views of emotion emphasize the role of anterior sectors of this circuit (shaded in green), including the amygdala, orbitofrontal cortex, ventromedial and orbital prefrontal cortex, and hypothalamus. These components were added later by MacLean, and their inclusion may help explain the longevity of the limbic system concept. By contrast, posterior components (shaded in blue)—including the hippocampus, posterior cingulate cortex, and their diencephalic connections—are more critical for other cognitive functions. (A from MacLean 1949.)

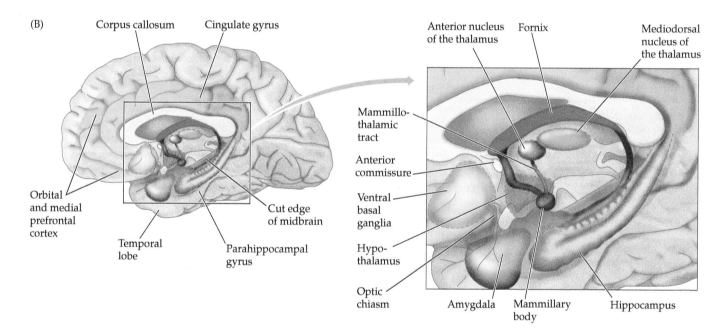

systems described in Chapters 3 and 4). In addition, several limbic system structures are now thought to have primarily cognitive rather than emotional or visceral functions. Most important, selective damage to the hippocampus, the cornerstone of the limbic system theory, yields profound impairments in declarative memory and spatial cognition (see Chapters 8 and 9), and has less impact on emotion.

Given the abundant evidence, described in earlier chapters, indicating that brain regions rarely, if ever, have a single function, a monolithic system is unlikely to be responsible for all aspects of emotional processing. Some investigators have taken the position that the limbic system theory should be abandoned altogether, arguing that a better strategy might be to decompose the overarching concept of emotion into constituent parts to look for more specific emotion systems in the brain (as has been done in other domains of cognitive neuroscience, such as memory; see Chapters 8 and 9). As discussed in the following section, research on fear has provided a good example of this approach.

Nonetheless, MacLean's concept of the limbic system has had a lasting impact, perhaps because it includes a number of brain regions whose emotional functions have stood the test of time, including the amygdala, the ventromedial and orbitofrontal cortex, and the rostral and ventral anterior cingulate gyrus (Figure 10.8B). The affective functions of these structures, as well as other paralimbic and neocortical regions not emphasized by the limbic system theory, are described in the following sections.

Contemporary Approaches to Studying the Neurobiology of Emotion

Methodological constraints have always made it a challenge to probe the affective function of limbic and diencephalic structures emphasized in early neurobiological theories, especially in human subjects. In the 1970s and 1980s, researchers focused on characterizing the affective functions of the neocortex, given the technological ability to record scalp EEG and to localize cortical lesions more accurately. With the advent of more advanced brain monitoring, imaging, and perturbation methods, researchers have made significant inroads into studying deeper brain regions and characterizing their relationships to cortical processing and concomitant changes in autonomic activity and emotional behavior. This surge in research activity has led to a number of different hypotheses about how specific aspects of emotion are mediated in the brain.

Hemispheric-asymmetry hypotheses

The marked expansion of neocortex in primate evolution affords complexity and flexibility not only in cognitive and executive functions but also in social and emotional behavior (see Chapters 11 and 13). As lateralization of cortical function has become a focus of investigation in recent decades, researchers have taken advantage of EEG, brain imaging, and lesion studies to examine the differential contributions of the right and left cerebral hemispheres to emotional processing.

Studies of neurological patients with unilateral damage to the neocortex suggest that the right cerebral hemisphere is specialized for mediating several aspects of emotion (sometimes called the **right-hemisphere hypothesis**). Patients with right-hemisphere damage tend to have more difficulty than patients with left-hemisphere damage in emotion perception tasks, as well as in the production of emotion in facial expression and speech prosody (Figure 10.9). As discussed in Chapter 12, language areas in the right hemisphere are organized for speech **prosody** (the inflections, rhythm, and stress in vocal sounds) in a way that parallels left-hemisphere organization for analysis of the content of speech. Healthy individuals are better able to discriminate vocal and facial affect when stimuli are presented to the left ear or left visual field and thus initially processed by the right hemisphere (but recall from Chapters 3 and 4

Figure 10.9 Lateralization of affective aspects of sound stimuli Neuropsychological studies reveal right-hemisphere lateralization of affective aspects of speech and other sound stimuli, such as music. (A) Anterior areas, centered near the right hemisphere (the homologue of Broca's area; see Chapter 12), are important for generating prosody in one's own speech. Damage to this region causes motor aphasia. (B) Posterior areas, centered near the right-hemisphere homologue of Wernicke's area (see Chapter 12), are important for perceiving and evaluating prosody in someone else's voice. Damage to this region causes sensory aphasia. (C) Patients with widespread damage to the right hemisphere lack both functions; they are unable to interpret affective intonation of the speech of others, and they speak with a flat affective tone. Damage to this region causes global aphasia. (After Ross 1997.)

(A) Motor

(B) Sensory

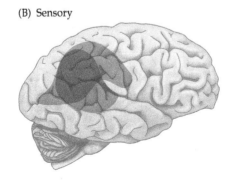

(C) Global

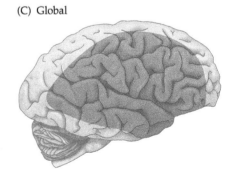

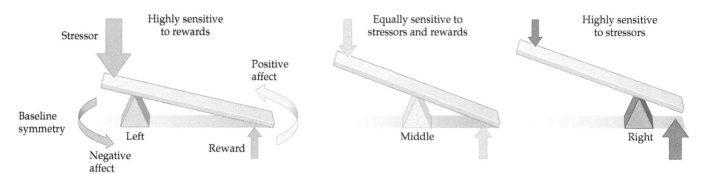

Figure 10.10 A schematic of prefrontal asymmetries in emotion This version of the hemispheric-asymmetry hypothesis argues that individuals vary in the degree to which they are sensitive to stressors and rewards. Across individuals, baseline differences in resting prefrontal EEG asymmetries promote motivational response tendencies upon an emotional trigger. Most individuals have an affective processing style that is relatively balanced, reflecting equal sensitivity to stressors and rewards in the environment (middle panel). Some individuals are predisposed to be highly sensitive to stressors, meaning that a small stressor will elicit a large change in negative affect and will trigger behavioral inhibition or avoidance (right panel). Conversely, these stress-sensitive individuals will need a relatively large reward to generate positive affect and approach behaviors. Still others show the opposite pattern: they are predisposed to react to rewards and generate positive affect/approach behaviors to small pleasures but need a much larger stressor to elicit negative affect/avoidant responses (left panel).

that lateralized sensory processing is not absolute). The left half of the face also tends to be more spontaneously expressive than the right, although this effect varies among individuals. Given that the right hemisphere has been associated with visuospatial and synthetic processing strategies, some of these findings may reflect lateralization of more basic functions, such as the holistic (global) processing of stimuli or the integration of information over longer timescales.

A different lateralization model—the **valence hypothesis**—proposes that the left and right hemispheres are specialized for positive and negative emotions, respectively. According to this hypothesis, positive emotions serve more linguistic and social functions (e.g., expressing romantic love, friendly affection, or pride) than do negative emotions, which tend to be reactive and survival-related. In this scheme, the left hemisphere is more adept at implementing the social-display rules of positive emotions and linking them with communicative functions. A more recent incarnation of the valence hypothesis restricts the hemispheric asymmetries to the experience and expression stages of emotional processing. According to this hybrid model, right posterior sensory regions are dominant for the *evaluation* of all emotions. However, the *experience* and *expression* of emotions is postulated to be asymmetrical, such that left frontal regions are dominant for positive emotions and right frontal regions for negative emotions.

EEG studies have provided some evidence for the valence hypothesis of emotion asymmetry. Recall from Chapter 2 that power in the alpha band (8 to 12 hertz) of the EEG is inversely related to cortical activity such that low values represent high activity levels. Alpha-band activity recorded over the prefrontal cortex tends to exhibit a leftward asymmetry (low values, high activity) in response to stimuli with positive valence, and a rightward asymmetry in response to negative stimuli. However, the emotion-related prefrontal asymmetry across the hemispheres varies considerably from one individual to the next (Figure 10.10). Interestingly, this asymmetry extends to baseline (resting) activity when no emotional stimuli are presented. Most individuals exhibit a symmetrical frontal EEG response and report having a more evenhanded affective disposition. Nonetheless, when it is found, the pattern of asymmetry is stable across

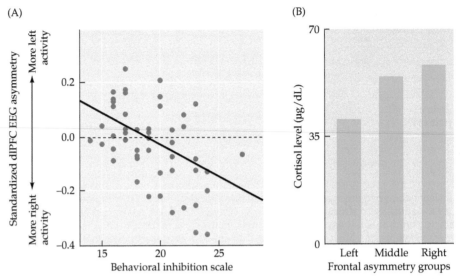

Figure 10.11 Emotional reactivity predicted by hemispheric asymmetries in EEG activity (A) The degree of behavioral inhibition in social contexts is correlated with the degree of rightward asymmetry in resting EEG activity recorded over dorsolateral prefrontal cortex (dlPFC). (B) In 1-year-old rhesus monkeys, basal stress hormone (cortisol) levels are also positively correlated with the degree of rightward prefrontal EEG asymmetry. (A after Shackman et al. 2010; B after Kalin et al. 1998.)

individuals over testing sessions. The asymmetry is thought to predispose an individual to react emotionally in a positive or negative way, given an appropriate elicitor. In shy or socially inhibited individuals, the pattern is skewed toward the right hemisphere (Figure 10.11A). In depression, a reduction of the leftward prefrontal asymmetry has been related to the accompanying **anhedonia**, an inability to experience positive affect as intensely as healthy individuals.

Because alpha-band EEG activity during resting conditions is relatively easy to measure in children, this neural index has also been used in developmental studies of temperament. The term **temperament** refers to the habitual emotional responses that characterize aspects of an individual's personality. One such personality factor is related to the degree of motoric and emotional reactivity to novel situations. Consistent with its role in social emotions, the degree of leftward prefrontal asymmetry predicts the extent to which toddlers engage in play behavior with novel toys and other children. Conversely, the degree of rightward prefrontal asymmetry predicts crying behavior when infants are separated from their mothers and placed in a room with novel toys or other children for a short period of time. In infant monkeys, the degree of rightward prefrontal asymmetry correlates with baseline stress hormone levels present during the morning diurnal peak in cortisol release (Figure 10.11B; see Box 10B for a description of the systems most affected by stress). This line of research emphasizes the **individual difference** approach to characterizing how variability in emotional behavior across individuals relates to brain function. This approach can uncover brain-behavior relationships that would otherwise be overlooked when data analysis techniques rely on averaging across all research subjects in a group.

Other studies have indicated that the prefrontal EEG asymmetry in the alpha band may reflect motivational tendencies of approach and avoidance rather than simply positive and negative valence. Whereas most positive emotions are associated with approach behavior, most negative emotions are associated with avoidance behavior. Anger is an exception to this general rule.

In offensive anger, one feels a sense of control over the outcome of the conflict and approaches the offender. Offensive anger is accompanied by a leftward prefrontal EEG asymmetry. This asymmetry is reduced if one feels empathic toward the offender because empathy diminishes approach tendencies associated with hostile attitudes. In contrast, rightward EEG asymmetry is found during defensive anger, when one feels a sense of helplessness over the conflict and tends to avoid the offender. Thus, the role of prefrontal asymmetries in studies of temperament and emotion may be better explained by dimensional theories that link specific emotions to fundamental motivational axes of approach and avoidance (see Figure 10.3A).

Vertical integration models: Fear acquisition

Whereas the limbic system theory emphasizes the contributions of deeper regions in the brain and hemispheric-asymmetry hypotheses emphasize neocortical contributions, some researchers have focused on relating these levels of processing with each other and with changes in the body. This approach defines **vertical integration models**, so called because they attempt to provide an integrative account of emotional processing across many levels of the nervous system. One of the best-characterized vertical integration models is based on studies of **fear conditioning**. As introduced in Chapter 8, the principles of classical and operant conditioning can explain in part how animals extract regularities that indicate when and where something positively or negatively reinforcing is likely to occur in the environment. Unlike the gradual acquisition of habits or motor skills, conditioning responses that entail emotion, particularly those involving fear, can be quite rapid, presumably because of their immediate consequences for survival. Understanding the mechanisms that mediate the acquisition and extinction of fear in response to environmental threats also has important implications for the treatment of anxiety disorders.

Studies in rodents have established a detailed understanding of the neuroanatomy, neurophysiology, and molecular signaling that underlie the acquisition of fear elicited by relevant cues and contexts. In a typical paradigm, rats are presented with an auditory conditioned stimulus (CS) that predicts the occurrence of a mild foot shock, which is the unconditioned stimulus (US). The testing chamber where conditioning occurs is the context. After a few CS-US pairings, rats exhibit a constellation of changes in physiology and behavior in response to the CS (the tone presented alone) that are adaptive in the sense of preparing the animal to deal with the impending threat. These changes indicate a state of fear and include the potentiation of startle reflexes, a cessation of exploratory behavior (freezing), and engagement of the sympathetic fight-or-flight response (pupillary dilation, increased blood pressure, increased heart and breathing rates; see Box 10A for a review of the autonomic nervous system). The conditioned response is elicited not only by the presence of the CS itself (cued fear) but also by features of the environment, such as the testing chamber where the conditioning episode took place (contextual fear).

The acquisition and expression of conditioned fear require the integrity of the **amygdala** (Figure 10.12). Rats with bilateral lesions to the basolateral and central nuclei of the amygdala are dramatically impaired in acquiring conditioned fear responses to both cues and contexts. To rapidly detect threats and other pertinent sensory stimuli, the amygdala gets direct input from the thalamus that bypasses the primary sensory cortical reception areas. Electrophysiological recordings from lateral amygdala neurons show conditioned increases in firing rates that occur within 15 milliseconds of CS onset in some cells, implying mediation via the direct thalamo-amygdala pathway. Long-term potentiation (LTP), a potential electrophysiological signature of learning (see Chapter 8), is also observed in this afferent pathway. Alterations in gene expression and

Figure 10.12 **Neuroanatomy of conditioned fear learning** A key station in this process is the amygdala, which integrates information from subcortical and cortical processing pathways (see the text). The hippocampus is important in contextual fear acquisition and the context-dependent recovery of fear after extinction training. The ventromedial prefrontal cortex suppresses fear responses when they are no longer adaptive (i.e., during extinction training) via inhibitory connections within specific subnuclei of the amygdala. Feedback connections between structures are not indicated. ITC, intercalated cells.

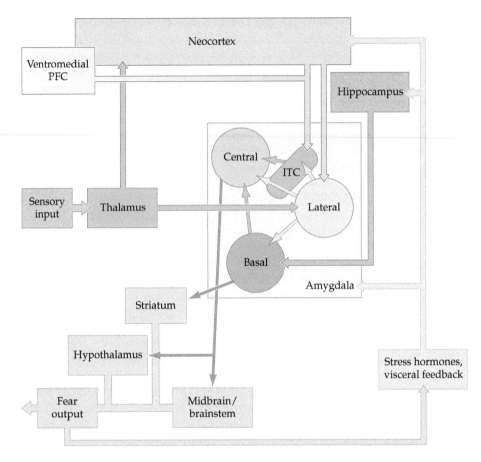

protein synthesis further strengthen synaptic connections related to this sort of conditioning as a means of consolidating memories of the associations that elicit fear. Studies in rodents indicate that activation of the rapid subcortical pathway is sufficient to evoke fear reactions to simple stimuli, although the extent to which this pathway contributes to emotions in primates, including humans, remains unclear.

This "fast" input route to the amygdala is capable of only crude sensory discrimination, however, and more sophisticated perceptual analysis reaches the amygdala somewhat later via cortical pathways. The rapid subcortical pathway may prime the amygdala to more effectively process the additional information that follows from the slower cortical route after the initial detection of a potentially significant stimulus arising from the environment. This parallel anatomical arrangement evolved presumably because of the advantages of triggering emotional responses more quickly than if information were processed solely by cortical sensory pathways. Synaptic plasticity in cortico-amygdala pathways following a threatening encounter permits alterations in long-term sensory representations that can facilitate the detection of similar threats in the future. Estimates of the number of primary, secondary, and tertiary cortical projections in macaque monkeys indicate that the amygdala is the most densely interconnected structure in the primate forebrain. Thus, the amygdala can exert a powerful influence over other cognitive, sensory, and motor systems of the brain to enable an organism to behaviorally adapt to and retain information about a threat to its survival.

The critical role of the amygdala in fear conditioning is also evident in humans. Patients with amygdala damage show diminished conditioned fear

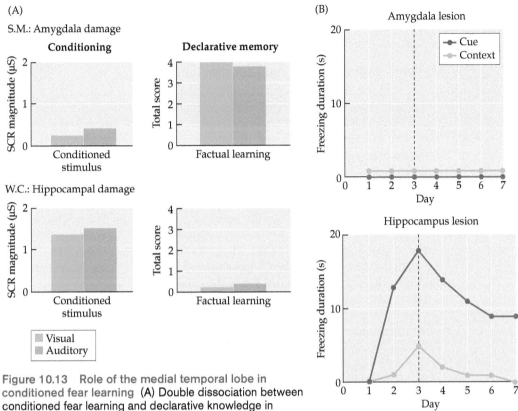

Figure 10.13 Role of the medial temporal lobe in conditioned fear learning (A) Double dissociation between conditioned fear learning and declarative knowledge in patients with selective damage to the amygdala and hippocampus. Patient S.M., who has bilateral amygdala damage, shows intact factual knowledge of the predictive relationship between the conditioned stimulus (CS) and the unconditioned stimulus (US) but fails to exhibit conditioned skin conductance responses (SCRs). In contrast, patient W.C. has bilateral hippocampal damage and shows the opposite pattern—that is, intact SCRs to conditioned fear cues but no factual knowledge about the predictive relationship between the CS and the US. (B) A similar dissociation is observed in rats. Rats with amygdala damage (top) fail to acquire conditioned freezing (immobility) responses to both cues and contexts that predict a foot shock. Rats with dorsal hippocampal damage (bottom) are selectively impaired on forming links between the reinforcement and the context in which it took place. Binding information to contextual cues is a hallmark of declarative memory. Dashed vertical line indicates change from acquisition training to extinction training. (A after Bechara et al. 1995; B after Phillips and LeDoux 1992.)

responses, including reduced fear-potentiated startle and **skin conductance responses**, or **SCRs** (see Box 10A). These deficits persist even when the patient is able to state the predictive properties of the CS, indicating that declarative knowledge about the learning parameters is not by itself sufficient to generate appropriate defensive behavior (**Figure 10.13**). This evidence suggests that simple forms of fear conditioning can be partly dissociated from declarative memory—a finding supported by the fact that fear-relevant stimuli (e.g., angry facial displays, or snakes) can be conditioned subliminally, without conscious awareness, in healthy participants.

Neuroimaging studies in humans show activity in the amygdala, thalamus, and anterior cingulate cortex (among other regions) during the acquisition phase of fear conditioning. Moreover, the degree of amygdala activation in individual participants correlates with the magnitude of fear learning expressed physiologically (usually in terms of skin conductance amplitude). Taken together, these findings provide strong evidence for the importance of the amygdala and related structures in warning animals of impending danger by associating the emotion of fear with potentially threatening circumstances and generating appropriate fight-or-flight responses through the activation of downstream subcortical structures.

Vertical integration models: Fear modification

Just as fear mandates changes in emotional response, it is also important to revise fear responses when experience indicates that potentially threatening circumstances are no longer present. Indeed, the persistence of fear responses to stimuli that are no longer real threats is a hallmark of some anxiety disorders, including phobias and posttraumatic stress disorder (see Introductory Box). This unwarranted persistence of fear has been termed **emotional perseveration** and is analogous to the continued deployment of cognitive strategies when they are no longer appropriate in problem-solving tasks (see Chapter 13). In fear-conditioning protocols, the fear value of a CS can be changed simply by removing the negative reinforcer during the ongoing training. Through repeated presentation of the CS without the US (e.g., foot shock), the animal learns that the meaning of the CS has changed. The conditioned fear responses then subside in a process called **fear extinction**.

Extinction depends on the integrity of the ventromedial prefrontal cortex (vmPFC). Rats with damage to this region, while able to acquire fear normally, take much longer to extinguish a conditioned fear response than do controls. This area influences the activity of neurons in the amygdala, and stimulation of this pathway in conjunction with presentation of a CS is sufficient to suppress amygdala responses and reduce conditioned fear behavior. In humans, vmPFC damage leads to difficulty reversing stimulus-reinforcer relationships, and fMRI activity in this region correlates with the retention of extinction behavior. Because of the important implications of these prefrontal-amygdala interactions for the suppression of irrelevant fears, clinicians have had a keen interest in targeting pharmacological agents to mimic or augment these effects in patients with anxiety disorders.

Given its role in spatial processing and declarative memory (see Chapter 9), the hippocampus is a likely site for the mediation of some aspects of **contextual fear conditioning**, in which fears are associated with specific places or circumstances. Rats with dorsal hippocampal lesions can be conditioned normally to discrete cues but fail to generate and retain fear responses to the context in which the training took place. Similarly, amnesia patients with hippocampal damage exhibit conditioned SCRs to a discrete CS that predicts shock delivery, but they do not retain information about the contextual details of the conditioning episode (see Figure 10.13). The hippocampus makes similar contributions to both emotional and nonemotional forms of learning and memory that depend on associating pertinent information with the contexts in which the learning occurs. This similarity makes it inappropriate to consider the hippocampus a structure specifically dedicated to emotional processing, as was hypothesized within the limbic system theory of emotion.

Interoception and the somatic marker hypothesis

As the tumor grew bigger, it compressed both frontal lobes upward, from below ... The surgery was a success ... What was to prove less felicitous was the turn in Elliot's personality ... He needed prompting to get started in the morning and prepare to go to work. Once at work he was unable to manage his time properly ... Or he might interrupt the activity he had engaged [in], to turn to something he found more captivating at that particular moment ... One might say that Elliot had become irrational concerning the larger frame of behavior ... Elliot's job was terminated ... Elliot charged ahead with new pastimes and business ventures. In one enterprise, he teamed up with a disreputable character. Several warnings from friends were of no avail, and the scheme ended in bankruptcy … There was a first divorce. Then a brief marriage … Then another divorce. Then more drifting, without a source of income … Elliot emerged as a man with a normal intellect who was unable to decide properly, especially when the decision involved personal or social matters.

A. R. DAMASIO 1994

Observations of patients like these with damage to the orbital and ventromedial prefrontal cortex led neurologist Antonio Damasio to propose a theory about the role of emotion in decision making. This somatic marker hypothesis attempts to explain how the brain and body signal affective information that is used to guide everyday decision making. Damasio argues that the vmPFC contains indexes that link factual knowledge and bioregulatory states associated with a particular event. When a similar situation is subsequently encountered, prior knowledge calls up the relevant somatic markers, which include autonomic, endocrine, and musculoskeletal changes that constitute a particular emotional state. The vmPFC triggers reactivation of the somatosensory pattern that describes the appropriate emotion through connections to emotion-eliciting structures, such as the amygdala. Such reactivation can occur directly through a body loop that includes expression of the appropriate visceral response, or indirectly by simulating the somatosensory pattern in the insula and somatosensory cortex but without necessarily evoking physical changes in the body (called an "as if" loop).

By evoking these somatosensory patterns, reasoning and decision-making processes are constrained to options that are marked as qualitatively good or bad. In this way, somatic markers serve as a heuristic rule of thumb that permits the organism to make optimal decisions efficiently, without elaborate logical weighing of the utility of various response options. This hypothesis makes the important claim that the reactivation of emotional states facilitates logical reasoning, and without guidance from these states, as in the case of Elliot, everyday decisions are costly. Note that this theory, like James's, emphasizes the important role of feedback from the body (or, at least, body representations) in the generation of emotional states.

Experimental evidence to support aspects of this hypothesis came from studies using the Iowa Gambling Task. In this task, participants are provided an endowment and are told to try to maximize their profit by choosing from one of four decks of cards that have different monetary gains or losses associated with them (Figure 10.14). Unbeknownst to the subjects, card decks A and B are disadvantageous in that selecting from them yields larger short-term rewards but also very large occasional punishers that lead to long-term losses. Decks C and D, by contrast, are advantageous in that they yield smaller short-term rewards but also smaller punishers, leading to higher long-term gains. Over 100 training trials, healthy subjects tend to stop choosing the high-risk decks and reap a monetary reward, whereas patients with vmPFC damage continue to select cards from the risky decks and lose their endowment. When selecting from the risky decks, healthy subjects exhibit an SCR, which Damasio argues is a somatic marker for risky actions in the context of this task, whereas vmPFC patients do not. According to the theory, patients with vmPFC damage have a compromised ability to learn from somatic marker links to risky actions, leading to nonoptimal choices and poor decision-making abilities.

In this scheme, the insula is a key brain region for monitoring the physiological state of the organism (called interoception), and for storing visceral and skeletomotor representations of emotional states that are reinstated

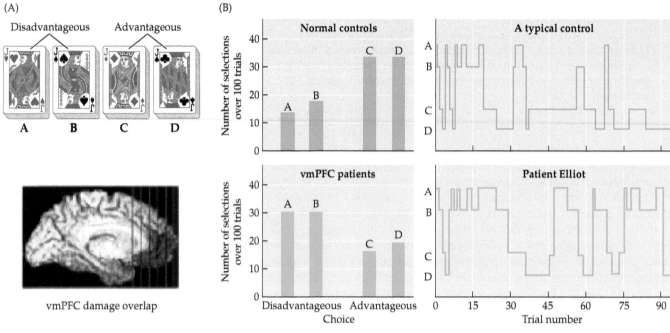

(A)

Disadvantageous   Advantageous

A   **B**   **C**   **D**

vmPFC damage overlap

(B)

Normal controls

vmPFC patients

A typical control

Patient Elliot

(C)

- Controls
- vmPFC patients

Anticipatory SCRs

Figure 10.14 **The Iowa Gambling Task** (A) Across 100 trials, participants turn over cards from four decks that are associated with monetary losses or gains. Selecting cards from decks A and B is disadvantageous, resulting in long-term monetary losses; choosing from decks C and D is advantageous, resulting in long-term monetary gains. (B) Healthy control subjects learn to adapt their choices over time, choosing mostly from the advantageous decks. In contrast, patients with vmPFC damage (inset) continue to choose from the disadvantageous decks throughout the task. (C) Choosing from the risky decks (A and B) elicits anticipatory skin conductance responses (see Box 10A for an explanation of the methodology) from control subjects but not patients. The somatic marker hypothesis argues that such visceral input to decision-making systems is important in order for the organism to learn the motivational value of response options. μS, microsiemens. (A brain image from Anderson et. al 1999; B,C after Bechara et al. 1994.)

during decision making. The insula is an evolutionarily older cortical region that lies hidden beneath the confluence of the frontal and temporal lobes on the brain's lateral surface. A posterior-to-anterior gradient in the insula provides a pathway for homeostatic regulation (Figure 10.15A). The posterior insula receives ascending information from pain and temperature pathways via the ventromedial thalamus, and parallel input from the cranial parasympathetic nerves, including the vagus and glossopharyngeal nerves, through brainstem projection sites. Information from the posterior insula is fed forward to the mid-insula, where it is integrated with exteroceptive input from somatosensory cortices and limbic regions, such as the amygdala. In primates, the anterior insula contains an additional level of integration, particularly in the right hemisphere, which is interconnected with the anterior cingulate cortex, orbitofrontal cortex, and dorsolateral prefrontal cortex. At each station along the way there is an increasingly complex rerepresentation of the body state that ultimately informs decision making and, in humans, conscious awareness of one's motivational and affective state.

Evidence supporting a role for the insula in body state monitoring and awareness includes studies that correlate anterior insula activation with the ability to detect one's own heartbeat (Figure 10.15B). Moreover, anterior insula activation during fMRI correlates with the subjective experience of temperature changes induced by a thermal probe applied to the hand. Insula damage in some patients who are smokers can even dampen internal cravings for cigarette

(A)

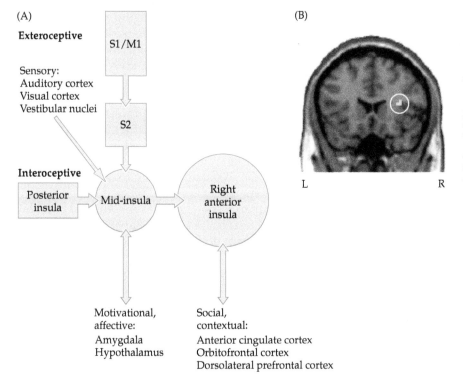

Exteroceptive

S1/M1

Sensory:
Auditory cortex
Visual cortex
Vestibular nuclei

S2

Interoceptive

Posterior insula → Mid-insula → Right anterior insula

Motivational, affective:
Amygdala
Hypothalamus

Social, contextual:
Anterior cingulate cortex
Orbitofrontal cortex
Dorsolateral prefrontal cortex

(B)

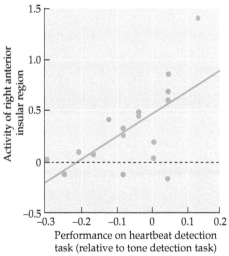

L   R

Activity of right anterior insular region

Performance on heartbeat detection task (relative to tone detection task)

Figure 10.15 Interoception and the insula (A) The insula receives information about the physiological state of the body from ascending visceral pathways to posterior sectors. These sectors then feed forward into the mid-insula, where exteroceptive inputs from somatosensory (S1, S2) and motor (M1) cortices are integrated with motivational and affective inputs. In primates, there is an additional body representation in the anterior insula, particularly the right hemisphere, which integrates visceral-state information with anterior cingulate and prefrontal cortex regions to guide goal-directed behaviors. Each level of body state representation is thought to be more complex and ultimately leads to the conscious experience of motivational and affective state in humans. (B) Across subjects, the magnitude of right anterior insula activity correlates with accuracy in detecting one's own heartbeat relative to a control task. During the heartbeat detection task, participants determined whether or not a series of tones was timed to be in synchrony with their heartbeat (which was achieved by a computer trigger from a pulse meter). The control task required participants to detect a tone that was deviant in pitch from its predecessors in a series. (A after Craig 2007; B after Critchley et al. 2004.)

smoking and promote abstinence; other patients lose their ability to appreciate music, presumably because of difficulties in evaluating the affective meaning of visceral responses to musical passages.

Although some researchers have argued for alternative interpretations of the Iowa Gambling Task and have criticized the "as if" loop clause, which makes the hypothesis hard to falsify, the somatic marker hypothesis is important in bringing the James-Lange idea of bodily feedback into contemporary neuroscience and in emphasizing the potentially beneficial effects of emotion, including negative emotion, in complex cognitive functions. Other contributions of the prefrontal cortex and insula to affective and risky decision making are covered in Chapter 14.

In search of categories of emotional experience

When humans consciously describe their affective state in response to the common question "How do you feel?" they often use verbal labels for specific emotional categories, such as those depicted in Figure 10.2. What information conveyed by the nervous system leads to this subjective experience of an emotion? While the interoceptive pathways just described suggest a general means of intuiting one's emotional state, whether specific emotions have unique autonomic or neural signatures remains unanswered.

The psychological theories reviewed at the beginning of the chapter predict different ways in which neuroscientists could proceed to answer this question. Recall that dimensional theories suggest that emotional categories emerge from points in a two-dimensional space formed by crossing axes of arousal and valence (or related motivational constructs of approach and avoidance; see Figure 10.3). According to these models, insights would be gained by characterizing brain regions that selectively code for these dimensions. The hemispheric-asymmetry models described earlier use this approach and have found some evidence, derived largely from alpha-band EEG recordings or observations of patients with larger cortical lesions, for the signaling of different valences across the hemispheres of the frontal lobe (with a preference for positive emotions in the left hemisphere and negative ones in the right). However, recall that most individuals do not show strong EEG asymmetries; indeed, neuroimaging studies of healthy individuals have failed to find a clear dichotomy between positive and negative affect signaling using more spatially refined hemodynamic measures.

In line with categorical theories of emotion, other studies support the idea of neural specialization for discrete emotions in limbic and paralimbic brain regions. For instance, the insula appears to be particularly important for the emotion disgust, which is related to its role in gustatory processing (see Chapter 4). As Figure 10.2 shows, facial reactions of disgust, which curl the upper lip, wrinkle the nose, and protrude the tongue, have evolved in part to facilitate the physical ejection of toxic substances from the oral cavity. Consistent with this idea, disgust is associated with the parasympathetic circuitry that mediates nausea and the vomiting reflex. Some patients with damage to the insula are specifically impaired in their ability to recognize facial and vocal expressions of disgust compared to other emotions (Figure 10.16A). Functional neuroimaging studies have confirmed involvement of the insula (and other brain areas) in disgust, including the recognition of someone else reacting to a disgusting situation. Investigators conducting other studies have argued that, given its role in interoception more generally, the insula contributes to the experience of many emotions, for which disgust is a particularly good example because of its evolutionary association with the rejection of toxic substances (see also the discussion of empathy in Chapter 11).

In a similar vein, the amygdala has been specifically linked to fear in numerous studies, including the fear-conditioning research described earlier. Further evidence comes from studies of facial-expression processing in amygdala-lesioned patients, such as S.M., a patient described by Antonio Damasio and his colleagues. In addition to her fear-conditioning deficits (see Figure 10.13A), S.M. has a specific deficit in recognizing fear in facial expressions. Patient S.M. has congenital damage to the amygdala caused by a rare disease (**Urbach-Wiethe syndrome**) that can sometimes produce calcification of structures in the medial temporal lobe. The recognition of facial affect in other amygdala-lesioned patients, while pronounced for fear, can extend to other negative emotions, such as anger and surprise (Figure 10.16B). S.M. has particular difficulty extracting information from the eye region of the face, which is critical for identifying the "wide-eyed" feature in expressions of fear. When directed to attend to the eyes alone, S.M.'s ability to identify fear in faces improves. Thus, her deficit in recognizing fear may be secondary to an underlying problem in attending to a facial feature relevant to the evaluation of some emotions. This insight makes strong claims about fear specificity difficult to defend, despite the clear relationship between the amygdala and defensive systems in the brain.

Neuroimaging studies that compare brain activity in response to discrete emotions have yielded mixed results regarding the signaling specificity in regions like the insula and amygdala. Recent meta-analytic studies that have pooled data from hundreds of research articles have failed to find obvious markers of specific emotions. Indeed, involvement of particular structures like the amygdala or insula seems to depend on the nature of the task (e.g., whether it emphasizes emotional evaluation versus experience), the intensity of the emotions elicited, and a host of other factors. Such context-dependent findings challenge efforts to identify neural correlates of emotion categories. Indeed, a lack of clear evidence has compelled some researchers to abandon the notion of emotion categories as having unique neural signatures.

Neuroscientists interested in emotion are now considering novel approaches to identifying the representation of specific emotional states. One strategy is to use multivariate statistics to reveal more complex patterns of neural and autonomic activity that carry information to differentiate emotions. Recall from Chapter 2 that statistical tools such as pattern classifiers can yield additional

(A)

Recognition of Emotion in Facial Expression

FACIAL EXPRESSION	FACIAL SET 1	FACIAL SET 2
Anger	9/10	5/8
Contempt	–	3/8
Disgust	5/10*	4/8**
Fear	7/10	8/10
Happiness	10/10	8/8
Sadness	8/10	8/8
Surprise	8/10	8/8

Recognition of Emotion in Vocal Expression

VOCAL EXPRESSION	NONVERBAL SOUNDS	EMOTIONAL PROSODY
Anger	10/20	7/10
Disgust	3/20***	4/10
Fear	14/20	8/10
Happiness	14/20	9/10
Sadness	18/20	7/10
Surprise	15/20	–

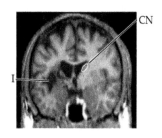

(B)

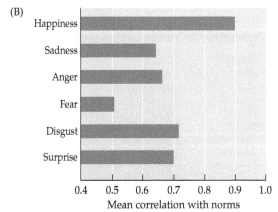

insights into complex data sets by analyzing the simultaneous interaction of many variables. Applying these tools involves training a pattern classifier on a set of biological data to discriminate specific states in response to emotional stimuli (such as responses to happy versus sad music). Once trained, the classifier is then tested on a new set of data (using new subjects or new music passages in the same subjects), and its discrimination accuracy is scored. How the data from different brain regions and autonomic indices are relatively weighted and grouped to correctly classify different emotions can provide important clues to their organizational structure. Emotion categories are likely to be "read out" by different combinations of activity patterns (including neural activity in cortical and limbic areas, as well as autonomic changes) that may be weighted in different ways across emotions to specify feelings. This approach could provide an analytic solution to the Cannon-Bard criticism that autonomic indices may be too undifferentiated to discriminate specific emotions.

Such approaches may help validate psychological theories of emotion that postulate different architectures underlying specific emotional experiences. This goal of affective neuroscience—explaining the basis of conscious feelings—depends on further refinement and integration of psychological theories and advanced neuroscientific methods.

Interactions with Other Cognitive Functions

Concomitant with body and brain responses to emotional elicitors, various cognitive processes are altered to help the organism understand, learn from, and cope with the situation at hand. In this section, we describe how emotional processing regions interact with other brain areas that contribute to perception and attention, learning and memory, and self-regulation.

Emotional influences on perception and attention

Processing sensory information that has emotional significance takes priority over processing inconsequential sensory information. Such prioritization is

Figure 10.16 Consequences of amygdala and insula damage to emotional evaluation (A) Recognition (by a patient known as N.K.) of emotions in facial and vocal expressions. The extent of the lesion in the left insula (I), caudate nucleus (CN), and putamen is indicated. N.K. correctly chooses the label "disgust" on only a small number of trials. Asterisks indicate accuracy levels significantly below those of healthy controls: *, $p < .05$; **, $p < .01$; ***, $p < .001$. (B) Amygdala damage alters ratings of the emotional intensity of facial expressions. Nine patients with damage to the medial temporal lobe, including the amygdala, were shown pictures of actors portraying each of the six basic emotions. They were asked to rate how intensely various emotions were expressed in each face. Their ratings were then correlated with ratings from healthy control participants. The correlations were high for happy faces but lower for several negative emotions, especially fear. (A after Calder et al. 2000; B after Adolphs et al. 1999.)

Figure 10.17 **Perception of fear without awareness** (A) The amygdala signals visually fearful facial expressions, even when stimuli are presented briefly (17 milliseconds) and masked to limit conscious awareness. In these stimuli, fear is conveyed solely by the whites of the eyes (the exposed area of which increases during fear as a result of sympathetically mediated contraction of the subcutaneous muscles in the skin surrounding the eye). (B) In this experiment, participants were shown images of a face projected to one eye and a house to the other eye, creating binocular rivalry (see Chapter 3). Participants indicated on each trial whether they perceived a face or a house. The amygdala exhibited greater activity for fearful than for neutral facial expressions, even when participants reported seeing only the house (i.e., when the fearful face was presumably processed only subcortically as a result of rivalry). (A after Whalen et al. 2004; B from Williams et al. 2004.)

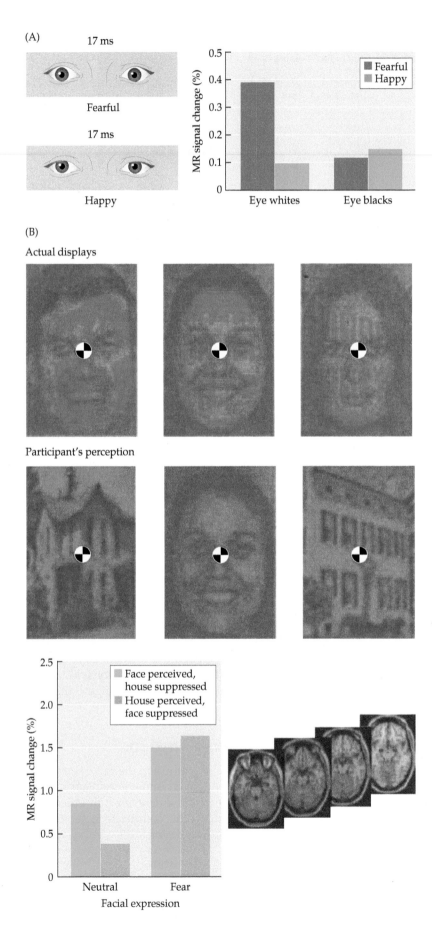

accomplished either by automatic (involuntary) detection of salient features in crowded environments, such as a gun at the scene of a crime; or by a voluntary attentional bias to process such emotional features, as when phobic patients constantly monitor their environment for sources of potential threats (the presence of spiders, for instance).

Experiments examining more automatic aspects of emotional detection typically investigate whether masked visual or auditory emotional stimuli elicit autonomic responses, modulate early-latency ERP components, or elicit hemodynamic responses in sensory and limbic brain areas in functional imaging studies. Of all the emotions, fear has received the most attention because threat in the environment must be detected quickly for defensive reflexes to be effective. Images of biologically relevant stimuli that have high threat value, such as a dangerous animal or the fearful facial expressions of others, elicit amygdala activity and skin conductance responses even when the participant is not consciously aware of the nature of the stimulus being presented (Figure 10.17). In patients with phobias and posttraumatic stress disorder, these patterns of autonomic and brain activity elicited by brief presentations of fear-inducing stimuli are exaggerated, particularly for threatening stimuli relevant to the individual's specific fear or traumatic experience. These findings underscore the contribution of covert perceptual processes to anxiety disorders.

Perceptual awareness can also be limited by *rapid serial visual presentation* (*RSVP*). Recall from Chapter 6 that when two target words are embedded in a rapidly presented stream of stimuli, reporting of the second stimulus is impaired, presumably because attention was still focused on the first one when the second one appeared ("attentional blink"). If only the second word in the pair is emotionally arousing, it can be detected at shorter lag times relative to neutral words (Figure 10.18). Importantly, this emotion-related improvement in performance is not found in patients with left-sided or bilateral lesions of the

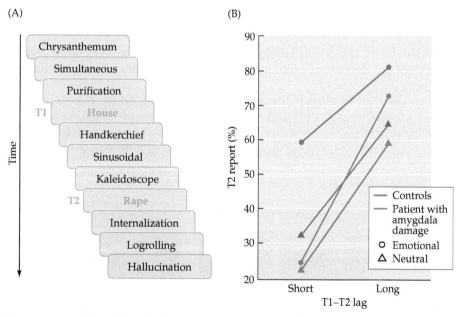

Figure 10.18 Emotional effects on the attentional blink paradigm (A) When target words (green) are embedded in a rapid stream of nontarget distracters (black), detection of the second target (T2) is impaired at short lag times. If the second target has emotionally arousing content, however, detection is facilitated. (B) A patient with bilateral amygdala damage (blue) does not show this effect. (After Anderson and Phelps 2001.)

Figure 10.19 Bidirectional communication between the amygdala and the ventral visual processing stream This drawing illustrates the macaque brain, but the same arrangement is assumed for humans. The amygdala receives input from late stages along this cortical pathway. However, it feeds back to multiple stages of the pathway, including the earliest stage of visual input, the primary visual cortex (V1). Such feedback projections provide a means for emotional states to access and tune perceptual representations.

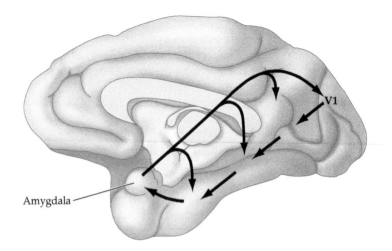

Amygdala

amygdala. The amygdala evidently overrides a capacity-limited perceptual encoding mechanism that allows emotional stimuli to reach awareness more readily.

The anatomical connections between the amygdala and sensory cortices also provide an avenue by which emotion might influence perception. These connections have been best described for vision. Whereas the amygdala receives input from only late stages of visual processing in the inferior temporal cortex, it provides feedback to most stations along the ventral visual stream, including the primary visual (striate) cortex itself (Figure 10.19). Evidence to support this feedback idea has come from an fMRI study of extrastriate responses to facial expressions in epileptic patients with damage to the medial temporal lobe. Although healthy controls and patients with hippocampal lesions showed enhanced activity in the fusiform gyrus and occipital cortex for fearful facial expressions relative to neutral expressions, patients with lesions of the amygdala did not (Figure 10.20). Furthermore, the amount of amygdala damage in the patients was correlated with the level of fusiform gyrus activity in response to fearful faces. These results suggest that the amygdala exerts a remote influence over perceptual processing in sensory regions, consistent with the idea of emotional feedback.

Even though emotional stimuli may initially elicit autonomic and neural responses relatively quickly and automatically, attentional and other cognitive functions are recruited to further evaluate the stimulus and initiate appropriate behavioral reactions. A first step in the allocation of attention is to alert and

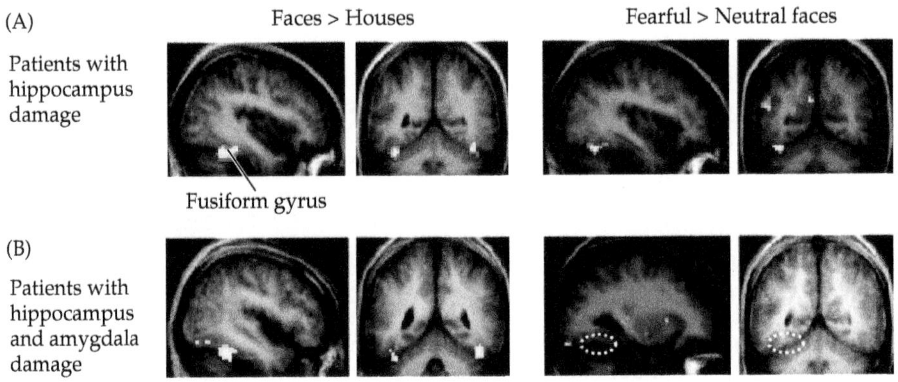

Figure 10.20 Fear-enhanced processing of faces in the fusiform gyrus is reduced in patients with amygdala damage Participants in this experiment were neurological patients with damage to the hippocampus (A) or to the hippocampus and amygdala combined (B). The face-selective area of the fusiform gyrus was first mapped in the patients by identifying where activity for neutral faces was greater than for houses. Then, patients were shown fearful and neutral faces. Patients without amygdala damage showed enhanced activity in the face-selective region of the fusiform gyrus for the fearful faces relative to the neutral ones. This emotional enhancement effect was absent in patients with amygdala damage (dashed ovals). The integrity of the amygdala appears to be important for enhancing representations of faces with emotional expression in visual areas, perhaps by feedback projections. (From Vuilleumier and Driver 2007.)

(A) Faces > Houses   Fearful > Neutral faces

Patients with hippocampus damage

Fusiform gyrus

(B)

Patients with hippocampus and amygdala damage

orient an individual to the emotional trigger. One way this is accomplished is to arrest ongoing behavior by engaging the autonomic nervous system. Automatic effects of emotional stimuli may be implemented directly in the subcortical and ventral cortical pathways connecting sensory and limbic regions, without engagement of the dorsal attentional control network. Indeed, patients with hemineglect syndrome arising from unilateral damage to the right parietal cortex (see Chapter 7) tend to preferentially detect social or predatory threats presented in the neglected hemifield. In other words, the patients' attention can be reflexively drawn toward emotional stimulus features presented in the neglected field, despite the impaired functioning of the frontoparietal attentional control system.

In addition to these automatic influences, limbic regions involved in emotional evaluation have several means of influencing goal-directed attentional processing. For instance, the amygdala can prompt the release of acetylcholine from the basal forebrain, which broadly increases cortical activity through its wide innervation of cortex. These modulatory actions of the amygdala boost various aspects of attention that contribute to appetitive conditioning in rodents and presumably serve similar functions in humans. Also influential are the prefrontal cortex and anterior cingulate interfaces that link the amygdala, insula, and other limbic areas to the dorsal frontoparietal attentional network (Figure 10.21).

Neurologist Helen Mayberg theorizes that the anterior cingulate and related regions in the medial and orbital PFC maintain a balance between ventral emotional and dorsal attentional functions in normal **mood regulation**. According to Mayberg, these activity patterns become skewed in mood disorders such that there is too much emphasis on somatic-emotional processing at the expense of cognitive-attentional operations. Consequently, individuals suffering from depression devote greater-than-normal resources to mulling over sad and stressful experiences, and they have difficulty refocusing attention on short-term behavioral goals. Recent evidence suggests that implanted stimulating

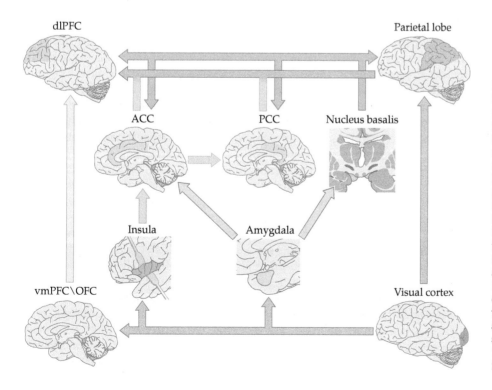

Figure 10.21 Attention-emotion interfaces Although the amygdala does not have many direct projections to the frontoparietal attentional control system, it can influence attention through several routes. The amygdala stimulates the release of acetylcholine from the nucleus basalis of Meynert, which enhances attention broadly in the neocortex. It also has projections to prefrontal interfaces in the anterior cingulate cortex (ACC), insula, and ventromedial and orbital frontal cortices (vmPFC/OFC). These regions, in turn, target other areas, such as the dorsolateral prefrontal cortex (dlPFC), parietal lobe, and posterior cingulate cortex (PCC). Finally, extensive feedback projections can enhance attention in sensory areas directly (not shown but illustrated for vision in Figure 10.19). (After Fichtenholtz and LaBar 2012.)

electrodes that target the subgenual portion of the anterior cingulate gyrus may help such patients restore balance across these systems and elevate their mood.

Emotional influences on memory consolidation

When we reflect on our lives, we tend to recall events that are emotionally salient and personally meaningful. These markers of life's ups and downs are often shared by family members and close friends, and they become the fabric of shared memories that facilitate social bonds. In some cases, unexpected tragedies experienced by individuals or communities leave long-lasting emotional traces that William James called "scars on the mind." The term **flashbulb memory** was introduced in the 1970s to refer to all the vivid details of an emotionally fraught episode that are registered graphically in the mind's eye. Although this analogy in the more literal terms in which it was originally proposed has not held up, salient experiences (both positive and negative) do tend to leave a more lasting memory than do mundane events.

Neurobiologist James McGaugh posits that emotionally arousing events enhance memory in part by engaging systems that regulate the storage of newly acquired information. His **memory modulation hypothesis** emphasizes the role of the amygdala in enhancing consolidation processes in other regions of the brain after an emotional episode. For declarative memory, these regions include structures in the medial temporal lobe and the dorsolateral and ventrolateral PFC, among others. McGaugh takes the arousal dimension of emotion to be the primary force behind the neuromodulatory influences of the amygdala. The amygdala's influence on the relevant brain areas is both direct by virtue of axonal projections, and indirect through the release of hormones into the bloodstream that have effects on the brain.

Although many neurotransmitters are used in the pathways that affect memory function, central to McGaugh's hypothesis are the actions of the catecholamine hormones **epinephrine** and **norepinephrine** and the corticosteroid hormone **cortisol** (called *corticosterone* in rodents). These **stress hormones** are secreted by the adrenal gland when stimulated by its sympathetic innervation, as described in **Box 10B**. Although cortisol can cross the blood-brain barrier and act on central receptor sites, epinephrine and norepinephrine activate beta-adrenergic receptors on visceral sensory endings in the periphery, which carry the information forward into the central nervous system. The influence of these two stress hormone systems in the basolateral amygdala is critical for modulating memory storage in the cortex in response to emotional events (Figure 10.22). Because the neuromodulatory action of stress hormones is relatively slow compared to neural signaling, such effects are maximal during a period of memory consolidation, after the events have actually occurred. The impact of the stress hormones thus reinforces whichever aspects of the episode are being consolidated in the relevant cortical storage sites.

Acute administration of cortisol or induction of psychosocial stress (e.g., via public speaking) generally enhances the retention of emotional memories. Because basal cortisol levels normally fluctuate during the day, influence a variety of receptor subtypes, and vary according to gender and other factors, the effects of cortisol on emotional memory have been somewhat inconsistent. A more striking effect is found when participants are administered the beta-adrenergic blocker **propranolol** before being exposed to an audiovisual narrative with emotional content (Figure 10.23). These participants remember fewer details of the emotional portion of the narrative than do placebo controls when memory is tested several weeks later. Interestingly, recognition memory for the neutral portions of the narrative is relatively unaffected by blocking of the adrenergic effects, implying a selective effect on emotional memory. Patients with amygdala lesions exhibit similar selective deficits, supporting the view that the drug effects in normal

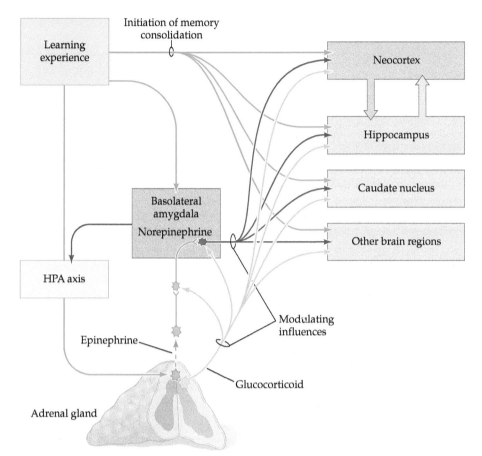

Figure 10.22 The memory modulation hypothesis As an emotionally arousing experience is being consolidated in memory, catecholamine and glucocorticoid stress hormone systems (along with other transmitters) influence the basolateral amygdala to enhance storage processes in other regions of the brain. (After McGaugh 2000.)

subjects may be mediated by the amygdala (see Figure 10.23). Although these findings suggest a possible pharmacological treatment for posttraumatic stress disorder (see Introductory Box), propranolol has not proved to be an effective treatment, perhaps because of the chronic and severe nature of PTSD compared to acute experimental manipulations in healthy subjects.

Further support of memory modulation by emotion comes from fMRI studies employing emotional versions of the *subsequent memory paradigm* (see Chapter 9). In this paradigm, participants undergo brain scanning while viewing words

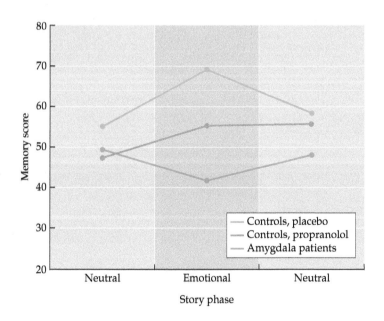

Figure 10.23 Pharmacological intervention and amygdala damage block the effects of emotional arousal on memory Participants are presented with an audiovisual narrative containing three parts. The first and last parts of the story are emotionally neutral, while the middle part of the story is emotionally arousing (describing a car accident). Healthy adults show long-term memory enhancement for the emotionally arousing (middle) portion of the story. This advantage is eliminated when propranolol, a beta-adrenergic blocker, is administered to healthy adults before they hear the story, as well as in patients with bilateral amygdala damage without drug administration. (After LaBar and Cabeza 2006.)

■ BOX 10B STRESS AND THE HYPOTHALAMIC-PITUITARY-ADRENAL AXIS

Stress is a complex term referring to the psychological and physiological changes that occur in response to a real or perceived threat to homeostasis. When encountering an aversive stimulus that is interpreted as potentially harmful to the individual (a *stressor*), the body initiates a complex pattern of endocrine, neural, and immunological activity (the *stress response*) in an attempt to cope with the elicitor and restore homeostatic balance. This *allostasis* (literally, "achieving stability through change") affects many bodily processes, including changes in cardiovascular function, respiration, glucose metabolism, muscle tone, and digestion.

Although the stress response evolved to handle physical threats such as extreme temperature changes or the appearance of a predator, psychosocial threats elicit similar response profiles. In the short term, the stress response is beneficial in that it mobilizes the body's resources to facilitate chances of survival. For instance, the stress response is activated during fear conditioning (see the text), which is an important mechanism for learning to predict when and where threatening events will occur in the environment. However, repeated or long-term stress increases the risk of developing a variety of physical and mental health problems, including peptic ulcers, hypertension, suppressed immune function, neuronal degeneration, reduced synaptic plasticity, cognitive impairment, obesity, and mood and anxiety disorders (see Introductory Box). Neuroscientist Bruce McEwen coined the term *allostatic overload* to refer to the cumulative wear and tear on the body that results from either too much stress or inefficient management of stress over time.

The principal stress response is mediated by a trio of organs—the paraventricular nucleus of the hypothalamus, the anterior lobe of the pituitary gland, and the cortex of the adrenal gland—commonly referred to as the **hypothalamic-pituitary-adrenal (HPA) axis** (see figure). Neurons in the paraventricular hypothalamus synthesize corticotropin-releasing factor (CRF) and vasopressin (AVP). In response to stress, CRF is released into hypophyseal portal vessels and binds to receptors in the anterior pituitary gland. Consequently, adrenocorticotropic hormone (ACTH) is released into the peripheral circulation (an action that is indepen-

dently facilitated by AVP), stimulating the synthesis and release of glucocorticoid steroid hormones (called *corticosterone* in rodents and *cortisol* in humans) in the adrenal cortex.

Glucocorticoids, in turn, regulate the downstream physiological changes associated with the stress response and have an inhibitory feedback action on the hypothalamus and pituitary gland to prevent further engagement of the HPA axis. Glucocorticoid hormones bind to two different receptor subtypes—the mineralocorticoid and glucocorticoid receptors—but have a lower affinity for the latter subtype, which is more implicated in the stress response. In contrast, mineralocorticoid receptors are occupied primarily during nonstressful states, and their activity regulates the basal tone of the system, which is highest on waking and gradually decreases over the day's activity cycle. Occupation of these receptors in cerebral sites is important for the modulatory effects of stress on memory consolida-

tion (see the text). The HPA axis is further modulated centrally and peripherally by neuropeptides (including substance P, neuropeptide Y, and galanin), serotonin, the catecholamines epinephrine and norepinephrine, and parasympathetic engagement.

Regions in the limbic forebrain and brainstem are important regulators of the HPA axis and are also targets of the long-term neurocognitive consequences of stress. The nucleus of the solitary tract in the brainstem integrates information from limbic and visceral sources to regulate CRF release in the hypothalamus through adrenergic and neuropeptide receptor-dependent mechanisms. The amygdala, particularly its central and medial nuclei, is sensitive to circulating glucocorticoids and initiates a positive feedback loop of HPA activation that promotes stress via connections with the bed nucleus of the stria terminalis, nucleus of the solitary tract, and hypothalamus. In contrast, the hippocampus and medial prefrontal

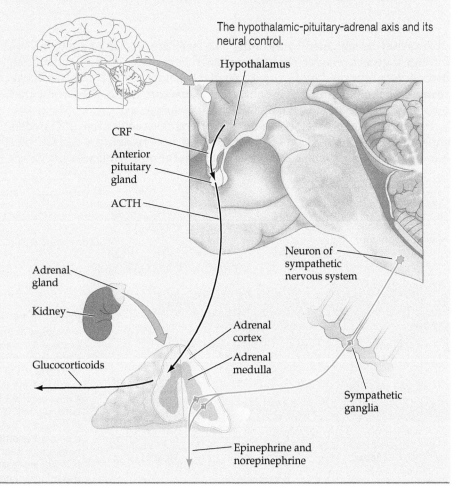

The hypothalamic-pituitary-adrenal axis and its neural control.

Hypothalamus

CRF

Anterior pituitary gland

ACTH

Adrenal gland

Kidney

Glucocorticoids

Neuron of sympathetic nervous system

Adrenal cortex

Adrenal medulla

Sympathetic ganglia

Epinephrine and norepinephrine

■ BOX 10B (continued)

cortex (PFC) exert inhibitory influences over the HPA axis through a similar set of anatomical intermediaries.

Interestingly, chronic stress treatments and/or glucocorticoid manipulations induce different cellular effects in these structures. Chronic restraint (immobilization) stress in a rat induces dendritic atrophy and reduces synaptic plasticity in the hippocampus and medial PFC, which are associated with impaired memory and fear extinction, respectively. But the same stressor will increase dendritic arborization and glutamatergic transmission in the amygdala, which is associated with greater fear conditioning. Deleterious effects of chronic stress on hippocampal volume and function in humans are especially pronounced in depression, posttraumatic stress disorder, development, and aging; and they are associated with low socio-economic status (as well as subordinate status in monkey dominance hierarchies).

Individuals differ widely in their stress tolerance (which is, in part, genetically influenced), and in the range of stimuli that they interpret as stressful. A key variable in coping with stress is perceived control of the situation. When aversive stimuli are perceived as uncontrollable, stress effects are exacerbated, and over the long haul, feelings of helplessness may emerge. The impact of stress on behavior and cognitive function also varies by sex and is related in part to the modulatory influence of oxytocin and estrogen on brain regions that regulate the HPA axis. Understanding how such individual differences translate into risk factors for stress-induced disease is an important area of current research.

References

BALE, T. L. (2006) Stress sensitivity and the development of affective disorders. *Horm. Behav.* 50: 529–533.

KOOLHAAS, J. M. AND 16 OTHERS (2011) Stress revisited: A critical evaluation of the stress concept. *Neurosci. Biobehav. Rev.* 35: 1291–1301.

MACHER, J. P. AND M. A. CROCQ, EDS. (2006) Stress. Special issue, *Dialogues Clin. Neurosci.* 8: 361–484.

MCEWEN, B. S. AND R. M. SAPOLSKY (1995) Stress and cognitive function. *Curr. Opin. Neurobiol.* 5: 205–216.

SAPOLSKY, R. M. (2005) The influence of social hierarchy on primate health. *Science* 308: 648–652.

SHORS, T. J. (1998) Stress and sex effects on associative learning: For better or for worse. *Neuroscientist* 4: 353–364.

TAYLOR, S. E., L. C. KLEIN, B. P. LEWIS, T. L. GREUENEWALK, R. A. R. GURUNG AND J. A. UPDEGRAFF (2000) Biobehavioral responses to stress in females: Tend-and-befriend, not fight-or-flight. *Psychol. Rev.* 97: 411–429.

---

or pictures that vary in emotional content. Memory is tested later, outside of the scanning environment. Recall that comparison of fMRI scans for items that are subsequently remembered versus forgotten enables the identification of brain regions that engage in successful encoding operations. Such effects are greater for emotional than for neutral material when activation is examined in the amygdala, hippocampus, entorhinal cortex, and ventrolateral and dorsolateral PFC, among other regions (Figure 10.24A). Moreover, activity that predicts successful recall is highly correlated between the amygdala and other regions of the medial temporal lobe (MTL) for emotional but not neutral stimuli (Figure 10.24B). These results indicate that the amygdala and adjacent MTL memory-processing

Figure 10.24 Interactions between the amygdala and memory-related regions of the medial temporal lobe These structures are functionally coupled during the successful encoding of emotional but not neutral memories. (A) Activity in the amygdala, hippocampus, and parahippocampal gyrus (PHG) is greater for emotional pictures that are subsequently remembered than for those that are forgotten. (B) Across individual participants, successful encoding activity (labeled "Dm" for "difference in memory") is correlated in the amygdala and entorhinal cortex for emotional stimuli, but not for neutral stimuli (similar effects occur in the hippocampus but are not shown). The entorhinal cortex is located in the anterior portion of the parahippocampal gyrus. (A from Murty et al. 2010; B after Dolcos et al. 2004.)

(A)

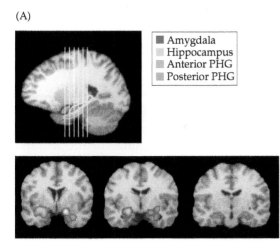

- ■ Amygdala
- ■ Hippocampus
- ■ Anterior PHG
- ■ Posterior PHG

(B)

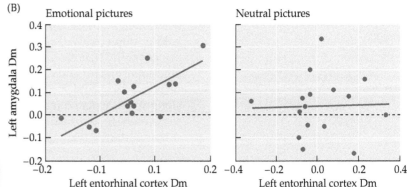

regions are functionally coupled during the encoding of emotional items that are later remembered, as predicted by the memory modulation hypothesis.

The memory modulation hypothesis addresses only one aspect of emotional memory: the enhancement of memory consolidation processes by emotional arousal and engagement of relevant stress hormones. It does not consider other aspects, such as the detrimental effects of stress on memory retrieval or the role of valence, which, as discussed earlier, tends to engage the prefrontal cortex (see the section on hemispheric-asymmetry models). Not surprisingly, given the complexity of the constructs involved, emotion affects memory in multiple ways.

Regulation of Emotion

The ability to regulate emotions in response to routine stressors is central to mental and physical health. Transient emotional episodes are often healthy reactions to environmental situations that permit adaptive behavioral actions. However, emotions that are socially inappropriate, displaced to irrelevant targets, or excessively prolonged, intense, or variable can lead to personal distress, interfere with daily activities, or even indicate psychopathology. Psychological studies of **emotion regulation** have shown many ways in which individuals consciously and unconsciously attempt to influence the intensity, duration, or quality of the emotions they feel, some of which are more effective than others. Central to this research is the fact that emotions are not experienced passively in response to elicitors but instead are active, subjective processes in humans (and presumably other animals). Therefore, cognitive-behavioral interventions are targeted at training individuals to generate new, adaptive responses to emotion elicitors, to modify existing thoughts or reactions as they unfold, or to be accepting (mindful) of their reactions and then let them go to avoid emotional perseveration. Although much research has focused on dampening negative affect, researchers are also examining the potentially beneficial effects of enhancing positive affect.

Psychologist James Gross proposed an influential model that classifies emotion regulation into different strategies according to the timing of their engagement (e.g., before or after an emotional response is elicited) and the regulatory target (e.g., controlling physiological expression or cognitive interpretations of the elicitor). At one extreme, individuals change their behavior patterns in an antecedent way to avoid the emotional encounter altogether (called **situation selection**), as when people with a fear of flying choose to travel by train. In a less extreme strategy, individuals engage in **cognitive reappraisal** to attend to or interpret the meaning of an elicitor in such a way as to alter its emotional impact.

One way of investigating cognitive reappraisal in the laboratory is to have participants use imagery to generate alternate hypothetical outcomes of emotional scenarios. When presented with pictures of combat, for instance, participants may be instructed to reinterpret the pictures to decrease the negative affect associated with viewing the picture, such as by imagining that a wounded soldier depicted will return home soon and get well. Reappraisal strategies are generally beneficial in reducing physiological arousal associated with the emotional elicitor and can facilitate explicit memory for the episode. In contrast, response-focused strategies in which individuals actively mask their facial expressions and associated feelings in response to emotion elicitors (called *expressive suppression*) tend to be maladaptive. Under these conditions, sympathetic arousal is inadvertently increased, unpleasant feelings are sometimes unaffected, and memory is worsened. Although these strategies are often studied individually, it is well recognized that people use a variety of interacting schemes, although some individuals tend to routinely engage in certain strategies more than others.

Neuroimaging research has detailed some of the ways in which conscious attempts to change emotional experience affect activity in the relevant frontolimbic

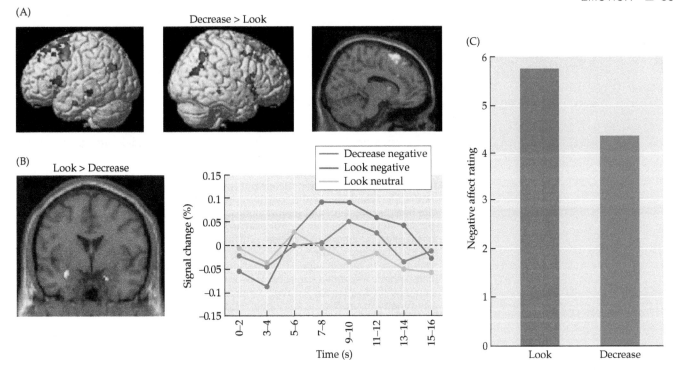

Figure 10.25 **Cognitive reappraisal of negative emotion** In this experiment, participants were instructed either to decrease negative emotions elicited by the presentation of aversive pictures or to passively look at the pictures. They decreased emotions by cognitively reappraising the stimulus either to imagine that things got better in the depicted scene (situation-focused reappraisal) or to cognitively distance themselves from the picture by viewing it from a detached third-person perspective (self-focused reappraisal). (A) Either way, when participants attempted to decrease their negative emotions, activity increased in the dorsal frontoparietal attentional network (relative to passive viewing) as well as in other regions in the inferior PFC and anterior cingulate. (B) In contrast, decreasing negative emotion reduced activity in the amygdala from the passive look condition, making it more similar to the activity observed when passively looking at neutral pictures. These patterns suggest that frontoparietal regions implement the regulatory strategy, while the amygdala is a target of the regulatory action on emotion generation. (C) The instructions were effective in decreasing emotion associated with the pictures, as indicated by reduced subjective reports of negative affect in response to the pictures. (After Ochsner et al. 2004.)

structures. When individuals engage in cognitive reappraisal of negative emotional stimuli, activity increases in the dorsal frontoparietal network as well as in other prefrontal regions, including the dorsal anterior cingulate cortex and ventrolateral PFC (Figure 10.25). Interestingly, some of these areas are responsive irrespective of whether the regulatory goal is to increase or decrease affect, suggesting that they are involved in selecting and applying the cognitive strategy. Conversely, other regions, including the amygdala and insula, are targets of the prefrontal modulation; accordingly, their activity is sensitive to the regulatory goal (e.g., increasing when negative affect is enhanced and decreasing when negative affect is dampened). Thus, attempts to cognitively alter emotional experience involve interactions between dorsal executive control and ventral emotion-processing regions of the brain.

Although much of this chapter described how emotions influence cognitive functions, studies of emotion regulation provide a good example of how executive control processes are recruited to modify emotional experience. This result is achieved by invoking other cognitive functions, including thinking, visual imagery, behavioral inhibition, and selection of information in working memory (see Chapter 13 for a similar discussion on self-regulation). Research in this area holds considerable promise for understanding individual differences in regulatory abilities, responsiveness to cognitive-behavioral therapy, and resilience to psychopathology.

Summary

1. Emotion is a complex set of regulatory and cognitive functions defined by related changes in physiology and behavior, accompanied by feelings that help humans and other animals respond flexibly to biologically significant stimuli. By focusing on aspects of emotion that are amenable to neurobiological investigation, researchers have begun to identify the neural circuits and systems involved in emotional evaluation, expression, and experience.

2. Some structures in the limbic forebrain, such as the amygdala, are critical for emotional information processing, in part because of their rich anatomical connections with both sensory and visceral motor regions.

3. The original limbic system theory put forward in the 1940s has been repeatedly revised to acknowledge the contributions of additional brain areas, along with the fact that some medial forebrain structures, such as the hippocampus, also participate in functions that are not primarily emotional. The involvement of some of these brain regions in emotion—including the amygdala, insula, orbitofrontal cortex, and ventral anterior cingulate gyrus—has been confirmed with modern techniques in humans and other species. Such studies have further identified hemispheric asymmetry in aspects of emotional processing, including a right-hemisphere dominance for affective prosody, and some evidence for prefrontal asymmetry in processing emotional valence.

4. The limbic and paralimbic regions implicated in emotional processing connect with cortical brain regions that mediate other cognitive functions, and these interactions guide goal-directed behavior.

5. Features of the environment that elicit emotional responses receive priority in perception and attention. The rapidity of such prioritization suggests subcortical as well as cortical processing.

6. In addition to facilitating the retention of information about emotional events, the amygdala detects regularities in the environment that predict aversive outcomes, as shown by fear conditioning. The association of conditioned fears with environmental contexts requires the hippocampus as well. The extinction of conditioned fear involves inhibitory interactions between the ventromedial prefrontal cortex and the amygdala.

7. Arousal enhances memory consolidation by way of the stress response systems, which interact with the amygdala and memory-processing regions of the medial temporal lobe, including the hippocampus.

8. Understanding the neural architecture and pharmacological substrates of emotion-cognition interactions provides potential targets for the treatment of affective disorders characterized by perceptual and attentional biases toward emotional stimuli, as well as intrusive traumatic and stressful memories.

9. The ability to regulate emotions is critical to mental and physical health. Decreasing negative emotions by reappraising the meaning of emotional stimuli—a core component of cognitive therapies—involves inhibitory interactions between executive control regions in the lateral prefrontal cortex and emotional processing regions in the limbic forebrain, including the amygdala.

Go to the **COMPANION WEBSITE**

sites.sinauer.com/cogneuro2e
for quizzes, animations, flashcards,
and other study resources.

Additional Reading

Reviews

BOROD, J. C., R. L. BLOOM, A. M. BRICK-MAN, L. NAKHUTINA AND E. A. CURKO (2002) Emotional processing deficits in individuals with unilateral brain damage. *Appl. Neuropsychol.* 9: 23–36.

CRAIG, A. D. (2007) Interoception and emotion: A neuroanatomical perspective. In *Handbook of Emotions*, 3rd Ed., M. Lewis, J. M. Haviland-Jones and L. F. Barrett (eds.). New York: Guilford, pp. 395–408.

DAVIDSON, R. J. AND W. IRWIN (1999) The functional neuroanatomy of emotion and affective style. *Trends Cogn. Sci.* 3: 11–21.

DAVIDSON, R. J., K. M. PUTNAM AND C. L. LARSON (2000) Dysfunction in the neural circuitry of emotion regulation—A possible prelude to violence. *Science* 289: 591–594.

DOLAN, R. J. (2002) Emotion, cognition, and behavior. *Science* 298: 1191–1194.

ELLSWORTH, P. AND K. R. SCHERER (2003) Appraisal processes in emotion. In *Handbook of Affective Sciences*, R. J. Davidson, K. R. Scherer and H. H. Goldsmith

(eds.). New York: Oxford University Press, pp. 572–595.

FICHTENHOLTZ, H. M. AND K. S. LABAR (2012) Emotional influences on visuospatial attention. In *Neuroscience of Attention: Attentional Control and Selection*, G. R. Mangun (ed.). New York: Oxford University Press, pp. 250–266.

HARMON-JONES, E., P. A. GABLE AND C. K. PETERSON (2010) The role of asymmetric frontal cortical activity in emotion-related phenomena: A review and update. *Biol. Psychol.* 84: 451–462.

HOLLAND, P. C. AND M. GALLAGHER (1999) Amygdala circuitry in attentional and representational processes. *Trends Cogn. Sci.* 3: 65–73.

JONES, C. L., J. WARD AND H. D. CRITCHLEY (2010) The neuropsychological impact of insular cortex lesions. *J. Neurol. Neurosurg. Psychiatry* 81: 611–618.

LABAR, K. S. AND R. CABEZA (2006) Cognitive neuroscience of emotional memory. *Nat. Rev. Neurosci.* 7: 54–64.

LEDOUX, J. E. (1991) The limbic system concept. *Concepts Neurosci.* 2: 169–199.

MAYBERG, H. S. (1997) Limbic-cortical dysregulation: A proposed model of depression. *J. Neuropsychiatry Clin. Neurosci.* 9: 471–481.

MCGAUGH, J. L. (2000) Memory: A century of consolidation. *Science* 287: 248–251.

OCHSNER K. N. AND J. J. GROSS (2005) The cognitive control of emotion. *Trends Cogn. Sci.* 9: 242–249.

PESSOA, L. (2005) To what extent are emotional visual stimuli processed without attention and awareness? *Curr. Opin. Neurobiol.* 15: 188–196.

ROSS, E. D. (1997) The aprosodias. In *Behavioral Neurology and Neuropsychology*, T. E. Feinberg and M. J. Farah (eds.). New York: McGraw-Hill, pp. 699–709.

VUILLEUMIER, P. AND J. DRIVER (2007) Modulation of visual processing by attention and emotion: Windows on causal interactions between human brain regions. *Phil. Trans. R. Soc. B: Biol. Sci.* 362: 837–855.

Important Original Papers

ANDERSON, A. K. AND E. A. PHELPS (2001) Lesions of the human amygdala impair enhanced perception of emotionally salient events. *Nature* 411: 305–309.

BARD, P. (1928) A diencephalic mechanism for the expression of rage with special reference to the sympathetic nervous system. *Am. J. Physiol.* 84: 490–515.

BECHARA, A., A. R. DAMASIO, H. DAMASIO AND S. W. ANDERSON (1994) Insensitivity to future consequences following damage to the human prefrontal cortex. *Cognition* 50: 7–15.

BECHARA, A., D. TRANEL, H. DAMASIO, R. ADOLPHS, C. ROCKLAND AND A. R. DAMASIO (1995) Double dissociation of conditioning and declarative knowledge relative to the amygdala and hippocampus in humans. *Science* 269: 1115–1118.

CAHILL, L., B. PRINS, M. WEBER AND J. L. MCGAUGH (1994) Beta-adrenergic activation and memory for emotional events. *Nature* 371: 702–704.

CALDER, A. J., J. KEANE, F. MANES, N. ANTOUN AND A. W. YOUNG (2000) Impaired recognition and experience of disgust following brain injury. *Nat. Neurosci.* 3: 1077–1078.

CRITCHEY, H. D., S. WIENS, P. ROTSHTEIN, A. ÖHMAN AND R. J. DOLAN (2004) Neural systems supporting interoceptive awareness. *Nat. Neurosci.* 7: 189–195.

DOLCOS, F., K. S. LABAR AND R. CABEZA (2004) Interaction between the amygdala and the medial temporal lobe memory system predicts better memory for emotional events. *Neuron* 42: 855–863.

KALIN, N. H., C. LARSON, S. E. SHELTON AND R. J. DAVIDSON (1998) Asymmetric frontal brain activity, cortisol, and behavior associated with fearful temperament in rhesus monkeys. *Behav. Neurosci.* 112: 286–292.

KLÜVER, H. AND P. C. BUCY (1939) Preliminary analysis of functions of the temporal lobes in monkeys. *Arch. Neurol. Psychiatry* 42: 979–900.

LANG, P. J., M. K. GREENWALD, M. M. BRADLEY AND A. O. HAMM (1993) Looking at pictures: Affective, facial, visceral, and behavioral reactions. *Psychophysiology* 30: 261–273.

MACLEAN, P. D. (1949) Psychosomatic disease and the "visceral brain": Recent developments bearing on the Papez theory of emotion. *Psychosom. Med.* 11: 338–353.

MILAD, M. R. AND G. J. QUIRK (2002) Neurons in medial prefrontal cortex signal memory for fear extinction. *Nature* 420: 70–74.

MURTY, V. P., M. RITCHEY, R. A. ADCOCK AND K. S. LABAR (2010) fMRI studies of emotional memory encoding: A quantitative meta-analysis. *Neuropsychologia* 49: 695–705.

OCHSNER, K. N. AND 6 OTHERS (2004) For better or for worse: Neural systems supporting the cognitive down- and up-regulation of negative emotion. *NeuroImage* 23: 483–499.

PAPEZ, J. W. (1937) A proposed mechanism for emotion. *Arch. Neurol. Psychiatry* 38: 725–743.

PHILLIPS, R. G. AND J. E. LEDOUX (1992) Differential contribution of amygdala and hippocampus to cued and contextual fear conditioning. *Behav. Neurosci.* 106: 274–285.

RUSSELL, J. A. (1980) A circumplex model of affect. *J. Pers. Soc. Psychol.* 39: 1161–1178.

SHACKMAN, A. J., B. W. MCMENAMIN, J. S. MAXWELL, L. L. GREISCHAR AND R. J. DAVIDSON (2010) Right dorsolateral prefrontal cortical activity and behavioral inhibition. *Psychol. Sci.* 20: 1500–1506.

VUILLEUMIER, P., M. RICHARDSON, J. ARMONY, J. DRIVER AND R. J. DOLAN (2004) Distant influences of amygdala lesion on visual cortical activation during emotional face processing. *Nat. Neurosci.* 7: 1271–1278.

WHALEN, P. J. AND 9 OTHERS (2004) Human amygdala responsivity to masked fearful eye whites. *Science* 306: 2061.

WILLIAMS, M. A., A. P. MORRIS, F. MCGLONE, D. F. ABBOTT AND J. B. MATTINGLEY (2004) Amygdala responses to fearful and happy facial expressions under conditions of binocular suppression. *J. Neurosci.* 24: 2898–2904.

Books

ARMONY, J. L. AND P. VUILLEUMIER (2012) *Handbook of Human Affective Neuroscience.* New York: Cambridge University Press.

BOROD, J. C. (2000) *The Neuropsychology of Emotion.* New York: Oxford University Press.

DAMASIO, A. R. (1994) *Descartes' Error.* New York: Putnam.

DAVIDSON, R. J., K. R. SCHERER AND H. H. GOLDSMITH (2003) *Handbook of Affective Sciences.* New York: Oxford University Press.

EKMAN, P. AND R. J. DAVIDSON (1994) *The Nature of Emotions.* New York: Oxford University Press.

GROSS, J. J. (2007) *Handbook of Emotion Regulation.* New York: Guilford.

NIEDENTHAL, P. M. AND S. KITAYAMA (1994) *The Heart's Eye: Emotional Influences in Perception and Attention.* San Diego, CA: Academic Press.

PANKSEPP, J. (1998) *Affective Neuroscience: The Foundations of Human and Animal Emotions.* New York: Oxford University Press.

PHELPS, E. A. AND P. J. WHALEN (2009) *The Human Amygdala.* New York: Guilford.

11

Social Cognition

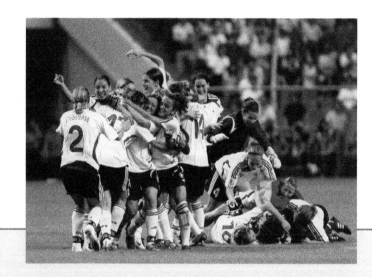

INTRODUCTION

A major goal of cognitive neuroscience is to identify the neural under-pinnings of the processes by which individuals understand themselves and their relationships to others. This subfield, known as social neuro-science, builds on the developments in affective neuroscience described in Chapter 10—in particular, the evidence that emotions serve important social functions. Emotions evident in facial expressions, body language, and speech are a means by which we communicate our intentions to others, and by which we interpret their actions. Humans and other species that live in social groups have evolved mechanisms for establish-ing hierarchies among members, for building kinship and other social bonds, and for setting acceptable norms of behavior.

Dysfunctional social processing can have profound consequences, as exemplified by autism spectrum disorders (see Introductory Box) and antisocial personality disorders. In many animals the basis for social behaviors is determined genetically, with individual experience playing a relatively minor role. In humans, however, culture, customs, and social learning markedly influence behavior throughout the life span. Because social psychologists and neuroscientists have joined forces only recently, many issues and observations in this field are contentious, and the an-swers to many questions remain open. This chapter summarizes some of the areas at the forefront of this new subfield, including self-referential processing, perception of nonverbal social cues, social categorization, theory of mind, empathy, and social competition. Social communication by means of language is taken up specifically in Chapter 12, and social influences on decision making are discussed in Chapter 14.

■ INTRODUCTORY BOX **AUTISM**

The term **autism spectrum disorder** refers to any of a range of neurodevelopmental problems characterized by functional deficits in communication and social interactions, and by repetitive, stereotyped behaviors. Epidemiological research suggests that some form of autism affects up to one in every 100 children. The severe form is highly heritable, with monozygotic twin studies indicating concordance rates from 60 to 90 percent.

Originally described by psychiatrist Leo Kanner in 1943, autism (from the Greek word *autos*, meaning "self, same, spontaneous; directed from within") is distinguished from other disorders by having social deficits as a core symptom. According to the American Psychiatric Association's *Diagnostic and Statistical Manual* (*DSM-IV*), the key criteria that define social deficits in autism include: (1) impairment in using nonverbal behaviors in social interactions such as eye-to-eye gaze, facial expression, and body posture/gestures; (2) failure to develop peer relationships appropriate for the individual's age level; (3) failure to spontaneously seek to share enjoyment, interests, or achievements with other people; and (4) lack of social or emotional reciprocity. For these reasons, researchers have been greatly interested in autistic individuals to gain insight into the brain regions specialized for social cognitive functions. Autism is often accompanied by mental retardation, and studies have tended to focus on high-functioning autistic individuals, defined as those with an IQ of 70 or higher.

Social perception deficits in autism include difficulty processing faces, emotional expressions, and biological motion. Studies using eye-tracking techniques show that people with autism allocate their attention to noncanonical facial features, such as the forehead, cheeks, or other features located near the face (e.g., earrings). By contrast, most people scan faces in a characteristic triangular pattern, looking back and forth between the two eyes and the mouth—the regions that convey the dynamic information used in social and emotional communication (Figure A). When making social judgments about others from facial features alone, individuals with autism tend to overestimate how trustworthy people appear. Such challenges in discriminating emotions and personal characteristics conveyed in facial displays, in turn, affect how these individuals relate to other people.

(A)

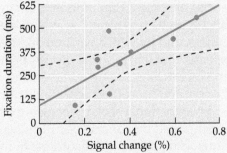

When viewing faces, autistic individuals show reduced activation in the fusiform gyrus, inferior temporal gyrus, superior temporal sulcus, and amygdala. The activation decrements in the fusiform gyrus and amygdala correspond to a reduction in attentional allocation to the faces as measured by eye fixations (Figure B). Individuals with autism usually do not exhibit enhanced activity in these brain regions when the faces that they are viewing express emotions. Finally, unlike controls, autistic individuals do not exhibit activity increases in the superior temporal sulcus when goal-directed biological motion sequences are violated, as when viewing animated characters whose reaching actions miss their intended targets.

Social impairments in autism extend beyond perceptual processes to include difficulties in extracting meaning from interpersonal interactions. The inability to follow the gaze of other individuals, which emerges early in development, contributes to later impairments in using gaze to understand other people's intentions and desires and in developing vocabulary skills, which are socially learned by using gaze, head, and pointing gestures to as-

(B)

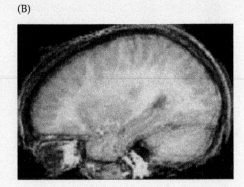

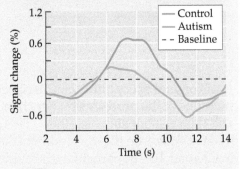

Face-processing deficits in autism. (A) In contrast to control subjects (left), individuals with autism (right) tend to focus on features of faces that are not critical for socioemotional communication, as the lines tracing eye movement in these photos indicate. (B) Faces elicit greater fMRI activity in the fusiform gyrus (indicated in the scan and the upper graph) in controls than in individuals with autism. The bottom plot shows that, in autistic individuals, fusiform activity is positively correlated with the duration of eye fixations on the face. (A from Pelphrey et al. 2002; B after Dalton et al. 2005.)

sociate objects in the environment with their names. Individuals with autism often fail theory-of-mind tasks (described later in the chapter), which require participants to distinguish their own views and beliefs from those of others.

■ INTRODUCTORY BOX (continued)

(C)

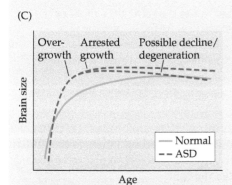

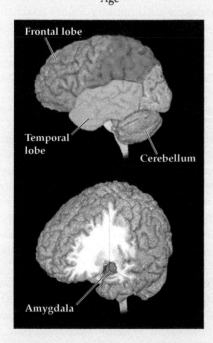

Brain growth in autism. (C) Across developmental stages, there is a general pattern of brain enlargement followed by arrested growth. This pattern is found in portions of the frontal and temporal lobes, cerebellum, and amygdala, among others. ASD, autism spectrum disorder. (C after Courchesne et al. 2011.)

Autistic individuals tend to have relatively larger brain volumes, perhaps arising from overgrowth of connections early in development. These alterations include more white matter in the cerebrum and cerebellum and larger cerebral gray matter, particularly in the frontal lobes and other regions implicated in social processing, as outlined already. However, by late childhood these global structural differences tend to become normal (Figure C). Aberrant wiring patterns nonetheless persist in autistic adulthood, including more short- and medium-range connections within the hemispheres, but fewer interhemispheric connections.

Thus, behavioral impairments in autism are most likely a result of altered processing and/or connectivity among interacting brain regions that mediate social cognition, communication, and executive motor functions. Consistent with this idea, autistic individuals sometimes have extraordinary talent in restricted domains like mental calculation, historical facts, or art—a phenomenon sometimes referred to as **savant syndrome** (see Introductory Box in Chapter 15). At the same time, individuals with autism have more difficulty integrating parts into wholes and synthesizing information across domains (called *central coherence*)—skills that require the normal operation of interacting large-scale networks. Their enhanced reliance on local task features and attention to detail often leads to a bias toward *systemizing*, the tendency of autistic individuals to analyze problems and construct knowledge by applying rigid, often mechanical, rules.

Rehabilitative training in autism focuses on exploiting this penchant for rules, mechanics, and focal attention to facilitate social and emotional competence. For instance, psychologists train autistic children to discriminate emotions by morphing human facial expressions onto animated mechanical characters that move rigidly and express emotions according to a specific set of rules. Initial short-term results of such rehabilitation exercises are promising, but the extent to which the eye-tracking and fMRI activation patterns improve following training is not known. With increased activity of advocacy groups, enhanced public awareness, and high-profile personal triumphs like those of Temple Grandin, research efforts are increasing to help understand this complex disorder.

References

BARON-COHEN, S., R. CAMPBELL, A. KARMILOFF-SMITH, J. GRANT AND J. WALKER (1995) Are children with autism blind to the mentalistic significance of the eyes? *Brit. J. Dev. Psychol.* 13: 379–398.

COURCHESNE, E., K. CAMPBELL AND S. SOLSO (2011) Brain growth across the life span in autism: Age-specific changes in anatomical pathology. *Brain Res.* 1380: 138–145.

DALTON, K. M. AND 7 OTHERS (2005) Gaze fixation and the neural circuitry of face processing in autism. *Nat. Neurosci.* 8: 510–526.

DiCICCO-BLOOM, E. AND 8 OTHERS (2006) The developmental neurobiology of autism spectrum disorder. *J. Neurosci.* 26: 6897–6906.

GOLAN, O. AND 6 OTHERS (2010) Enhancing emotion recognition in children with autism spectrum conditions: An intervention using animated vehicles with real emotional faces. *J. Autism Dev. Disord.* 40: 269–279.

GRANDIN, T. (2011) *The Way I See It: A Personal Look at Autism and Asperger's*, 2nd Ed. Arlington, TX: Future Horizons.

HAPPÉ, F. AND U. FRITH (2006) The weak coherence account: Detail-focused cognitive style in autism spectrum disorders. *J. Autism Dev. Disord.* 36: 5–25.

KANNER, L. (1943) Autistic disturbances of affective contact. *Nerv. Child* 2: 217–250.

MOLDIN, S. O. AND J. L. R. RUBENSTEIN, EDS. (2006) *Understanding Autism: From Basic Neuroscience to Treatment.* Boca Raton, FL: CRC Press.

PELPHREY, K. A., N. J. SASSON, J. S. REZNICK, G. PAUL, B. D. GOLDMAN AND J. PIVEN (2002) Visual scanning of faces in autism. *J. Autism Dev. Disord.* 32: 249–261.

SCHUMANN, C. M. AND 8 OTHERS (2009) The amygdala is enlarged in children but not adolescents with autism; the hippocampus is enlarged at all ages. *J. Neurosci.* 24: 6392–6401.

The Self

Distinguishing oneself from others is a necessary first step in establishing fluent social interactions. Understanding the nature of the self has long perplexed philosophers, psychologists, and laypeople alike. In his treatise on psychology written at the end of the nineteenth century, William James described the self as follows:

> Whatever I may be thinking of, I am always at the same time more or less aware of myself, of my personal existence. At the same time it is I who am aware; so that the total self of me, being as it were duplex, partly known and partly knower, partly object and partly subject, must have two aspects discriminated in it.
>
> W. James 1890, p. 176

Despite the conceptual difficulties in defining what constitutes the entity we all consider the **self**, a core cognitive ability described by James is the ability to consider one's own being as an object, and thus subject to objective consideration. This ability is called **self-reflexive thought**.

Non-human animals presumably possess a rudimentary ability to distinguish themselves from other animals because of its obvious biological value. However, more complex aspects of self-awareness that characterize humans provide the ability to think of oneself in abstract and even symbolic terms, including the creation of mental images to imagine alternative outcomes in complex social situations.

As described in Chapter 15, the capacity for self-awareness evolved in mammals and other animals in conjunction with related social, emotional, and cognitive skills. Animals with small brains and less complex nervous systems seem to operate in the world primarily by responding to external cues. But even rodents can navigate in their environment using either egocentric or allocentric frames of reference, indicating an ability to explore the world either in terms of their own place in it (egocentric, or first-person, view) or simply in terms of external reference points (allocentric, or third-person, view). Head direction cells in the hippocampus, thalamus, and retrosplenial cortex help rodents navigate in an egocentric framework, and shifting between these frames of reference involves transformations in the parietal cortex.

Some non-human animals can recognize themselves in a mirror. At first sight, great apes regard the individual reflected in the mirror as a conspecific and display interpersonal social signals. Over time, however, self-directed behaviors, such as self-grooming in response to the reflection become apparent. A hallmark of such self-recognition is the "mark test," in which an experimenter places a mark on the face or forehead of the animal that is viewable only in the mirror. The mark test is "passed" if the animal repeatedly palpates the mark while viewing itself in the mirror (relative to a comparable baseline period with no mirror present). In addition to great apes, elephants conduct self-examinations by using their trunks to touch a mark visible to them only in the mirror.

Despite these rudimentary abilities, self-recognition and self-reflexive behaviors are markedly more advanced in humans. The archaeological record suggests that the rapid development of culture with a focus on the importance of individuals (and thus the self) emerged in the evolution of humans approximately 50,000 years ago, as evidenced by ritualized burials and artifacts of self-ornamentation. The value of symbolic self-reflexive thought is not difficult to imagine. This ability enables an appraisal of one's personality traits, strengths, and weaknesses in comparison to others and to cultural norms. Such evaluation is essential to successful social behavior by generating self-esteem, regulating one's actions in social contexts, and abiding by social rules.

Whereas humans normally possess a sense of a unitary self across both time and space, the stable concept of the self breaks down in some clinical disorders. For example, **fugue states** are defined as transient states of confusion in which self-relevant knowledge is temporarily unavailable to consciousness, and uncharacteristic and often self-destructive behaviors ensue. Fugue states can arise following some types of epileptic seizures, but how the sense of self is lost is unknown. In **dissociative identity disorder**, individuals have recurrent, multiple identities that emerge to control behavior at different points in time. This disorder typically originates following exposure to a highly traumatic event, and therapies are directed toward integrating the identities into a unified stream of consciousness. While we take a continuous sense of self in our personal lives for granted, these rare disorders highlight the profound social and behavioral impairments that can arise when discontinuities in self-awareness emerge.

Self-reflection

Only recently have the approaches of cognitive neuroscience been brought to bear on these philosophical and clinical concerns by identifying brain areas that mediate aspects of the self, including self-reflexive thoughts and self-directed feelings. Self-reflection requires an initial redirection of attentional focus from external sensory events to internal thoughts, memories, feelings, and visceral sensations. Two sets of brain regions have been broadly implicated in these functions—midline cortical regions involved in the **default mode** of brain processing, and limbic/paralimbic regions involved in **interoception**.

Recall from Chapter 7 that neuroimaging studies have identified brain areas whose activity *decreases* during tasks that require attention to external stimuli. This default-mode activity thus provides a basis for beginning to understand the brain regions that are more active during internal self-reflection and self-projection into another place or time unrelated to the current sensory environment. This spontaneous, coordinated activity occurs in the dorsal and ventromedial prefrontal cortex (PFC), posterior cingulate, and medial and lateral parietal cortex. Some researchers have speculated that this activity reflects an ongoing stream of consciousness. Indeed, some of these same brain regions are sensitive to variations in consciousness associated with different levels of self-awareness (e.g., stages of sleep, the effects of anesthesia, or recovery from vegetative states; see Chapter 7).

Building on these observations of resting-state activity, researchers have directed participants to explicitly engage in self-reflection during brain scanning. For instance, participants are asked to indicate how well adjectives referring to personal traits (e.g., *ambitious*) and sentences (e.g., "I tend to worry a lot") describe themselves (self-endorsement tasks), or to compare their personality traits with those of famous people or individuals they know well (social comparison tasks). Activity in the anterior medial PFC and parietal regions is increased when identifying attributes of oneself relative to those of a stranger (Figure 11.1A). Moreover, TMS applied to the medial parietal cortex has been reported to temporarily block the retrieval of some self-relevant knowledge. The degree of anterior medial PFC activity in response to trait words during self-endorsement tasks also predicts their later recall. Because this finding does not generalize to nonsocial encoding tasks, such as those involving perceptual or semantic processing, a particular type of self-referential encoding process is implied.

These observations are consistent with studies of autobiographical memory retrieval, which implicate the same default-mode processing regions. For example, successful memory retrieval for spatial landmarks cued by photos taken by an individual elicits greater medial PFC activity than does successful retrieval cued by photos of the same landmark that were taken by others (Figure 11.1B). As described in Chapter 10, the medial PFC has been implicated more generally in mental processes needed to reflect on autobiographical memories, such as monitoring for their accuracy, and in generating the mental imagery required in working memory tasks that project actions of the self into the future.

Figure 11.1 Role of the medial PFC in self-referential processing (A) Greater activity in the anterior medial PFC (yellow circle) is found when participants make trait judgments about themselves relative to trait judgments about a best friend or perceptual judgments about the appearance of the trait word (i.e., whether it is upper- or lowercase). (B) Activity in the same brain area during autobiographical memory retrieval. College students were instructed to take pictures of campus landmarks; they then viewed these photos, as well as pictures of the same landmarks taken by other people. Successful recollection of photos taken by the students themselves was associated with greater activity in the anterior medial PFC than was successful recollection of photos taken by others. In both (A) and (B), a self-referential effect is inferred from the lack of a deactivation pattern typically seen in midline cortical regions that constitute the "default mode" of brain processing. (A after Heatherton et al. 2006; B after Cabeza et al. 2004.)

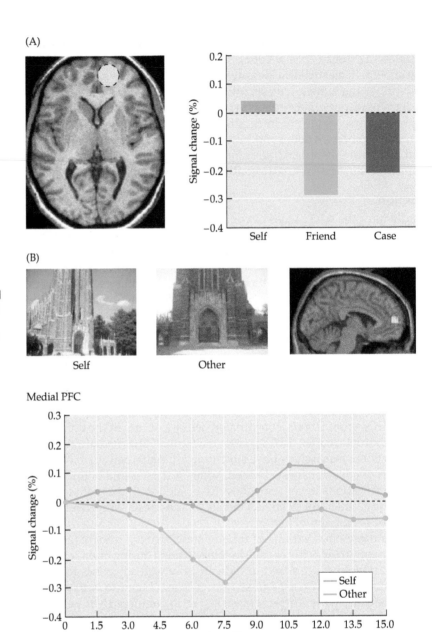

While default-mode research has focused on judgments of personality traits or past experiences, other work has focused on the subjective feelings that accompany emotional or painful stimuli. These studies have implicated not only the brain regions involved in self-reflexive thought, but also brain regions implicated in interoception and empathy, such as the anterior cingulate and insula (see Chapter 10 and the discussion later in this chapter). Greater activity in the rostral anterior cingulate is found when participants are instructed to report their own arousal in response to emotionally aversive scenes than when they focus on the spatial layout of the scenes. Focusing on spatial layout, on the other hand, elicits greater activity in the posterior parietal cortex. Thus, the same emotional images can engage different brain regions depending on whether attention is on an internal evaluative response to the images or an analysis of their sensory features.

Anterior cingulate responses to emotional stimuli and emotional memories are further enhanced by individual differences in performance on the Levels of

Emotional Awareness Scale, which assesses how deeply and complexly emotions are experienced. Anterior cingulate activity increases with autonomic measures of arousal and the subjective experience of the unpleasantness of pain, and it is implicated in the regulation of pain modulation. This work further reinforces the idea that the anterior cingulate integrates attentional and emotional functions (see Chapter 10), but with the more specific goal of directing attention to one's own emotional responses in order to motivate plans of action.

The anterior insula signals awareness of bodily sensations, such as alterations in respiration and heart rate during arousing states. As reviewed in Chapter 10, the posterior and mid-insula are part of a visceral processing network that includes brainstem autonomic centers, the hypothalamus, the mediodorsal and ventromedial thalamus, and the anterior cingulate. Multiple afferent pathways converge on the anterior insula, particularly in the right hemisphere, which, in turn, projects to the orbitofrontal cortex. The cortical components of this hierarchy are hypothesized to represent body state in an integrated way. An awareness of body states signaled by these cortical regions presumably provides a basis for self-reflective feelings that involve affective and visceral components of self-awareness.

Embodiment

Embodiment refers to the sense of being localized within one's own body. The psychologist Ulrich Neisser has referred to this aspect of self-knowledge as the "ecological" self because the physical abilities of the body constrain how individuals interact with other agents and objects in the environment. The sense of embodiment gives rise to self-location (the feeling of being at a particular location and position in space) and egocentric frame of reference (navigating in the world with reference to one's own viewpoint and spatial location). The ability of humans to use symbolic analogues of themselves also permits mental imagery of the position of the body from a non-egocentric frame of reference (e.g., imaging the view of oneself from behind). In dreams and memories, experiences are sometimes transformed from a first-person to a third-person perspective, and some memories, such as the memory of giving a public address, tend to have a canonical third-person perspective (e.g., from the vantage point of the audience).

Although most individuals experience a spatial unity of self and body, in certain conditions individuals lose this routine sense. As described in Chapter 7, patients with right parietal damage may ignore or deny the existence of the left side of their body (neglect syndrome). Others experience sensations from an amputated body part (phantom limb sensations; see Chapter 4). Still other patients deny that their body is suffering from a particular ailment (agnosognosia) or may experience a feeling of being located outside their body (disembodiment). Out-of-body experiences can also be elicited by psychotropic drugs such as ketamine.

Two brain regions have been implicated in body representations and disembodiment phenomena. A region of extrastriate visual cortex, sometimes called the *extrastriate body area*, is engaged when individuals visually process human bodies or body parts, imagine changes in the position of a body part, or adopt a third-person perspective for visualizing their own body (Figure 11.2A). In addition, out-of-body experiences have been linked to the **temporoparietal junction**, a multisensory area at the border between the temporal and parietal lobes and surrounding the posterior aspect of the Sylvian fissure (Figure 11.2B).

The Swiss neurologist Olaf Blake examined these phenomena in epileptic patients undergoing neurosurgery, as well as in healthy adults during mental imagery tasks. One patient reported out-of-body experiences, illusory changes in arm and leg position, and whole-body displacements following stimulation of

(A)

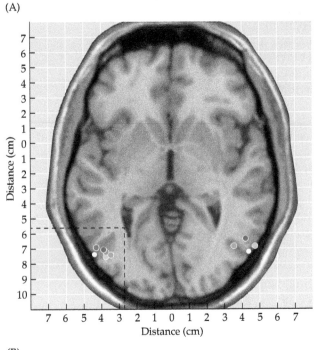

(C)

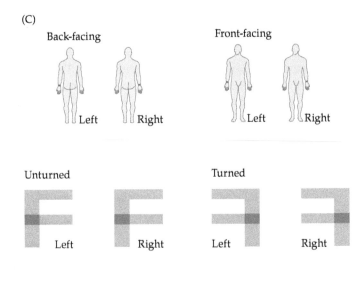

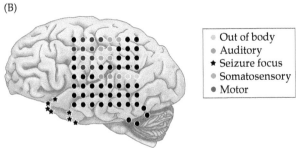

Body task

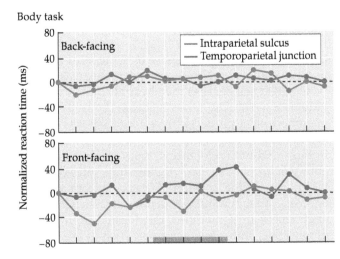

(B)

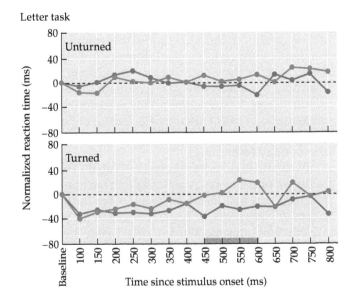

Letter task

Figure 11.2 **Brain regions implicated in body perception and imagery tasks** (A) A region of visual cortex is sensitive to visual features of body parts and is active during the genesis of body imagery. Each dot represents the peak activation from a different functional imaging study. (B) The temporoparietal junction is implicated in body illusions and mental transformations of body position. Cortical stimulation sites are centered on the right angular gyrus of a patient with epilepsy. Stimulation at these sites reliably elicited illusions of body movement and out-of-body experiences. (C) In healthy adults, TMS applied over the right temporoparietal junction 350 to 550 milliseconds after stimulus onset (gray-shaded area in the body task graphs) produced slower reaction times in making judgments of hand location (red wrists) using a mentally rotated, front-facing body frame of reference, but not when making similar dot location judgments on rotated letters. TMS applied over the intraparietal sulcus 450 to 600 milliseconds after stimulus onset (gray-shaded area in the letter task graphs) impairs performance in the letter rotation task, demonstrating a double dissociation between the brain areas underlying body and object mental rotation tasks. (A from Arzy et al. 2006; B after Blanke et al. 2005.)

the right angular gyrus in the vicinity of the temporoparietal junction. Another patient was asked to mentally rotate her body to mimic the viewpoint of her seizure-induced out-of-body experience, and in this case increased activity was recorded near the seizure focus at the left temporoparietal junction. Similarly, healthy adults who imagine rotations of their body axis show enhanced ERP responses localized by source modeling to the temporoparietal junction bilaterally, but with a right-sided bias.

When TMS is applied to this region, judgments of body rotations are affected, but not judgments of mentally rotated objects (Figure 11.2C). Recall that areas near the temporoparietal junction in the right hemisphere have also been implicated in neglect syndrome (see Chapter 7). Given its multisensory input, this region may integrate visual attention with vestibular and somatosensory information to track body positions in space, establish an egocentric visual perspective, and help create a spatial unity of self and body.

In summary, focusing on oneself relies on processing in particular brain areas. The midline PFC, cingulate, and parietal regions contribute to aspects of self-reflexive thought; the insula and anterior cingulate contribute to the representation of central feelings, visceral sensations, and autonomic arousal; and the sense of embodiment relies on visual processing in the extrastriate visual processing areas and on multisensory integration in the temporoparietal junction. Other aspects of the self, including a first-person perspective during social interactions, a capacity for self-regulatory control, and the experience of ownership of intentional actions (agency), build on these basic processes that mediate focusing one's attention on the self and on a body representation of the self.

Perception of Social Cues Evident in the Face and Body

In primates, nonverbal cues in facial expressions and body language provide an abundance of information that influences interpersonal exchanges. Consider your reaction to greeting an acquaintance who fails to make eye contact, whose head and shoulders are turned down, and whose facial expression is unreactive during your conversation. Much information about the personality, mood, and intentionality of others can be inferred from such cues, even unconsciously. Comparisons of these cues with cultural schemas pertinent to social contexts and with prior encounters with the same individual allow you to infer the appropriateness of behavior, to detect changes in comportment, and thus to make appropriate responses. Decoding the nuances of these social signals requires the development of specialized perceptual skills, for an inability to extract such information can cause debilitating social deficits, as is evident in autism (see Introductory Box). The discussion that follows describes the analysis of facial and body movements; for a discussion of vocal affect, see Chapter 12.

Face perception

Human faces present particularly salient and complex social cues that we use to infer the mental states of others (a receptive function) and to influence someone else's thoughts and behavior (a communicative function). A prominent neuropsychological model of face perception (Figure 11.3A) includes a core system for the visual analysis of facial information that begins by parsing facial features in the occipital lobe. Following this initial stage, face processing is divided into two parallel but interacting processing streams. A ventral pathway—including portions of the fusiform gyrus and associated inferior temporal cortex—is specialized for the processing of invariant aspects of face perception in order to discriminate faces from other objects and to individuate

(A)

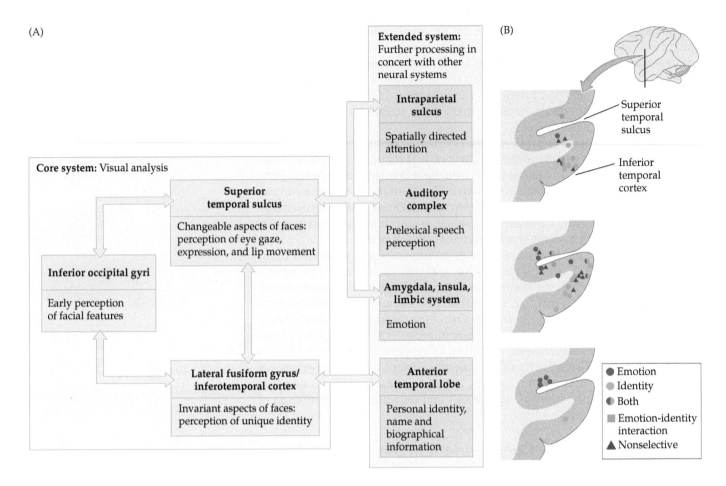

(B)

Figure 11.3 **Pathways for face processing in the temporal lobe** (A) Visual information flows along an inferior temporal–hippocampal route for facial identity, person recognition, and name retrieval. By contrast, a superior temporal–amygdala route processes dynamic feature encoding of facial information, including analysis of eye gaze and emotional expression. (B) Single neurons in the monkey temporal lobe code for facial expression and identity. Macaque monkeys were shown three faces of conspecifics that expressed three different emotions. Recordings were obtained from 45 neurons that showed selective responses to faces relative to other objects. Whereas most emotion-selective neurons were located in the superior temporal sulcus, most identity-selective neurons were located in the inferior temporal cortex. (C) Similar dorsal-ventral dissociations in the temporal lobe are apparent in human subjects when participants are presented with faces that changed in either emotional expression or personal identity. aSTS, anterior superior temporal sulcus; ITG, inferior temporal gyrus; pSTS, posterior superior temporal sulcus. (A after Haxby et al. 2000; B after Hasselmo et al. 1989; C from LaBar et al. 2003.)

(C)

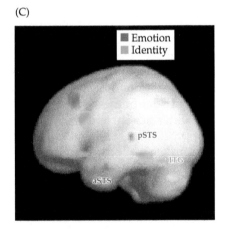

particular people. Recall from Chapter 3 that a region in the fusiform gyrus called the **fusiform face area** is to some degree specialized for encoding such information about faces. Face representations of this ventral pathway are then linked with semantic and episodic knowledge about individuals (such as their names, personalities, and memories of shared experiences) through additional processing stages in the anterior temporal lobe, including the hippocampus and surrounding cortex. In this way, the ventral pathway forms the basis for person recognition.

Another pathway routed through more dorsal sectors of the temporal lobe, including the superior temporal sulcus (STS), is thought to process dynamic facial features, such as changes in emotional expression, mouth movements, and gaze shifts (see Figure 11.3A). The detection of these attributes of biological motion is relayed to the amygdala and other limbic forebrain structures for the analysis of emotion, to multisensory areas for the integration of mouth movements with speech, and to the parietal lobe for spatially directed attention in response to head movements or gaze shifts. The two pathways must interact (e.g., detecting your sister's quirky smile can facilitate her identification), and later processing stations are assumed to feed back onto earlier ones to enhance attention to particular facial features as necessary (e.g., to focus attention on specific face parts in order to resolve ambiguous facial expressions).

Evidence for the partial independence of invariant and dynamic featural processing of faces comes from studies of prosopagnosic patients who have suffered damage to ventral regions of the temporal lobe (see Introductory Box in Chapter 3). These patients have difficulty recognizing individuals by their facial features, but they often identify emotional facial expressions correctly. In contrast, patients with damage to the amygdala or STS have difficulty evaluating emotional expression and/or eye gaze direction, but they can recognize and name individuals normally. Electrophysiological recordings from neurons in the temporal lobe in non-human primates confirm that different populations of cells are specialized for signaling facial identity versus facial expression (Figure 11.3B), in accord with neuroimaging observations in normal humans (Figure 11.3C).

Evidence for the integration of dynamic social information in faces has also come from electrophysiological studies of non-human primates. When monkeys watch images of conspecifics, neurons of the STS tend to increase their firing rate when there is a correspondence between the direction of head movement and the direction of eye gaze, suggesting a preference for a spatial alignment of these two signals (e.g., face forward with eye contact, or both face and eyes averted). In the human amygdala, activity in response to facial expressions also varies according to whether the direction of gaze is forward or averted (Figure 11.4). Responses in both of these regions are enhanced to stimuli that present dynamic shifts in facial configurations compared to static displays.

Decoding rapid changes in facial movements facilitates quick reactions during personal interactions and helps predict the impending actions of others. The ability to extract signals from the position of the eyes may have been helped by an evolutionary change in the color of the sclera, from the darker color in non-human primates to white in hominids. The whites of the eyes make it easier to discern the direction of gaze, and they are important for detecting a person's emotional state. For example, in response to the sympathetic nervous system activity elicited by fear, the palpebral fissure widens markedly, showing more scleral white, and the pupils dilate.

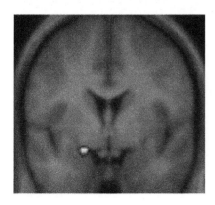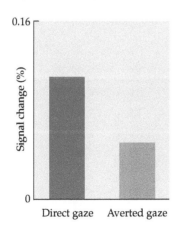

Figure 11.4 The importance of eye features in socioemotional communication The amygdala responds with more intense fMRI activation to threatening faces when eye gaze is direct compared to when it is averted. Individuals tend to judge direct eye contact in the context of a negative social interaction as being more threatening. (After Adams et al. 2003.)

Perception of biological motion

Nonverbal communication entails much more than analyzing faces; as already implied, body movements and gestures are equally important. In parallel with face processing, visual information about the position and status of other body parts is relayed from visual areas (including the specialized extrastriate body area) to similar person recognition and biological motion pathways in the temporal lobe.

Neuroimaging and intracranial recording studies of body part gestures and whole-body ambulation indicate that the posterior STS, particularly in the right hemisphere, discriminates biologically plausible from implausible motion (Figure 11.5). Responses of the STS are greater to human and robotic walking relative to either coherent mechanical motion, such as pendulum swings, or fragmented biological motion (moving but detached body parts). This brain area also responds to human walking even when body parts are partially occluded, which is important for tracking biological motion in natural circumstances.

The STS shows a preference for body actions that are meaningful and goal-directed. For instance, hand and arm gestures that complete intentional action

(A)

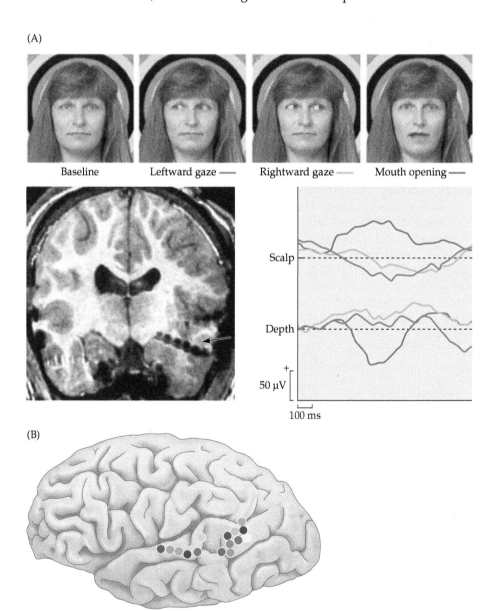

Figure 11.5 Perception of biological motion activates the STS (A) Intracranial recordings were taken from an epilepsy patient with electrodes implanted in the temporal lobe to monitor seizures (electrode locations indicated by arrow in MRI scan). Depth electrodes in the STS respond strongly to mouth movements (red line) relative to shifts in gaze direction (blue and green lines) or static faces ("baseline"). ERPs recorded from the scalp of a healthy participant over the temporal lobes indicate a similar response pattern arising from a source in the vicinity of the STS. μV = microvolts. (B) A summary of neuroimaging studies of biological motion reveals a focus of activity in the STS and adjacent cortical surface. Each colored dot represents a different experiment. (From Allison et al. 2000.)

sequences, such as grabbing a coffee cup and lifting it to the lips, are signaled more robustly than are meaningless or scrambled action sequences. In accord with this observation, sign language gestures that complete grammatically appropriate sentences engage this region more in studies of congenitally deaf individuals than do nonsense gestures.

Activity in the STS further indicates when body movements violate expectations set up by the social circumstance or conflict with other cues (Figure 11.6). For instance, when watching an animated figure direct eye movements in response to the appearance of a visual target, participants' activation in the STS are stronger when the figure's gaze fails to track the object than when it succeeds (Figure 11.6A). In most natural situations, a person's gaze tracks

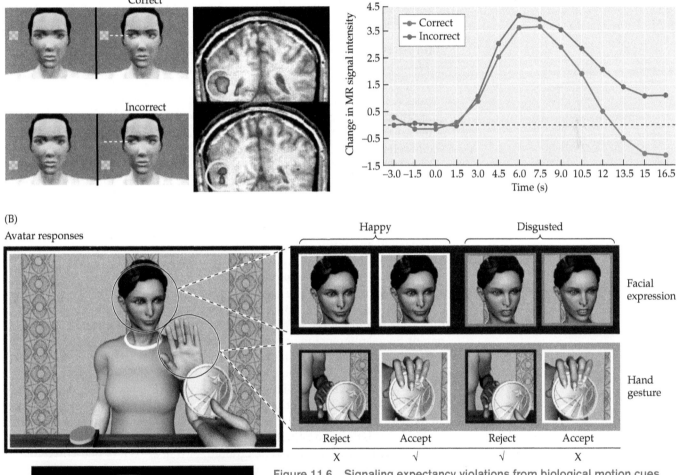

Figure 11.6 Signaling expectancy violations from biological motion cues in the STS (A) Participants watched an animated character whose eyes moved in response to the sudden appearance of a peripheral target. Activation in the STS was greater when the gaze direction deviated from the target than when it correctly tracked the target. (B) Participants interacted with a virtual character by offering her a virtual gold coin. The character reacted to the participant's action through a combination of a change in facial expression (happy, disgusted) and an arm gesture (accept the coin, reject the coin). Activation in the STS and inferior frontal gyrus (IFG) was greater when the facial expression and gesture were incongruent (e.g., happy expression combined with rejection gesture, or disgusted expression combined with acceptance gesture) than when they were congruent. Signaling conflicting nonverbal cues in the context of goal-directed actions helps individuals track when the behavior of others is inconsistent with their intentions or is internally inconsistent. (A after Pelphrey et al. 2003; B from Zucker et al. 2011.)

objects that suddenly appear in the environment, so gaze tracking failures are considered a violation of expected behavior. In addition, the STS preferentially signals when animated characters display conflicting information between their arm gestures and facial affect during a social exchange compared to when these cues are congruent (Figure 11.6B). Such studies highlight the importance of prior knowledge about how people typically behave in social settings (generally or individually) in gleaning insight into the meaning of their current actions.

Interpretation of body language is effective only insofar as it leads to appropriate planning of actions in social settings. The readout of gestural information from regions like the STS feeds into attentional and executive systems in the parietal lobe and premotor areas of the frontal lobe to plan appropriate behavior. The output of the STS is conveyed to frontoparietal cortices for attentional modulation and action planning, as well as to limbic brain structures for further interpretation of the emotional and motivational significance of the motion patterns.

Interpersonal attention and action direction

In social groups, changes in body posture, head orientation, direction of gaze, and facial expression are combined with vocalizations to communicate the attitudes of individuals toward one another and to signal the presence of significant stimuli in the environment. How these cues are used to interpersonally direct attention and initiate group actions has been investigated in studies of social referencing and joint attention.

Social referencing refers to the use of body gestures and facial and vocal expressions of others to determine how to deal with an ambiguous or novel situation. During development, social referencing is critical for learning how to appropriately behave in particular situations, given the lack of social knowledge and self-regulation abilities of young children. For instance, when confronted by a visual cliff apparatus that gives the illusion of a sudden drop in height, 10- to 12-month-old infants will cross the cliff only if guided by positive emotions and encouraging gestures expressed by the parent. In this case, the nonverbal signals communicate to the child whether approach or withdrawal behavior is appropriate in a given context. The emotions in this situation are used to direct the actions of the infant rather than to express the internal state of the parent. Social referencing occurs in a variety of interpersonal contexts to glean information from others to help select appropriate actions.

Joint attention refers to the allocation of processing resources toward an object cued by another individual. This ability emerges in infants around 1 year of age. Gaze direction, head orientation, and body and trunk position all indicate where an individual is focusing attention, making it easy for others to take advantage of this information, particularly to make inferences about features of the environment that otherwise would be ignored, or that are out of one's own field of view. Non-human primates can also exploit joint attention through deception, presenting misleading displays to others and then directing their own actions elsewhere. In humans, this behavior is exemplified by pickpockets, magicians, and athletes, who fake an intended action to facilitate a different one.

Such abilities require knowledge about how others cue spatial locations in the environment. Electrophysiological studies of the monkey STS show that some neurons are tuned to multiple body features to signal the information conveyed by the orientation of a conspecific animal. For example, a neuron might fire in much the same way in response to downward deflection of the eyes or head, or a crouched body position of another monkey, all of which indicate the other animal's attention to something on the ground.

A variant of the Posner attentional cuing task (see Chapter 6) has been used to investigate how gaze shifts can direct visual spatial attention in monkeys and humans. Recall that in this task a central cue is used to direct attention toward a peripheral location in space where an upcoming target may appear. For faces, the position of the eyes serves as a salient cue about where someone is focusing attention in space (even more so than head direction or body posture in some circumstances). To model such behaviors experimentally, subjects in a gaze-directed attentional cuing paradigm are shown a face and are required to respond to a subsequent target that appears either in a location cued by the gaze of the face (valid trials) or in the opposite hemifield (invalid trials) (**Figure 11.7**). The subject's reaction time to detect or discriminate the target is then compared for validly cued and invalidly cued trials to quantify whether the gaze shift was attended by the participant (who is given no other explicit instruction about where to attend). Compared to the use of arrow cues in the standard Posner task, subjects are more willing to follow gaze even when its predictive value is low, suggesting more automaticity in following gaze than in using other symbols to guide attention.

Valid gaze cues improve target detection performance and lead to larger-amplitude early ERP components (P1 and N1) to those targets, implying

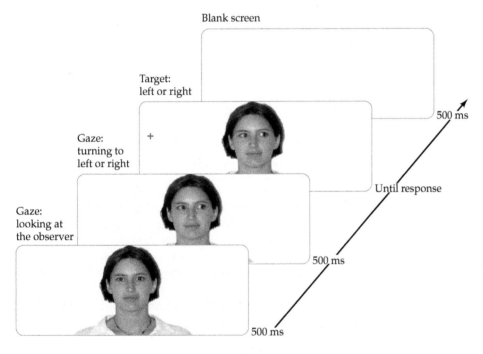

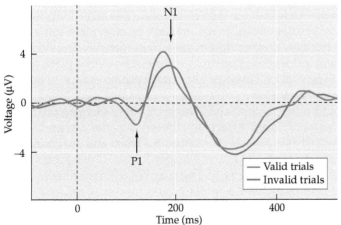

Figure 11.7 Modulation of attentional orienting by gaze cuing Participants view a face with a sudden onset of a particular direction of gaze. Targets subsequently appear either in the location at which gaze is directed (valid trials) or in the opposite visual field (invalid trials). Reaction times are faster on valid trials (the illustration above the graph shows only an invalid trial), and ERP amplitudes are enhanced for early-latency potentials (P1 and N1) that indicate attentional enhancements in extrastriate cortex. μV = microvolts. (After Schuller and Roisson 2001.)

attentional modulation of visual processing in extrastriate regions of cortex (see Chapter 6). Invalidly cued targets show slower reaction times and elicit later enhancement of a P300 component, suggesting a need to update information in working memory because the target appears in an unexpected location. Violations of expectancy based on gaze direction also modulate fMRI activity in the STS, further supporting the important role of this region in using biological motion cues to guide attention in social settings.

In sum, nonverbal cues from the face and body provide a wealth of information that facilitates social interaction. Analysis of this information aids person recognition, provides insight into an individual's emotional state, and guides interpersonal behavior through social referencing and joint attention. Several brain regions contribute to the perception of social cues, including face- and body-processing regions of the visual cortex, the amygdala, and the STS. Some of these areas, such as the amygdala and STS, are sensitive to multiple communicative signals. Stronger responses are elicited in the STS when perceived actions violate expectations, which helps to indicate when the behavior of others doesn't align with their goals or when they are expressing mixed messages.

Social Categorization

The perception of people's identifying features is also used to gauge the characteristics of individuals and place them into social groups. Resource models in social psychology argue that such processes are useful because they facilitate our ability to form impressions and make sense of those around us, especially given the large social network size of humans. For instance, if you are introduced to someone who claims to be a member of a particular political party or religious sect, this information can provide some clues as to the person's core values. Categorizing individuals in this way involves both automatic and controlled processes and is influenced by cultural norms, knowledge of stereotypes, and personal attitudes.

From an evolutionary perspective, social categorization serves important survival functions in defending territories from invading groups, identifying and protecting kin, and selecting mates. In human cultures, however, it is all too clear that prejudicial reactions based on stereotypes of individuals according to their gender, race, and other factors can and do lead to social injustice. As a result, there is much interest in using neuroscientific approaches to inform theories and identify mechanisms of stereotyping and social categorization, and to determine the extent to which these phenomena can be voluntarily regulated and changed by social interactions with others.

Perception of social category information

Research using ERPs has identified the earliest stages of neural processing that are influenced by social category information such as race. ERPs have been the favored method because their temporal sensitivity permits an investigation of rapid, automatic influences of category information before participants can engage deliberate control processes to alter their responses (e.g., to appear more egalitarian). In a typical study, subjects view faces that vary in ethnicity (along with gender and other factors) and categorize those faces according to either racial or nonracial features. Effects attributed to racial categorization generally appear within 200 milliseconds of stimulus onset and are characterized by larger frontocentral N1 and P2 amplitudes for racial out-group faces than for racial in-group faces (Figure 11.8). These early ERP components index attentional orienting responses (see Chapters 2 and 6) and may reflect greater vigilance to unfamiliar out-group members. Later in time the racial category effects reverse, such that enhanced frontocentral N2 responses are observed to

(A) Implicit Association Test (IAT)

(B) Startle eye-blink

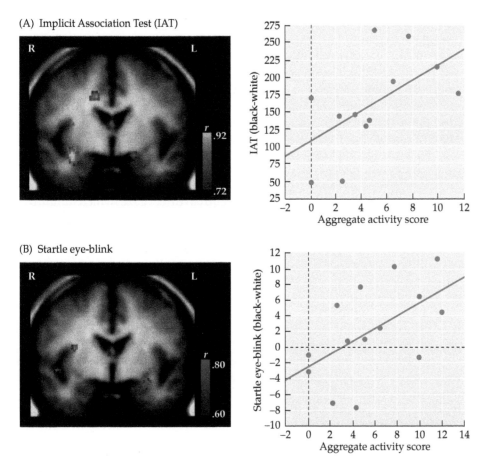

Figure 11.8 Amygdala activity and racial bias Amygdala activity in response to novel African American faces correlates with implicit measures of racial bias in Caucasian participants. Although the amygdala did not exhibit an overall difference between African American (black) and Caucasian (white) faces when averaged across all participants, the degree to which the amygdala differentiated African American and Caucasian faces in individual participants is correlated with (A) Implicit Association Test performance and (B) differential startle eyeblink responses to the faces obtained outside the scanning environment. Correlation coefficients (r) are displayed in the fMRI scans (left), and aggregate scores of significant activity are displayed in the graphs (right). (After Phelps et al. 2000.)

in-group faces, perhaps indicating a shift toward greater individuation of the faces (see Figure 11.8). The impact of social category on early ERP amplitudes is greater when viewing racially unambiguous compared to ambiguous (biracial) faces, and when viewing faces relative to other body parts.

These ERP effects are present regardless of whether the task requires an overt racial categorization or not. Other studies have replicated these findings using tasks known to reduce stereotyping effects, such as detecting a particular visual feature in the stimulus (feature detection task) or judging whether the person depicted is likely to be introverted or to exhibit a particular food preference (individuation task). Such observations indicate that the early processing of social category information may be relatively obligatory, even when that information is not critical to the context of the social interaction.

Stereotypes and automatic racial biases

In addition to the analysis of perceptual features that indicate social categories, interpersonal exchanges can be affected by stereotypes, prejudicial emotional responses, and, ultimately, overt discrimination. In racially biased individuals, executive processing resources are often recruited in an effort to control the expression of automatic negative attitudes toward out-group members. Even in individuals with more egalitarian social views, automatic activation of familiar cultural stereotypes must be overcome to guide social behavior according to one's own attitudes. Building on a foundation of research on emotion processing, emotion regulation, and cognitive control (see Chapters 10 and 13), researchers have begun to identify brain regions whose activity relates to measures of racism and interracial interactions.

One such study reported a correlation in Caucasian participants between amygdala activity in response to unfamiliar African American faces and two implicit indices of racial bias: the Implicit Association Test (IAT; Box 11A) and startle eyeblink responses (see Figure 11.8). Because potentiated eyeblink responses are indicative of negative evaluations (see Box 10A), this study provided additional validation of the IAT as a measure of implicit racial attitudes. The results did not extend to explicit measures of racial bias as assessed by the Modern Racism Scale (see Box 11A), implying that the brain imaging findings may be more specifically associated with implicit racial biases. Subsequent research has also related startle responses and amygdala activation to implicit racial bias but has also shown that these effects are attenuated when the faces are familiar, when the faces have averted rather than direct gaze (which minimizes their threat value; see Figure 11.4), when the task emphasizes individuated rather than categorical processing of people, or when the faces are shown for prolonged durations (presumably reflecting engagement of control processes).

Additional evidence suggests that face-processing regions of the fusiform gyrus show enhanced activity for faces of one's own race, perhaps because of greater individuation and/or familiarity with in-group members. Together, these findings highlight the plasticity, contextual modulation, and regional specificity of neurophysiological activity when members of stigmatized cultural groups are evaluated in various ways.

Such work presents numerous ethical and experimental challenges, and the results must be interpreted cautiously. For instance, functional brain imaging is inherently correlational, and the causal role of brain activity in a given region for behavior as complex as social biases can only be suggestive. A brain scan cannot definitively indicate whether someone is racially biased, whether the activity patterns represent a source or a consequence of behavior, or whether the activity has been shaped by prior exposure to stereotyped messages or by personal experiences. Brain imaging provides only a snapshot of activity in an experimental setting during the performance of a particular cognitive task, and the results may not generalize to behavior during real-world social exchanges. Finally, such measures rarely distinguish between activation of semantic knowledge related to cultural stereotypes versus a personal, evaluative attitude toward members of a social category.

Monitoring and controlling racial bias

Additional work has focused on neural mechanisms engaged when group stereotypes induce response conflicts and motivate a need for voluntary control over biases that might be expressed. A two-stage model of cognitive control (see Chapter 13) supposes the following: (1) that anterior cingulate activity reflects continual monitoring of conflict during information processing; and (2) that prefrontal regions are subsequently recruited to implement regulatory responses once a need for conflict resolution has been detected. This framework has been combined with knowledge about sources of ERP components to make predictions regarding when and how cognitive control is engaged in interracial scenarios. For this objective, a key ERP component is the **error-related negativity (ERN)**, which is sensitive to information-processing conflicts that lead to response errors. The ERN has been localized to the anterior cingulate gyrus and offers a potential neural index of ongoing conflict monitoring that can be applied to studying personal interactions that lead to self-regulation failures (see Chapter 13 for other interpretations of the ERN).

As an example, the ERN has been used to investigate conflict monitoring of racial stereotypes on a weapons identification task. In this rapid classification task, Caucasian participants had to decide whether briefly presented pictures of objects on a computer screen were weapons or tools. Prior to each presentation,

■ BOX 11A MEASURING IMPLICIT AND EXPLICIT RACIAL ATTITUDES

To measure implicit racial attitudes, investigators commonly use the *Implicit Association Test (IAT)* developed by social psychologist Anthony Greenwald and his colleagues. In one version of this test, participants are presented with a series of faces (either African American or Caucasian) intermixed with positively and negatively valenced words that represent good or bad concepts (e.g., *friend*, *enemy*). One set of trials requires the same button-press response for both African American faces and negative words, whereas another response is given for both Caucasian faces and positive words. The response requirements are then reversed so that participants make the same button-press response for both African American faces and positive words, and another response for both Caucasian faces and negative words. Participants are instructed to respond as quickly as possible.

Implicit racial biases are quantified as a difference in reaction time for the second condition compared to the first, such that higher scores reflect greater difficulty (response cost) when pairing African

American faces with positive words and Caucasian faces with negative words than the reverse. Alternate versions assess attitudes toward other social groups based on characteristics such as age, gender, sexual orientation, and political or religious affiliation (you can test yourself at http://www.implicit.harvard.edu).

Although the reasons for the reaction-time costs are debated (including suggestions that they reflect knowledge of cultural stereotypes rather than personal attitudes), the IAT has good test reliability. Furthermore, the IAT has been validated with a psychophysiological index of evaluative emotional responding (see the text). Performance on this test is compared to other paper-and-pencil assessments that test racial attitudes explicitly, such as the Modern Racism Scale. Other tests determine whether subjects are motivated to respond to out-groups in a way that appears more socially appropriate to others. Often, IAT performance reveals biases in processing that are not captured by the explicit measures and can be related to electrophysiological signatures of automatic evaluative processes (see text).

References

CUNNINGHAM, W. A., K. J. PREACHER AND M. R. BANAJI (2001) Implicit attitude measures: Consistency, stability, and convergent validity. *Psychol. Sci.* 12: 163–170.

GEHRING, W. J., A. KARPINSKI AND J. L. HILTON (2003) Thinking about interracial relations. *Nat. Neurosci.* 6: 1241–1243.

GREENWALD, A. G., D. E. MCGHEE AND J. K. L. SCHWARTZ (1998) Measuring individual differences in implicit cognition: The Implicit Association Test. *J. Pers. Soc. Psychol.* 74: 1464–1480.

MCCONAHAY, J. B. (1996) Modern racism, ambivalence, and the Modern Racism Scale. In *Prejudice, Discrimination, and Racism*, J. Dovidio and S. Gaertner (eds.). Orlando, FL: Academic Press, pp. 91–125.

PLANT, E. A. AND P. G. DEVINE (1998) Internal and external motivation to respond without prejudice. *J. Pers. Soc. Psychol.* 69: 811–832.

an African American or Caucasian face was flashed on the screen. Priming of objects by African American faces tended to facilitate detection of weapons and impair detection of tools, whereas priming by Caucasian faces had no differential effect. The ERN that was time-locked to the response showed not only sensitivity to performance (larger for errors than for correct object classifications) but also stereotype incongruity on error trials (larger for tools primed by African American faces than for the other face-object combinations; Figure 11.9).

The ERN stereotyping effects were larger in individuals who characterized themselves as being primarily internally motivated to regulate prejudiced reactions than in those who acknowledge avoidance of social disapproval as part of the motivation to regulate their reactions. If the two-stage model of cognitive control is correct, this finding suggests that internally motivated individuals exhibit greater online monitoring of stereotype conflict as a potentially biased response is generated. Because the behavioral and ERN results occur in individuals with low levels of racial bias, they implicate a Stroop-like response conflict due to automatic activation of learned cultural stereotypes in relation to aggression and hostility (see Chapters 7 and 13 for a discussion of the Stroop effect). Internally motivated, low-bias individuals have greater motivation to override these automatic stereotypes in order to behave in accordance with their own egalitarian principles.

Prefrontal responses to out-group faces may also mediate the relationship between implicit racial attitudes and cognitive consequences following an interracial encounter. In one study, researchers gave Caucasian participants the IAT test followed by a staged encounter with either an African American or a Caucasian experimenter, who asked them to comment on social topics of racial profiling and the college fraternity system. A classic Stroop color-naming interference task (see Chapter 13) was then administered. In a separate session, the participants underwent fMRI scanning while being presented with either African American or Caucasian faces. Performance on the Stroop task was quantified as a function of implicit racial attitudes and the race of the experimenter in the social encounter, and compared with the fMRI activity to out-group faces.

As **Figure 11.10** shows, individuals characterized by implicit racial biases based on IAT performance exhibited greater Stroop interference following the

(A)

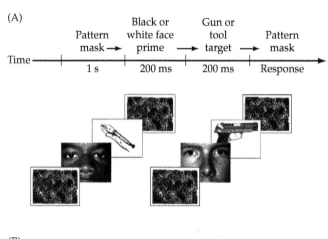

(B)

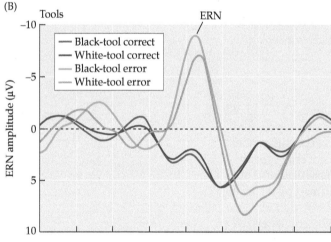

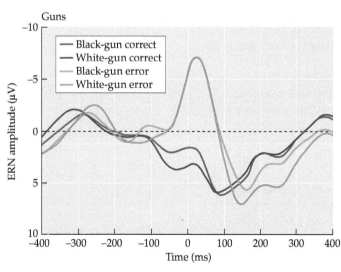

Figure 11.9 Error-related negativity (ERN) and social stereotypes (A) Participants had to categorize whether the objects presented were guns or tools. These objects were primed by brief presentations of black or white male faces. (B) Presumably because of cultural stereotypes linking black males with hostility, participants made more errors in identifying tools when primed by a black face (behavioral data not shown), and these errors were associated with larger ERN responses than when tools were primed by a white face. No differences due to the priming manipulation were found on gun trials. (C) ERN activity to tools primed by black male faces was larger for individuals who were internally motivated to respond without prejudice (good regulators) than for those not motivated (nonregulators) or those motivated by external factors to appear unbiased in social contexts (poor regulators). This ERN pattern suggests that individuals who are internally motivated to respond without prejudice have greater demands placed on automatic control processes when cultural stereotypes are activated. μV = microvolts. (A,B after Amodio 2008; C after Amodio et al. 2008.)

(C)

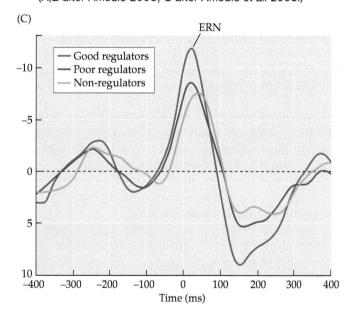

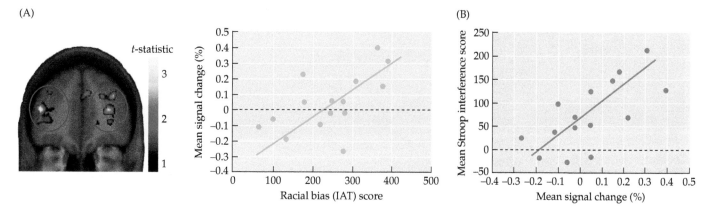

Figure 11.10 Implicit racial attitudes and cognitive performance (A) Individuals who had greater dorsolateral PFC activity (circled) in response to out-group faces also had greater implicit racial biases as assessed by the IAT. (B) The same individuals exhibited a strong relationship between right dorsolateral PFC activity and color Stroop task interference following an interracial encounter. (After Richeson et al. 2003.)

interracial encounter, but not following the encounter with an in-group member. Functional MRI analyses revealed a positive correlation between performance on the IAT test and activity in the anterior cingulate and dorsolateral prefrontal cortex (dlPFC) to African American faces relative to Caucasian faces. The magnitude of dlPFC activity also predicted the relationship between IAT and Stroop task performance. These results suggest that individuals with implicit racial biases exert greater effort in controlling reactions to out-group members in part by engaging prefrontal circuitry.

This initial body of research has laid the groundwork for discovering the relationships between social behavior and brain correlates of the psychological constructs underlying racial bias. To guard against the influence of cultural stereotypes, internally motivated, low-bias individuals experience greater demand on executive resources than do high-bias individuals. In contrast, high-bias individuals experience greater demand during interracial encounters. Such endeavors inform debates about the role of neuroscience in contributing to an understanding of racial and other social prejudices.

Impression formation and trust

In addition to social category information, other personal attributes are readily judged from physical features and inferred from nonverbal behaviors to form general impressions of individuals. One such personality trait is trustworthiness. Many individuals end up in bankruptcy because they are susceptible to financial scams. People who find themselves in this predicament may be poor at evaluating the trustworthiness of those who are trying to get their money.

Neuroimaging studies have found that assessment of trustworthiness based on facial appearance alone is associated with activity in brain regions involved in other aspects of social cognition and emotional evaluation. In particular, enhanced activity is observed in the insula when participants are shown faces of individuals whom others have judged to have an untrustworthy appearance, and enhanced activity is observed in the medial PFC, orbitofrontal cortex, and caudate for faces deemed trustworthy. The amygdala responds to both highly trustworthy and highly untrustworthy faces; however it is more sensitive to differences in untrustworthy faces (**Figure 11.11A**). These patterns are evident even when the faces are not explicitly appraised for trust, indicating automatic evaluative processes. Confirming the neuroimaging findings, autistic individuals

(A)

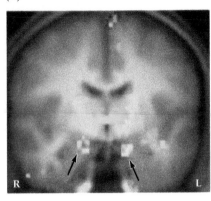
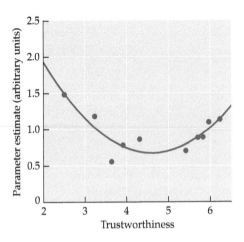

(B)

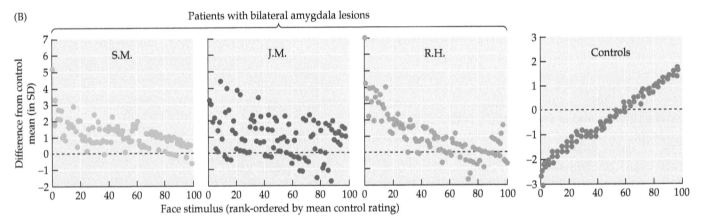

Figure 11.11 Evaluating trust in faces (A) A region of the amygdala (arrows) responds strongly to both very untrustworthy and very trustworthy faces, with weak responses to intermediate values of trustworthiness. However, this region is more sensitive to detecting subtle differences in untrustworthy faces than in trustworthy faces, as indicated by the shape of the function depicted in the right-hand panel (plotted data come from the right amygdala). (B) Trustworthiness ratings from three patients with bilateral amygdala damage (S.M., J.M., R.H.). Values plotted in the left three panels depict each patient's standard deviation (SD) from the mean ratings of control subjects, which are illustrated in the far-right panel. Each patient rated untrustworthy faces as more trustworthy than controls did, but the patients' performance became normal for more trustworthy faces. (A after Said et al. 2008; B after Adolphs et al. 1998.)

(see Introductory Box) and patients with bilateral amygdala damage (Figure 11.11B) tend to judge untrustworthy faces as more trustworthy.

The impression of trustworthiness is gleaned from a rapid, global impression of the face that occurs within 100 milliseconds and improves little with longer exposure. This pattern indicates the importance of a "first glance" prior to initiation of saccades to specific facial features. Behavioral studies have shown that judgments of trustworthiness are related to competence and facial attractiveness—a fact exploited by Hollywood casting agents, politicians, and business managers who hire salespeople. Analysis of shifts in eye gaze and body movements also contributes to trustworthiness appraisals in that individuals who are "shifty-eyed" and restless are rated as less trustworthy because of apparent nervousness. Such cues are also used by airline security officers to identify potentially suspect passengers. These findings reveal how the basic building blocks of social perception, which are based on nonverbal cues related to gaze analysis, joint attention, and emotional evaluation, can be combined to infer personality attributes of others. Studies of trust in economic games are described in Chapter 14.

Understanding the Actions and Emotions of Others

To successfully navigate the social environment, it is important to link social and affective cues with behavioral outcomes during interpersonal interactions. This ability ranges from mere mimicry of motoric and emotional gestures to more complex forms of goal-directed imitation behavior, and ultimately to modeling one's behavior after the behavior of others to transmit learning and establish cultural practices. In humans, social competence is further facilitated by inferring mental states in others, and attributing the actions of others to their beliefs, goals, desires, and feelings. This multifaceted capacity is called **mentalizing** or **theory of mind**.

Scholars debate about whether mentalizing occurs though simulation of the behaviors and internal states of others (e.g., mentally representing potential actions, feelings, or thoughts of others as if they were one's own) or by the building of theories (scripts) of how others typically behave in particular contexts. The philosopher Daniel Dennett suggests that social interactions benefit when one adopts an **intentional stance**—that is, assuming that others are agents motivated to behave in a way that is consistent with their current mental state, which may differ from one's own mental states and/or the reality of the situation. As detailed in the discussion that follows, coding and interpreting the actions and mental states of others are complex processes involving both dedicated neural systems and the co-opting of domain-general functions like working memory and symbolic representation.

Mirror neurons

To interpret behaviors meaningfully, it is useful to code actions performed by others in a way that is related to one's own actions. In the 1990s, the discovery of **mirror neurons** in the premotor cortex of the macaque monkey brain sparked much interest and debate about possible neural mechanisms underlying action representation. These neurons in and around the inferior frontal gyrus (area F5, presumably homologous to the inferior frontal convexity in humans) increase their activity not only when a grasping action is selected and performed, but also when that action is passively viewed while it is being performed by another animal or a human experimenter (**Figure 11.12**).

Such mirror responses are more robust when participants are observing goal-directed biological actions compared to non-goal-directed biological actions (mimes) or goal-directed mechanical actions (e.g., a hammer hitting a nail). The responses often track the general goal of the motor act (e.g., putting food into a bucket) rather than the specific features of the movement, such as the initial starting position or orientation of a hand executing the action. A smaller proportion of F5 neurons respond to both visual and auditory features of a unique goal-directed biological action (e.g., ringing a bell).

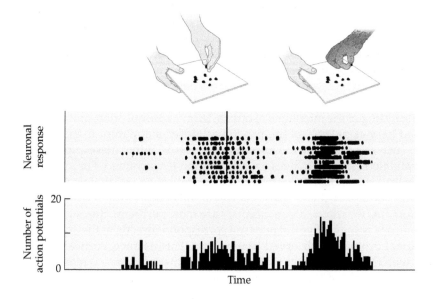

Figure 11.12 **A mirror neuron in the premotor cortex of a macaque monkey** The experimenter places and removes a food morsel from a tray while the monkey watches. The raster plot shows the neuronal responses (the vertical line indicates the time the morsel was placed on the tray), which are compiled in the histograms below. The neuron activates both when the monkey watches passively (left panel) and when the monkey itself retrieves the morsel (right panel). (After Rizzolatti et al. 1996.)

(A)

(B)

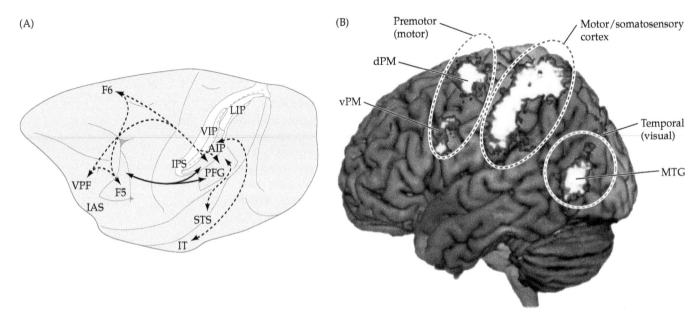

Figure 11.13 The monkey and human mirror systems (A) Schematic of the key components in the macaque brain (shaded in yellow). This system includes the ventral premotor cortex (F5), ventral parietal regions (PFG, AIP) and their interconnections (solid lines). Connections between the mirror system and some other brain areas are indicated by dashed lines. AIP, anterior intraparietal area; F6, dorsal premotor cortex; IAS, inferior limb of the arcuate sulcus; IPS, intraparietal sulcus; IT, inferior temporal lobe; LIP, lateral intraparietal area; STS, superior temporal sulcus; VIP, ventral intraparietal area; VPF, ventral prefrontal cortex. (B) The putative human mirror system. Data are from an fMRI study that identified reliable activations across individual subjects for both action observation and action execution. dPM, dorsal premotor cortex; MTG, middle temporal gyrus; vPM, ventral premotor cortex. (A after Rizzolatti and Sinigaglia 2010; B from Keysers et al. 2010.)

Mirror neurons have also been found in a region of rostral inferior parietal cortex that projects to premotor area F5, implicating an interconnected fronto-parietal mirror system (Figure 11.13). Some neurons in this circuit also exhibit context specificity of the action sequences related to the end goal (e.g., selectively responding to grasping actions that lead to eating rather than grasping actions that simply move an object from one place to another). Neurons in the superior temporal sulcus (STS) relay perceptual information about biological motion to the parietal component of this system but do not exhibit mirroring responses themselves. Because the observation of actions does not automatically elicit an analogous motor response, activity in this premotor circuit is inhibited to prevent obligatory copying behavior.

A number of investigators have used this neurophysiological evidence to speculate about the importance of these areas of the primate brain in generating an understanding of the intentions of others, language acquisition, and empathy (discussed below), as well as the functional deficits apparent in behavioral disorders such as autism (see the Introductory Box). Whether these implications will be validated remains to be seen, and caution is warranted. For one thing, adult monkeys do not learn much by direct imitation—a fact that undermines what would perhaps be the simplest interpretation of the role of mirror neurons. And in humans, where these speculations are most pertinent, the evidence for mirror neurons is suggestive but does not correspond directly to the anatomical or functional properties observed in monkeys. For instance, cortical activity detected with fMRI in response to similar paradigms in humans is more widely distributed throughout the motor system and STS; moreover, similar activity occurs when people mime. Unlike the monkey electrophysiological data, most of the human evidence has come from brain imaging studies. These studies do not have the spatial resolution to determine whether the executed and observed actions are being signaled by the same neurons (a key criterion for defining a mirror neuron) or by adjacent ones within the same general brain area.

Some researchers taking an embodied cognition perspective (see Chapter 9) have suggested that mirror neurons provide a means for understanding social actions through direct perceptual-motor links. Others believe such linkages are simply established by experience through general associative learning processes and do not represent a unique social cognitive function. Whatever the correct interpretation, these observations indicate that viewing actions pertinent to particular behavioral goals influences the activity of some frontoparietal neurons in the same way as performing those actions does.

Perspective taking and mental-state attribution

Although mirroring functions help establish shared representations used for understanding agent-directed actions, they do not readily distinguish the execution of one's own actions from the observation of similar actions executed by others. Moreover, actions do not map onto intentions in a one-to-one manner. Mirroring depends on another agent being present in the immediate environment and cannot account for other forms of mental simulation, such as self-projection into past or future circumstances. In short, differentiating one's actions from those of others and understanding the reasons behind others' actions clearly require cognitive abilities and mechanisms that go beyond mirroring.

Key among these is the ability to flexibly adopt the perspective of another individual (third-person perspective) and distinguish that viewpoint from one's own (first-person perspective). Because an egocentric view of the world may be part of a default mode of information processing, adopting other people's perspectives and inferring their beliefs, motives, or feelings requires a disengagement of self-directed thoughts, a redirection of attention to the mental and physical states of others, and a decoupling of knowledge of the actual unfolding of events from other people's perceptions of those events. Memory is also important in this process because prior knowledge about the personality traits and response patterns of others in similar contexts refines one's own interpretation of the current social context and the possible responses to it.

Neuroimaging studies have compared first- and third-person **perspective taking** across different cognitive, emotional, and motoric domains. For instance, participants might imagine themselves or someone else performing specific actions, responding to a painful stimulus, or reacting to an emotional scenario. Other studies of mental-state attributions have asked participants to consider the viewpoints of different characters in stories or cartoons, to guess what an opponent might do during an interactive game, or to judge whether historical figures had access to knowledge about specific artifacts. While many studies have used explicit instructions to adopt the perspective of another agent, in social situations often the intentions and mental states of others are inferred spontaneously.

In all these domains, taking the perspective of others and inferring their mental states elicits activity in a set of brain regions that includes the medial PFC (most consistently the paracingulate cortex), temporal polar cortex, right inferior parietal cortex, temporoparietal junction, and superior temporal sulcus (Figure 11.14). Because of the complexity of the mentalizing construct, heterogeneity of the tasks involved, and variety of the control conditions employed, it is difficult to ascribe specific functions to these brain areas. Nonetheless, the temporoparietal junction may be particularly concerned with transient inferences based on the current context, whereas the medial prefrontal cortex may be more

(A) Temporal pole

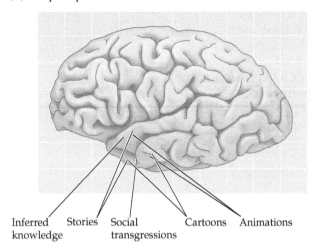

Inferred knowledge   Stories   Social transgressions   Cartoons   Animations

(B) Superior temporal sulcus

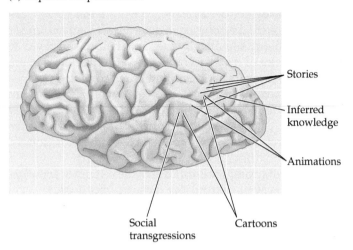

Stories

Inferred knowledge

Animations

Social transgressions   Cartoons

(C) Paracingulate cortex

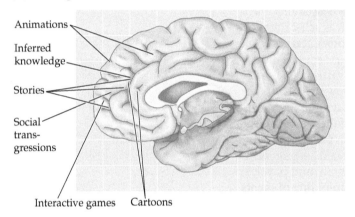

Animations

Inferred knowledge

Stories

Social transgressions

Interactive games   Cartoons

Figure 11.14 **Brain regions implicated in mentalizing tasks** Across various domains, activity in the temporal pole (A), superior temporal sulcus (B), and paracingulate cortex (C) is elicited when participants adopt the perspectives of other individuals and infer their mental states. (After Frith and Frith 2003.)

concerned with inferences based on more enduring traits or qualities. Although some view these regions as simply supporting domain-general cognitive operations needed to solve the mentalizing tasks (the functions needed to retrieve memories or semantic knowledge, reallocate attentional resources, manipulate internal representations, etc.), recent evidence indicates some specificity in the relevant brain activity for solving social problems. For instance, the medial PFC activation during mentalizing tasks is greater than during general reasoning tasks that do not involve social evaluations.

Theory of mind in children and apes

In the late 1970s, psychologists David Premack and Guy Woodruff raised the question of whether chimpanzees and other great apes have the capacity to represent and understand the mental states of conspecifics in the same general way that humans do. Observations of great apes in the wild indicate that they engage in deception (to hoard food sources, for example), which requires at least some understanding of where conspecifics are orienting their attention and what they expect to happen in a given social context.

To ask whether chimpanzees have basic mentalizing abilities, experimenters paired subordinate and dominant chimpanzees in a large chamber (Figure 11.15). The subordinate chimp was shown food items that the dominant chimp could either see or not see, or was shown that the location of a food item had or

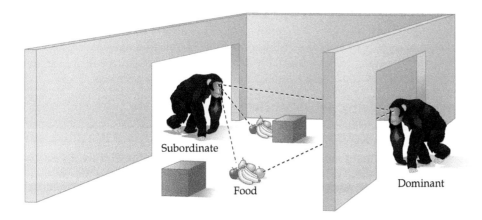

Figure 11.15 **Testing mentalizing ability in chimpanzees** This socially competitive paradigm tests what chimpanzees know about the viewpoint of a conspecific. A subordinate chimp is shown multiple food caches that are either out of the view or in the view of a dominant chimp. Subordinate chimps prefer to move toward the food cache that is out of view of the dominant chimp, conferring a behavioral advantage. Chimps exhibit similar behavior when a food cache is switched to a different location, again unbeknownst to a dominant chimp. These observations imply that, in socially competitive situations, chimps have rudimentary mentalizing abilities. (After Hare et al. 2001.)

had not been switched out of view of the dominant chimp. In either case, the subordinate chimp showed a preference for moving toward food items about which the dominant chimp either had no knowledge or could be assumed to hold a false belief about its location. Such behavior clearly imparts an advantage to the subordinate chimp in the context of competition for food with a dominant conspecific, and could be interpreted as relying on some degree of third-person perspective taking.

However, the acid test of a theory of mind is the capacity to predict others' behavior according to false beliefs that they hold. Understanding the false beliefs of others requires making a distinction between knowledge about a true state of affairs and what another individual falsely believes to be true. False-belief experimental tasks come in two major flavors: location-change tasks and unexpected-contents tasks (see also Chapter 15). In *location-change tasks*, an object is placed in one location, and unbeknownst to a third party, the position of the object is switched to an alternate location. The participant then must indicate where the third party would look for the object (its true location or the location where the third party last viewed the object). In *unexpected-contents tasks*, an object is placed in a container, and unbeknownst to a third party, the object is replaced by another one. The participant must then indicate which object the third party thinks is in the container.

Humans develop false-belief attributions to characters in animated vignettes by about 4 years of age. However, because these tasks require complex narrative and action sequence comprehension, working memory, and inhibition of rapid responses, there is some debate about the specificity of the findings. Some investigators have proposed that children between 3 and 4 years old simply learn to select the correct responses in the task rather than depending on theory-of-mind abilities. Nonetheless, children of this age routinely use words like *pretend*, *think*, *know*, *want*, and *like*, implying some knowledge about mental states. In contrast, autistic children (and autistic adults) generally fail false-belief tests, although some investigators find the evidence to be equivocal because of the potentially confounding deficits in language abilities and executive function present in autism.

Given the controversy over whether children and chimpanzees possess theory-of-mind abilities, some investigators have turned to the distinction made in memory research between implicit and explicit processes (see Chapter 8). Most researchers believe that young children and great apes can implicitly (i.e., unconsciously) track another individual's mental state. However, they also admit that there is currently no convincing evidence that young children and apes can explicitly represent the mental contents of another individual, as in the ability to have thoughts such as "I know my friend thinks that the food is in location A when I know it is really at B." This ability to abstract the mental contents of agents in a social situation and represent them symbolically, also called *metarepresentation*, presumably requires further cognitive development and is unlikely in young children, let alone non-human primates.

Empathy, sympathy, and prosocial behavior

Understanding another individual's beliefs, goals, and intentions also extends to emotion. Although sometimes incorporated into the concept of theory of mind, understanding others' emotional states recruits brain regions that are not necessarily used for making inferences about other mental states. A better descriptor of understanding someone else's emotional state is *empathy*. **Empathy** is the capacity to comprehend and resonate with another's emotional experience, which leads to a sharing of that person's feelings. Once an empathic feeling arises, individuals must distinguish their own emotional responses from those of the other individual and regulate their responses accordingly. This ability requires knowing that the other person's feelings are the source of the shared emotional state.

Rather than exemplifying a specific emotion, empathy can be considered a process by which any emotion is shared according to the social context. For instance, having a conversation about a friend's nervousness before a job interview may lead to shared feelings of anxiety. When the conversation shifts to the outcome of the interview, feelings of disappointment may be shared upon hearing that the job was not obtained. Eliciting empathy is critical for effective storytelling and advertising.

Empathy differs from **sympathy** in that a sympathetic reaction does not entail a sharing of emotional experience. Rather, a person who is sympathetic may feel concerned or sorry for the plight of another person but does not feel the actual emotion felt by the other. In the job interview example, for instance, one may feel sympathetic toward a friend's situation without actually experiencing anxiety or disappointment of one's own.

Empathy has both automatic and controlled components and builds on basic social cognitive and emotion-processing mechanisms. Early in development, human infants will cry in reaction to another infant's cry and will mimic basic facial emotions expressed by a parent. At about 2 years of age, when self-versus-other distinctions and social emotions such as shame begin to emerge, children express sympathetic concern, such as gestures of consolation to family members in distress. Although initially such gestures are egocentric (e.g., offering a gift such as a doll to an adult whom the child likes), the offerings gradually become other-focused (e.g., offering a gift that the adult family member likes). With increased cognitive and emotional capacities for perspective taking later in childhood, more complex forms of empathy are conveyed. Forms of empathy observed in apes presumably rely on more automatic aspects of emotion interpretation and somatic activation, which contribute to helping, affiliative, and cooperative behaviors.

Psychologist Jean Decety developed a model of empathy that encompasses several of the social and emotional processes, as well as the concepts of mental representation, discussed earlier (Figure 11.16). According to the model, a full empathic response, which can be initiated either automatically or voluntarily, requires the coordinated operation of four component processes:

1. *Emotion sharing* between individuals is based on automatic perception-action coupling and shared somatic-emotional representations that rely on processing in the somatosensory cortex, insula, and anterior cingulate cortex.

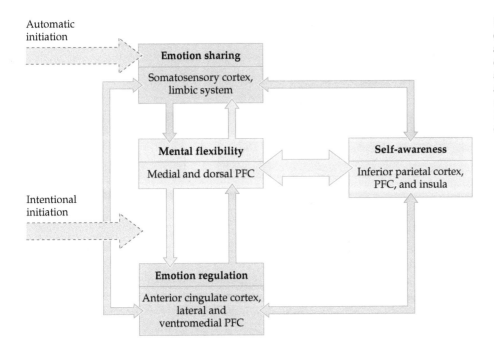

Figure 11.16 **A proposed model of empathy** A full empathic response to another individual is thought to depend on brain regions involved in sharing somatic and emotional responses, self-awareness and self-other distinctions, mental flexibility in social contexts (including perspective taking), and emotion regulation.

2. *Self-awareness* and the distinction between self and other are also thought to entail processing in the parietal lobes, prefrontal cortex, and insula.

3. *Mental flexibility* to adopt the perspective of another individual recruits medial and dorsolateral prefrontal regions, among others.

4. *Emotion regulation* operates on the emotional and somatic states generated by engaging executive control mechanisms in the anterior cingulate and lateral and ventromedial prefrontal cortex.

Evidence to support the emotion-sharing component comes from studies that ask participants to observe another individual experience an emotion and to experience the same emotion themselves (or imagine their own emotional reaction to the same situation). The logic of these studies is similar to the mirroring tasks described earlier, but it concerns emotional states rather than motor actions. The brain regions involved in these tasks include the insula, anterior cingulate cortex, and secondary somatosensory cortices (Figure 11.17A), which are thought to represent a shared feeling state with another individual and promote a motivation to act. These areas are distinct from those that mediate the self-awareness (see Figure 11.1) and mental flexibility (Figure 11.17B; see also Figure 11.15) components of empathy, as well as the mirror neuron circuit for action understanding (see Figure 11.13). Brain regions that support emotion-regulating processes are discussed in Chapter 10.

Although it is generally assumed that empathy leads to helping others and altruistic actions, additional factors influence such prosocial behaviors. For instance, high levels of arousal associated with observing another's troubled emotional state can lead to personal distress, a lack of emotion regulation, and thus an inability to take action other than to alleviate one's own distress. Prosocial behaviors are more likely when an individual is in a positive mood, when the action required is not unpleasant or onerous, and when the person to be helped is not a direct competitor. Adults (but not young children) may also engage in helpful behaviors to repair sad moods because they understand the social rewards associated with the actions. Nonetheless, in some circumstances

Figure 11.17 Brain regions that mediate emotion sharing (A) Empathy tasks entail asking participants to consider the emotional state of others and themselves in response to emotion-eliciting situations, such as those that evoke pain. The tasks may require watching another individual's emotional reaction or imaging the reaction of others or oneself in response to a painful action. Brain regions common to both self- and other-focused painful reactions include the anterior cingulate cortex (ACC) and insula. (B) Brain regions that mediate the emotion-sharing component of empathy (orange) are distinct from those that mediate the cognitive ability to flexibly adopt the perspective of another individual (green). AI, anterior insula; MFC, medial prefrontal cortex; SII, secondary somatosensory cortex; STS, superior temporal sulcus; TP, temporal pole; TPJ, temporoparietal junction. (From Hein and Singer 2008.)

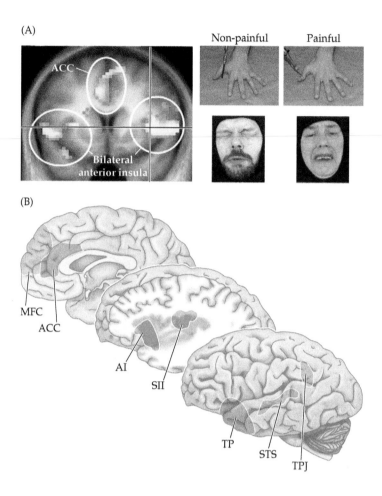

empathy can lead to antisocial behavior, as when an accomplice is empathic toward the motives of a fellow criminal.

Social Competition

Competition among members of a species' social group establishes hierarchies that affect the distribution of wealth, resource allocation, mating opportunities, and division of labor. Leaders of the social group are responsible for defending against intruders and for establishing acceptable norms of behavior. Members who do not adhere to the rules face punishment or ostracism. Provided that governance and rank are not entirely inherited, group dynamics can influence the maintenance of the hierarchy, leading to social upheaval and a change in social structure. The biobehavioral processes that mediate social competition and its consequences for the individual are described here.

Of course, social competitive forces must be balanced by social cooperation and affiliative functions that promote social bonds among a particular group's members. Some evolutionary anthropologists believe that the drive for social cooperation was particularly influential in the evolution of advanced intellectual skills in humans. These topics are covered in Box 11B and Chapter 15.

Social rank and stress

For species that live in social groups, the relative dominance ordering (rank) of individuals has important implications for physical and mental health. In Westernized human societies, lower socioeconomic status is associated with increased risk of cardiovascular, respiratory, rheumatoid, and psychiatric

■ BOX 11B SOCIAL BONDS AND KINSHIP

Social signals related to mating, bonding, and kinship are important for the maintenance and survival of social groups. Some primate species analyze secondary sex coloration in the face and anogenital regions to select mates. Female rhesus monkeys prefer looking at males whose faces are redder, and this coloration is in turn related to the amount of circulating testosterone in males during the mating season. In mandrills, a male's social dominance rank is accompanied by continually updated changes in secondary sexual characteristics such as testicular volume and reddening of anogenital skin. These characteristics facilitate the mating success of the most dominant members of a species.

In some species, such as prairie voles, mating leads to the establishment of monogamous partner preferences. A breeding pair of prairie voles shares the same nest, intruders of either sex are rejected, and males contribute to care of the young. Even following death, a new mate is accepted by either sex only rarely (about 20 percent of the time). Offspring remain sexually immature until they leave the natal group, and females undergo puberty only when exposed to the urine of an unrelated male, at which time they mate repeatedly with the same male and form a selective and long-lasting pair bond. During mating, oxytocin and vasopressin are released in mesolimbic pathways, including the nucleus accumbens, where they interact with the dopaminergic reward system (see Chapter 14). This neurochemical interaction presumably links social information of the partner with reward circuits to reinforce the sexual preference and solidify the social bond. If oxytocin receptors are blocked during mating, long-term partner preferences are not established.

In other species, oxytocin and vasopressin also play important roles in social recognition. Rats given vasopressin show increased social recognition abilities by olfactory cues, as measured by habituation in sniffing behavior toward a recently introduced partner. Vasopressin and oxytocin knockout mice exhibit a form of social amnesia in which they fail to habituate to the presence of a recently introduced partner, despite normal habituation to the repeated presentation of other odorants. These social recognition abilities in rodents have been linked to activity in mesolimbic structures, including the amygdala and septum. For instance, oxytocin administration in the central nucleus of the amygdala engages inhibitory neurons to decrease fear signaling, increase parasympathetic tone, and reduce release of the stress hormone corticosterone in social contexts.

Many primates, particularly arboreal species, distinguish kin from non-kin by vocal characteristics alone. Female vervet monkeys distinguish the cries of juvenile monkeys in their troop. A mother vervet will respond selectively to the cry of her own infant and will look preferentially at other mothers in the troop when their own infants cry. Auditory characteristics of primate calls, such as the acoustic structure and number of vocalizations, are also used to indicate social rank and physical health to other members of the group.

References

Ghazanfar, A. A. and L. R. Santos (2004) Primate brains in the wild: The sensory bases for social interactions. *Nat. Rev. Neurosci.* 5: 203–216.

Insel, T. R. and R. D. Fernald (2004) How the brain processes social information: Searching for the social brain. *Annu. Rev. Neurosci.* 27: 697–722.

diseases, as well as increased mortality rates (including infant mortality). Both physical and psychosocial stressors contribute to these effects (see Box 10B for a description of the stress system). The impact of rank remains significant even when other lifestyle factors, such as higher incidence of alcohol use or poor diet, are taken into consideration. Although socioeconomic status indicates rank at a macro level of social organization, the complex, nested structure of human cultures yields ranks at multiple social scales (e.g., within one's family, place of employment, or peer group).

Across species, the relationship between rank and stress further depends on the characteristics of the culture. For despotic social groups—in which resource access is skewed and dominance is attained through intimidation—stress is particularly high for subordinates. Stress, however, can shift among group members depending on how dominance is maintained. Dominant group members can experience high stress when their rank must be maintained by constant physical aggression (as in ring-tailed lemurs), or during times of major hierarchical reorganization when their rank is at risk of being lost. Thus, stress is associated with both lower rank and life "at the top" (Figure 11.18).

Subordinates have greater physiological indices of stress relative to dominant members when dominance is asserted through psychological intimidation (e.g., eye contact, vocalizations) or for social groups with stable, inherited social hierarchies, as in female rhesus macaques. Subordinates can reduce their stress if coping strategies are available. In non-human primates, these activities include forming social coalitions through grooming and roaming to avoid encounters

Figure 11.18 Rank and stress in baboons By observing wild male baboons over a 9-year period, researchers characterized the relationship between dominance rank and biomarkers of stress. Measures of fecal glucocorticoids increased with lower dominance rank, with the exception of the most dominant baboons, who also experienced higher stress levels. (After Gesquiere et al. 2011.)

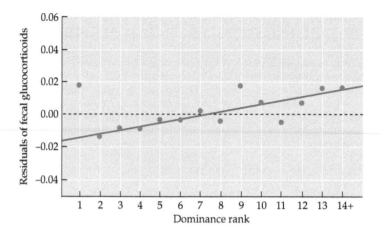

with dominant members. Rank-induced stress is evident across a variety of physiological measures, including hyperactive glucocorticoid secretion (see Figure 11.18), hypertension, impaired reproduction, immunosuppression, inhibition of neurogenesis, reduced synaptic plasticity and dendritic atrophy in brain regions such as the hippocampus. Given that the hippocampus provides negative feedback to the hypothalamic-pituitary-adrenal axis (see Box 10B), the physical consequences are prolonged in situations of chronic stress.

Power motivation and dominance contests

To usurp status in a social hierarchy and ascend in rank, an individual has to be both physically able to win dominance competitions and psychologically motivated to achieve power and status. In non-human animals, dominance contests are typically determined through physical battles between dominant and subordinate members. In humans, dominance contests can take the form of political debates, sporting events, or battles of wit, intellect, or talent.

Power motivation in humans is defined as an enduring preference for having impact on other people or the world at large. Individuals who express a need for power find this impact on others rewarding, and they are motivated to seek out opportunities to exert social influence. Power motivation can be implicitly measured through performance on a picture story exercise. In this exercise, participants are shown ambiguous pictures of people and are asked to write hypothetical narratives about them. The stories are then coded for the presence of power motivation themes, including descriptions of situations involving control or influence over others, fame or prestige, offers of unsolicited help, or actions that evoke an emotional response in others. Individual differences in the degree to which these themes are present in the stories is used as a trait marker of implicit power motivation. Power can also be explicitly primed prior to the picture story exercise by having participants listen to powerful presidential speeches, movies, or stories of achievement.

Power motivation is associated with levels of the sympathetic catecholamines epinephrine and norepinephrine, which promote the release of testosterone in men (Figure 11.19). Testosterone, in turn, facilitates dopamine release in the nucleus accumbens, a key component of the brain's circuitry for reward learning (see Chapter 14). The neuroendocrine profile of power motivation in women is less clear but has been related to elevated levels of estradiol. Individuals who score high on measures of power motivation tend to engage in more risky behaviors, attain higher positions in corporate management, and be more sexually active. However, these individuals also tend to use alcohol more and to enter into more complicated domestic relationships, including abusive ones.

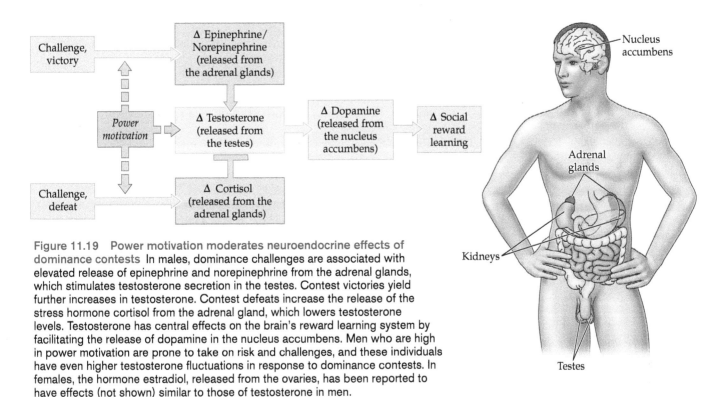

Figure 11.19 Power motivation moderates neuroendocrine effects of dominance contests In males, dominance challenges are associated with elevated release of epinephrine and norepinephrine from the adrenal glands, which stimulates testosterone secretion in the testes. Contest victories yield further increases in testosterone. Contest defeats increase the release of the stress hormone cortisol from the adrenal gland, which lowers testosterone levels. Testosterone has central effects on the brain's reward learning system by facilitating the release of dopamine in the nucleus accumbens. Men who are high in power motivation are prone to take on risk and challenges, and these individuals have even higher testosterone fluctuations in response to dominance contests. In females, the hormone estradiol, released from the ovaries, has been reported to have effects (not shown) similar to those of testosterone in men.

Endocrine markers further indicate the outcome of a dominance contest. Victory is associated with a surge in testosterone in men and estradiol in women. In contrast, the stress hormone cortisol is elevated following defeat. These effects of winning and losing are even present in social observers who are not direct participants in the competition, as in the case of sports fans observing a team match, or voters participating in a political election.

Summary

1. Social interactions engage a distributed set of brain regions involved in self-referential processing, perception of biologically relevant cues such as body stance and biological motion, social categorization, and emotion interpretation.

2. Whether social interactions are an emergent property of the cognitive functions described in other chapters or a core set of specialized brain structures and processes has been widely debated. A reasonable view is that both domain-specific and domain-general factors contribute to social cognition.

3. The ability to think reflexively about the self and our sense of embodiment depends on processing in the temporoparietal junction, medial parietal, and prefrontal cortical regions, as well as specialized sectors of the visual association cortex.

4. The perception of socially relevant cues arising from the faces and bodies of others depends on the fusiform gyrus, superior temporal sulcus, amygdala, and orbitofrontal cortex.

5. The categorization of individuals as members of social groups is rapid and automatic, and it depends in part on evaluative processes in the amygdala. Automatic influences of social stereotypes engage conflict-monitoring and self-regulation functions of the anterior cingulate gyrus and dorsolateral prefrontal cortex.

6. Theory-of-mind abilities, though present implicitly in great apes and young children, increase in complexity in late human development and depend on processing in the medial prefrontal cortex, temporal polar cortex, inferior parietal cortex, temporoparietal junction, and superior temporal sulcus, as well as areas that mediate symbolic representation more broadly.

7. Empathizing with the emotional state of others involves regions implicated in somatic and emotional state representation (including the insula), self-awareness, perspective taking, and emotion regulation.

8. Balancing the opposing forces of competition and cooperation is important for the stability and advancement of any social group. These forces affect the functioning of diverse physiological systems, including stress-related agents, hormonal markers of victory (testosterone) or defeat (cortisol), and agents related to social bonds (oxytocin/vasopressin).

9. Insights into the ways we perceive and make inferences from social cues have led to new treatments of autism spectrum disorders, as well as new developments in computer animation and human-machine interactions.

Additional Reading

Reviews

ALLISON, T., A. PUCE AND G. MCCARTHY (2000) Social perception from visual cues: Role of the superior temporal sulcus region. *Trends Cogn. Sci.* 4: 267–278.

BROTHERS, L. (1990) The social brain: A project for integrating primate behavior and neurophysiology in a new domain. *Concepts Neurosci.* 1: 27–51.

GALLESE, V., C. KEYSERS AND G. RIZZOLATTI (2004) A unifying view of the basis of social cognition. *Trends Cogn. Sci.* 8: 396–403.

HAXBY, J. V., E. A. HOFFMAN AND I. GOBBINI (2000) The distributed human neural system for face perception. *Trends Cogn. Sci.* 4: 223–233.

HEIN, G. AND T. SINGER (2008) I feel how you feel but not always: The empathic brain and its modulation. *Curr. Opin. Neurobiol.* 18: 153–158.

KEYSERS, C., J. H. KAAS, AND V. GAZZOLA (2010) Somatosensation in social perception. *Nat. Rev. Neurosci.* 11: 417–428.

NORTHOFF, G. AND F. BERMPOHL (2004) Cortical midline structures and the self. *Trends Cogn. Sci.* 8: 102–107.

RIZZOLATTI, G. AND C. SINIGAGLIA (2010) The functional role of the parieto-frontal mirror circuit: Interpretations and misinterpretations. *Nat. Rev. Neurosci.* 11: 264–274.

STANTON, S. J. AND O. C. SCHULTHEISS (2009) The hormonal correlates of implicit power motivation. *J. Res. Person.* 43: 942–949.

TODOROV, A. (2008) Evaluating faces on trustworthiness: An extension of systems for recognition of emotions signaling approach/avoidance behaviors. *Ann. N. Y. Acad. Sci.* 1124: 208–224.

VAN OVERWALLE, F. (2011) A dissociation between social mentalizing and general reasoning. *NeuroImage* 54: 1589–1599.

Important Original Papers

ADAMS, R. B., JR., H. L. GORDON, A. A. BAIRD, N. AMBADY AND R. E. KLECK (2003) Effects of gaze on amygdala sensitivity to anger and fear faces. *Science* 300: 1536.

ADOLPHS, R., D. TRANEL AND A. R. DAMASIO (1998) The human amygdala in social judgment. *Nature* 393: 470–474.

AMODIO, D. M., P. G. DEVINE AND E. HARMON-JONES (2008) Individual differences in the regulation of intergroup bias: The role of conflict monitoring and neural signals for control. *J. Pers. Soc. Psychol.* 94: 60–74.

BLANKE, O., S. ORTIGUE, T. LANDIS AND M. SEECK (2002) Stimulating illusory own-body perceptions. *Nature* 410: 269–270.

BLANKE, O. AND 7 OTHERS (2005) Linking out-of-body experience and self processing to mental own-body imagery at the temporoparietal junction. *J. Neurosci.* 25: 550–557.

BRUCE, V. AND A. YOUNG (1986) Understanding face recognition. *Br. J. Psychol.* 77: 305–327.

GESQUIERE, L. R., N H. LEARN, C. M. SIMAO, P. O. ONYANGO, S. C. ALBERTS AND J. ALTMANN (2011) Life at the top: Rank and stress in wild male baboons. *Science* 333: 357–360.

HASSELMO, M. E., E. T. ROLLS AND G. C. BAYLIS (1989) The role of expression and identity in the face-selective responses of neurons in the temporal visual cortex of the monkey. *Behav. Brain Res.* 32: 203–218.

LABAR, K. S., M. J. CRUPAIN, J. B. VOYVODIC AND G. MCCARTHY (2003) Dynamic perception of facial affect and identity in the human brain. *Cereb. Cortex* 13: 1023–1033.

PELPHREY, K. A., J. D. SINGERMAN, T. ALLISON AND G. MCCARTHY (2003) Brain activation evoked by perception of gaze shifts: The influence of context. *Neuropsychologia* 41: 156–170.

PERRETT, D. I., J. K. HIETANEN, M. W. ORAM AND P. J. BENSON (1992) Organization and functions of cells responsive to faces in the temporal cortex. *Philos. Trans. R. Soc. Lond. B.* 335: 23–30.

PHELPS, E. A. AND 6 OTHERS (2000) Performance on indirect measures of race evaluation predicts amygdala activation. *J. Cogn. Neurosci.* 12: 729–738.

RICHESON, J. A. AND 6 OTHERS (2003) An fMRI investigation of the impact of interracial contact on executive function. *Nat. Neurosci.* 6: 1323–1328.

RIZZOLATTI, G., L. FADIGA, V. GALLESE AND L. FOGASSI (1996) Premotor cortex and the recognition of motor actions. *Cogn. Brain Res.* 3: 131–141.

SAID, C. P., S. G. BARON AND A. TODOROV (2008) Nonlinear amygdala response to face trustworthiness: Contributions of high and low spatial frequency information. *J. Cogn. Neurosci.* 21: 519–528.

SCHULLER, A. M. AND B. ROSSION (2001) Spatial attention triggered by eye gaze increases and speeds up early visual activity. *Neuroreport* 12: 2381–2386.

ZUCKER, N. L. AND 6 OTHERS (2011) Neural signaling of mixed messages during a social exchange. *Neuroreport* 22: 413–418.

Books

CACCIOPPO, J. T., P. S. VISSER AND C. L. PICKETT, EDS. (2006) *Social Neuroscience: People Thinking about Thinking People.* Cambridge, MA: MIT Press.

HARMON-JONES, E. AND P. WINKIELMAN, EDS. (2007) *Social Neuroscience: Integrating Biological and Psychological Explanations of Social Behavior.* New York: Guilford.

JAMES, W. (1890) *Psychology: Briefer Course.* New York: Holt.

12

Language

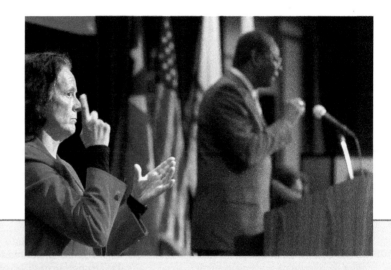

INTRODUCTION

A standard dictionary definition of *language* is "the particular form of speech of a group of people." For cognitive neuroscience, however, a better definition is something along the lines of "a symbolic system used to communicate concrete or abstract meanings, irrespective of the sensory modality employed or the particular means of expression." This broader definition includes spoken and heard language, language communicated in written form, and sign (gestural) language. Because of their enormous importance in all human societies, speech and language have been intensively studied by linguists, philologists, anthropologists, sociologists, psychologists, neurologists, and of course, cognitive neuroscientists. Although speech differs widely among the estimated 6000 to 7000 languages in use around the world today, any given language includes a vocabulary, a grammar, and rules of syntax. For languages that have a written form (estimated to be about 200), how the brain processes this visual form of language is also of interest. Finally, vocal and auditory communication systems in non-human primates and other animals have been intensively examined to explore how these systems compare with human language, and what this information implies about the origins of language.

Speech

Since language is defined by speech, it makes sense to begin the chapter with a brief review of speech production and comprehension.

Producing speech

The human vocal tract includes the vocal apparatus from larynx to lips (Figure 12.1A). The air expelled from the lungs streams through the opening between the vocal cords in the **larynx** (the *glottis*). As the airstream accelerates through this narrowing, the decreased pressure that results causes the cords to come together until the pressure buildup in the lungs forces them open again (the physical principle involved is what generates the lift given an airplane by the faster movement of air over the top surface of the wings; it is called *Bernoulli's*

■ INTRODUCTORY BOX DYSLEXIA

Dyslexia is a common problem that affects a child's ability to read. Despite having normal or above-normal intelligence, people afflicted with dyslexia are poor readers and have difficulty more generally in processing speech sounds and translating visual to verbal information, and vice versa. Thus, in addition to suffering reading problems, people with dyslexia often have difficulty writing, are poor spellers, and are prone to errors of letter transposition. Because there is no specific diagnostic criterion, estimates of the prevalence of dyslexia vary widely; an estimated 5 to 15 percent of children are affected, with greater occurrence in boys and a strong tendency for the problem to run in families. Although dyslexia is generally accepted as a learning disability, its cause is unclear, and some investigators have argued that this disorder is simply the lower tail of the distribution of performance in learning to read.

Given these facts, dyslexia probably has a number of causes. Nonetheless, researchers have understandably focused on areas of the brain concerned with reading. Functional MRI studies indicate that a specific set of left-hemisphere brain areas is activated during reading. Some of these areas are also activated by spoken language, but one of them, the *visual word form area* (VWFA) located in the region of the left occipitotemporal sulcus, is selectively activated by written characters and not by spoken words or low-level visual stimuli (see figure). The VWFA appears to develop with experience, and activation levels in this area in children and adolescents predict word-phoneme decoding abilities. People with dyslexia tend to have a weaker blood oxygenation level–dependent (BOLD) signal in this general area compared to normal subjects, as well as underdevelopment of the associated cortex and white matter tracts.

Evidence for a functionally specific brain region is surprising, given that until recently, few humans were literate. Thus, the VWFA could not have evolved to support reading per se. To make sense of these observations, cognitive neuroscientists Stanislas Dehaene and Laurent Cohen have argued that brain circuits that evolved to serve one purpose can be "recycled" to serve a new, culturally specified function. An extension of this idea is that cultural inventions like reading and writing are constrained to specific brain circuits across cultures. For example, in all alphabets, letters are made up of roughly three strokes, which might in turn be related to the efficient use of receptive fields by neurons at successively higher levels of visual cortex. The argument is that by matching the appearance of letters to the inherent functions of neurons involved in recognizing elementary objects, writing and reading systems are similarly determined across cultures.

There is no accepted treatment for dyslexia, but investigators now agree that identifying the problem early and implementing remediation through extra training and effort is helpful in most people with this disorder.

References

DEHAENE, S. AND L. COHEN (2007) Cultural recycling of cortical maps. *Neuron* 56: 384–398.

EDEN, G. F. AND D. L. FLOWERS (2008) Developmental dyslexia. In *Encyclopedia of Neuroscience*, L. S. Squire, T. Albright, F. Bloom, F. Gage, and N. Spitzer (eds.). Oxford: Elsevier, pp. 741–747.

EDEN, G. F. AND T. A. ZEFFIRO (1998) Neural systems affected in developmental dyslexia revealed by functional neuroimaging. *Neuron* 21: 279–282.

GABRIELI, J. D. E. (2009) Dyslexia: A new synergy between education and cognitive neuroscience. *Science* 235: 280–283.

GALABURDA, A. M., J. LoTURCO, F. RAMUS, R. H. FITCH AND G. D. ROSEN (2006) From genes to behavior in developmental dyslexia. *Nat. Neurosci.* 9: 1213–1217.

GRIGORGENKO, E. L. (2001) Developmental dyslexia: An update on genes, brains and environment. *J. Child Psychol. Psychiatry* 42: 91–125.

SHAYWITZ, S. E. (1998) Dyslexia. *New Engl. J. Med.* 338: 307–312.

TALLAL, P., R. L. SAINBURG AND T. JERNIGAN (1991) The neuropathology of developmental dysphasia: Behavioral, morphological, and physiological evidence for a pervasive temporal processing disorder. *Read. Writ.* 3: 363–377.

VINCKIER, F., S. DEHAENE, A. JOBERT, J. P. DUBUS, M. SIGMAN AND L. COHEN (2007) Hierarchical coding of letter strings in the ventral stream: Dissecting the inner organization of the visual word-form system. *Neuron* 55: 143–156.

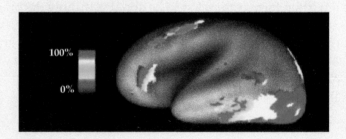

Location of the VWFA in the left occipitotemporal cortex of a normal subject. The colors from blue to red indicate an anterior-posterior gradient of BOLD signal intensity as read stimuli are progressively changed from single letters to complete words. (From Vinckier et al. 2007.)

principle). This process gives rise to a vibration whose frequency is determined primarily by the muscles that control the tension of the vocal cords. The fundamental frequency of these oscillations ranges from about 100 to 400 hertz, depending on the gender and size of the speaker. The rest of the vocal tract is

(A)

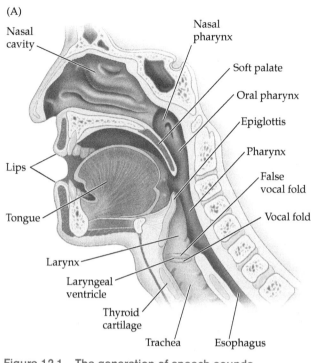

Nasal cavity

Nasal pharynx

Soft palate

Oral pharynx

Epiglottis

Pharynx

False vocal fold

Vocal fold

Lips

Tongue

Larynx

Laryngeal ventricle

Thyroid cartilage

Trachea

Esophagus

(B)

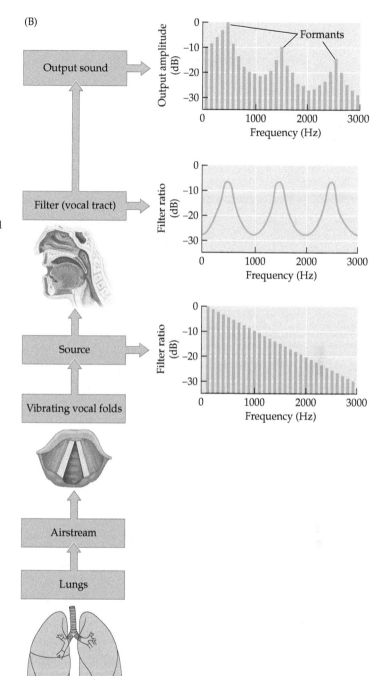

Output sound

Filter (vocal tract)

Source

Vibrating vocal folds

Airstream

Lungs

Formants

Figure 12.1 The generation of speech sounds
(A) The human vocal tract includes the vocal apparatus from the larynx to the lips. The structures above the larynx, including the pharynx, soft palate, and nasal cavity, shape and filter the harmonic series that are generated by the vocal cords when they vibrate. (B) The source-filter model of speech sound production. Using air expelled by the lungs, the vocal cords of the larynx are the source of the vibrations that become speech stimuli. Other components of the vocal tract, including the pharynx and the structures of the oral and nasal cavities, filter the laryngeal harmonics by the superposition of their own resonances, thus creating the speech sound stimuli that we ultimately hear. (B after Miller 1991.)

effectively an attached *resonating body*. Much like the body of a guitar, the vocal tract above the larynx shapes and filters the power in the harmonic series produced by vibration of the vocal cords.

The natural resonances of the vocal tract that filter the sound pressure oscillations generated by the larynx produce speech **formants**, defined as the peaks of power that are produced by this source-filter mechanism (**Figure 12.1B**). To generate different speech sounds, the shape of the vocal tract is actively changed by the musculature of the pharynx, tongue, and lips, in this way producing different natural resonances, and thus different formant frequencies. The relative frequencies of the formants create the variety of voiced speech sound stimuli that humans routinely produce in their native language.

The **source-filter model** of speech illustrated in Figure 12.1B was proposed in the nineteenth century by the German anatomist and physiologist Johannes Müller and has been generally accepted ever since. The lungs serve as a reservoir of air, and the muscles of the diaphragm and chest wall provide the motive force. The vocal cords then provide the periodic vibration that characterizes **voiced** (tonal) sounds such as those made when vowels are spoken. The pharynx, oral and nasal cavities, and their included structures (e.g., tongue, teeth, and lips) are the filter. These dynamically changing spaces and their natural resonances modify the periodic energy generated by the laryngeal source, thus determining speech sounds that eventually emanate from the speaker. Of course, not all human vocalizations are speech, and nonspeech vocalizations such as laughing, crying, grunting, and so on are important in their own right.

Comprehending speech

The basic speech sound stimuli in any language are called **phones**, and the perceptions they elicit are called **phonemes**. One or more phones make up syllables in speech, which in turn make up words, which ultimately make up sentences. Considering languages worldwide, most linguists estimate the number of phones (and phonemes) to be about 200, of which roughly 30 to 100 are used in any given language. The use of different subsets of these speech sound stimuli in different languages helps explain why people have trouble learning a new language (they have to produce and comprehend unfamiliar phones), and why they retain accents characteristic of their native language unless the second language is learned before the age of 8 or so (the familiar ways of producing phones and hearing phonemes are deeply entrenched in the organization of the adult brain, as we'll see later in this discussion).

Phones can be divided into **vowel** and **consonant** speech sound stimuli. The approximately 40 phones that characterize English are nearly equally divided between vowels and consonants, but other languages vary greatly in this respect. Vowel sounds comprise most of the *voiced* elements of speech—the elemental speech sounds that are generated by oscillations of the vocal cords in any language (see the preceding section). Because these oscillations are periodic, vowel sounds have a **tonal** quality, eliciting the perception of pitch in both speech and song. The majority of the acoustic power in speech is in the vowel sounds.

Consonant sound stimuli are phones that typically begin and/or end syllables, in contrast to vowel phones, which typically form the nucleus of each syllable. Consonant sounds are usually briefer than vowel sounds, involve more rapid changes in sound energy over time, and are acoustically more complex. Consonants are categorized according to the site in the vocal tract that determines them (*place of articulation*) or the physical way they are generated (*manner of articulation*). The click languages of southern Africa, of which about 30 survive today, show another variation in the production of consonants. Each of these languages has four or five different click sounds that are double consonants (the consonant equivalent of diphthongs) made by sucking the tongue down from the roof of the mouth (everyone can make such sounds, but they are rarely incorporated in speech). Somewhat surprisingly, consonants are the main carriers of information in speech. Thus, in interpreting spoken sentences from which either the vowels or the consonant sounds have been artificially removed, it is much easier to understand utterances without vowels than without consonants.

Interpreting speech sounds

Although our impression is that speech is physically divided into words, syllables, and phones—and, by implication, that the neural analysis of speech operates on these elements as such—this expectation is not borne out. Recordings of speech, such as the example in Figure 12.2, show that the sense we have that

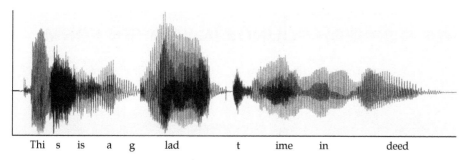

Figure 12.2 Recording of the spoken sentence "This is a glad time indeed" The intensity of the sound signal is plotted against time, with the elements of the sentence indicated on the time axis (which represents about 2 seconds). Such recordings of human speech show no clear or consistent physical distinction between the various components of speech (phones, syllables, and words), as might be assumed by the discrete way we seem to hear these components of speech. (From Schwartz et al. 2003.)

speech consists of a string of discrete words is false, at least in acoustic terms. Although this is the way we hear speech, our perception is at odds with the lack of any physical distinction or breaks between different syllables or even words. Thus, it is impossible to decipher what a speaker has said simply by looking at recordings of speech.

The neural processing—and ultimately cognitive understanding—of speech evidently proceeds in a more holistic way. Consistent with the generation of other classes of percepts described earlier, speech percepts are actively created by the human auditory and language processing systems, and are not simply neural translations or representations of physical stimuli at the ear (see Chapter 4). Underscoring this general point, studies of eye movements as people read a text indicate that syllables, words, and even distinct phrases are not the elements being processed during normal reading. As our eyes fixate sequentially while reading, the movements do not follow syllabic or word boundaries (see Introductory Box and Box 12A). Thus, syllables and words are not natural units of speech processing.

These facts present an additional challenge to understanding the neural underpinnings of language comprehension. How and why do we hear speech sounds in ways that bear little resemblance to the physical characteristics of the stimuli? One approach to resolving this puzzle was suggested by speech psychologist Alvin Liberman in the 1970s. Liberman proposed that what we perceive in speech sounds are the underlying "vocal gestures." By this he meant that what we hear corresponds much more closely to what the vocal tract is doing as speech is uttered than to the acoustic signal as such (see Figure 12.2).

This perspective should not, however, be taken too literally. One problem is that vocal-tract changes during speech overlap in time and influence one another—a phenomenon called coarticulation. Another problem is that the acoustic characteristics of the phones associated with different vocal gestures overlap in the natural speech of men, women, and children, making it difficult to imagine how sound stimuli could be unambiguously associated with configurations of the vocal tract. Nonetheless, Liberman's idea points in the right direction, implying that what we hear in speech is more closely related to vocal intention and contextual meaning than to the physical characteristics of the sound signal as such.

Sentences, grammar, and syntax

Words are combined in most forms of speech to make *sentences*, defined as sequences of words that express a complete and meaningful thought. The

■ BOX 12A REPRESENTING SPEECH SOUNDS IN WRITTEN FORM

Among the approximately 200 written forms of the 6000 to 7000 extant languages, three major types of graphical systems have been used to represent speech symbolically: symbols that represent *words*, symbols that represent *syllables*, and symbols that represent *phonemes*. Taken together, these visual tokens are called *graphemes*. Chinese *logograms* (Figure A) are examples of graphemes that represent words (in some cases with features that are visually similar to an object word). This is a difficult system from a practical perspective; Chinese children must learn about 8000 graphemes to be fully literate, and knowledge of at least 2000 is the definition of literacy in China. This system has persisted presumably because Chinese words are generally monosyllabic. In any event, the system obviously has worked for a significant fraction of the world's population for thousands of years.

Egyptian *hieroglyphs* evidently began as logograms but eventually came to correspond to syllables. Representing syllables in writing is still evident in modern languages like Japanese (Figure B).

(A) Words (e.g., Chinese)	(B) Syllables (e.g., Japanese)	(C) Phonemes (e.g., English)
汉漢字	ザ	A B C

The three major ways of representing speech visually with graphemes. (A) Representing entire words (Chinese; each of the three symbols here is a different word). (B) Representing syllables (Japanese). (C) Representing phonemes (English).

The most flexible system, however, is one representing phonemes—the basic heard sounds of speech (Figure C). The phonetic system arose in the Semitic languages of the early Phoenicians, Arabs, and Hebrews; the English alphabet is effectively one of the progeny of this symbolic approach. There is, however, no one-to-one correlation between the letters of a phonetic alphabet (e.g., the graphemes in English) and phonemes, just as there is no one-to-one correlation of phonemes to the acoustic stimuli (phones) underlying the heard sounds in language.

References

MILLER, G. A. (1991) *The Science of Words.* New York: Scientific American Library.

organization of speech at this level is described in terms of grammar and syntax. **Grammar** is the system of rules by which words are properly formed and combined in any given language. **Syntax** refers to the more general set of rules describing the combinations of grammatically correct words and phases that can, in turn, be used to make meaningful sentences.

The rules of grammar and syntax are conventions that change continually over the history of any language, and vary enormously among languages. Speakers of English today use the word order subject-verb-object (e.g., "The boy threw the ball") and might well imagine that this seemingly natural and logical order is characteristic of all languages. In fact, all possible arrangements are found among the world's languages, and more languages today use the order subject-object-verb ("The boy ball threw") than the familiar English order.

The importance of context

The meanings of phones, syllables, words, phrases, and sentences, even when used with grammatical and syntactical correctness, are fraught with ambiguity. In addition to the acoustic ambiguity of phones already alluded to, this uncertainty raises challenges for understanding how speech is comprehended. Consider, for example, the prevalence in any language of homonyms and homophones. *Homonyms* are words represented by the same spelling and sound stimulus that have multiple meanings; the word *bank*, for example, has several meanings as both a noun and a verb. *Homophones* are words that are also represented by the same sound stimulus but have different meanings and spellings—the words *kernel* and *colonel*, for instance. As a result of these additional ambiguities, understanding the meaning of a given word in speech is deeply

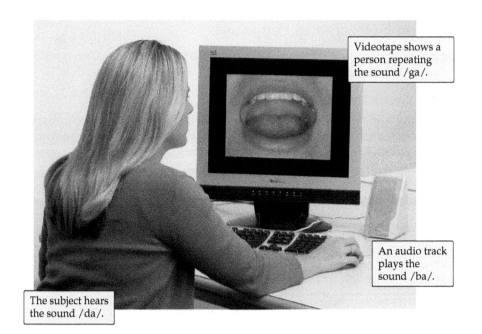

Videotape shows a person repeating the sound /ga/.

An audio track plays the sound /ba/.

The subject hears the sound /da/.

Figure 12.3 **What we see influences what we hear** This phenomenon, known as the McGurk effect, was demonstrated in studies that presented videos of a person's face while speaking coupled with speech sound stimuli controlled by the experimenter. Here the position and visibility of the lips, teeth, and tongue are those that would normally accompany the sound /ga/; however, the synchronized sound was /ba/. When looking at a video of the speaker in these circumstances, most people hear /da/, a speech sound that, in visual terms, lies more or less between the visible vocal-tract configurations for the sounds /ga/ and /ba/. This type of altered perception is known as the *fused response*. When observers close their eyes, however, they hear /ba/, the stimulus that is actually being presented to the ears.

dependent on context. Because these disambiguating contexts must be learned, the comprehension of speech—and the underlying neural processing—necessarily relies on the accumulated experience of the listener.

The early-twentieth-century American teacher and educator William Bagley was one of the first investigators to carry out experimental work on the importance of context in understanding speech. By cutting up and rearranging words (an approach he referred to as "word mutilation"), Bagley showed that the ability to correctly identify and understand syllables depends critically on the acoustic characteristics of their immediate surroundings in a word or sentence. Much work since has shown that words are easier to recognize in sentences than in isolation, and that the ability to recognize words increases monotonically with their frequency of use in the relevant language, confirming the conclusion that familiarity based on past experience is how speech is disambiguated.

A different demonstration of the importance of context in understanding speech is the **McGurk effect**. More than 30 years ago, psychologists Harry McGurk and John McDonald showed that the speech sounds we hear are strongly influenced by what we see. As illustrated in Figure 12.3, the effect arises when subjects see movements of a speaker's lips and tongue that have been experimentally changed so that they no longer accord with the speech sound stimuli that are heard simultaneously. Such experiments reinforce the conclusion that what a listener hears is not simply determined by the sound signal processed by the auditory system, but a more complex construct elaborated by language-processing regions of the brain. Both fMRI and transcranial magnetic stimulation (TMS) indicate that this integration occurs in the region of the superior temporal sulcus.

The simplest interpretation of these several lines of evidence is that speech perception is based on the *empirical significance* of speech sounds derived from the broader context of the speech signal, whether considered in terms of phonemes, syllables, words, phrases, sentences, or even entire passages. Indeed, the importance of context and the consequences for the empirical meaning of a stimulus apply not only to speech sounds, but to sound stimuli generally (see Chapter 4). Given this range of complexities, the success of computational systems now widely used for recognizing and producing speech is remarkable.

Acquiring Speech and Language

A great deal of investigation over the years has been aimed at understanding the enormously complex skein of information that any language entails.

Learning a vocabulary

Learning any one of the thousands of human languages is obviously a remarkable feat. There is, first of all, the need to know the meanings of a significant number of words—that is, the acquisition of a vocabulary. About 500,000 words are included in the current edition of the *Oxford English Dictionary* (OED), a monumental project that began in the mid-nineteenth century.

The compilation of a dictionary is bedeviled by the fact that vocabulary, like grammar and syntax, is in continual flux, with words being lost and added at a prodigious rate. Think, for instance, of all the words now in use that have been generated by the rapid rise of digital computation in the last few decades (*byte*, *website*, *laptop*, *blog*, and *wiki*, to name just a few). Think, too, of all the obscure words in the dictionary that are, for all intents and purposes, extinct and will eventually be dropped, although they were once used and are still included for reasons of completeness and etymology (much to the delight of Scrabble players and crossword puzzle addicts).

A highly verbal person with a college-level education knows perhaps 50,000 of the words in the OED, although many fewer (approximately 10,000) are used in ordinary discourse. The challenge of learning a language, however, is not just acquiring an adequate vocabulary. Speakers must also learn grammar and syntax—tasks that are greatly complicated by the importance of context in speech, as just discussed. This wealth of linguistic information is normally learned through an enormous amount of trial and error in infancy and childhood—a process that continues to some degree throughout life.

The shaping of phonemes and phones

Much research in linguistics and cognitive neuroscience has shown that the speech sounds an infant hears begin to shape and indeed to limit the child's perception and production of speech from the earliest days of postnatal life. The various languages that exist today use quite different subsets of the approximately 200 phones that humans employ to produce speech of languages worldwide. Infants can initially perceive and discriminate among all these speech sounds and are not innately biased toward any particular phonemes, as the fact that an infant can become fluent in any language makes clear. However, this ability at birth to appreciate and then produce the full range of human phones does not persist, eventually giving rise to the difficulties that older children and adults have in perceiving and uttering the phones that are not used in their native language.

One of the most thoroughly studied examples of this phenomenon concerns the phonetic differences between Japanese and English. Native Japanese speakers cannot reliably tell the difference between the /r/ and /l/ sounds in English because this phonetic distinction is not made or used in Japanese. Nonetheless, 4-month-old Japanese infants can make this discrimination as reliably as 4-month-old babies raised in English-speaking households. Researchers infer what infants perceive by measuring sucking frequency on a pacifier or the duration of looking at a stimulus source. Sucking rate and eye fixation time increase in the presence of a novel stimulus and can thus indicate whether an infant perceives two speech stimuli as the same or different. By 6 months of age, infants already show preferences for phonemes in their native language compared to those in foreign languages, and by the end of the first year they no longer respond to phonetic elements peculiar to a non-native language.

Interestingly, the "baby talk" that adults instinctively use when speaking to very young children (sometimes called *motherese*) emphasizes the phonetic distinctions in a language to a greater degree than normal speech among adults does, presumably helping the infant to hear the phonetic characteristics of the language that it is struggling to learn. Moreover, losing the ability to discriminate these acoustic differences is specifically related to speech sounds; adult Japanese and Americans are equally good at discriminating nonspeech sounds that include the acoustic characteristics of the phones that give them so much trouble in the context of spoken language.

A critical period for language acquisition

Although a maturing child begins to lose the ability to hear non-native phonetic distinctions at a remarkably early age, the ability to learn another language fluently persists for some years. As is apparent from the experience of learning a new language in school or from observing friends and family who began learning a second language at various ages, becoming fluent nevertheless requires linguistic experience relatively early in life. This fact reflects a broader generalization about neural development—namely, that neural circuitry is especially susceptible to modification during early development, and that this malleability gradually diminishes with maturation. The window for extensive neural modification supporting a behavior is referred to as the *critical period* (also called the *sensitive period*), and it is evident in the acquisition of language, as it is in many other cognitive behaviors (see Chapter 15).

Psycholinguists Jacqueline Johnson and Elissa Newport undertook a detailed study of this aspect of language learning, examining the critical period for the acquisition of a second language in Asian Americans who had come to the United States at various ages (**Figure 12.4A**). Using a battery of grammatical and other tests of fluency, they found that learning a second language before about age 7 results in adult performance that is indistinguishable from that of native speakers, although the details for second-language learning are debated.

The requirement for experience during a critical period is also apparent in studies of language acquisition in children who become deaf at different ages. The effects on language skills tend to be more marked when the onset of deafness occurs early in life than when the onset occurs later in childhood or in adult life. Younger children who have acquired some speech but then lose their hearing suffer a substantial decline in spoken language because they are unable to hear themselves speak and thus cannot refine their initial efforts at speech by testing the relative adequacy of what they are trying to say through auditory feedback. Differences in brain activation observed in children and adults doing

Figure 12.4 The critical period for language learning (A) The critical period for fully fluent language learning is apparent in studies of the fluency of Chinese Americans as a function of the age of their arrival in the United States, marking the onset of significant exposure to English. Ultimate fluency starts to drop off when language learning begins after about age 7. **(B)** Areas in the brains of children and adults that are differently active during language-based tasks are shown in yellow. These differences provide a possible neural basis for the diminishing ability to learn a new language with increasing age, although more specific interpretation of this evidence is not yet possible. (A after Johnson and Newport 1989; B from Brown et al. 2005.)

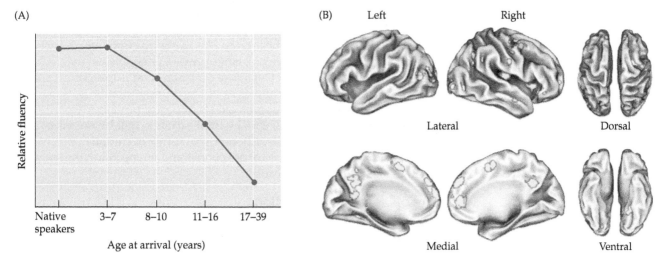

(A)

Relative fluency

Native speakers | 3–7 | 8–10 | 11–16 | 17–39

Age at arrival (years)

(B) Left | Right

Lateral | Dorsal

Medial | Ventral

language-based tasks provide some indication of the neural regions pertinent to diminished language-learning skills in adults (**Figure 12.4B**).

In sum, researchers agree that the normal acquisition of human language is subject to a critical period of approximately a decade; exposure and practice must occur within this time for a person to achieve full fluency. Of course, some ability to learn language persists into adulthood, but at a reduced level of efficiency and ultimate performance. This generalization is consistent with much other evidence from neural development that underscores the special importance of early experience in the full development of cognitive abilities (see Chapter 15).

Mechanisms of language learning

The most obvious aspects of the biological mechanisms that underlie language learning are extensive exposure and practice. Like other complex skills, language proficiency requires repeated activation of the relevant neural circuits, presumably because of the neural associations made by altering the relative strengths of synaptic connections (see Chapters 8 and 9). Many neurobiological studies in simple model systems suggest that exposure and practice would selectively preserve and strengthen the brain circuits pertinent to phonetic distinctions of the language in which a child is immersed daily. At the same time, the absence of exposure to non-native phones would presumably result in a gradual weakening of the connections representing sound stimuli that are not heard and practiced, which would in turn be reflected in a declining ability to distinguish and enunciate these phones correctly.

In this conception, the language circuitry that is used is retained, whereas circuits that are unused weaken and, after some years, cease to be functional or are perhaps lost altogether. Given what is known about developmental neurobiology more generally, these changes arise from the influence of neural activity or the lack of it on the cellular and molecular mechanisms that regulate the strength and prevalence of synaptic connections. That is not to say, however, that all language learning is necessarily based on extensive repetition. Psychologist Paul Bloom and others have suggested that children are also capable of "fast mapping" new words with only a few exposures, or even just one. Although this question is currently debated, Bloom has proposed that this rapid acquisition is the result of fitting a new word into an existing schema of language associations that makes use of the full range of cognitive information that the child is learning.

Some more detailed insight into speech sound learning has emerged from work by cognitive neuroscientist Patricia Kuhl and her colleagues. Kuhl's studies show that adults have a strong tendency to group speech sounds. For example, when asked to categorize a continuous spectrum of artificially constructed phones between /r/ and /l/, native English speakers tend to perceive the intermediate stimuli as all sounding like either /r/ or /l/. These perceptions are based on core phonemic preferences in different languages—a phenomenon that Kuhl has likened to a "perceptual magnet" (a more common term is categorical speech perception). A similar effect is apparent in developing infants, as illustrated in **Figure 12.5**: infants only 6 months old tend to group phones according to the biases in their native language. The implication is that by means of such grouping, related but acoustically different sounds are eventually perceived as representing the routine variations of the phones and phonemes in the language to which the learner is being exposed.

Effects of language deprivation

An issue complementary to normal language learning concerns the effects of language deprivation, a topic already touched on earlier when we briefly

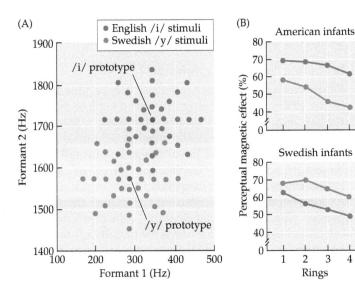

Figure 12.5 The "perceptual magnet" concept of phonemic grouping (A) Formant frequencies associated with a prototypical American English /i/ are shown in red; those with a Swedish /y/ prototype, in blue. (B) Six-month-old American and Swedish babies show greater generalization for the speech sound stimulus to which they have been exposed in their native language than to the foreign phone when tested with the range of stimuli in (A), supporting the perceptual magnet idea. ("Rings" refers to areas included in the prototype regions in [A]). (After Kuhl et al. 1992.)

discussed the deterioration of language in hearing-deficient individuals as a function of age. A broader question, asked since antiquity, is what would happen if an otherwise normal child were never exposed to language. Would the child remain mute, or could it develop some ability to speak, and if so, what sort of language would it have?

The closest approximation to a realization of this sort of "thought experiment" is a handful of unfortunate cases in which children have been deprived of significant language exposure as a result of having been raised by deranged parents. In the most fully documented case, a girl in a Los Angeles suburb was raised from infancy until age 13 under conditions of almost total language deprivation (she is known in the literature as "Genie"). Genie was brought to the attention of social workers in 1970, who found her locked in a small room, where she had been isolated and allegedly beaten if she made any noise. She was removed from these desperate conditions and taken to the children's hospital at UCLA, where she was found to be in adequate general health.

Given these highly unusual circumstances, a team of psychologists and linguists at UCLA studied Genie's language and other cognitive skills during the subsequent 5 years. Although Genie had little or no language ability initially, the investigators found no evidence of brain damage or mental retardation in the usual sense, and they described her overall personality as rather docile and generally pleasant. As might be expected, Genie also received extensive remedial training to teach her the language skills that she had never learned as a child. Despite these efforts, as well as daily life in more or less normal conditions in foster homes, Genie never acquired more than rudimentary language skills. Although she eventually learned a reasonable vocabulary, she could not put words together grammatically, saying things like, "Applesauce buy store?" when she wanted to ask whether she might buy some applesauce at the store.

Genie's case and a few similar examples starkly define the importance of adequate early experience for successfully learning any language, in accord with the more abundant evidence of a critical period for learning a second language.

Theories of Language

Given the enormous diversity of speech sounds, grammar, and syntax among the world's many spoken languages and the profound dependence of speech comprehension on context in any language, the idea of an encompassing "theory of language" would seem a daunting if not impossible goal. Nevertheless, some

TABLE 12.1 Frequency of Words Associated with the Probe Word *Chair*

RESPONSE TO PROBE WORD *CHAIR*	FREQUENCY[a]
Table	191
Seat	127
Sit	107
Furniture	83
Sitting	56
Wood	49
Rest	45
Stool	38
Comfort	21
Rocker	17
Rocking	15
Bench	13
Cushion	12
Legs	11
Floor	10
Desk; room	9
Comfortable	8
Ease; leg	7
Easy; sofa; wooden	6
Couch; hard; Morris; seated; soft	5
Arm; article; brown; high	4

Source: KENT, G. H. AND A. J. ROSANOFF (1910) A study of association in insanity. *J. Insanity* Jul/Oct: 37–96.

[a]Number of times the probe word elicited the response indicated, based on a survey of 1000 men and women.

important theoretical generalizations about languages have received much attention over the years.

Is there a "universal grammar"?

Beginning with linguist Noam Chomsky and his students in the 1950s, many investigators have explored the idea that all languages must share some basic rules—a concept referred to as a *universal grammar*. Chomsky argued that all languages must have "deep structures" that are "transformed" into the "surface structures" of particular languages as expressed in speech.

Finding a universal grammar, if indeed there is one, proved elusive in the decades that followed Chomsky's introduction of this idea. From what has already been said, any such structures would have to be deeply buried indeed, since fundamental grammatical features such as subject-verb-object order; the use of past, present, and future verb tenses; and pretty much every other structural feature that has been examined vary widely across languages. Nonetheless, human infants—as well as the young of other vertebrate species—come into the world with a great deal of preprogrammed circuitry pertinent to social communication, including, in the case of humans, a very strong predisposition to learning language.

In addition, studies of congenitally deaf individuals living in relatively isolated communities have shown that idiosyncratic sign languages that allow the affected children to communicate with their families emerge quickly and spontaneously. This preparation of neural circuitry for language in specialized brain regions implies a basis for the deep structures that Chomsky imagined, but no one has so far been able to say much about these preparatory circuits, let alone translate their organization into grammatical or syntactical terms.

Connectionist theory

Another general approach to understanding language across the idiosyncrasies of particular languages has focused on its associational character. When someone is presented with any word (e.g., *chair*), other words automatically come to mind (e.g., *table*)—some far more frequently than others (Table 12.1). This sort of word association is the basis of various psychological tests described in previous chapters, has strong effects on reaction time, and arises at least in part from the statistical co-occurrence of words in normal speech and language-based thought (the latter is presumably the primary reason that *table* pops to mind in response to *chair*).

Whatever the focus of psychological interest, the associative nature of language indicates something fundamentally important about the underlying neural basis of languages—namely, that they entail linkages that must depend on the relative strength of synaptic connections in the relevant parts of the brain. In this conception, words like *table* and *chair* are associated because their common co-occurrence in language use has strengthened the neuronal circuitry between their respective representations in the language areas of the cortex. A more specific extension of this general idea about the organization of language in associational networks is a broadly hierarchical cascade of related categories. Such associations can diverge in very different directions, as illustrated for the

(A)

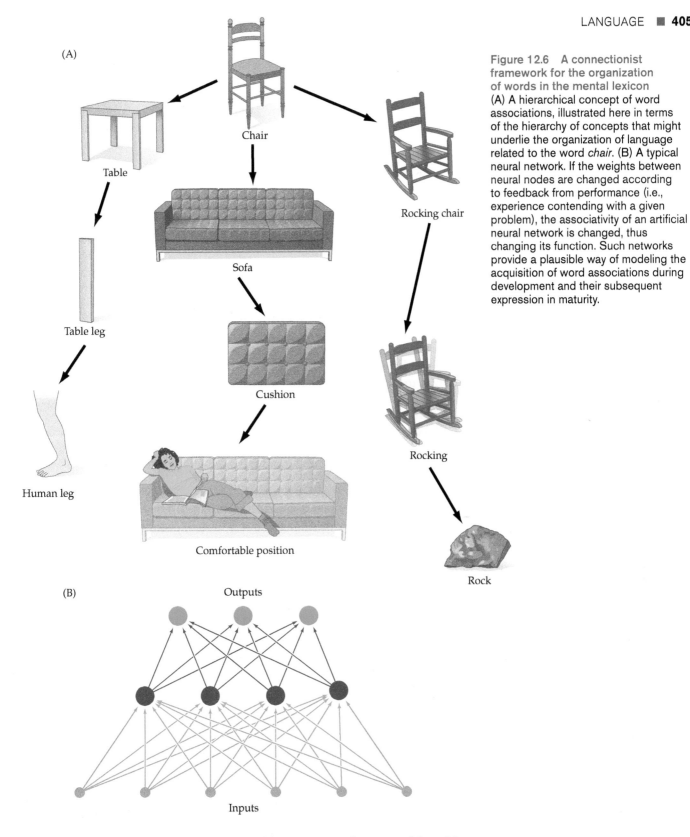

Chair

Table

Table leg

Human leg

Sofa

Cushion

Comfortable position

Rocking chair

Rocking

Rock

Figure 12.6 A connectionist framework for the organization of words in the mental lexicon (A) A hierarchical concept of word associations, illustrated here in terms of the hierarchy of concepts that might underlie the organization of language related to the word *chair*. (B) A typical neural network. If the weights between neural nodes are changed according to feedback from performance (i.e., experience contending with a given problem), the associativity of an artificial neural network is changed, thus changing its function. Such networks provide a plausible way of modeling the acquisition of word associations during development and their subsequent expression in maturity.

(B)

Outputs

Inputs

category "chair" in Figure 12.6A, presumably accounting for some of the odder associations in Table 12.1.

This general idea of associational linkages as a model for the lexical aspects of language (and many other cognitive functions) has found more specific expression in **connectionist** theories (see Box 8C) of how such associations might work, and their simulation in artificial **neural networks** whose properties are changed by alteration of the weightings (*synaptic connections*, in biological terms) of the relevant nodes (neurons) in such networks (**Figure 12.6B**). Although the history of neural networks goes back to the 1940s, the major figures in the modern connectionist approach are David Rumelhart and James McClelland, who began their work in the 1970s. A particular attraction of a connectionist view of language organization is its foundation in statistical association—a powerful mechanism that accords with neural mechanisms for encoding and storing information discussed in Chapter 9 in the context of semantic memory.

The Neural Bases of Language

Much is now known about the neural foundations of language, and until recently most of this information has come from clinical studies carried out by neurologists and neurosurgeons. The most general features of the language regions described in the following sections are their broad division into regions in the frontal lobe (where other motor functions are carried out; see Chapter 5) that have become specialized for the *production* of speech, and regions in the temporal lobe (where other auditory functions are carried out; see Chapter 4) that are specialized for its *comprehension*.

The initial evidence that the production and comprehension of language are localized to significantly different regions of the brain was provided by *clinical-pathological correlations*. Such studies were first reported by the French anatomist and neurologist Paul Broca and the German neurologist and psychiatrist Carl Wernicke—both of whom made many basic contributions to understanding the relationship of a variety of neurological lesions and their clinical consequences. Broca and Wernicke examined the brains of patients who had suffered brain damage (typically from a stroke or a tumor), had difficulty with language as a result, and later died (Broca's most famous patient actually suffered from tertiary syphilis, a common cause of brain lesions in the days before penicillin and other antibiotics). The term given to such problems with language is **aphasia**, which describes difficulty producing and/or comprehending speech, even though the vocal apparatus and hearing mechanisms are intact (difficulty speaking because of a lesion involving an aspect of the vocal musculature and its control is called *dysarthria*).

Neural bases for producing speech and language

Correlating the clinical picture and the site of brain damage in his patients, Broca concluded that loss of the ability to produce normal speech arose from damage to the ventral posterior region of the frontal lobe (**Figure 12.7**). Equally important, he observed that this sort of aphasia is typically associated with damage to the *left* hemisphere. The preponderance of aphasic syndromes associated with damage to various parts of the left hemisphere noted by neurologists ever since has supported Broca's nineteenth-century claim that "one speaks with the left hemisphere."

Patients with classic **Broca's aphasia** (caused by damage to the ventral posterior region of the frontal lobe, which is also called **Broca's area**), cannot express thoughts appropriately, because the rules of grammar and syntax have been disrupted by the lesion in the frontal lobe. These rules of language are closely related to the overall organization of other motor behaviors that depend

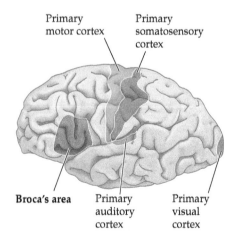

Primary
motor cortex

Primary
somatosensory
cortex

Broca's area

Primary
auditory
cortex

Primary
visual
cortex

Figure 12.7 Broca's area Broca took this region of the brain to be the basis for the production of language. The primary sensory, auditory, visual, and motor cortices are indicated to show the relation of Broca's area in the left hemisphere to these other areas that are necessarily involved in the production and comprehension of speech, albeit in a less specialized way.

on the general region of the frontal cortex anterior to the primary motor cortex in the prefrontal gyrus (the *premotor cortex*; see Chapter 5). The typical effects of damage in this area are evident in the following example reported by the neurologist Howard Gardner (who is the author in the following quoted passage). The patient was a 39-year-old Coast Guard radio operator named Ford, who had suffered a stroke that affected his left posterior frontal lobe.

> "I am a sig … no … man … uh, well, … again." These words were emitted slowly, and with great effort. The sounds were not clearly articulated; each syllable was uttered harshly, explosively, in a throaty voice. With practice, it was possible to understand him, but at first I encountered considerable difficulty in this. "Let me help you," I interjected. "You were a signal …" "A sig-nal man … right," Ford completed my phrase triumphantly. "Were you in the Coast Guard?" "No, er, yes, yes, … ship … Massachu … chusetts … Coastguard … years." He raised his hands twice, indicating the number nineteen. "Oh, you were in the Coast Guard for nineteen years." "Oh … boy … right … right," he replied. "Why are you in the hospital, Mr. Ford?" Ford looked at me strangely, as if to say, Isn't it patently obvious? He pointed to his paralyzed arm and said, "Arm no good," then to his mouth and said, "Speech … can't say … talk, you see."
>
> HOWARD GARDNER 1974
> *The Shattered Mind: The Person after Brain Damage*, pp. 60–61

Despite the structural disorder of the patient's speech, a listener would be impressed that this individual knew what he was trying to say. The lack of ability to organize and/or control the linguistic content of utterances indicates that such patients continue to comprehend language and know what they want to say. Even though they transpose words and generally produce structurally incorrect utterances, some sensible meaning can still be discerned. Thus, this type of aphasia is also called *production aphasia* or *motor aphasia*.

Neural bases for comprehending language

Broca was basically correct in his assertion about the location and laterality of the lexical and syntactical aspects of language. Modern studies have confirmed that damage in the vicinity of Broca's area is indeed responsible for many production aphasias, and that in roughly 97 percent of individuals the circuitry for both the production and comprehension of the lexical and semantic aspects of language is located primarily in the left cerebral hemisphere. However, Broca was off the mark in implying that language is a unitary function whose neural infrastructure is limited to a single brain region, or even a single hemisphere for that matter. As is evident in the discussion that follows, laterality is a far more complicated phenomenon than Broca imagined.

It was Wernicke who first made clear that the instantiation of language in the brain is indeed more complex. Wernicke distinguished between the locations of lesions in patients who had lost the ability to *produce* language and locations in those who could no longer *comprehend* language.

From his own clinical observations, Wernicke concluded that some patients with aphasia retain the ability to produce utterances with appropriate grammar and syntax but don't understand what is being said to them (or what they read). In addition, they generate utterances that, although structurally coherent, convey little or no meaning. In general, the patients that fit Wernicke's description are found at autopsy to have lesions of the posterior and superior temporal lobe, almost always on the left side (Figure 12.8). These findings have led to the generalization that damage to the posterior and superior regions of the temporal lobe on the left causes a deficiency referred to as *sensory aphasia*

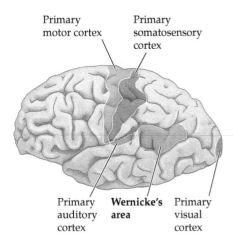

Primary motor cortex Primary somatosensory cortex

Primary auditory cortex **Wernicke's area** Primary visual cortex

Figure 12.8 **Wernicke's area** The brain area described by Wernicke defines a major part of the neural substrate for the comprehension of language.

or *receptive aphasia*. (Deficits of reading and writing—*alexias* and *agraphias*—are related disorders that can arise from damage to other brain areas; most people afflicted with aphasia, however, also have difficulty with these closely linked abilities if the language that they speak has a written form; see Introductory Box.) This region is referred to as **Wernicke's area** in honor of its discoverer, and the corresponding deficiency is called **Wernicke's aphasia.**

In contrast to a production (Broca's) aphasia, the major difficulty in a sensory (Wernicke's) aphasia is putting together objects or ideas and the words that signify them, and subjectively comprehending this relationship. Thus, in a sensory aphasia, speech is superficially fluent and well structured but makes little or no sense because words and meanings are not correctly linked, as is apparent in the following example. The patient in this case (again from Gardner) was a 72-year-old retired man who had suffered a stroke affecting his left posterior temporal lobe.

> Boy, I'm sweating, I'm awful nervous, you know, once in a while I get caught up, I can't get caught up, I can't mention the tarripoi, a month ago, quite a little, I've done a lot well, I impose a lot, while, on the other hand, you know what I mean, I have to run around, look it over, trebbin and all that sort of stuff. Oh sure, go ahead, any old think you want. If I could I would. Oh, I'm taking the word the wrong way to say, all of the barbers here whenever they stop you it's going around and around, if you know what I mean, that is tying and tying for repucer, repuceration, well, we were trying the best that we could while another time it was with the beds over there the same thing.
>
> GARDNER 1974, p. 68

Unlike the example of a Broca's aphasia, this example would cause a listener to conclude that the patient had little understanding of what he was trying to say. Table 12.2 summarizes the primary differences between these major sorts of aphasias.

More complex aphasias can arise from lesions to the pathways connecting the relevant temporal and frontal regions; as might be expected, patients with these aphasias often show an inability to produce appropriate responses to heard communication, even though the communication is understood.

Additional evidence from neurosurgery

This classical description of the localization and lateralization of language functions might give the impression that two well-defined regions of the brain

TABLE 12.2 Characteristics of Broca's and Wernicke's Aphasias

BROCA'S APHASIA[a]	WERNICKE'S APHASIA[b]
Halting speech	Fluent speech
Tendency to repeat phrases or words (perseveration)	Little spontaneous repetition
Disordered syntax	Syntax adequate
Disordered grammar	Grammar adequate
Disordered structure of individual words	Contrived or inappropriate words
Comprehension intact	Comprehension not intact

[a]Also called motor, expressive, or production aphasia.

[b]Also called sensory or receptive aphasia.

are responsible for language production and comprehension, and that these regions are in the left hemisphere. Not surprisingly, matters are a good deal more complex. During the 1950s and early 1960s, neurologist Norman Geschwind undertook a major effort to refine the earlier categorization of aphasias. Clinical and anatomical data from a large number of patients, along with a better understanding of cortical connectivity gleaned by that time from animal studies, led Geschwind to conclude that several other regions of the parietal, temporal, and frontal cortices are involved in human language abilities. A variety of subsequent studies using a range of approaches have confirmed that many additional regions of the brain in both hemispheres contribute to language.

The most dramatic additional evidence about the organization of language and other brain functions has come from ongoing studies of patients in whom the connections between the two hemispheres have been severed during neurosurgery to relieve intractable epileptic seizures. Interrupting these connections is an effective way of treating epilepsy in a small minority of patients who do not respond to conventional medical treatments of this common disorder. This surgical treatment is used much less today than it was several decades ago; the procedure is now done only in patients who suffer frequent seizures that cause a sudden loss of consciousness and are thus quite dangerous, and as other treatments improve may soon not be done at all.

In patients whose hemispheres have been surgically separated by cutting the corpus callosum and the anterior commissure that normally connect the right and left hemispheres, the function of the two cerebral hemispheres can be assessed independently. The first studies of these so-called **split-brain patients**, carried out by neuroscientist Roger Sperry and his colleagues in the 1960s and 1970s, established the hemispheric lateralization of language beyond any doubt. This work also gave much insight into the role of the *right* hemisphere in language and demonstrated many other functional differences between the left and right hemispheres. Sperry's studies continue to stand as an extraordinary contribution to understanding the cognitive organization of the brain, in particular, the relative roles of the two hemispheres.

To evaluate the range of cognitive and other functions of each hemisphere in split-brain patients, it is essential to provide information to one side of the brain only. Sperry, his student Michael Gazzaniga, and others devised several ways to do this. The simplest method was to ask the subject to use each hand independently to identify objects without visual assistance (Figure 12.9A). Recall that somatosensory information from the right hand is processed by the left hemisphere, and vice versa. By asking the subject to describe an item being manipulated by one hand or the other, researchers were able to examine the language capacity of the relevant hemisphere. Such testing showed that the two hemispheres indeed differ in their language ability, as expected from the postmortem correlations described earlier. Using the left hemisphere, split-brain patients were able to name objects held in the right hand without difficulty. Using the right hemisphere, however, most subjects could produce only an indirect description of the object that relied on rudimentary words and phrases rather than the precise lexical tokens for the object (e.g., "a round thing" instead of "a ball"), and some could not provide any verbal account of what they held in their left hand.

Presenting visual information to the right or left visual fields too rapidly for eye movements to follow (called *tachistoscopic presentation*) is another way to evaluate the two cerebral hemispheres independently. Such studies have shown that the right hemisphere can respond to pictorial instructions to carry out an action or, in some cases, to rudimentary written commands (Figure 12.9B).

Table 12.3 summarizes the major functional differences between the cerebral hemispheres determined in split-brain studies. These distinctions in the language

(A)

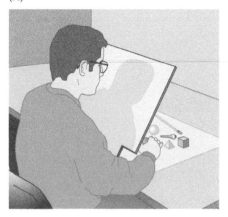

Figure 12.9 Hemispheric specialization of language Such specialization was confirmed by studies of patients in whom the connections between the right and left hemispheres had been surgically severed. (A) The task of recognizing shapes using one hand hidden from view is a means of evaluating the language capabilities of each hemisphere. Split-brain subjects are unable to name objects that they identify by feeling with the left hand. The right hand provides somatosensory information to the left hemisphere, so objects felt with the right hand are easily named. Objects held in the left hand, however, cannot generally be named accurately, because the tactile information processed in the right hemisphere cannot access the language areas in the left hemisphere, and the relevant language areas in the right hemisphere do not have this ability. (B) Visual stimuli or simple instructions can be given independently to the right or left hemisphere in normal and split-brain individuals. Since the left visual field is perceived by the right hemisphere (and vice versa), a briefly presented (tachistoscopic) instruction in the left visual field is appreciated only by the right brain (assuming that the individual maintains fixation on a mark in the center of the viewing screen). In normal subjects, activation of the right visual cortex leads to hemispheric transfer of visual information via the corpus callosum to the left hemisphere. In split-brain patients, information presented to the left visual field cannot reach the left hemisphere, and patients are unable to produce a verbal report regarding the stimuli. However, such patients *are* able to provide a verbal report of stimuli presented to the right visual field. A wide range of hemispheric functions can be evaluated using this tachistoscopic method, even in normal subjects.

(B)
Normal individual

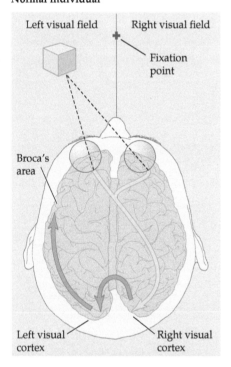

Split-brain individual

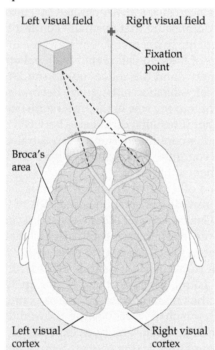

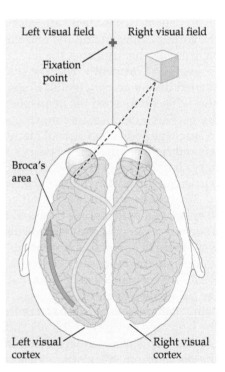

TABLE 12.3 Major Distinctions between the Language and Other Functions of the Left and Right Hemispheres	
LEFT-HEMISPHERE FUNCTIONS	**RIGHT-HEMISPHERE FUNCTIONS**
Analysis of right visual field	Analysis of left visual field
Stereognosis (right hand)	Stereognosis (left hand)
Lexical and syntactical language	Emotional coloring of language
Writing	Spatial abilities
Speech	Rudimentary speech

■ BOX 12B LANGUAGE, HANDEDNESS, AND CEREBRAL DOMINANCE

The evidence that language and some other cognitive functions are strongly lateralized has led to the popular idea that the left cerebral hemisphere is dominant over the right. In addition, clinicians refer to the hemisphere that serves as the substrate for the explicitly verbal aspects of language as the "dominant hemisphere." Another factor underlying the idea of a dominant hemisphere is handedness. Approximately 9 out of 10 people are right-handed in all human cultures. A superficial implication of the predominance of right-handedness is that the left hemisphere, which controls the right hand, is stronger or better than the right.

This unwarranted bias spills over into the sense many people have that being left-handed is somehow not as good as being right-handed. A century ago, many parents in the United States (and elsewhere) routinely tried to discourage emerging left-handed behavior in children. In most countries, however, such attempts to change a child's natural behavior have waned, largely in response to the empirical evidence that being left-handed is a disadvantage only in that many objects have been created for the right-handed majority (e.g., scissors, guitars, manual can openers, and so on; see figure). However, four out of five recent U.S. presidents were left-handed, and on average, left-handers actually do somewhat better in school than right-handers do. Being left-handed is also an advantage in sports like fencing (because opponents are less practiced in dealing with the thrusts and parries of left-handers).

The fact that language and handedness are typically represented in the left hemisphere is not that the left half of the brain is in any sense superior. Indeed, there is no evidence for a deep link between the lateralization of language and handedness. Consider, for example, the

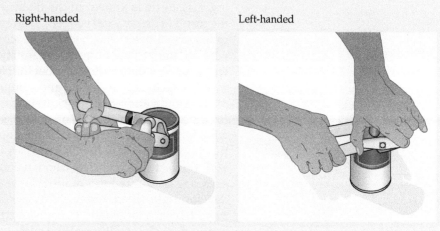

Right-handed   Left-handed

The nature of objects and the ease of using many of them in the world reflects the prevalence of right-handers.

results obtained over many years from the so-called *Wada test*, in which a short-acting anesthetic is injected into one of the carotid arteries to determine the hemisphere in which language function is primarily located (the patient will become transiently mute if language function is in the anesthetized hemisphere). The large number of such tests carried out for clinical purposes has shown that, in the vast majority of humans—including a large majority of left-handers—major language functions are in the left hemisphere. Because most left-handers have language function on the side of the brain opposite the right-hemisphere control of their preferred left hand, there is clearly no strict relationship between these two lateralized functions (although language in the right hemisphere is more common among left-handers).

The lateralization of language and hand preference is presumably a result of the advantage of having any highly specialized function on one side of the brain or the other to make the most efficient use of the neural circuitry available for cognitive and other functions in a brain of limited size. A belief that the neural circuitry on one side of the brain is less well developed, less useful, or less effective than the cerebral circuitry on the other is simply unwarranted.

References

BAKAN, P. (1975) Are left-handers brain damaged? *New Scientist* 67: 200–202.

COREN, S. (1992) *The Left-Hander Syndrome: The Causes and Consequences of Left-Handedness*. New York: The Free Press.

DAVIDSON, R. J. AND K. HUGDAHL (EDS.) (1995) *Brain Asymmetry*. Cambridge, MA: MIT Press.

SALIVE, M. E., J. M. GURALINIK AND R. J. GLYNN (1993) Left-handedness and mortality. *Am. J. Pub. Health* 83: 265–267.

abilities of the two hemispheres appear to reflect broader hemispheric differences summarized by the statement that the left hemisphere in most humans is specialized for (among other things) the more explicit aspects of the verbal and symbolic processing that are important in communication, whereas the right hemisphere is specialized for (among other things) processing visuospatial and, as described in the next section, emotional information (see also Chapter 10). Box 12B makes the additional point that this detailed evidence for lateralization of function does not support the pop psychology notion that one hemisphere dominates the other in any simple sense. The hemispheres are simply dedicated to significantly different but complementary functions.

One particular patient in Sperry's original split-brain series also gives some insight into the latent potential of the right hemisphere for language processing. L.P., as he is known in the literature, was highly exceptional in that, as the result of an unusual congenital anomaly, he had never developed a corpus callosum—a defect that had been discovered incidentally. Unlike the patients who had undergone surgery in maturity, L.P. was shown to have good bilateral language function, indicating that the right hemisphere in such circumstances is fully capable of producing and comprehending language.

This indication that the right hemisphere can do the same job as the left under some conditions is, of course, supported by the 3 percent of people who, for reasons that are not understood, normally have the major language functions in the right hemisphere (see Box 12B). This observation also agrees with the fact that children who have undergone left hemispherectomy at an early age for a rare form of intractable and life-threatening epilepsy can also develop right-sided verbal skills, as can children who, during the perinatal period, have a large left-hemisphere stroke that includes the language areas. In adults, such insults would be permanently crippling to language and many other functions, in keeping with much other evidence that neural plasticity decreases progressively with age.

Given the radical nature of split-brain surgery, it is not surprising that the inability of the two halves of the brain to communicate also has significant, if subtle, effects on the overall cognitive functioning of the affected individuals. Split-brain subjects are reported to be less efficient than control subjects in carrying out coordinated bimanual tasks (threading a needle or playing the guitar, for example), and they have been described by Sperry and others as being less able to generate imaginative ideas and express them verbally. Although these latter observations are more difficult to document, they support the idea that communication between the hemispheres is important for the fullest expression of language and language-based thought.

Further insight into the ways language is organized in the brain has come from the detailed mapping of language areas that has long been carried out in patients undergoing surgical procedures that involve (or are simply near) the language areas of the brain. Neurosurgeons typically map language functions by electrically stimulating the cortex during surgery to refine their approach to the problem at hand. In removing a brain tumor or an epileptic focus, for instance, the surgeon must pinpoint the language (and other) areas so that the procedure causes minimal subsequent impairment. Because the brain has no pain receptors, such surgery can be done under local anesthesia (i.e., with the patient conscious), allowing the surgeon to assess the location of sites that cause interference with speech when stimulated.

The legendary neurosurgeon Wilder Penfield and his colleagues initiated this approach in the 1930s (see Introductory Box, Chapter 2). Using electrical mapping techniques adapted from work that had been done since the late nineteenth century in experimental animals, Penfield specifically delineated the language areas of the cortex (among many other functional regions) before removing diseased brain tissue (Figure 12.10A). This general approach has been employed ever since, with increasingly sophisticated stimulation and recording methods, to guarantee that the effects of surgery will not be worse than the effects of the disorder being treated. Over the years this neurosurgical safeguard has yielded a wealth of additional information about the organization of language.

Penfield's observations, together with more recent studies performed by neurosurgeon George Ojemann and others, have amply confirmed that large regions of the perisylvian frontal, temporal, and parietal cortices in the left

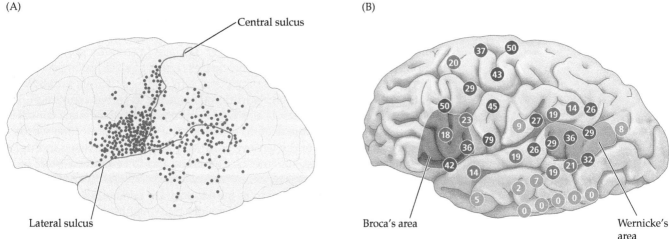

Figure 12.10 Cortical mapping of language areas in the left cerebral cortex (A) The red dots indicate sites of stimulation that caused interference with speech in Penfield's original study, based on neurosurgeries performed in the 1930s. **(B)** More recent evidence for the variability of language representation among individuals. This diagram summarizes data from 127 patients whose language areas were mapped by electrical recording at the time of surgery by Ojemann and his colleagues. The number in each circle indicates the percentage of the patients who showed interference with language in response to stimulation at that site. Note both that the percentages vary considerably, and that many of the sites that elicited interference in both Penfield's and Ojemann's series fall outside the classic language areas described by Broca and Wernicke. (A after Penfield and Roberts 1959; B after Ojemann et al. 1989.)

hemisphere are involved in language production and comprehension. A surprise, however, has been the variability in language localization from patient to patient in such studies (**Figure 12.10B**). Ojemann and his colleagues found that the cortical regions involved in language are only approximately those indicated by most textbook treatments of the "classic" language areas (see Figures 12.7 and 12.8); the exact locations differ widely among individuals. Indeed, the exact location and size of any functional brain system (the primary visual cortex is a good example) vary substantially among individuals.

Equally unexpectedly, bilingual patients do not necessarily use the same region of cortex for storing the names of the same objects in two different languages. Moreover, although neurons in the temporal cortex in and around Wernicke's area respond preferentially to spoken words, they do not show preferences for a particular word. Rather, a wide range of words can elicit a response in any given cortical location; in addition, single-unit recordings in humans have shown that selected words and related pictures evoke activation in the same neurons. All these observations have broadened classical and simpler concepts of language organization in the brain.

Contributions of the right hemisphere to language

Although split-brain studies, mapping during neurosurgery, and other avenues of evidence have shown unequivocally that the left hemisphere in most individuals is the major seat of semantic and lexical language functions, it would be wrong to suppose that the right hemisphere has little or no importance for language. As already described, the right hemisphere in some split-brain individuals can produce rudimentary words and phrases. More significantly, clinical and other observations have long suggested that the right hemisphere is normally the source of the emotional coloring of language—an idea introduced in Chapter 10. This evidence is consistent with the studies described in

Chapter 4 showing that the right hemisphere is also primarily responsible for the processing of musical information and its emotional effects.

It should not be surprising, then, that language deficits of a different and more subtle sort are apparent following damage to roughly corresponding regions of the right hemisphere. The clearest effect of such lesions is a deficit in the emotional and tonal components of language—called its **prosodic** elements—which normally impart additional meaning to verbal expression. This emotional coloring of speech is a critical component of the message conveyed, and in most languages it is used to modulate the significance of the words or phrases uttered (think of the variety of inflections commonly used in English to distinguish questions, statements, demands, and the emotional state of the speaker).

These deficiencies, referred to as **aprosodias**, are generally associated with right-hemisphere damage to the cortical regions that roughly correspond to Broca's and Wernicke's areas in the left hemisphere. The aprosodias are characterized by monotonic, or "robotic," speech that listeners find hard to interpret from the perspective of understanding the speaker's emotional state and intentions. Imagine the loss of meaning when statements such as "I love you!" are uttered in a monotone. These deficits following right-hemisphere damage emphasize that, although the left hemisphere figures more prominently in the comprehension and production of language for most humans, other regions, including areas in the right hemisphere, are needed to generate the full richness of everyday speech and language.

In sum, Broca's conclusion that we speak with the left brain is not strictly correct. It would be more accurate to say that we understand language and communicate its explicit semantic content much better with the left hemisphere than with the right, but that the right hemisphere makes a major contribution to the overall significance of spoken and heard communication. Language processing in both hemispheres supports the overall goals of social communication, but in different ways.

A number of theories have been proposed over the years to explain the hemispheric differences in language and other functions. Some investigators have argued that the left hemisphere is specialized for analytic and sequential processing, and that the right hemisphere is concerned with spatial and synthetic processing. Others have suggested that the left hemisphere is specialized mainly for voluntary motor functions (including speech production). Still others have offered the idea that the left hemisphere is specialized for rapid information processing and the right hemisphere for slower processing. In this view the left hemisphere is more adept at the rapid associations involved in lexical and syntactical processing; and the right, at the somewhat less time-dependent emotional features of speech. There is as yet no consensus about the relative merit of these ideas.

Noninvasive Studies of Language Organization

For much of the twentieth century, the bulk of the evidence about the organization of language in the brain came from neurologists and neurosurgeons, as described in the previous sections. The advent of noninvasive brain imaging in the late 1970s and ongoing improvements in recording event-related potentials, however, opened the door to studies of the neural organization of language in normal subjects.

Initially, recording event-related potentials (ERPs) was especially useful in exploring how the language areas of the brain respond to semantic stimuli, where words and meanings normally follow each other in quick succession. Psychologists Marta Kutas and Steven Hillyard pioneered such language studies.

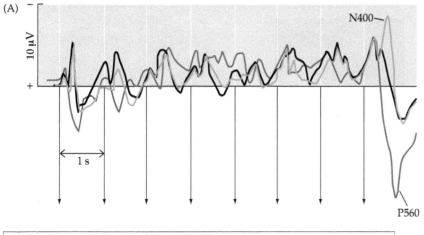

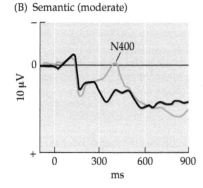

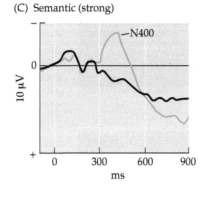

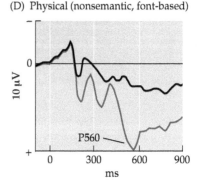

Figure 12.11 Semantic processing (A) ERP recordings show the average responses of subjects to silent reading of the three sentences indicated. The seventh words in the first two sentences (*work* and *socks*) are semantically sensible and nonsensical, respectively; in the third sentence, the seventh word (*shoes*) is printed in a larger font, providing a nonsemantic anomaly as a control. The N400 wave in the ERP response is increased by the nonsensical word, but not by the larger font. (B–D) These graphs show average responses to moderate violation of semantic expectation (B), strong semantic violation (C), and a physical rather than semantic violation (D). Note the absence of an N400 response in (D). (After Kutas and Hillyard 1980.)

In a paper published in 1980, they showed that when people read sentences, ERP responses vary quite strikingly as a function of the nature of the semantic material (Figure 12.11). In particular, they found that the N400 component of the response to a word in a sentence read silently was enhanced if the word was semantically inappropriate, and thus unfamiliar or unexpected (e.g., "The *table* chased the cat"; recall from Chapter 6 that the N400 is observed in response to unexpected semantic events like this). This effect was not seen, however, if the test word was semantically appropriate but printed in a different font, showing that this ERP response is specific to language anomalies and not simply a reflection of anything unusual in the material being read. On the basis of these and other observations, Kutas and Hillyard suggested that the N400 wave reflects a sort of "stumbling over" and reprocessing of language information that does not make sense in comparison to the semantic flow that is usually experienced.

Kutas and others went on to show that words used frequently in speech elicit *smaller* N400 waves than uncommon words do, suggesting that processing familiar language information requires less (or more distributed) neural engagement than does processing more difficult material—a finding that also holds for processing sentences and more complex material. A related finding is that homonyms (e.g., words like *bank* that have multiple meanings) elicit a smaller N400 wave when embedded in a sentence that clarifies the intended

(A) Passively viewing words

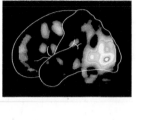

Listening to words

"Table"

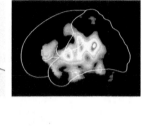

Speaking words

Table

"Table"

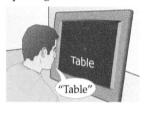
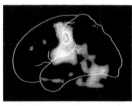

Generating word associations

Table

"Chair"

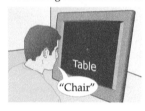
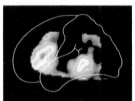

(B)

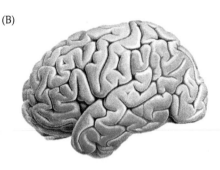

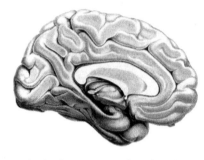

Figure 12.12 Language-related regions of the left hemisphere mapped by PET and fMRI (A) In human subjects, language tasks such as listening to words and generating words elicit activity in Broca's and Wernicke's areas, as expected. However, primary and association sensory and motor areas are also activated in both the active and passive language tasks. These observations indicate that language processing involves many cortical regions in addition to the classic language areas. (B) Language areas activated in the left hemisphere are summarized here in a meta-analysis of more than 100 fMRI studies of normal subjects. (A from Posner and Raichle 1994; B from Binder et al. 2009.)

meaning compared to a context that does not (e.g., "She was waiting for her cashier's check at the bank" versus "She was waiting for her friend at the bank").

Thus, language processing in the relevant cortical regions appears to depend on an individual's prior experience with word frequencies and contextual meanings. This evidence accords with the conclusions reached on other grounds—that is, that the strategies of language processing are fundamentally associational, and that probabilities conveyed by contextual information are used to disambiguate the inherently uncertain information in speech sound stimuli.

Although ERP approaches to language continue to be used by many investigators, much work is now based on imaging techniques. The initial brain imaging studies of language based on PET, like the mapping studies done during neurosurgery, challenged older concepts about the representation of language in the brain. Although high levels of activity were found in the expected regions with both PET and fMRI, large areas of both hemispheres were activated in various language tasks, indicating that language processing involves far more of the brain than was initially supposed (Figure 12.12)—a result that accords with the electrophysiological evidence derived from neurosurgical mapping (see Figure 12.10).

In certain circumstances, language-related tasks can involve even more brain areas. For instance, blind individuals reading Braille show extensive activation of the visual cortex with fMRI, implying that nonlanguage regions can be brought into play when needed, and that these regions may normally be involved in some aspects of language and reading (in accord with the evidence mentioned earlier that the right hemisphere can develop language capabilities when the corpus callosum fails to develop or the left hemisphere is removed in young children).

TMS has also made a contribution to this broader picture of the way language is processed. An example is the work of Alvaro Pascual-Leone and his collaborators. These investigators showed that TMS can suppress the function of various language regions, thus providing a way of determining language laterality that is less invasive than the Wada test mentioned in Box 12B, which carries a significant morbidity and mortality rate. In keeping with other evidence that language is more broadly supported in the brain than was thought in earlier decades, TMS causes significant interference with language processing when processing in either hemisphere is disrupted in this way.

Other studies using noninvasive brain imaging have focused on the categorization of words and meanings by neural networks in the temporal lobes, showing that some lexical and conceptual categories activate overlapping but appreciably different cortical regions within the areas of the brain that mediate these aspects of language (i.e., Wernicke's area and surrounding regions). For instance, PET studies have shown that distinct regions of the temporal cortex are activated by tasks in which subjects are asked to name particular people, animals, or tools. This work has been extended using fMRI, which shows that category-specific patterns of activity are elicited in the temporal cortices when subjects view, name, or read category-specific material (Figure 12.13).

These studies are consistent with Ojemann's electrophysiological studies, which also suggest that language is organized according to categories of meaning rather than individual words. They are also consistent with the work described in Chapter 3 indicating that visual objects are represented in overlapping but distinguishable areas of the temporal lobe. With respect to language, this evidence for a more specific organization by categories within the general cortical region first described by Wernicke helps explain the clinical finding that, when a relatively limited region of the temporal lobe is damaged (usually by a stroke

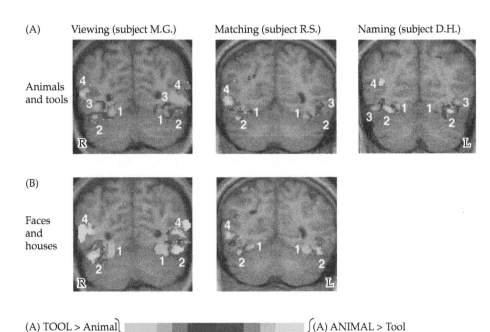

Figure 12.13 Lexical and conceptual categories activate overlapping but different cortical regions Functional MRIs show activation of different regions in the temporal lobe in three normal subjects during viewing, matching, and naming tasks that involved different object categories—either animals and tools (A) or faces and houses (B). The color code at the bottom indicates the category-specific activations; numbers indicate anatomical regions: 1, medial fusiform gyrus; 2, lateral fusiform; 3, middle and inferior temporal; 4, superior temporal sulcus. Notice that the activity elicited is bilateral, implying a significant role for both right and left temporal lobes in this aspect of language processing. (From Chao et al. 1999.)

on the left side), language deficits are sometimes limited to particular sorts of objects. For instance, some patients show impaired knowledge for animals but normal knowledge for nonliving objects such as tools. The reverse pattern has also been described but is much less common. Although the location of the damage in these conditions is variable and to a degree controversial, deficits in animate knowledge are more often associated with lesions of the temporal cortex, and deficits in inanimate knowledge are more often associated with left-sided damage that is more anterior, extending into the parietal and frontal lobes.

Some researchers have attempted to rationalize this evidence about categorization in various theoretical frameworks. One theory, proposed by psychologist Elizabeth Warrington and collaborators, suggests that conceptual or category knowledge is organized according to *sensory* features such as form, motion, and color, as well as according to *functional* properties such as the motion and/or the location of objects. Another idea, advocated by Alfonzo Caramazza and his colleagues, entails a *domain-specific* theory, which argues that ecological relevance has led to the evolution of specialized brain mechanisms for processing classes of objects. The fact that activation patterns for different stimulus categories are distributed and overlapping is more easily reconciled with property-based theories because the regions involved in processing different properties are distributed and thus shared across categories.

In any event, these studies leave little doubt that the temporal cortices (and very likely other cortical regions) include overlapping neural networks that represent various objects and concepts, or at least aspects of them, and that these areas are not exclusively devoted to categorizing language.

Evidence that the neural basis of language is fundamentally symbolic

Another informative approach to understanding what the language areas in the brain actually do has been to examine the neural substrate of sign language in congenitally deaf individuals. The basic question asked in this work is whether the major language areas in the brain are devoted specifically to processing speech sounds, or are more generally concerned with symbolic processing.

American Sign Language has all the elements—vocabulary, grammar, and syntax—of spoken and heard language, and it clearly serves the same purposes of social communication. Moreover, signers can express emotional coloring and most, if not all, of the nuances that are conveyed by speech. In an important addition to work on sign language, linguist Ursula Bellugi and her colleagues examined the cortical localization of signing abilities in patients who had suffered lesions of either the left or right hemisphere. All these individuals had been deaf since birth, had been signing throughout their lives, had deaf spouses, were members of the deaf community, and were right-handed.

The patients with left-hemisphere lesions, which in each case involved the language areas of the frontal and/or temporal lobes, had measurable deficits in sign production and comprehension when compared to normal signers of similar age (Figure 12.14). In contrast, the patients with lesions in approximately the same areas in the right hemisphere did not have signing "aphasias." Instead, as might be expected from evidence in hearing patients with similar lesions, right-hemisphere language functions such as emotional processing and expression were impaired in the signing of these individuals. Although the number of subjects studied was necessarily small (deaf signers with lesions of the language areas are difficult to find), the capacity for signed and seen communication is evidently represented predominantly in the left hemisphere, in much the same areas as spoken language. This evidence indicates that the language regions of the brain are specialized for the representation of social communication by means of *symbols*, rather than for heard and spoken language per se.

(A) Patient with signing deficit

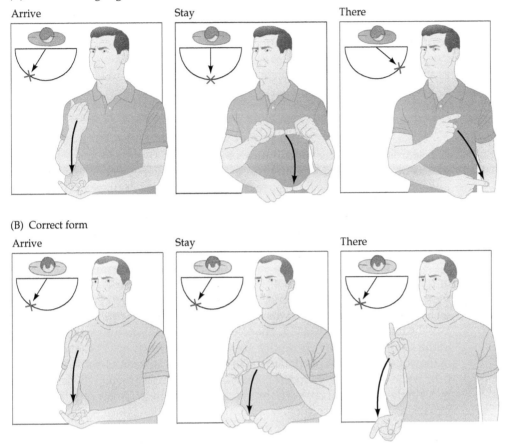

(B) Correct form

Figure 12.14 Signing "aphasia" Signing deficits are seen in congenitally deaf individuals who learned sign language from birth and later suffered lesions of the left-hemisphere language areas. Left-hemisphere damage produced signing problems in these patients analogous to the aphasias seen after comparable lesions in hearing, speaking patients. In this example, the patient in (A) is expressing the sentence "We arrived in Jerusalem and stayed there." Compared to a subject lacking the deficit (B), he cannot properly control the spatial orientation of the signs. The aberrant direction of "aphasic" signs (A) and the direction of the correct signs (B) are indicated in the upper left corner of each panel. (After Bellugi et al. 1989.)

In line with this conclusion, the capacity for seen and signed communication, like that for spoken language, emerges in early infancy. Observations of early language practice (called *babbling*) in hearing and eventually speaking infants shows the production of a predictable pattern of sounds related to the ultimate acquisition of fluent language. Thus, babbling prefigures mature language. The congenitally deaf offspring of deaf, signing parents "babble" with their hands in gestures that are evidently the forerunners of fluently expressed signs. Like verbal babbling, the amount of manual babbling increases with age until the child begins to form accurate, meaningful signs. These observations imply that the strategy for acquiring the rudiments of symbolic communication from parental or other social cues—regardless of the means of expression—is similar in deaf and hearing individuals.

These developmental facts are also pertinent to the possible antecedents of language in the nonverbal communication of other animals, and they suggest a continuum across species between spoken language and other symbols or tokens of meaning, such as gestures, facial expressions, and body language.

Despite this contentious question, the organization of language areas in the brain does not simply reflect specializations for hearing and speaking; rather, these areas are more broadly organized for processing the variety of symbols pertinent in human communication (see Box 12C for a consideration of numerical symbols). This conclusion again emphasizes that the brain areas supporting the production and comprehension of speech are by no means exclusively dedicated to these cognitive tasks.

Genetic Determination of Language Functions

The search for genetic contributions to cognitive functions and their disorders is being pursued in many contexts. Because genes play some role in all phenotypic features, and because the propensity for language acquisition by infants is obvious, exploring the genes involved is plausible. Furthermore, the occurrence of language and/or reading problems that run in families makes plain that genetic anomalies can play a role in the normal development of these cognitive functions (see also the Introductory Box).

Another inherited but rare disorder has more specifically raised the question of the genetic determination of language and, in popular accounts, whether there might be a "language gene." The gene of interest, called *FOXP2*, is located on human chromosome 7. It was discovered in 1990 in a family in which about half the members are afflicted. The affected individuals in the pedigree, known in the literature as the K.E. family, are unable to fluently select the movements of the vocal apparatus needed to make appropriate speech sounds. Thus, what they try to say is largely incomprehensible. The impairment, which is caused by a single autosomal recessive mutation, is thus one of motor organization as it pertains to speech production rather than comprehension. IQs in the afflicted family members, however, also are lower than the IQs of their unafflicted relatives, indicating that the defect is not specific for language.

The mechanism by which the gene defect exerts these effects is not known, but the protein that it encodes is a transcription factor, meaning that the gene product is an agent that binds to the promoter regions of other genes to control their expression. The *FOXP2* gene is expressed in other animals, including mice, where it affects many aspects of development, including the ultrasonic vocalization of these animals.

Interesting though this gene may be, reports about the discovery of a language gene were clearly unwarranted. Because it encodes a transcription factor, *FOXP2* affects many other genes with a range of developmental consequences, some evidently influencing the neural circuits that support the motor organization and expression of language via speech.

Is Human Language Unique?

Over the centuries, theologians, natural philosophers, and a good many neuroscientists have argued that language is uniquely human; in this view, human language sets us apart from our fellow animals. However, evidence of sophisticated forms of vocal or other symbolic communication in species as diverse as bees, birds, monkeys, and whales has made this anthropocentric point of view untenable.

Nonetheless, some aspects of human language appear to have no equivalent in the communication systems of other animals. One such aspect is that, whereas other animals have only a limited repertoire of vocal sounds whose acoustic patterns have specific and fixed meanings, humans arbitrarily link phones to an indefinitely large set of meaningful words. By the same token, only human language has appeared to use a recursive grammar. By this, linguists and others

■ BOX 12C REPRESENTING NUMBER

We routinely use numbers to make judgments about sets of items, to measure continuous quantities, to order priorities by rank, and more generally to label objects in the world around us. The most familiar forms of number use in humans—such as the arithmetic and math that we learn in school—depend on explicit symbols and words used to describe them. To solve even a simple problem, such as determining the sum of 17 + 12, requires a good deal of cognitive processing. People solving such problems must understand the meaning of the symbol for addition and the meaning of the arbitrary symbols that represent number. They must then retrieve or calculate the answer, using either declarative memory systems if the answer has been worked out earlier and is remembered, or working memory if the answer must be calculated.

A precise, symbolically mediated system for understanding numbers appears to be built, in part, on the fuzzier sense of quantities generally referred to as *numerosity*—an approximation of the number of things or events to be counted. This sense must have evolved well before language for numbers or arithmetic, since monkeys, rats, birds, bees, and other animals also have this ability. And like research in non-human animals, human behavioral studies show that, in the absence of explicit symbols for numbers, both adults and preverbal children estimate quantities as analog magnitudes in much the same way that physical quantities such as weight, length, or even loudness are estimated (Figure A).

The *numerosity sense* is apparent even when adult humans make relatively precise judgments using Arabic numerals or number words. When given pairs of numbers and asked to choose the symbol that represents the larger magnitude (see Figure A), accuracy increases and latency (reaction time) decreases with increasing numerical distance (Figure B). For example, people take more time to say that 5 is larger than 3 than to say that 8 is larger than 3. Furthermore, when numerical distance is held constant, performance decreases with increasing numerical magnitude (Figure C). In this case, people take more time to indicate that 9 is larger than 7 than to indicate that 7 is larger than 5.

These distance and size effects indicate that accuracy and latency are modulated by the ratio of the quantities that the numerals represent. The effects have been replicated in many languages and cultures, with different representational formats, with double-digit stimuli, and in children as young as 5 years old. Ratio dependence means that numerical discrimination, like time discrimination, follows the Weber-Fechner law (see Box 3B). For example, if an individual required a 3:4 ratio to discriminate a value from 12 (e.g., could differentiate 12 from 16 but not 12 from 14), then if presented with a larger value (such as 24), the subject would be able to differentiate it from 32 but not from 28, even though 24 and 28 have the same numerical difference as 12 and 16 have.

Thus, culturally specific systems for dealing with numbers appear to tap into a phylogenetically ancient sense. The presence of a numerosity sense in a diversity of animals implies that estimating quantities is highly useful for most species—in foraging for food, avoiding predators, and making social decisions such as whether or not to challenge another group. The biological importance of number has evidently favored hardwiring a numerosity sense into the nervous system.

References

BRANNON, E. M. (2006) The representation of numerical magnitude. *Curr. Opin. Neurobiol.* 16: 222–229.

DEHAENE, S., N. MOLKO, L. COHEN AND A. J. WILSON (2004) Arithmetic and the brain. *Curr. Opin. Neurobiol.* 14: 218–224.

FEIGENSON, L., S. DEHAENE AND E. SPELKE (2004) Core systems of number. *Trends Cogn. Sci.* 8: 307–314.

GELMAN, R. AND B. BUTTERWORTH (2005) Number and language: How are they related? *Trends Cogn. Sci.* 9: 6–10.

MOYER, R. S. AND S. T. DUMAIS (1978) Mental comparisons. In *The Psychology of Learning and Motivation*, Vol. 12, G. H. Bower (ed.). New York: Academic Press, pp. 117–155.

MOYER, R. S. AND T. K. LANDAUER (1967) Time required for judgments of numerical inequality. *Nature* 215: 1519–1520.

The numerosity sense in numerical judgment. (A) In experiments designed to measure numerical distance and size effects, subjects are posed questions like the one illustrated here. (B) The time taken to choose the larger of two numerical symbols is a function of the numerical distance between them. (C) Reaction time when the task is to choose the larger of two numerical symbols increases as a function of numerical size when the numerical distance is held constant. (B after Moyer and Landauer 1967; C after Moyer and Dumais 1978.)

(A)

Which is larger?

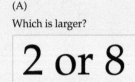

(B)

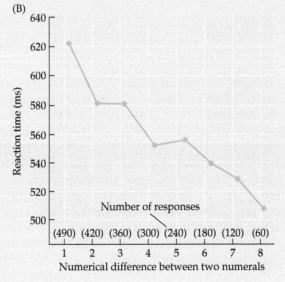

(C)

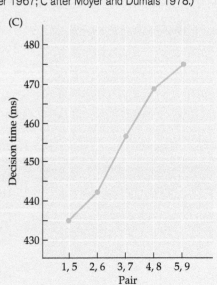

■ BOX 12D LEARNED VOCAL COMMUNICATION IN NON-HUMAN SPECIES

Humans are not the only animals that learn to communicate during a critical period of development, and studies of non-human species have added greatly to a better understanding of social communication by vocalization. Many animal vocalizations are innate in the sense that they require no experience to be correctly produced and interpreted. For example, quails raised in isolation or deafened at hatching so that they never hear conspecific vocal stimuli nonetheless produce the full repertoire of species-specific vocalizations. Some species of birds, however, *learn* to communicate by vocal sounds—a process that is in some respects similar to the way humans learn language. Particularly well characterized is vocal learning in song sparrows, canaries, and finches. These and other bird species use songs to define their territory and attract mates (Figures A and B).

As with human language, early sensory exposure and practice are key determinants of subsequent perceptual and behavioral capabilities. Furthermore, the developmental period for learning these vocal behaviors, as for learning language, is restricted to early life. (Canaries are exceptional in that they continue to build their song repertoire from season to season, which is one reason these birds have been such popular pets over the centuries.) Song learning in these species entails an initial stage of *sensory acquisition*, when the juvenile bird listens to and memorizes the song of an adult male "tutor" of its own species. This period is followed by a stage of vocal learning through practice, when the young bird matches its song to the memorized

(A)

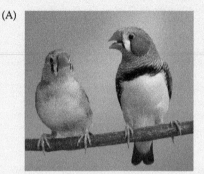

(B)

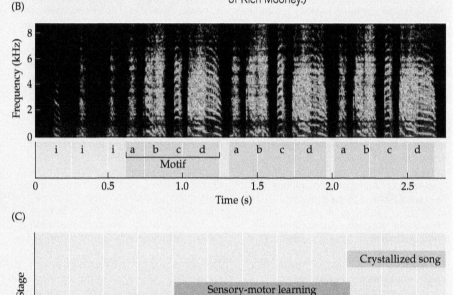

Birdsong learning. The spectrogram in (B) shows the song of an adult male zebra finch—the bird on the right in (A)—that is used in courting the female (as a general rule, only male songbirds sing). The recording plots the frequency of the song against time, showing the syllables and motifs that characterize the song of this species. Color indicates the intensity of the vocal signal, with red representing higher intensity and blue, lower. (C) The stages of song learning in the zebra finch (0 indicates the time of hatching). (Courtesy of Rich Mooney.)

mean the ability to embed clauses meaningfully in sentences, and to iterate these additions ad infinitum (in principle) in a manner that still makes sense. For example, for any particular sentence of the type "Jane knows cognitive neuroscience," it is possible to embed another similar phrase to make a meaningful sentence, such as "Bob knows that Jane knows cognitive neuroscience," and to embed the same sort of phrase yet again to make a sentence like "Bill knows that Bob knows that Jane knows cognitive neuroscience," and so on. Humans routinely use recursion and easily recognize the meaning of such constructions. The progressive addition and back-referencing is why such embedment is called *recursive*, a term borrowed from logic.

This sort of grammar is referred to as a context-free grammar by linguists because the addition of "Z knows that …" to "X knows Y" will work for any specific terms X and Y. A context-free grammar is thus distinct from a finite-

■ BOX 12D *(continued)*

tutor model by auditory feedback. This *sensory-motor learning* stage ends with the onset of sexual maturity, when songs become acoustically stable (i.e., *crystallized*; Figure C).

In the species typically studied, young birds are especially impressionable during the first 2 months after hatching and become refractory to further exposure to tutor songs as they age, thus defining a critical (or sensitive) period for song learning, much as for human language. The early exposure to the tutor (typically the father) generates a memory that can remain intact for months (or longer) in some species before the onset of the vocal practice phase. Moreover, juveniles need to hear the tutor song only 10 to 20 times to vocally mimic it months later, and exposure to other songs after the sensory acquisition period does not affect this memory. The songs heard during this time, but not later, are the only ones that the young bird mimics. Songbirds also exhibit learned regional dialects, much as human infants learn the language that is

characteristic of the region in which they are raised.

Other studies indicate that birds have a strong intrinsic predisposition to learning the song of their own species. Thus, when presented during maturation with a variety of recorded songs that include their own species' song, together with the songs of other species, juvenile birds preferentially learn the song of their own species. This observation shows that juveniles are not really naïve, but are innately biased to learn conspecific songs relative to those of other species. Other evidence suggests that songbirds have a rough template of their species song that is expressed in the absence of any exposure to that song or any other. Thus, birds raised in isolation produce highly abnormal "isolate" songs that have some characteristics of the song they would normally have learned. Such songs, however, are biologically ineffective in that they fail to attract mates.

In sum, the vocally relevant parts of the bird brain are already prepared dur-

ing early life to learn the specific vocal sounds of the species, much as the brains of human infants are prepared at birth to learn language. Although the similarities with human language acquisition can be exaggerated, at least some aspects of human language have analogues in the learned communicative abilities of other animals.

References

Brenowitz, E. A. and M. D. Beecher (2005) Song learning in birds: Diversity and plasticity, opportunities and challenges. *Trends Neurosci.* 28(3): 127–132.

Doupe, A. and P. Kuhl (1999) Birdsong and human speech: Common themes and mechanisms. *Annu. Rev. Neurosci.* 22: 567–631.

Marler, P. and H. W. Slabbekoorn (2004) *Nature's Music: The Science of Birdsong.* New York: Academic Press.

state grammar, in which the pattern as such determines the significance of the stimulus. In general, communication among non-human animals has long been thought to depend on this simpler finite-state grammar. In the dance of the honeybee, for example, each symbolic movement made by a foraging bee that returns to the hive encodes only a single meaning about resource location, whose expression and interpretation has been hardwired into the nervous system of the actor and the respondents. The same general point has long been made for birdsong, in which vocal stimuli are presumably attached to a fixed biological meaning (e.g., "I own this territory" or "Here I am, if you're looking for a mate"; Box 12D).

Other investigators examined this issue in a songbird, the European starling. They took advantage of the fact that the starling song has two components—a rattle and a warble—both of which occur in the starling's song motifs. They could thus synthesize recursive $a^n b^n$ vocal stimulus forms such as *ab* (rattle, warble), *aabb* (rattle, rattle; warble, warble), *aaabbb* (rattle, rattle, rattle; warble, warble, warble), and so on, as well as nonrecursive $(ab)^n$ forms such as *ab* (rattle, warble), *abab* (rattle, warble; rattle, warble), *ababab* (rattle, warble; rattle, warble; rattle, warble), and so on. The investigators found that, after a great deal of training, most of the birds tested could reliably distinguish the two forms in an operant conditioning paradigm in which only the recursive grammatical form was rewarded. Although starlings presumably make no use of this ability in vocal communication, the researchers concluded that the rudiments of the ability to use recursive grammars are present in some non-human animals.

This and other evidence does not, of course, settle the centuries-old debate about the uniqueness of human language. However, it challenges those who want to claim that human speech and language are fundamentally different from vocal communication in other species.

Figure 12.15 **Rhesus monkey calls** The *coo* call (A) is relatively long and drawn out, as indicated by the sound signal and spectrographic recordings. It is quite different from the more pulsatile *threat* call (B). (From Ghazanfar and Logothetis 2003.)

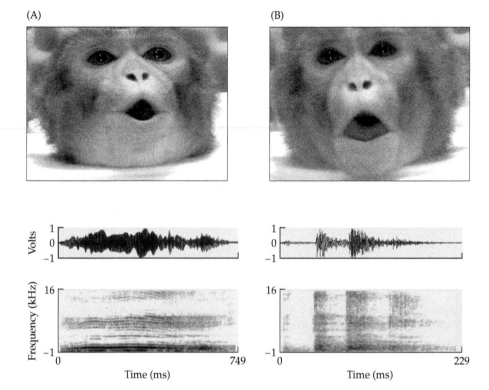

The Origins of Human Language

The fact that human language is similar in a number of ways to systems of vocal communication in some other species raises the question of how human language originated. Although it should be clear that no one knows the answer, some clues are worth considering.

Field studies in a variety of non-human primate species have shown a surprising degree of vocal communication that seems a plausible antecedent for human speech. One well-studied example is the alarm calls of vervet monkeys, which differ according to the nature of the perceived threat. Ethologists Dorothy Cheney and Robert Seyfarth found that a specific alarm call uttered when a leopard had been spotted by one animal caused other nearby monkeys to climb a tree. In contrast, the different alarm call given when a monkey saw an eagle caused the other members of the group to look skyward.

This work has now been augmented by detailed studies of the vocalizations of rhesus monkeys. These animals utter at least five food-related vocalizations that are referred to respectively as *warble, harmonic arch, chirp, coo,* and *grunt,* as well as a threat call (**Figure 12.15**). Different vocalizations had appreciably different effects on the monkeys that were listening (assessed, for example, by the degree to which other monkeys turned toward the monkey uttering a particular call). They also showed that the animals integrated visual and auditory information in doing so, much as humans do (see Figure 12.3). Moreover, studies in the field indicated that the different vocalizations were specifically related to the motivational state of the monkey uttering the call, as well as to the affective state and even to the particular qualities of food that had been discovered by the "speaker" during foraging.

More controversial studies in great apes going back several decades have sought to show more directly that the rudiments of abstract symbolic communication are present, or at least latent, in our closest relatives. Others have suggested that language may have arisen from primate gestures. Although techniques

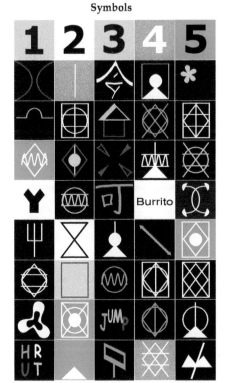

Symbols

Meanings

1	2	3	4	5
Car	Raisin	Hamburger	Sherman	Egg
Sue's office	Groom	Log cabin	Chow	Stick
Outdoors	Rose	Fire	TV	Rock
Yes	Milk	Hotdog	Burrito	Criss-cross
Orange	No	Can opener	Pine needle	Ice
Bread	Hug	Water	Straw	Hide
Hose	Get	Jump	Turtle	Goodbye
Hurt	Look	Tree house	Come	Midway

Figure 12.16 Abstract symbols used to assess the ability of chimpanzees to communicate The animals are trained to manipulate tiles (left) with symbols that represent words and syntactical constructs (right) in order to communicate demands, questions, and even spontaneous expressions. (From Savage-Rumbaugh et al. 1998.)

have varied, most such studies have used some form of symbols that can be arranged to express ideas in an interpretable manner. For example, chimpanzees have been trained to manipulate tiles to represent words and syntactical constructs, allowing them to communicate simple expressions (Figure 12.16). With extensive training, chimps can choose from as many as 400 different symbols to construct what appear to be meaningful statements or questions. The more accomplished of these animals are alleged to have "vocabularies" of several thousand words or phrases. Compared to children, however, the way chimps use these words is far less impressive; moreover, children can learn new words and how to use them very rapidly (as discussed earlier). Indeed, whether the chimps are using symbols in the same way that humans use words as tokens is much debated, and many cognitive neuroscientists remain skeptical of how analogous such usage is to human language.

Summary

1. The human vocal tract and its controlling neural apparatus have become highly specialized over evolutionary time, allowing this system to produce approximately 200 distinct speech sounds (phones), which produce corresponding auditory percepts (phonemes). A few tens of these speech sounds are used in any given language to produce the syllables, words, phrases, sentences, and ultimately the narratives that humans use to communicate verbal information.

2. Language must be learned in early life, and if such experience does not occur, then a person's linguistic ability is severely and permanently limited. Nonetheless, an infant's brain, like the vocally relevant brain regions of some other species, is already prepared to incorporate the speech information that the infant hears.

3. Virtually all researchers studying the neural bases of language are now agreed that most of the semantic, grammatical, and syntactical processing of language comprehension and expression resides in a number of interconnected regions of the left frontal, temporal, and parietal cortices in the majority of humans.

Nevertheless, there is a great deal of individual variation, including variation in the degree of lateralization and the location of the relevant areas.

4. Most researchers also agree that the corresponding cortical regions in the right hemisphere contribute importantly to language by adding the emotional coloring evident in speech prosody, and presumably by interpreting this and other nonverbal aspects of language. The right hemisphere also has the rudiments of the processing abilities that exist in the left hemisphere, as evidenced by split-brain patients, again with wide variation among individuals.

5. Electrophysiological recording, brain imaging, and other techniques have gradually made clear that the language-processing areas initially identified by clinical-pathological correlations are components of a widely distributed set of brain regions that allow humans to communicate effectively by means of tokens that can be attached ad infinitum to objects, concepts, and feelings deemed important, and that these same areas are involved in other functions.

6. Comparison of the neural substrates of sign language in congenitally deaf individuals shows further that the cortical representation of language is independent of the means of its expression and perception (spoken and heard versus gestured and seen). Thus, the neural bases of language represent a system for symbolic processing that transcends verbal expression as such.

7. Although phenomenally well developed in humans compared to other animals, language has many basic similarities with systems of social communication in other species, which appear to entail the same general scheme of constructing acquired neural associations within a framework of dedicated brain circuitry that has already been put in place by inherited developmental programs.

Go to the **COMPANION WEBSITE**

sites.sinauer.com/cogneuro2e
for quizzes, animations, flashcards, and other study resources.

Additional Reading

Reviews

BACHOROWSKI, J.-A. AND M. J. OWREN (2003) Sounds of emotion: The production and perception of affect-related vocal acoustics. *Ann. N. Y. Acad. Sci.* 1000: 244–265.

BELIN, P., S. FECTEAU AND C. BEDARD (2004) Thinking the voice: Neural correlates of voice perception. *Trends Cogn. Sci.* 8: 129–135.

BELLUGI, U., H. POIZNER AND E. S. KLIMA (1989) Language, modality, and the brain. *Trends Neurosci.* 12: 380–388.

BINDER, J. R., H. RUTVIK, W. DESAI, W. GRAVES AND L. CONANT (2009) Where is the semantic system? A critical review and meta-analysis of 120 functional neuroimaging studies. *Cereb. Cortex* 19: 2767–2796.

BLOOMFIELD, T. C., T. Q. GENTNER AND D. MARGOLIASH (2012) What birds have to say about language. *Nat. Neurosci.* 14: 947–948.

BUHUSI, C. V. AND W. H. MECK (2005) What makes us tick? Functional and neural mechanisms of interval timing. *Nat. Rev. Neurosci.* 6: 755–765.

DAMASIO, A. R. (1992) Aphasia. *New Engl. J. Med.* 326: 531–539.

DAMASIO, A. R. AND N. GESCHWIND (1984) The neural basis of language. *Annu. Rev. Neurosci.* 7: 127–147.

EVANS, N. AND S. C. LEVINSON (2009) The myth of language universals: Language diversity and its importance for cognitive science. *Behav. Brain Sci.* 32: 429–492.

FRIEDERICI, A. D. (2009) Pathways to language: Fiber tracts in the human brain. *Trends Cogn. Sci.* 13: 175–181.

GAZZANIGA, M. S. (1998) The split brain revisited. *Sci. Am.* 279(1): 50–55.

GAZZANIGA, M. S. AND R. W. SPERRY (1967) Language after section of the cerebral commissures. *Brain* 90: 131–147.

GHAZANFAR, A. A. AND M. D. HAUSER (2001) The auditory behavior of primates: A neuroethological perspective. *Curr. Opin. Neurobiol.* 12: 712–720.

GIBBON, J., C. MALAPANI, C. L. DALE AND C. R. GALLISTEL (1997) Toward a neurobiology of temporal cognition: Advances and challenges. *Curr. Opin. Neurobiol.* 7: 170–184.

HAUSER, M. D., N. CHOMSKY AND W. T. FITCH (2002) The faculty of language: What is it, who has it, and how did it evolve? *Science* 298: 1569–1579.

KUHL, P. K. (2000) A new view of language acquisition. *Proc. Natl. Acad. Sci. USA* 97: 12850–12857.

KUTAS, M., C. K. VAN PETTEN AND R. KLUENDER (2006) Psycholinguistics electrified II (1924–2005). In *Handbook of Psycholinguistics*, 2nd Ed., M. A.

Gernsbacher and M. Traxler (eds.). New York: Elsevier, pp. 659–724.

MAYBERRY, R. I. (2010) Early language acquisition and adult language ability: What sign language reveals about the critical period for language. In *The Oxford Handbook of Deaf Studies, Language, and Education*, M. Marschark and P. E. Spencer (eds.). Oxford: Oxford University Press, pp. 281–291.

MILES, H. L. W. AND S. E. HARPER (1994) "Ape language" studies and the study of human language origins. In *Hominid Culture in Primate Perspective*, D. Quiatt and J. Itani (eds.). Niwot: University Press of Colorado, pp. 253–278.

NEWPORT, E. L., D. BAVELIER AND H. J. NEVILLE (2001) Critical thinking about critical periods: Perspectives on a critical period for language acquisition. In *Language, Brain, and Cognitive Development: Essays in Honor of Jacques Mehler*, E. Dupoux (ed.). Cambridge, MA: MIT Press, pp. 481–502.

OJEMANN, G. A. (1983) The intrahemispheric organization of human language, derived with electrical stimulation techniques. *Trends Neurosci.* 4: 184–189.

POLLICK, A. S. AND F. B. M. DE WAAL (2007) Ape gestures and language evolution. *Proc. Natl. Acad. Sci. USA* 104: 8184–8189.

SEYFARTH, D. M. AND D. I. CHENEY (1984) The natural vocalizations of non-human primates. *Trends Neurosci.* 7: 66–73.

SPELKE, E. S. (2003) What makes us smart? Core knowledge and natural language. In *Language in Mind: Advances in the Study of Language and Thought*, D. Gentner and S. Goldin-Meadow (eds.). Cambridge, MA: MIT Press, pp. 277–312.

ZUBERBUHLER, K. (2005) Linguistic prerequisites in the primate lineage. In *Language Origins: Perspectives on Evolution*, M. Tallerman (ed.). New York: Oxford University Press, pp. 262–282.

Important Original Papers

ABE, K. AND D. WATANABE (2012) Songbirds possess the spontaneous ability to discriminate syntactic rules. *Nat. Neurosci.* 14: 1067–1074.

BAGLEY, W. C. (1900–1901) The apperception of the spoken sentence: A study in the psychology of language. *Am. J. Psychol.* 12: 80–130.

BROWN, T. T., H. M. LUGAR, R. S. COALSON, F. M. MIEZIN, S. E. PETERESEN AND B. L. SCHLAGGAR (2005) Developmental changes in human cerebral functional organization for word generation. *Cereb. Cortex* 15: 275–290.

CHAO, L. L., J. V. HAXBY AND A. MARTIN (1999) Attribute-based neural substrates in temporal cortex for perceiving and knowing about objects. *Nat. Neurosci.* 2: 913–919.

DELONG, K., T. URBACH AND M. KUTAS (2005) Probabilistic word pre-activation during language comprehension inferred from electrical brain activity. *Nat. Neurosci.* 8: 1217–1221.

FROMKIN, V., S. KRASHEN, S. CURTIS, D. RIGLER AND M. RIGLER (1974) The development of language in Genie: A case of language acquisition beyond the "critical period." *Brain Lang.* 1: 81–107.

GENTNER, T. Q., K. M. FENN, D. MARGOLIASH AND H. C. NUSBAUM (2006) Recursive syntactic pattern learning by songbirds. *Nature* 440: 1204–1207.

GHAZANFAR, A. A. AND N. LOGOTHETIS (2003) Facial expressions linked to monkey calls. *Nature* 423: 937.

GIL-DA-COSTA, R., A. MARTIN, M. A. LOPES, M. MUNOZ, J. FRITZ AND A. R. BRAUN (2006) Species-specific calls activate homologs of Broca's and Wernicke's areas in the macaque. *Nat. Neurosci.* 9: 1064–1070.

JOHNSON, J. S. AND E. L. NEWPORT (1989) Critical period effects in second language learning: The influence of maturational state on the acquisition of English as a second language. *Cogn. Psychol.* 21: 60–99.

KUHL, P. K., B. T. CONBOY, D. PADDEN, T. NELSON AND J. PRUITT (2005) Early speech perception and later language development: Implications for the "critical period." *Lang. Learn. Dev.* 1: 237–264.

KUHL, P. K., K. A. WILLIAMS, F. LACERDA, K. N. STEVENS AND B. LINDBLOM (1992) Linguistic experience alters phonetic perception in infants 6 months of age. *Science* 255: 606–608.

KUTAS, M. AND S. A. HILLYARD (1980) Reading senseless sentences: Brain potentials reflect semantic incongruity. *Science* 207: 203–205.

MILLER, G. A. AND J. C. R. LICKLIDER (1950) The intelligibility of interrupted speech. *J. Acoust. Soc. Am.* 22: 167–173.

NIEDER, A. AND E. K. MILLER (2004) A parieto-frontal network for visual numerical information in the monkey. *Proc. Natl. Acad. Sci. USA* 101: 7457–7462.

OJEMANN, G. A. AND H. A. WHITAKER (1978) The bilingual brain. *Arch. Neurol.* 35: 409–412.

PICA, P., C. LEMER, W. IZARD AND S. DEHAENE (2004) Exact and approximate arithmetic in an Amazonian indigene group. *Science* 306: 499–503.

POLLICK, A. S. AND F. B. M. DE WAAL (2007) Ape gestures and language evolution. *Proc. Natl. Acad. Sci. USA* 104: 8184–8189.

SCHLAGGAR, B. L., T. T. BROWN, H. M. LUGAR, K. M. VISSCHER, F. M. MIEZIN AND S. E. PETERSEN (2002) Functional neuroanatomical differences between adults and school-age children in the processing of single words. *Science* 296: 1476–1479.

SHULMAN, G. L., J. M. OLLINGER, M. LINENWEBER, S. E. PETERSEN AND M. CORBETTA (2001) Multiple neural correlates of detection in the human brain. *Proc. Natl. Acad. Sci. USA* 98: 313–318.

TOMASELLO, M. (2004) What kind of evidence could refute the UG hypothesis? *Stud. Lang.* 28: 642–644.

WHITEN, A. AND 8 OTHERS (1999) Cultures in chimpanzees. *Nature* 399: 682–685.

XU, F. AND E. SPELKE (2000) Large number discrimination in 6-month-old infants. *Cognition* 74: B1–B12.

Books

BLOOM, P. (2002) *How Children Learn the Meanings of Words*. Cambridge, MA: MIT Press.

CHOMSKY, N. (1957) *Syntactic Structures*. The Hague, Netherlands: Elsevier.

DARWIN, C. (1872) *The Expression of the Emotions in Man and Animals*. Reprint, Chicago: University of Chicago Press, 1965.

GARDNER, H. (1974) *The Shattered Mind: The Person after Brain Damage*. New York: Vintage.

GELMAN, R. AND C. GALLISTEL (1978) *The Child's Understanding of Number*. Cambridge, MA: Harvard University Press.

GOODALL, J. (1990) *Through a Window: My Thirty Years with the Chimpanzees of Gombe*. Boston: Houghton Mifflin.

GRIFFIN, D. R. (1992) *Animal Minds*. Chicago: University of Chicago Press.

HAUSER, M. (1996) *The Evolution of Communication*. Cambridge, MA: MIT Press.

LENNEBERG, E. (1967) *The Biological Foundations of Language*. New York: Wiley.

LIBERMAN, A. M. (1996) *Speech: A Special Code*. Cambridge, MA: MIT Press.

MCNEIL, D. (2000) *Language and Gesture*. Cambridge: Cambridge University Press.

MILLER, G. A. (1991) *The Science of Words*. New York: Scientific American Library.

PLOMP, R. (2002) *The Intelligent Ear: On the Nature of Sound Perception*. Mahwah, NJ: Erlbaum.

POSNER, M. I. AND M. E. RAICHLE (1994) *Images of Mind*. New York: Scientific American Library.

PROVINE, R. R. (2000) *Laughter: A Scientific Investigation*. New York: Penguin.

ROGERS, T. T. AND J. L. MCCLELLAND (2004) *Semantic Cognition: A Parallel Distributed Processing Approach*. Cambridge, MA: MIT Press.

SAVAGE-RUMBAUGH, S., S. G. SHANKER AND T. J. TAYLOR (1998) *Apes, Language, and the Human Mind*. New York: Oxford University Press.

VON FRISCH, K. (1993) *The Dance Language and Orientation of Bees*. (Translated by Leigh E. Chadwick.) Cambridge, MA: Harvard University Press.

WINCHESTER, S. (2003) *The Meaning of Everything: The Story of the Oxford English Dictionary*. Oxford: Oxford University Press.

13

Executive Functions

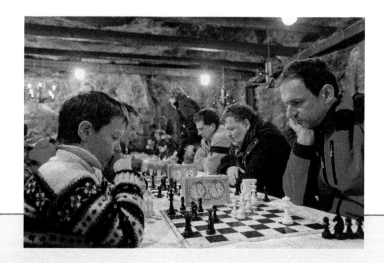

INTRODUCTION

The human brain must coordinate an array of complex functions to achieve desired goals. In many situations, **executive functions** modulate the activity of other cognitive functions in a flexible and goal-directed manner. As the name implies, executive functions perform supervisory or regulatory roles. In some cases, they involve measured and thoughtful processing, as when we mentally simulate an opponent's strategies in a complex game. Or they may operate rapidly and largely unconsciously to guide the flow of sensory information or to initiate a motor action.

Half a century ago, executive functions were given relatively short shrift in psychology textbooks, typically being discussed as minor aspects of a chapter on "thinking." Over the past two decades, however, research into the brain mechanisms underlying executive function has become one of the most active areas of cognitive neuroscience. A primary target for research on executive functions has been the **prefrontal cortex.** Patients with prefrontal damage may seem to have normal cognitive functions: they can identify objects and sounds, can comprehend and carry on conversations, and can perform motor tasks with dexterity. Yet, when faced with real-world challenges, they may have difficulty selecting the right action for the current context (see Introductory Box). Despite the importance of the prefrontal cortex for many executive processes, no single part of the brain—no "homunculus"—can be identified as the neural equivalent of a chief executive. Instead, executive functions arise from a distributed set of brain regions that also includes parietal cortex, the basal ganglia, and other brain areas.

A Taxonomy of Executive Function

Central to nearly all definitions of executive function are two concepts: *rules* and *control*. The rules that guide human behavior—and the behavior of many other but not all organisms—are abstract and flexible. Consider the seemingly simple rule "Drive on the right-hand side of the road." That rule applies to a very wide range of contexts (e.g., all of the physically and perceptually distinct

■ INTRODUCTORY BOX ENVIRONMENTAL DEPENDENCY SYNDROME

In the mid-1980s, French neurologist François Lhermitte identified a set of behaviors associated with damage to the anterior and medial parts of the frontal lobe. Lhermitte was an unusual clinician in that he made a point of observing his patients in complex, open-ended interviews and in real-world situations. He found that patients with this sort of frontal lobe damage, but not those with damage to other brain regions, exhibited a remarkable sort of inflexibility in their behavior: their actions were based not on their own goals, but on what they observed in the surrounding environment. Lhermitte called this pathological inflexibility an *environmental dependency syndrome*.

Patients with this syndrome had two striking features. The first was *imitation behavior*. If, for example, the interviewer unexpectedly touched his nose with his thumb, the patients mimicked this behavior, touching their own noses. Such imitation was evident not only for physical movements such as common hand gestures or changes in body posture, but also for actions with objects, such as drawing, combing hair, or chewing on a pencil. Imitation also extended to vocalizations like singing or speaking simple phrases. Most such patients imitated the interviewer from the outset, and they continued to do so even after being told to stop. When their behavior was questioned, patients reported feeling compelled to imitate. In testing many neurologically normal subjects in a similar fashion, not surprisingly Lhermitte found no such imitation (although many were amused by his actions).

The second feature of the environmental dependency syndrome was *utilization behavior*, an abnormal reliance on immediate environmental stimuli to trigger behavior (see the examples in Figures A and B). For instance, if a glass and pitcher were placed on a table, patients might repeatedly pour water into the glass and drink it, whether or not they were thirsty. If patients walked down a hallway and saw a set of stairs, they might walk up those stairs, regardless of whether they wanted to go in that direction. Utilization behavior was present in about half of the patients with imitation behavior, and it is

considered a more severe expression of the same underlying deficit.

Patients with environmental dependency syndrome, like those with other frontal lobe syndromes, lack insight into the causes and consequences of their actions. Lhermitte suggested that, because such patients do not initiate actions of their own accord, their behavior is excessively determined by social or environmental cues. The patients simply perform whatever actions are most strongly associated with an object or stimulus in the local environment, much like the patient shown in Figure B, who,

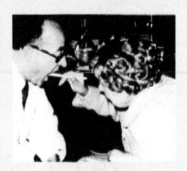

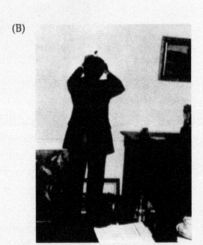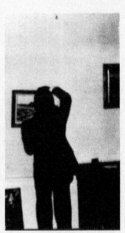

Overdependence on immediate sensory cues to guide behavior after damage to the ventromedial prefrontal lobe. The patient in (A) was brought into a room where several pieces of medical equipment lay on a table. Without prompting, she picked up the equipment and began examining the doctor. When on a social visit to the apartment of his doctor, the patient in (B) encountered a picture that was lying on the floor. He grabbed a nearby hammer and nailed a bracket into the wall to hang the painting. (Photos from Lhermitte 1986.)

when he saw a hammer, used it to drive a nail.

References

LHERMITTE, F., B. PILLON AND M. SERDARU (1986) Human autonomy and the frontal lobes. Part I: Imitation and utilization behavior: A neuropsychological study of 75 patients. *Ann. Neurol.* 19: 326–334.

LHERMITTE, F. (1986) Human autonomy and the frontal lobes. Part II: Patient behavior in complex and social situations: The "environmental dependency syndrome." *Ann. Neurol.* 19: 335–343.

environments that we categorize as "roads"), constrains the complex set of motor actions that constitute driving, and generalizes to qualitatively distinct sorts of behavior (e.g., forward and backward driving, direction of travel on roundabouts). Control processes allow us to engage rules appropriate to a particular context. When we travel to a new location—say, from the United States to the United Kingdom—we now adopt the rule for driving in that location, as well as for all it implies for our behavior. These two aspects of executive function—(1) creating and modifying rules for behavior and (2) engaging the appropriate rule for a particular context—represent the highest levels of a taxonomy for executive function and thus reflect major sections of this chapter (Figure 13.1).

Under these major divisions, further differentiation is possible. Effective use of rules for behavior requires several sorts of functions: *initiating* rules that match stimuli to actions based on behavioral goals, *inhibiting* (or discarding) rules that are not relevant to behavior, *shifting* (or *task-shifting*) functions that facilitate the transition from one rule for behavior to another more appropriate rule, and *relating* rules to each other to form higher-order contingencies for behavior. These four functions are considered as subsections within the section on rule processing. Control functions are often considered to include **monitoring** the current state of the environment to guide the engagement of other executive functions; if the environment is changing rapidly, for example, then rules should be updated more frequently than would be the case in a more stable environment. All executive functions are considered to rely on capacity-limited short-term information stores—often called *working memory*—that enable the maintenance of rules and of the information that guides the execution of those rules.

This taxonomy reflects one of several ways of conceptualizing executive function. More than for any other area within cognitive neuroscience, research on executive function has led to an explosion of theoretical frameworks, each with its own set of postulated functions. How terms are used can differ dramatically across those frameworks. A given term (e.g., *cognitive control*) sometimes defines a specific operation within a task but other times loosely characterizes a psychological process—or even serves as a synonym for *executive function* itself. Trying to adjudicate between the many existing models of executive function is a challenge well beyond the scope of this chapter. The main goal here is to introduce the basic executive functions and to consider ways in which new research in cognitive neuroscience is influencing the conception of executive function.

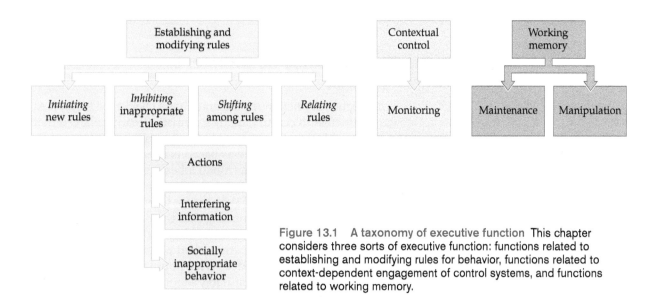

Figure 13.1 A taxonomy of executive function This chapter considers three sorts of executive function: functions related to establishing and modifying rules for behavior, functions related to context-dependent engagement of control systems, and functions related to working memory.

■ BOX 13A COMPARATIVE ANATOMY OF THE PREFRONTAL CORTEX

Despite some unsavory uses, the measurement of brain size across species remains an important tool in cognitive neuroscience. Investigators recognized early on that overall brain size is a poor index of intelligence or other cognitive functions. The average adult human brain, for example, is only about a fourth as large as the brain of an adult elephant, and the brains of orangutans and cows are of roughly similar size. Most research has thus focused on the *relative* size of specific regions. With respect to the prefrontal cortex, there are clear differences across a range of mammals. The early-twentieth-century German physiologist and anatomist Korbinian Brodmann estimated that only 7 percent of the dog's cortex, and less than 4 percent of the cat's, is prefrontal. In contrast, Brodmann found that the prefrontal cortex constitutes about 10 percent of total brain volume in monkeys (e.g., gibbon, macaque), 20 percent in the great apes (e.g., chimpanzee), and 30 percent in humans (Figures A and B).

Although this ranking is plausible, given what is known about the relative capabilities of these species, contemporary researchers have modified Brodmann's original estimates. Neuroanatomist Katerina Semendeferi and her colleagues used structural MRI to measure the frontal lobes in a wide variety of primate species. They found that the proportional size of the frontal lobes in humans is actually about the same as that in great apes, occupying about 35 percent of the brain volume (Figure C). In addition, there were no significant differences between humans and other great apes in the extent

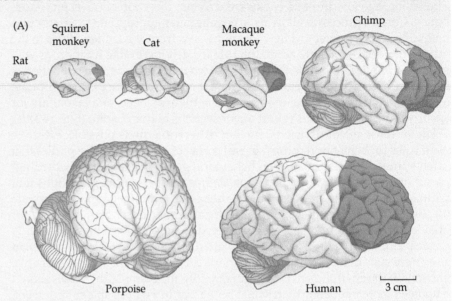

(A) Comparative anatomy of the prefrontal cortex. Not only is absolute brain size greater in primates compared to other mammals, but there is also a disproportionate increase in the size of the prefrontal cortex (blue). The porpoise brain is provided for size comparison; its prefrontal cortex is not indicated, because there are no clear homologies between the prefrontal cortices of primates and cetaceans.

of the prefrontal cortex, defined as the cortex anterior to the precentral sulcus. In all the species tested, the prefrontal cortex accounted for 26 to 33 percent of total brain volume.

Although the proportion of prefrontal cortex generally tracks cognitive competence across mammals, these modern results indicate that the relative size of the frontal lobes does not, by itself, explain the different cognitive capabilities of humans and other great apes. It would

seem that humans are distinctive from other apes because of their relatively large brains and not because of their large prefrontal cortices.

References

BRODMANN, K. (1912) Neue Ergebnisse über die vergleichende histologische Lokalisation der Grosshirnrinde mit besonderer Berücksichtigung des Stirnhirns. *Anat. Anzeiger* 41: 157–216.

Prefrontal Cortex: A Key Contributor to Executive Function

The localization of executive functions in the brain has a checkered history. At the beginning of the nineteenth century, many scientists already believed that the frontal lobes were critical for controlling behavior and for higher cognitive functions generally. This conviction was based on very limited evidence, such as the gross anatomical fact that the frontal lobes are relatively larger in humans and great apes than in other mammals (Box 13A). By studying the skulls of different species and individual humans, German physician and anatomist Franz Gall went further, speculating that the brain comprised different faculties that could be discerned by the way they had shaped the surface features of the skull—a theoretical framework called **phrenology** (see Chapter 1 for historical context). Although these ideas were popular at the time, many of Gall's scientific contemporaries were justifiably skeptical. The phrenologists'

■ **BOX 13A** *(continued)*

(B) Prefrontal cortex scaling according to Brodmann (1912)

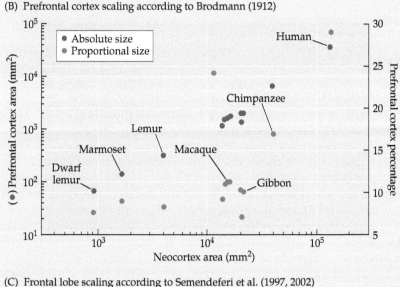

(B) The prefrontal cortex is particularly well developed in primates. Largely because of Brodmann's work, it was thought that the proportional size of the prefrontal cortex was greater in humans than in other great apes. (C) More recent studies indicate that the frontal lobes and the prefrontal cortex occupy about the same proportion of overall brain volume in great apes and humans. (B after Brodmann 1912; C after Semendeferi et al. 1997, 2002.)

DEANER, R. O., K. ISLER, J. BURKART AND C. VAN SCHAIK (2007) Overall brain size, and not encephalization quotient, best predicts cognitive ability across non-human primates. *Brain Behav. Evol.* 70: 115–124.

SEMENDEFERI, K., H. DAMASIO, R. FRANK AND G. W. VAN HOESEN (1997) The evolution of the frontal lobes: A volumetric analysis based on three-dimensional reconstructions of magnetic resonance scans of human and ape brains. *J. Hum. Evol.* 32: 375–388.

SEMENDEFERI, K., A. LU, N. SCHENKER AND H. DAMASIO (2002) Humans and great apes share a large frontal cortex. *Nat. Neurosci.* 5: 272–276.

STRIEDTER, G. F. (2005) *Principles of Brain Evolution.* Sunderland, MA: Sinauer.

(C) Frontal lobe scaling according to Semendeferi et al. (1997, 2002)

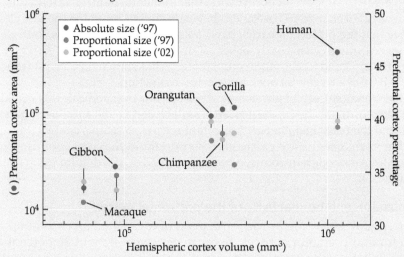

speculations did, however, have two salutary effects. They encouraged exploration of how different cognitive processes might be localized in the brain, and they encouraged the idea that higher cognitive functions may be specifically localized in the frontal lobes.

By the latter half of the nineteenth century, physiologists had developed experimental techniques that could investigate cortical function in animals. The first studies of the frontal lobes in an animal were conducted by German physiologist Eduard Hitzig and his colleague Gustav Fritsch in the late 1860s. When they electrically stimulated the posterior parts of the frontal lobes in a dog, the animal moved its limbs on the opposite side; conversely, damage to the posterior frontal lobe led to a lack of voluntary control over motor actions, although the animal could still engage in reflexive movements like walking. Together, these results provided evidence that the more posterior portions of the frontal lobes are associated with motor function (see Chapter 5). Damage to

(A)

Dorsolateral
prefrontal cortex

Posterior
parietal cortex

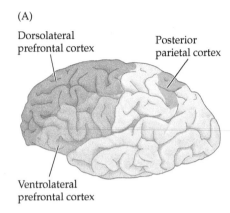

Ventrolateral
prefrontal cortex

(B)

Dorsomedial
prefrontal cortex

Anterior
cingulate gyrus

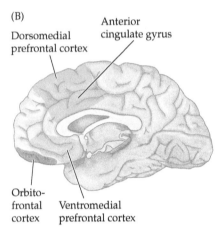

Orbito-
frontal
cortex

Ventromedial
prefrontal cortex

(C)

Caudate nucleus

Putamen

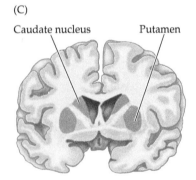

Figure 13.2 **Major brain regions that support executive control** The brain regions that mediate executive control are (A) lateral structures including the lateral prefrontal cortex (PFC), which is split into dorsal and ventral aspects, and the posterior parietal cortex; (B) midline and inferior structures including the ventromedial PFC, orbitofrontal cortex (which continues to the ventral surface of the frontal lobes, not shown), and dorsomedial PFC, which includes the anterior cingulate gyrus; and (C) the caudate nucleus and putamen within the basal ganglia.

the anterior frontal lobes, in contrast, caused neither paralysis nor any obvious sensory deficits; moreover, electrical stimulation of those regions evoked no discernible movements or muscle activity. With mainly this limited evidence, Hitzig and Fritsch speculated that the anterior frontal lobes are associated with higher cognitive functions rather than with sensation or motor control.

This experimental approach was extended and refined over the succeeding decades by British physiologist David Ferrier and Italian physiologist Leonardo Bianchi, each of whom created various prefrontal lesions and followed up with careful observations of behavior. Bianchi found that, in monkeys, bilateral prefrontal damage caused deficits in a range of cognitive functions: failure to recognize known objects, inability to use past experience to guide behavior, deficits in initiative, loss of affective responses, and lack of coherent behavior. He also made the important observation that unilateral damage rarely caused these behavioral changes. These and other early studies provided the first clear evidence that the prefrontal cortex plays a key role in the executive control of behavior. Although these early observations of Hitzig, Fritsch, Ferrier, and Bianchi remain valid today, more recent research has shown that the prefrontal cortex is part of a larger network for executive function.

Modern anatomical and physiological studies, however, indicate that in addition to the prefrontal cortex, the **posterior parietal cortex**, the **anterior cingulate cortex**, and the **basal ganglia** play important roles in executive control (**Figure 13.2**). The basal ganglia are particularly important in the context of decision making; thus, although introduced here, they are discussed more extensively in Chapter 14.

Organization and connectivity of the prefrontal cortex

The prefrontal cortex comprises those parts of the frontal lobes anterior to the motor and premotor cortices. Because of its size—about 35 percent of the human brain—the prefrontal cortex is typically subdivided into several functional regions. Its lateral surface, as spanned by the inferior, middle, and superior frontal gyri, is usually called **lateral prefrontal cortex**. In some topographical systems, the lateral prefrontal cortex is separated into upper and lower parts, termed the **dorsolateral prefrontal cortex** and **ventrolateral prefrontal cortex**, respectively. The ventral surface of the frontal lobes is often called **orbitofrontal cortex** (i.e., the part of the brain above the orbits of the eyes), and regions along the ventral midline are specifically called **ventromedial prefrontal cortex**. The medial surface of the prefrontal cortex can be roughly divided into anterior and posterior aspects. The anterior aspect is often associated with social cognition, as introduced in Chapter 11. The posterior, dorsal parts—collectively called **dorsomedial prefrontal cortex** and including the anterior cingulate gyrus—are important for executive function and considered in this chapter. Finally, the most anterior parts of the prefrontal cortex are often called **frontopolar cortex**.

The anatomical connections of various cortical regions are good, if imperfect, indicators of the functional interactions among those regions, as is clearly evident in the frontal lobes. More than any other part of the cortex, prefrontal

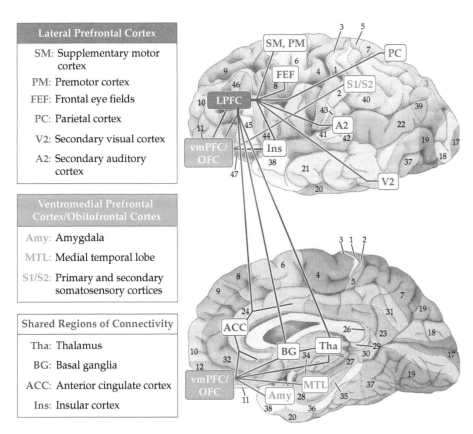

Figure 13.3 Connectivity of the prefrontal cortex Neurons in the prefrontal cortex project to and receive input from secondary sensory cortices, motor preparatory structures, and parietal cortex. This schematic diagram shows some of the major connections for lateral prefrontal cortex (LPFC) and for ventromedial prefrontal cortex and orbitofrontal cortex (vmPFC/OFC, combined here for simplicity). All indicated connections are bidirectional, with the important exception of a unidirectional projection from LPFC to the basal ganglia (which projects back to LPFC via the thalamus).

regions have numerous, diverse, and bidirectional connections with other brain regions (Figure 13.3). The prefrontal cortex has substantial bidirectional connectivity with the thalamus, particularly to its mediodorsal nucleus. Generally, the prefrontal cortex exhibits direct connectivity with secondary (rather than primary) sensory cortices. For example, the inferior temporal cortex, which supports higher-level object processing (see Chapter 3), projects to the lateral prefrontal cortex, while the primary visual cortex does not. The one notable exception to this rule is the orbitofrontal cortex, which receives projections from primary taste, olfactory, and somatosensory cortices.

Other key connections include the strong link between posterior parietal cortex and dorsolateral prefrontal cortex; the projection of the hippocampus throughout prefrontal cortex; the bidirectional connections between the amygdala and primarily the ventromedial regions of prefrontal cortex; and the projection of the ventral tegmental area of the midbrain to primarily ventromedial prefrontal regions. Important exceptions to the typical bidirectionality are the basal ganglia, which are a target of prefrontal cortex but connect back to it only indirectly, via the substantia nigra and thalamus. This arrangement may reflect the role of the basal ganglia in the control of motor output, since it is similar to the pathway pattern between prefrontal cortex and premotor regions (see Chapter 5).

In summary, the broad connectivity of the prefrontal cortex is consistent with the diversity of processes required for adaptive, goal-directed behavior. Understanding how subdivisions of the prefrontal cortex (in conjunction with other brain regions) guide complex behaviors remains a major challenge for cognitive neuroscience.

Consequences of damage to the prefrontal cortex

An individual with damage to the prefrontal cortex—whether from stroke, trauma, surgery, or a degenerative disease—may appear normal when first encountered. Perceptual, language, and motor abilities are usually unimpaired, and the ability to recall events or facts from memory is typically intact. Yet the patient may have profound difficulty carrying out simple activities and may have greatly diminished quality of life. These subtle yet profound deficits suggest that a deeper examination of the functional properties of prefrontal cortex is needed to understand its role in cognition, both normal and disordered.

Broadly considered, prefrontal cortex damage can lead to either of two general syndromes, depending on the affected region. Damage to the lateral prefrontal cortex can lead to the constellation of symptoms called **dysexecutive syndrome** (or **frontal dysexecutive syndrome**). Individuals with this syndrome—like others with frontal lobe damage—do not present with obvious deficits in intelligence. They can use language normally and can remember events and facts. But they have great difficulty managing their daily lives. They fail to plan for the future, rarely initiate new projects or set long-term goals, leave tasks uncompleted if initiated, and have a limited span of attention. They may have difficulty interacting with others, both because of these deficits and because of impairments in understanding the goals and thoughts of others. They show a lack of insight into their own and others' actions. They may even deny the existence of any problem—or create implausible explanations for those problems (i.e., **confabulate**) as their life deteriorates around them. As introduced in the next sections, these difficulties dealing with the real world are accompanied by impairments in specific tasks that can be carried out in a laboratory.

Damage to ventral and medial portions of the frontal lobe, in contrast, gives rise to what has been termed **disinhibition syndrome** (or **frontal disinhibition syndrome**). Patients with this syndrome, like dysexecutive syndrome patients, present with what generally appear to be normal cognitive functions. But unlike dysexecutive syndrome patients, they tend to perform normally on laboratory tests of response selection and working memory. Nonetheless, their lives outside of the laboratory are often chaotic. Patients with disinhibition syndrome often exhibit constant movement not channeled toward productive activities, and they may be euphoric or manic with an abnormal sense of humor. Thus, they may laugh at inappropriate times in simple social situations, fail to respond to normal social cues, or reveal embarrassing personal information. Their outward expressiveness stands in sharp contrast to the quietness and apathy associated with lateral prefrontal damage.

The famous case of Phineas Gage (Figure 13.4) has been historically considered an example of disinhibition syndrome, although recent investigation of Gage's life history suggests a more complex picture. Despite the accident that destroyed much of his ventral frontal lobes, Gage remained employed for most of his remaining life and failed to show some typical personality markers of this type of prefrontal damage (e.g., he was reported to be a good storyteller and could communicate with socially appropriate affect).

The deficits associated with prefrontal damage may seem diverse and disjointed, and different individuals may present with idiosyncratic deficits in some or all of these functions. But these deficits share a common core:

(A)

(B)

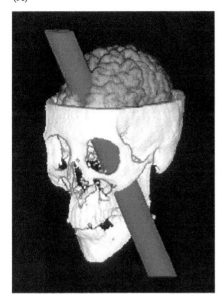

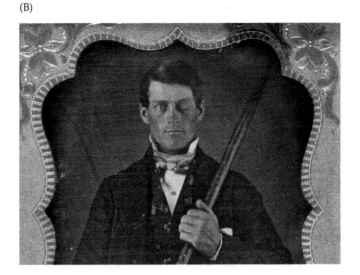

Figure 13.4 **The case of Phineas Gage** In 1848, Phineas Gage was a foreman on the team constructing a new railway in Vermont. While he was tamping down some blasting powder in a hole in the rock, the powder unexpectedly exploded, driving the tamping iron (a metal rod about 2 meters in length and 3 centimeters in diameter) through his left cheek and out the top of his skull. (A) This modern reconstruction based on the damage to Gage's skull illustrates that the most likely path of the rod was through the middle of the frontal lobes, leading to significant damage to the orbitofrontal and medial prefrontal cortex. (B) The traditional narrative about Phineas Gage reports that this damage had dramatic effects on his personality; for instance, he changed from being responsible and conscientious to being profane, reckless, and impulsive. Recent research suggests that this narrative is exaggerated. For example, Gage was hardly itinerant and unproductive; after the accident, he traveled independently to South America and remained employed there for several years. This photograph of Gage after his accident was recently discovered. (A from Damasio et al. 1994; B from Wilgus and Wilgus 2009.)

impairments in the forming, updating, and implementing of rules for appropriate or effective behavior.

Establishing and Modifying Behavioral Rules

No simple division exists between executive functions and a number of other cognitive functions considered in this book. Like attentional and mnemonic functions, executive functions enhance some aspects of neural activity while lessening or suppressing others. These different functions are usually separated, both in the larger literature and, as described in this book, by what sorts of processing they modulate. Modulation of incoming sensory information and perceptual representations (e.g., imagery, mnemonic content) is typically considered within the domain of "attention," for example, whereas executive functions act primarily on rules for behavior.

A useful metaphor for executive function is a switch operator who controls the pattern of tracks in a busy railroad yard. In many circumstances in such a yard, such as when a single train travels along frequently used tracks, no action from the operator is required. But when two trains are on a collision course, the operator must set up a new pattern of tracks to maximize the efficiency and success of what might follow. Cognitive neuroscientists Earl Miller and

Figure 13.5 A conceptual framework for executive functions In the framework advanced by Miller and Cohen, control processes in the prefrontal cortex inhibit or strengthen rules for behavior to fit the current context. Thus, when a person hears a phone ringing, there is a strong tendency (indicated here by the thick connecting lines) to answer it, especially at home. However, this behavior is inappropriate in other contexts, such as at a neighbor's house. The prefrontal cortex is postulated to model the current context and possible actions, so that the necessary action can be potentiated (thick lines) and undesirable actions can be inhibited (dashed lines). In this conception, the prefrontal cortex allows information to flow along some paths but not others to facilitate effective behavior. (After Miller and Cohen 2001.)

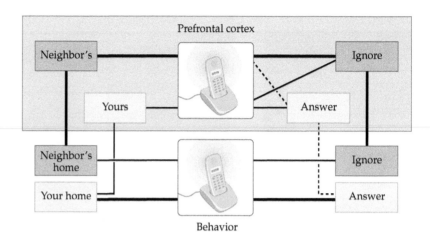

Jonathan Cohen suggested that executive processes in prefrontal cortex, like a railroad switch operator, set up rules for the patterns of information flow in other brain regions, in order to meet immediate demands and achieve future goals (Figure 13.5).

Nothing in this metaphor or in any other description of executive function requires that control be exerted consciously. Consider the simple thermostat. It detects temperature changes in the environment and adjusts the output of heating and cooling systems, in accordance with some simple rules. More complex systems—like those that regulate traffic on highway systems or the movements of trains in modern railroad yards—use very sophisticated algorithms to regulate large numbers of interacting components in changing environments. Such algorithms and the devices they modulate are described by engineers as *control systems*, even though there is no single controller. The following sections introduce three sorts of information processing that are common to a wide range of control systems, conscious or otherwise (see Figure 13.1): initiating new rules for action, inhibiting rules that are no longer valid, and relating rules to support more complex forms of control.

Initiating rules for behavior

Damage to the lateral prefrontal cortex typically impairs the ability of an individual to initiate motor movements, complex actions, and mental plans. Like Hitzig's dogs and Bianchi's monkeys, human patients with lateral prefrontal damage do not readily change their behavior in response to the world around them. Rather, they tend to show little spontaneity of thought or action, even if verbal and motor abilities are spared; and they may withdraw from society, losing contact with friends and family. This reclusiveness is the result of not only blunted affect, but also a loss of interest in maintaining social relationships. Furthermore, when questioned about their abnormal personality and lifestyle, patients with lateral prefrontal damage show little concern. They may know that they should feel sad following the loss of a job or a loved one, but they do not seem to experience the corresponding emotion.

Of course, different individuals may exhibit some but not all of these impairments. For example, motor deficits are characteristic in the clinical condition known as **abulia**, which is characterized by lethargy and quiet withdrawal. Abulia can result from strokes or lesions that damage lateral aspects of the frontal lobes but spare ventral and medial aspects. Patients with this condition can perform movements or answer questions in response to commands, but they act slowly and are easily distracted. They also have difficulty sustaining attention or continuing a motor action for an extended period of time (e.g., following the instruction "Stick out your tongue for 20 seconds"). As in the more general dysexecutive syndrome, patients with abulia are apathetic about the surrounding environment and about their future.

In light of these symptoms of frontal damage related to initiating and following behavioral rules, how might such rules be encoded in the brain? Single-unit electrophysiology in non-human primates has provided evidence that prefrontal cortex neurons carry information about rules in a distributed manner. That is, populations of neurons carry information about different rules, and the relative activity of neurons depends on which rules are relevant to the current context. In one electrophysiological study, monkeys associated sets of cues with particular behavioral rules (**Figure 13.6**). On each trial, a visual stimulus and a cue (e.g., a juice reward or an auditory tone) were presented simultaneously. The cue indicated whether a matching or a nonmatching rule was active on that trial. About 2 seconds later a second stimulus was presented. The monkeys had been trained to respond to the second stimulus if it was consistent with the cued rule or, if it was not consistent, to respond instead to a third stimulus presented immediately afterward. The single-unit recordings showed that neurons in prefrontal cortex responded as if they were selective for particular rules, independent of the cues signaling which rule to follow, as well as the stimuli on which the rules acted.

Figure 13.6 Evidence for rule specificity in prefrontal cortex Monkeys were trained to follow particular rules—either matching rules (A) or nonmatching rules (B)—that varied according to a sensory cue (e.g., a juice reward or a high tone). The experimenters recorded from neurons in the lateral prefrontal cortex. Some neurons exhibited increased activity to particular rules, regardless of which picture was presented as the sample or which cue was used to signify the rule. (C) These graphs plot data from a neuron whose firing rate increased when the cue indicated a match-to-sample trial, but whose firing rate remained low on non-match-to-sample trials. Each line indicates a different rule cue. (After Wallis et al. 2001.)

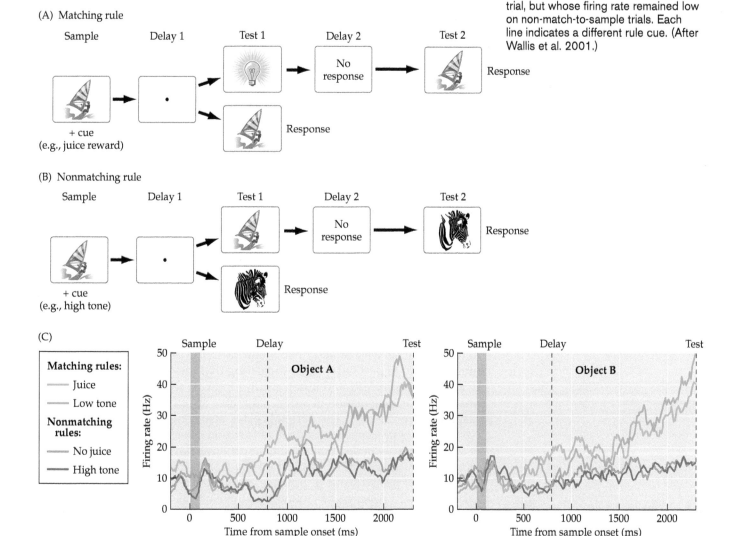

Figure 13.7 **Basal ganglia control of behavior** (A) Inputs to and projections from basal ganglia contribute greatly to motor control. (B,C) Basal ganglia loops in the prefrontal cortex affect nonmotor behavior and support particular forms of cognitive control.

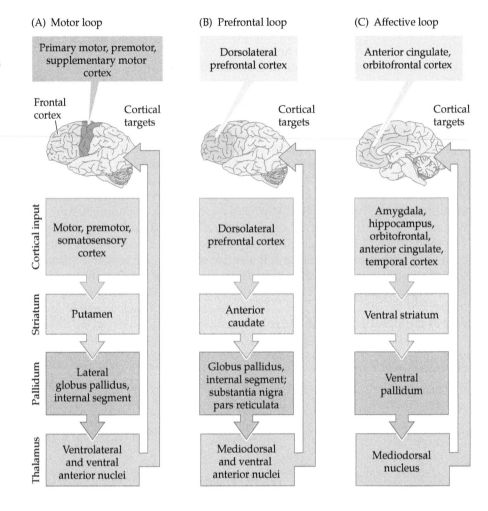

Rule-selective neurons have now been found throughout prefrontal cortex, most prevalently along the principal sulcus in lateral prefrontal cortex. Note, however, that when a rule involves a complex sequence of actions, then a given neuron may code for only part of the rule, such as for a particular action or even for a particular action only when it occurs at one point in a sequence (see Figure 5.18 for an example).

Creating new rules for behavior does not rely on the prefrontal cortex alone. The basal ganglia, for example, interact with prefrontal cortex to support particular forms of cognitive control (Figure 13.7). More specifically, in category learning tasks, subjects must form abstract rules that match categories of stimuli to responses. As we just described, neurons in the prefrontal cortex respond preferentially to particular rules, indicating that they code such abstractions. In contrast, both fMRI and lesion studies indicate that the basal ganglia are important for the creation of rules that map a specific stimulus to a specific response (Figure 13.8). The parietal cortex also contributes to rule creation, particularly with aspects of executive function closely tied to the generation of actions. Studies of decision making in primates have indicated that neurons along the intraparietal sulcus (called the lateral intraparietal area, or LIP) encode the expected value of possible actions related to a potential decision. Likewise, fMRI research has found that the parietal cortex is activated when subjects create and maintain the set of possible actions that might be required in a given situation.

(A)

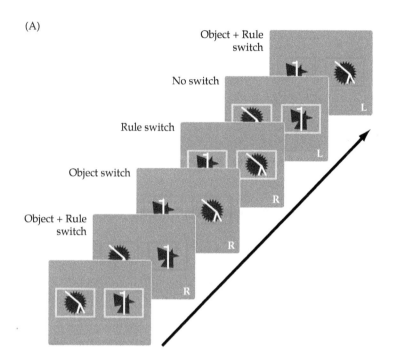

Object + Rule switch

No switch

Rule switch

Object switch

Object + Rule switch

Figure 13.8 Contributions of basal ganglia and prefrontal systems to executive control (**A**) Subjects were shown pairs of complex, difficult-to-name objects, each surrounded by a box. If the boxes were outlined in yellow, the subjects were to choose the same object they chose on the previous trial and hold it in working memory. If the boxes were outlined in blue, subjects were to choose the other object and hold it in working memory instead. Thus, each trial could involve no switch at all; a switch in rule but not object; a switch in object but not rule; or a switch in both object and rule. The correct responses–left (L) or right (R)–are indicated at the lower right of each display. (**B**) Signal change in each switch condition is compared here to trials with no switching at all. The key finding was that the basal ganglia were activated only for object switches and not for rule switches. In contrast, the dorsolateral prefrontal cortex was activated for all types of switches. (After Cools et al. 2004.)

(B)

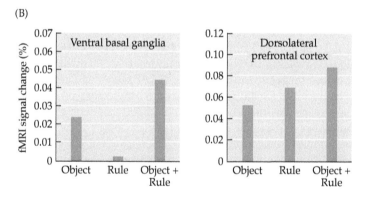

Inhibiting rules for behavior

Inhibition is the suppression of unimportant or distracting information or behavior. Although typically discussed separately, inhibition and initiation are complementary aspects of executive control. In both cases, executive functions change the relative strength of different rules in order to bring about appropriate or effective changes in behavior. There are four primary forms of inhibition: (1) halting behaviors that are well trained or previously valid; (2) preventing irrelevant information from interfering with other processing; (3) restraining actions that are inappropriate in a given social context; and (4) removing irrelevant information from working memory. The first two of these processes are considered in this section; the third is introduced in the following section; and the fourth is discussed later, in the section on working memory.

Studies using ERPs and fMRI have implicated lateral prefrontal cortex in processes of inhibition. For example, in the *oddball task*, subjects attend to a continuous sequence of stimuli, most of which require a standard response (e.g., pressing a button with the left hand) or require no response at all, depending on the variant of the task (**Figure 13.9A**). On a fraction of trials, typically about 5 to 10 percent, a target stimulus appears that requires the selection of a different response (e.g., pressing a button with the right hand) and thus also

(A) Oddball

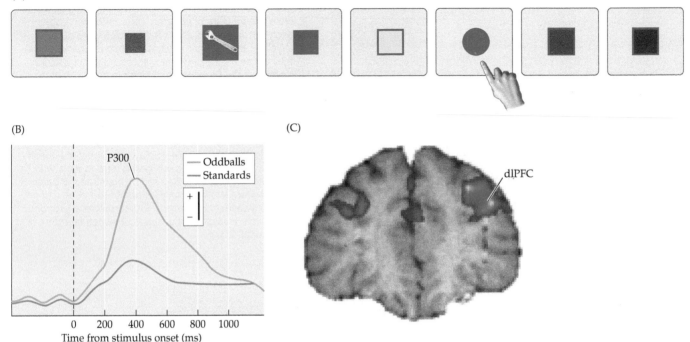

(B)

P300

— Oddballs
— Standards

Time from stimulus onset (ms)

(C)

dlPFC

Figure 13.9 The oddball task
(A) In the visual oddball task, participants watch a stream of rapidly presented standard stimuli (e.g., squares varying in size and color), looking for infrequent target stimuli (e.g., circles). Some versions of the task include distracter stimuli (such as the picture of the wrench in the third stimulus shown here) that occur with the same frequency as the targets but do not require a change in response from the standard stimuli. (B) Compared to the common standards, the oddball targets evoke a positive ERP response known as the P300 that begins around 300 milliseconds. (C) Oddball targets tend to evoke activation in dorsolateral prefrontal cortex (dlPFC). (A from Huettel et al. 2004; B after Polich 2007; C from Huettel and McCarthy 2004.)

requires inhibition of the standard response. Such target oddballs evoke a well-characterized ERP component known as the **P300**, a positive deflection in the scalp-recorded EEG waveform that begins approximately 300 milliseconds following the onset of the target stimulus (Figure 13.9B; see also Chapter 6). Through recording of the EEG signal from electrodes implanted intracranially, both in humans and in non-human animals, the P300 has been shown to arise from a distributed set of generators that include parietal cortex, medial prefrontal cortex, and lateral prefrontal cortex, with concurrent activity also observed in subcortical regions including the hippocampus. As shown first by cognitive neuroscientist Gregory McCarthy and colleagues, oddball stimuli evoke fMRI activation in dorsolateral prefrontal cortex, as well as in the parietal cortex (Figure 13.9C).

The converse of the oddball task is the *go/no-go task*, which requires subjects to respond to most stimuli ("go"), but to inhibit responding to particular infrequently presented stimuli ("no go"). Like the target stimuli in the oddball task, the no-go stimuli evoke activation in the lateral prefrontal and parietal cortices. Some brain disorders are associated with deficits in this form of inhibitory control. In particular, patients with **schizophrenia** perform normally on go trials but are greatly impaired on no-go trials. These behavioral impairments are accompanied by abnormal ERP and fMRI responses, suggesting a frontal lobe deficit in schizophrenia.

In a *stop-signal task*, participants respond to stimuli whenever they are presented but must inhibit those responses if a signal to stop is presented shortly thereafter. Patients with damage to the posterior ventrolateral frontal cortex in the right hemisphere, but not those with damage to other prefrontal regions, have difficulty inhibiting their responses following the signal to stop. Similar problems are observed in patients with impulse control disorders, such as **attention deficit hyperactivity disorder** (**ADHD**). Moreover, deficits in basal ganglia function associated with Parkinson's disease can also lead to difficulty inhibiting behavior in the stop-signal task (and similar tasks), independently of the effects of that disease on generalized motor function. Such results suggest that motor inhibition relies not just on lateral prefrontal cortex, but on circuits that connect lateral prefrontal cortex with the basal ganglia (and likely other brain regions).

Inhibitory processes are also important for preventing task-irrelevant information from interfering with the ongoing performance of a primary task. Patients with lateral prefrontal damage have difficulty in such inhibition of task-irrelevant sensory information. At sensory stages of neural processing, this deficiency is evident as increased amplitude—or disinhibition—of early-latency ERP components generated in the sensory cortices (see Chapter 6 for discussion of how attention modulates activity in these regions). One consequence of sensory disinhibition may be that irrelevant information is not effectively filtered, impairing the ability of prefrontal patients to keep task-relevant information online in the presence of distracting inputs.

The importance of the prefrontal cortex for suppressing distracting information is also apparent in a delayed match-to-sample task. In a typical version of that task, participants hear a single tone, maintain that tone in working memory over a delay of a few seconds, and then indicate whether a second presented tone matched the first. Despite having normal working memory, prefrontal patients make many more errors when the delay includes distracting auditory stimuli than when no distraction is present; that is, they are also more impaired by distraction than are patients with damage in other brain regions.

Inhibiting socially inappropriate behaviors

In social contexts, such as interactions within groups of people in casual conversation, some sorts of behavior are more appropriate than others. Coarse language and physical horseplay might be reasonable when you're interacting with friends from college, but not when you're interacting with a potential employer at a job interview. Interacting successfully with others requires matching one's behavior to the current social context, and most people naturally inhibit behaviors when they are inappropriate.

People with damage to ventral prefrontal cortex often exhibit a generalized failure to match their behavior to typical rules for social interactions. In severe cases, patients with the disinhibition syndrome introduced earlier in this chapter can be argumentative, profane, aggressive, violent, and/or unable to control sexual impulses. Their behavior becomes self-indulgent and directed toward desires of the moment, even as family responsibilities, work demands, and future plans languish. All the while, these patients show a lack of insight. Even when they recognize that their behavior is self-destructive, they seem neither concerned about its consequences nor motivated to seek a solution.

Neurologist Antonio Damasio has called the most severe form of frontal disinhibition syndrome **acquired sociopathy** (i.e., antisocial behavior that arises because of trauma or disease). As in congenital sociopathy, people with acquired sociopathy have blunted emotional affect punctuated by extreme emotional outbursts; make poor decisions, especially in social situations; and have difficulty interacting with others. However, there are differences between acquired and congenital sociopathy. Patients with acquired sociopathy can state the rules for reasonable behavior and can distinguish good actions from bad, even if their impulsivity leads them to select the latter. Similarly, they may feel remorse for their actions, although that remorse may not be followed by behavioral change. Patients with congenital sociopathy, by contrast, have difficulty expressing the reasoning behind social rules, explain moral dilemmas in terms of simple actions and consequences, and rationalize any problematic consequences of their actions (especially the consequences for others). Moreover, their behavior is goal-directed rather than impulsive, and they are rarely remorseful.

One explanation of these differences is that ventromedial prefrontal damage impairs social behavior, but not necessarily the cognitive appreciation of

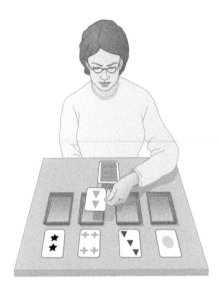

Figure 13.10 The Wisconsin Card Sorting Test This test uses a deck of cards whose faces differ in color, shape, and number of the symbols depicted. On each trial, subjects are given a rule by which they sort each card into one of four piles. The correct rule periodically changes without warning during the course of the experiment, and patients with prefrontal damage are often poor at inhibiting the previously valid rule.

rules for behavior that were established during development with acquired sociopathy. Clinical and neuropsychological studies of young adult patients who have suffered damage to ventromedial prefrontal cortex in infancy are particularly revealing. These patients have troubled histories that include habitual misbehavior, shunning by peers, problems maintaining employment and living independently, risky sexual behavior, and criminal activity. Importantly, such early-damage patients are similar to those with congenital sociopathy in their inability to comprehend social rules (although their impulsivity differs from the goal directedness of those with congenital sociopathy); moreover, they are impaired in moral reasoning tasks, treating social dilemmas in a superficial and self-centered manner.

Shifting among rules for behavior

In many real-world and laboratory settings, goal-directed behavior requires the formation of a set of rules—any one of which might be relevant at a given time—and then shifting among those rules as one's goals change. One widely used task for rule shifting used in the laboratory and in clinical assessment is the **Wisconsin Card Sorting Test** (Figure 13.10). Each card in the deck contains one to four images of a simple shape (e.g., circle, star, triangle, or cross), all of the same color (e.g., black, green, yellow, or blue). The subject's task is to sort the cards into piles according to one of the three stimulus attributes—number, shape, or color. For example, suppose that the first card in the deck has one yellow star. The subject might sort it according to its shape (the star). If feedback reveals that sorting to be incorrect, the participant might try to sort the next card according to its color. Using trial and error, subjects can determine the correct rule and begin to sort the cards correctly. Unbeknownst to the subject, however, after a predetermined number of consecutive correctly sorted cards, the sorting rule changes. Individuals with an intact prefrontal cortex recognize this change fairly quickly and shift their sorting to the new rule.

As first reported by Canadian neuropsychologist Brenda Milner in 1963, patients with prefrontal damage continue to use the previously valid rule, despite receiving negative feedback. This persistence of behavior is known as **perseveration**, which is considered a hallmark of impaired prefrontal function. Perseveration does not simply reflect an inability to follow new behavioral rules; if the previously valid rule is unavailable—for example, if the previous rule was to sort by color and all the cards now share the same color—prefrontal patients learn the new rule at the same rate that neurologically normal individuals do. Thus, perseveration reflects difficulty shifting away from the previous rule that still could be used, even if there is evidence it is no longer valid. Note that adaptive performance on the Wisconsin Card Sorting Test in normal adults is correlated also with measures of inhibition, not just shifting—which shows how a single task can rely on multiple executive functions. Nor is there a one-to-one mapping between prefrontal cortex damage and perseverative behavior. Prefrontal patients make more random errors on the Wisconsin Card Sorting Test (i.e., not using either the previous or current response rules), presumably because of an increased susceptibility to distraction. Furthermore, some studies suggest that damage to other brain regions, including the medial prefrontal cortex and the temporal lobe, can also cause perseverative behavior.

The ventral frontal lobes, especially the orbitofrontal cortex, also facilitate shifting between rules for behavior—particularly in situations involving reward and punishment (see Chapter 14 for evidence from the domain of decision making). The orbitofrontal cortex is heavily interconnected with sensory regions (including primary taste, olfactory, and somatosensory cortices), with regions of the brainstem that track body states, and with object-processing areas in the ventral visual stream. These connections point to the important role of this frontal region for incorporating affective information into plans for behavior (see Chapter 10 for discussion of the **somatic marker hypothesis** for ventral frontal lobe function).

Damage to the orbitofrontal cortex also causes impairments in learning the relationship of stimuli and rewards. This kind of deficit is particularly apparent in **reversal learning** tasks. Animals with orbitofrontal lesions learn stimulus-reward contingencies (e.g., a bright light predicts food, whereas a dim light predicts no food) about as well as control animals do. But when the rule mapping stimuli to rewards is unexpectedly switched (e.g., a dim light now predicts food), the lesioned animals are slower to learn the new relationships. Neuroimaging studies have also found that orbitofrontal cortex is activated when neurologically normal subjects switch to a new stimulus-reward contingency. Conversely, patients with damage to orbitofrontal cortex are impaired in reversal learning tasks, frequently switching their responses following large rewards, while not switching responses following losses.

Although some patients with lateral prefrontal damage show deficits in reversal learning, those problems seem to be associated with failures to remain engaged in the task (consistent with dysexecutive syndrome), rather than problems with learning about rewards. As long as lateral prefrontal patients attend to the reward feedback, performance is normal. The impairment in reversal learning is reminiscent of the perseverative behavior seen in the Wisconsin Card Sorting Test. In both cases, prefrontal damage leads to an inability to recognize a context change, and thereby to the inappropriate persistence of a previously relevant behavior.

Relating rules to create higher-order models of the world

The ability to create complex mental models of the world has long been championed as a fundamental feature of human cognition (**Box 13B**). German neuropsychologist Kurt Goldstein, writing with Martin Scheerer, argued in the early twentieth century that the inability to create higher-order abstract representations is a core feature of frontal lobe damage:

> What [frontal damage] affects and modifies is the *way of manipulating and operating with ideas and thoughts*. Thoughts do, however, arise but can become effective only in a concrete way. Just as the patient cannot deal with outer world objects in an abstract manner, he has to deal with ideas simply as "things" … This lack of abstract frame of reference holds also for the patient's inner experiences; it manifests itself in his inability to arouse and organize, to direct and hold in check ideas or feelings by conscious volition.
>
> K. GOLDSTEIN AND M. SCHEERER 1941 (emphasis in original)

The force of this argument is apparent when considering specific examples of frontal lobe damage. For example, Goldstein describes a patient who is asked simply to repeat the phrase "the snow is black." The patient tells the interviewer that he cannot repeat that phrase, because it is untrue. Only after the experimenter explains that phrases can be spoken even if false does the patient repeat the phrase—but immediately thereafter disclaiming, "No, the snow is white." The same patient would not repeat the phrase "the sun is shining" when the sun was hidden behind clouds. More generally, when presented with pictures that tell a story, patients with prefrontal lesions are often unable to integrate the pictures into a coherent narrative. They also give literal responses when asked to interpret simple proverbs. For instance, when given the proverb "People who live in glass houses should not throw stones," one frontal lobe patient explained the sense of the metaphor to be: "Otherwise they will break the walls around them."

■ BOX 13B THE NEUROBIOLOGY OF INTELLIGENCE

The questions of how to measure and explain differences in intelligence have a long and controversial history. Some conceptions suggest that intelligence reflects the ability to reason and solve problems. The great thinkers of the ages, such as Leonardo da Vinci and Benjamin Franklin, are thus considered to have possessed very great intelligence. Other perspectives extend intelligence to include more specific cognitive abilities (like vocabulary, mathematical skills, and memory), artistic talent, emotional and empathic traits, or even athletic excellence. From these broader perspectives, a talented pianist or a world-famous painter or even a champion basketball player might be considered intelligent. In all of these domains, from art to sports, outstanding individuals are described by terms, such as *brilliant* or *gifted*, that are often synonyms for *intelligent*.

Given the breadth of ways in which behavioral and intellectual competence can be expressed, it seems an impossible task to characterize intelligence using a single measure. Even so, intelligence testing has a long history, whose best-known example is the IQ test developed by French psychologist Alfred Binet in the early twentieth century. This test and its descendants ask a broad set of questions that tap reasoning, logic, math, vocabulary, and general knowledge, resulting in an intelligence quotient, or IQ. The specific interpretation of an IQ score depends on the test that is used; in a typical scaling system, a mean score would be 100 with a standard deviation of 15 points.

Even though IQ scores seem authoritative, a person with an IQ of 130 may not necessarily be better at any particular task requiring intelligence than is someone else with an IQ of 120. One contemporary of Binet, English psychologist Charles Spearman, recognized that there were still individual differences in specific contributors to intelligence. Some people may have very strong verbal aptitude but poor math skills; others may have exceptional spatial skills but poor memory. Nevertheless, Spearman believed strongly in the existence of a central intelligence factor (which he labeled "g," for *general ability*). Although considerable disagreement

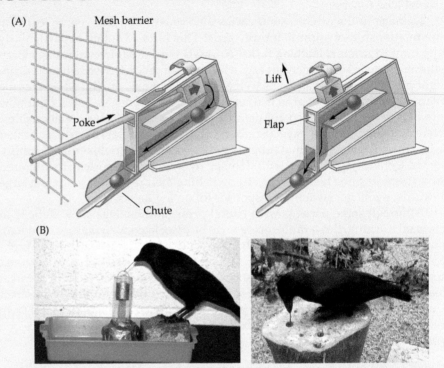

(A) Dominant female chimpanzees were taught to obtain food from a complex apparatus like the ones shown here either by poking a stick through a hole (left) or by lifting a hook (right) to dislodge a barrier and get a food pellet. When a trained female returned to her group, the other chimpanzees observed her operating the apparatus and successfully mimicked her method for obtaining the food. (B) New Caledonian crows spontaneously shape natural materials (or wires, in the laboratory) into hooks that can be used to extract food. Brain changes associated with the development of intelligence.

about the specific constituent factors remains, there is now broad recognition that intelligence comprises at least several separate components (e.g., verbal abilities, mathematical abilities) that tend to be partially correlated across individuals.

The features of the human brain that correspond to intelligence have been equally contentious. Humans and other primates have large brains, modern adult humans have larger brains than our evolutionary ancestors had, and genes that control brain size are still evolving rapidly. Yet brain size does not predict intelligence among individuals; for example, males have larger brains than females, even though the average intelligence of males and females is essentially identical. Nor does brain size predict intel-

ligence across species (see Chapter 15), as demonstrated by examples of intelligent behavior both in species that have a brain structure similar to our own (chimpanzees; Figure A) and in species with a brain structure that is not like ours (crows; Figure B).

What seem to matter more for intelligence are the relative size of the brain compared to the rest of the body and specific differences within the parts of the brain that organize complex behaviors. Unlike other mammals, humans and great apes have large frontal lobes (see Box 13A); the executive and other functions of these brain regions fit nicely with the idea that the frontal lobes are especially (although certainly not uniquely) important in mediating intelligence. Converging

■ BOX 13B *(continued)*

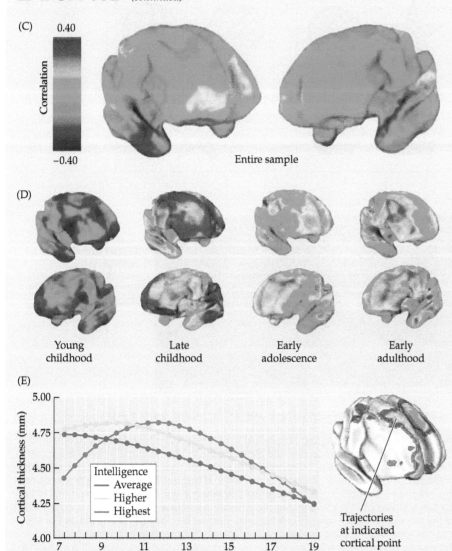

to assess whether IQ scores could be predicted from the thickness of the cerebral cortex in particular brain regions. Taking the entire age range as a whole, intelligence was only weakly related to the thickness of any particular brain region (Figure C). In specific age ranges, however, strong patterns were evident (Figure D). For example, the children who eventually became the most intelligent tended to show a rapid increase in cortical thickness until early adolescence (11 to 12 years of age), particularly in the prefrontal cortex, followed by a rapid thinning thereafter (Figure E). This result suggests that adult intelligence is not simply a function of the size of the frontal lobes, but of the specific aspects of development of the frontal lobes and the rest of the brain, perhaps reflecting how synaptic connectivity is modulated by experience.

References

EVANS, P. D. AND 8 OTHERS (2005) Microcephalin, a gene regulating brain size, continues to evolve adaptively in humans. *Science* 309: 1717–1720.

GRAY, J. R., C. F. CHABRIS AND T. S. BRAVER (2003) Neural mechanisms of general fluid intelligence. *Nat. Neurosci.* 6: 316–322.

KENWARD, B., A. A. WEIR, C. RUTZ AND A. KACELNIK (2005) Behavioural ecology: Tool manufacture by naive juvenile crows. *Nature* 433: 121.

LEE, K. H. AND 6 OTHERS (2006) Neural correlates of superior intelligence: Stronger recruitment of posterior parietal cortex. *Neuroimage* 29: 578–586.

SHAW, P. AND 8 OTHERS (2006) Intellectual ability and cortical development in children and adolescents. *Nature* 440: 676–679.

THOMPSON, P. M. AND 12 OTHERS (2001) Genetic influences on brain structure. *Nat. Neurosci.* 4: 1253–1258.

WEIR, A. A., J. CHAPPELL AND A. KACELNIK (2002) Shaping of hooks in New Caledonian crows. *Science* 297: 981.

WHITEN, A., V. HORNER AND F. B. DE WAAL (2005) Conformity to cultural norms of tool use in chimpanzees. *Nature* 437: 737–740.

(C) The color map indicates the strength of the correlation between the thickness of the cortex in a particular brain region and intelligence in children and adolescents. Note that few regions exhibited significant correlations across the age range. (D) More revealing were the correlations at specific age points, with young children of the highest intelligence having thinner cortices overall, and the adolescents of the highest intelligence having relatively thick prefrontal cortices. (E) The individuals of the highest intelligence exhibited a relatively late thickening and subsequent thinning of prefrontal cortex. (C–E after Shaw et al. 2006.)

evidence comes from fMRI studies that have found links between general intelligence (i.e., Spearman's "g") and differences in activation of the frontal and parietal cortices during reasoning tasks.

Variations in how the brain matures may also predict differences in intelligence across individuals. A developmental study scanned a large sample of children, adolescents, and young adults

(A) Relational ("change")   (B) Control ("texture")

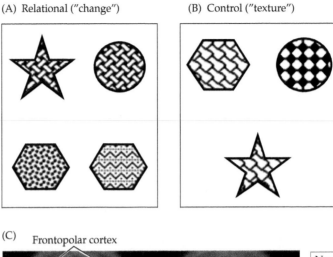

(C)   Frontopolar cortex

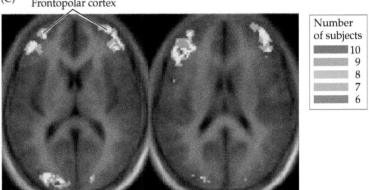

Number of subjects	
	10
	9
	8
	7
	6

Figure 13.11 Frontopolar cortex supports the higher-order integration of rules Participants in an fMRI experiment made a series of judgments about simple stimuli that varied in shape and texture. (A) In the relational condition, participants had to determine whether the top pair and the bottom pair of objects differed on the same dimension. Shown here is a "mismatch" trial, since the two objects in the top pair differ in shape but the objects in the bottom pair differ in texture. To perform this task requires the integration of two lower-level judgments to reach a higher-order judgment. (B) In the control condition, the participant judged whether a stimulus at the bottom matched either of the top stimuli on the specified dimension. Shown is a "match" trial because the star and hexagon share the same texture. (C) Significantly greater activation was found in frontopolar cortex in the relational condition compared to the control condition, and this activation was highly consistent across task participants. (After Smith et al. 2007.)

The ability to relate simple rules forms the basis of classic tests for deficits in frontal lobe function. In the Raven's Progressive Matrices test, subjects view a matrix of shapes that progress along one or more dimensions (e.g., a three-by-three matrix with one dot in each cell of the left column, two dots in the cells of the middle column, and three dots in the cells of the right column). The subject's task is to identify the shape that best completes a pattern by filling in a blank cell. Depending on the complexity of the matrix, the task may require only simple logic or it may require complex relational and integrative processes. Patients with damage to frontopolar cortex, in particular, exhibit greatly reduced performance when solving complex patterns, although they often show normal performance when dealing with simpler patterns. Converging data come from fMRI studies demonstrating that frontopolar activation is observed when abstract information from different sources must be integrated to form a more general rule (Figure 13.11).

(A)

(B)

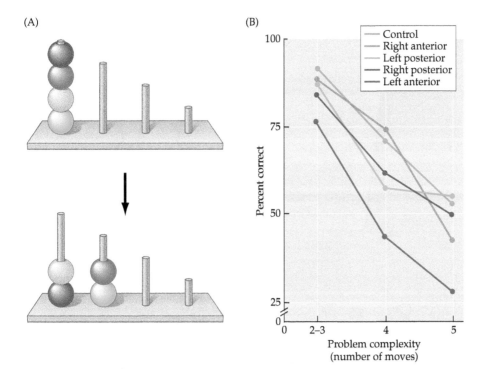

Figure 13.12 Testing executive function with the Tower of London puzzle (A) In this puzzle, subjects must mentally determine the fewest number of moves required to transform one arrangement of colored elements (e.g., all stacked on one of a set of posts, as above) to a different arrangement (below). (B) Patients with damage to the left anterior frontal lobe perform much more poorly at this task than normal subjects do, especially when the puzzles are more complex. (After Shallice 1982.)

Simulation deficits are also evident in tasks that require planning or processing the future consequences of actions. Commonly used to test this aspect of executive function are the Tower of London and Tower of Hanoi manipulation puzzles (Figure 13.12). In these puzzles, subjects view a starting configuration of balls stacked on rods and must move one ball at a time to reach a goal configuration. To solve the puzzle efficiently, the subject must simulate the consequences of a series of moves: "If I move the red ball to the right pole, then I will be able to move the blue ball to the center pole. That will free up the yellow ball. ..." Patients with prefrontal damage—especially of the left hemisphere—have difficulty with these puzzles, reflecting their deficits in planning into the future and reasoning (Box 13C).

Furthermore, frontopolar cortex may be critical for implementing higher-order goals. In real-world behavior, organisms often must balance two types of goals. Reward-seeking (*exploitative*) goals involve choosing the actions that will lead to the greatest immediate reward, given what is already known about the environment. Information-seeking (*exploratory*) goals involve taking actions that will provide new information about the environment, often at the expense of short-term rewards. When people engage in exploratory behavior to gain new information, activation of the frontopolar cortex and the intraparietal sulcus increases; in contrast, when people choose to receive a sure reward, activation of key subcortical reward-related regions increases (see Chapter 14). Taken together with prior studies, this finding indicates that frontopolar cortex contributes to longer-term and higher-order goals—a conclusion echoed in the hierarchical models introduced next.

Hierarchical models for executive function

The research described so far indicates that the lateral prefrontal cortex makes critical contributions to several executive functions. Left unanswered are questions about the larger functional organization of prefrontal cortex: In what ways do different subregions contribute to distinct executive functions, and are those different functional roles organized into any sort of topography? Neurologists

■ BOX 13C **REASONING**

More than any other abilities, reasoning and problem solving embody what are commonly called thinking and intelligence. Indeed, the capacity to reason is often considered the essence of humanity—a point made most famously by René Descartes' dictum "I think, therefore I am." The fact that reasoning and problem-solving skills are central to the cognition of *Homo sapiens* is clear, although similar abilities—albeit not so well developed—are apparent in non-human primates and in some other mammals and birds. Understanding the mechanisms that underlie reasoning and problem solving remains an extraordinary challenge for cognitive neuroscience.

The simplest case of reasoning involves argument from premises to conclusions; an example is Aristotle's syllogism "All men are mortal. Socrates is a man. Therefore, Socrates is mortal." This sort of progression in thinking is known as deductive reasoning because the truth of a given conclusion must be deduced solely from a set of premises that is already in hand. Like other executive processes, deductive reasoning requires functionally intact frontal lobes, with the lateral prefrontal cortex appearing to be the most critical brain region. Studies of split-brain patients by cognitive neuroscientist Michael Gazzaniga and colleagues have led to the idea of a left-brain interpreter that can form inferences and associations among multiple concepts (Figure A). Interestingly, patients with damage to the left frontal lobe perform similarly to control subjects in some reasoning tasks, but unlike controls, their performance does not improve when social information is present. Although the bulk of the evidence indicates that deductive reasoning is a primarily left-hemisphere ability, some neuroimaging data suggest that deduction may also involve right-hemisphere

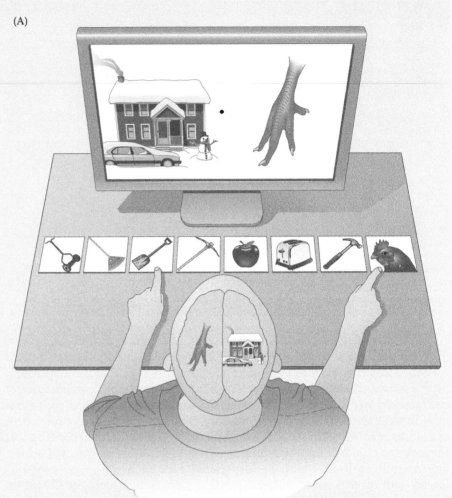

(A)

(A) Evidence for the left-brain interpreter. In patient P.S., most of the corpus callosum had previously been severed, so visual information could not travel between the two hemispheres. Compound images such as the one shown were flashed briefly while he looked at the center of the screen (black dot). Thus, each half of the image was processed within the contralateral hemisphere. When asked to explain why his left hand pointed to a picture that seemed unrelated to his verbal report, the patient's left hemisphere created a plausible, albeit inaccurate, story about shoveling the chicken coop. (A after Gazzaniga and LeDoux 1978.)

have long recognized that more posterior regions in the frontal lobes are related more closely to motor behavior, while more anterior regions of the frontal lobes support processes related to reasoning and mental simulation. Furthermore, the posterior frontal regions mature relatively early during human development and share more similarities with our evolutionary relatives, whereas the anterior regions like the frontopolar cortex develop late in both the ontogenetic and phylogenetic senses.

A natural speculation, therefore, is that there is a rostral-caudal organization of the frontal lobes according to increasing abstraction of executive functions, such that posterior regions support simple functions associated with matching

■ **BOX 13C** *(continued)*

(B)

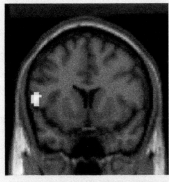

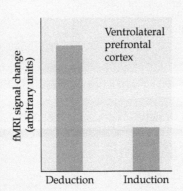

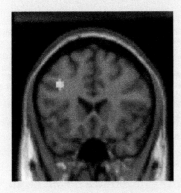

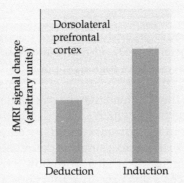

(B) Prefrontal activation during deduction and induction tasks. Although both inductive and deductive reasoning involve the left prefrontal cortex, deduction evokes greater activation in an ventrolateral region (top), and induction evokes greater activation in a dorsolateral region (bottom). (B after Goel and Dolan 2004.)

critical for inductive reasoning (but not needed for deductive reasoning). Neuro-imaging studies show that deduction and induction both activate the left prefrontal cortex, although the specific foci of activation differ. In particular, when directly compared in an experiment undertaken by cognitive neuroscientists Vinod Goel and Raymond Dolan, induction activated dorsolateral prefrontal cortex, and deduction activated ventrolateral prefrontal cortex (Figure B). This difference may reflect greater demands for generating and testing hypotheses during induction, but greater syntactic and linguistic demands during deduction.

References

CRONE, E. A., C. WENDELKEN, L. VAN LEI-JENHORST, R. D. HONOMICHL, K. CHRISTOFF AND S. A. BUNGE (2009) Neurocognitive development of relational reasoning. *Dev. Sci.* 12: 55–66.

FANGMEIER, T., M. KNAUFF, C. C. RUFF AND V. SLOUTSKY (2006) fMRI evidence for a three-stage model of deductive reasoning. *J. Cogn. Neurosci.* 18: 320–334.

GAZZANIGA, M. S. AND J. E. LEDOUX (1978) *The Integrated Mind.* New York: Plenum.

GOEL, V. AND R. J. DOLAN (2004) Differential involvement of left prefrontal cortex in inductive and deductive reasoning. *Cognition* 93: B109–B121.

regions that are anatomically homologous to Broca's area. The conditions under which right-hemisphere activation is observed are not yet well established and may depend on the type of deduction being performed.

However, few challenges of daily life require deduction (adherence to laws and taboos is the best example). Much more common is inductive reasoning, in which one determines the likely truth of a conclusion from a set of probabilistic, often imperfect premises: "House cats purr when they are happy. Lions are related to house cats. Therefore, lions purr when they are happy." The left lateral prefrontal cortex is particularly important for the generation of new hypotheses, which is

behavior to stimuli, whereas anterior regions support complex functions related to higher-order behavioral goals (Figure 13.13).

Two main theories have been proposed. The first theory, championed by cognitive neuroscientist Etienne Koechlin, argues that executive functions are organized according to their level of temporal abstraction. Specifically, executive functions that implement rules about the current time with respect to a particular circumstance are represented in posterior regions like premotor cortex; functions that implement rules about how changes in behavior associate with changing contexts are supported by middle regions; and functions pertaining to long-term goals for behavior are associated with the most anterior regions.

Figure 13.13 Evidence for a topographical organization in lateral prefrontal cortex Across a number of studies, growing evidence suggests that posterior regions support relatively simple forms of rule processing (e.g., selecting an action in response to a stimulus), whereas anterior regions support more complex associations (e.g., higher-order rules, tracking of goals and subgoals). Shown here are the key regions included in one model for lateral prefrontal cortex, along with examples of the types of processes that have been linked to each region. PFC, prefrontal cortex. (After Badre and D'Esposito 2009.)

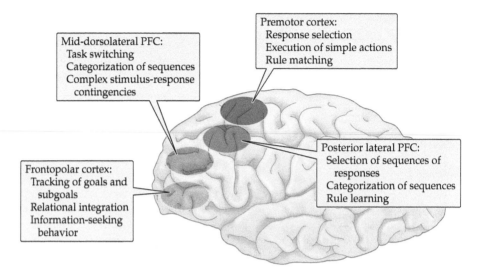

Mid-dorsolateral PFC:
Task switching
Categorization of sequences
Complex stimulus-response
contingencies

Premotor cortex:
Response selection
Execution of simple actions
Rule matching

Frontopolar cortex:
Tracking of goals and
subgoals
Relational integration
Information-seeking
behavior

Posterior lateral PFC:
Selection of sequences of
responses
Categorization of sequences
Rule learning

An alternative organization, called policy abstraction, is advocated by cognitive neuroscientists David Badre and Mark D'Esposito. Like Koechlin, they recognize that posterior regions support the formation and execution of simple rules linking stimuli to behavior (e.g., "Press the button when you see a red square"). But they contend that the more anterior regions support higher-order policies for behavior, which are needed to determine which of several simple rules applies in the current context. By embedding several levels of increasingly complex rules into a single experiment—from simple stimulus-response mapping to metarules that govern how a task should be approached—their research suggests that executive functions are organized in a hierarchy, such that more complex processing of the anterior regions shapes the functioning of the posterior regions.

Other complementary organizations of executive functions remain possible. The regions shown in Figure 13.13 are relatively dorsal, running roughly along the middle frontal gyrus. Some researchers have postulated that more ventral regions along the inferior frontal gyrus also contribute to a range of executive functions, but with a different topographical organization. Still other research is investigating dorsal-ventral differences within the frontal lobes based on stimulus domain or other nonexecutive factors. How regions outside of prefrontal cortex fit into these hierarchical models within prefrontal cortex is also an important area of ongoing study. For at least some sorts of rules (e.g., cues for spatial locations, or numerical rules), evidence from single-unit recordings indicates that neurons within the parietal cortex show selectivity for simple stimulus-action rules similar to that of prefrontal cortex neurons.

Control: Matching Behavior to Context

A general question about executive function is what triggers the brain to engage particular processes. For example, what determines whether the current stimulus-response rules are sufficient to achieve a goal, or whether new rules are needed? Executive functions carry a cost. Attempting to engage an executive function consciously (i.e., to think about the rules underlying one's behavior) can slow down or disrupt automatic processing—a problem familiar to athletes, musicians, or other skilled performers. For executive functions to be implemented effectively, the brain must spend resources to monitor the success of behavioral actions and resolve conflicts between actions that might be taken; thus, it is important to allocate these resources efficiently. Adopting the term from engineering, cognitive neuroscientists often label processes related to monitoring and conflict resolution as *control systems*.

Conflict monitoring

An early perspective on behavioral control was introduced in 1990 by Michael Posner and Steven Petersen (see Chapter 7 for its relationship to attention). They hypothesized the existence of three general systems: one for maintaining alertness/vigilance, one for orienting to sensory stimuli, and one for detecting and identifying events that require additional resources for their processing. The last of these functions, which came to be called conflict monitoring, was postulated to depend on the anterior cingulate gyrus in the midline frontal lobe. Evidence in support of this conjecture came from PET and fMRI studies showing that activation in the anterior cingulate gyrus increased under conditions of high conflict between responses. Response conflict arises when information that points to an incorrect response is available earlier than or simultaneously with information indicating the correct response. The Stroop task is a good example of a paradigm that generates such conflicts (**Figure 13.14A**). Because reading words is so much faster than naming ink colors, the irrelevant color words automatically evoke rules for responding that can interfere with production of the correct ink name.

Over the past decade, numerous functional neuroimaging studies using the Stroop task, as well as other paradigms, have implicated regions within the dorsomedial prefrontal cortex in monitoring and allocating resources for cognitive control. For example, activation of the anterior cingulate cortex (**Figure 13.14B**) during a Stroop task is greater when the ink color mismatches the color name (incongruent trials), compared to when the ink and name refer to the same color (congruent trials). Furthermore, this activation (and the associated slowing in response time) is greater when the previous trial is a congruent trial rather than an incongruent trial, supporting the idea of a conflict monitoring process rather than behavioral selection. Increased activation in the anterior cingulate cortex on one trial results in increased activation in the dorsolateral

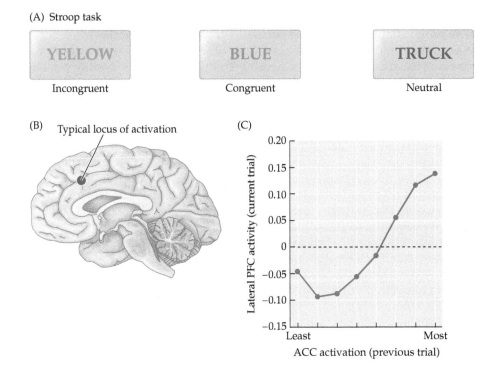

(A) Stroop task

YELLOW — Incongruent

BLUE — Congruent

TRUCK — Neutral

(B) Typical locus of activation

(C)

Lateral PFC activity (current trial) vs. ACC activation (previous trial) — Least to Most

Figure 13.14 The anterior cingulate cortex exhibits increased activation when a stimulus evokes conflicting responses (A) The Stroop task. Subjects are able to read color words very quickly, and the color of ink in which those words are printed has little effect on the speed of reading those words (or pressing a button indicating the color name). But when asked to name the color of the ink in which the word is printed (or press a button indicating the ink color), subjects are slower when the ink color is incongruent with the printed word than when the ink color is congruent or the word is neutral. (B) Neuroimaging studies that use Stroop tasks show increased activation in the anterior cingulate gyrus on incongruent trials. (C) When activation in the anterior cingulate cortex (ACC) is high on one trial, activation in the lateral prefrontal cortex (PFC) increases on the next trial. (B after Bush et al. 1998; C after Kerns et al. 2004.)

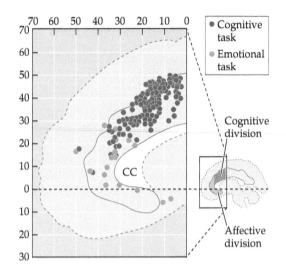

Figure 13.15 **Executive processing in the dorsal anterior cingulate gyrus** Meta-analysis shows that the dorsal part of the anterior cingulate gyrus responds to cognitive control demands, while more ventral regions support emotional processing. Numbers along the axes represent the distance, in millimeters, from the origin of a stereotactic space centered on the anterior commissure. CC, corpus callosum. (After Bush et al. 2000.)

prefrontal cortex on the next trial (Figure 13.14C); this finding supports the idea that control processing in cingulate cortex shapes rule application in dorsolateral prefrontal cortex. Converging data from many neuroimaging studies indicates that executive processes tend to evoke activation in the dorsal part of the anterior cingulate gyrus and other dorsomedial regions, whereas affective processes tend to evoke activation in more anterior and ventral parts of the anterior cingulate gyrus (Figure 13.15).

Electrophysiological recordings have provided further evidence for the role of the anterior cingulate cortex in monitoring behavior, notably in the processing of feedback. The **error-related negativity** (**ERN**) is a negative-polarity scalp electrical potential that follows either of two sorts of mistaken actions: a motor movement that a participant realizes is incorrect (response ERN) or feedback indicating that an action did not result in a desired outcome (feedback ERN). A similar electrophysiological response is evoked following feedback about a monetary loss in a gambling paradigm (see Figure 14.8). The amplitude of this potential is positively correlated with response time on the subsequent trial, suggesting that it is associated with the engagement of control processes. Source localization of the ERP data led to the speculation that the error signal arises from activity in the anterior cingulate gyrus—an idea later supported by fMRI. More recent work using MEG, however, suggests that the posterior cingulate cortex may also contribute to the ERN.

Challenges to the conflict-monitoring model

Although the idea that neurons within the anterior cingulate gyrus support the monitoring and resolution of conflict has substantial support, recent studies have raised challenges. One open question is what sort of monitoring occurs. Whereas activation in this region is typically observed when two potential rules for behavior are in conflict (e.g., naming an ink color versus reading a color word), activation has also been observed to feed back about correct responses or other rewarding outcomes. Conflict monitoring might also occur at processing stages earlier than the one underlying the response itself. Thus, the medial prefrontal cortex may monitor forms of conflict at stages of processing other than response generation.

Another question is whether the increased activation on error trials has to do with errors themselves or with another process. Neuroimaging data indicate that when subjects are allowed to choose whether to guess on a trial of a visual search task, dorsomedial prefrontal activation is greatest when the subjects choose not to guess, but it does not differentiate between correct and error trials. This observation suggests that, when cognitive control processes are dissociated from error monitoring, this region supports the avoidance of mistakes, not necessarily the detection of errors.

Data from electrophysiological and lesion studies have also been difficult to reconcile with a conflict-monitoring explanation. When monkeys are trained to perform a stop-signal task of the sort described earlier in the chapter, the activity of cingulate gyrus neurons does not increase when the animals must stop a previously initiated movement (i.e., the condition in which maximal

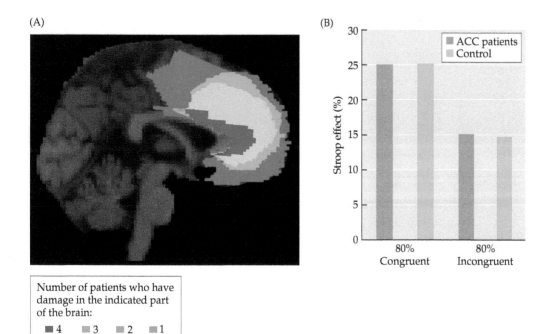

(A)

(B)

Number of patients who have damage in the indicated part of the brain:

■ 4   ■ 3   ■ 2   ■ 1

Figure 13.16   Evidence against the idea that the anterior cingulate gyrus is necessary for conflict monitoring The information here is based on a study of patients with damage to the anterior cingulate gyrus. (A) Color maps indicate the areas of lesion overlap. All patients had damage to the dorsal aspect of the cingulate cortex. (B) Although patients responded more slowly than neurologically normal control subjects, the magnitude of the Stroop effect (incongruent > congruent) was similar. This similarity was present in both congruent and incongruent trials. These results suggest that an intact anterior cingulate gyrus is not necessary for normal interference effects in the Stroop task, at least under the conditions tested. (After Fellows and Farah 2005.)

response conflict would be expected), even though fMRI activation is observed in such tasks. Another paradigm used cue-induced conflict: a cue that signaled whether to move the eyes to the left or right was sometimes presented on the same side of the display as the cued direction (low conflict) or on the opposite side of the display (high conflict). Again, no conflict-related signals were observed in neurons within the anterior cingulate gyrus. Likewise, patients with damage to the dorsal anterior cingulate gyrus (Figure 13.16) perform normally on tasks involving response conflict, despite having significant damage to the region that is most frequently activated in neuroimaging studies of conflict. These patients have normal conflict-related adjustments of performance in both the Stroop and the go/no-go tasks. Similarly, in a study of macaque monkeys, lesions to the cingulate cortex did not influence their abilities to detect errors or to modify their behavior in response to those errors. Instead, the monkeys had difficulty learning the optimal behaviors in response to a series of rewards.

More recent work recasts the dorsomedial prefrontal cortex activation as involving a mismatch between new information and expectations. For example, when performing simple psychological laboratory tasks (e.g., the Stroop paradigm), participants typically expect to respond accurately to each stimulus; when errors occur, activity can be observed in dorsomedial prefrontal cortex using any of a number of cognitive neuroscience methods. That activity, it is argued, can serve as a learning signal that changes predictions about the task, such as one's estimates about which stimulus might occur next or how much executive control is required to perform at an acceptable level. Notably, signals about unexpected mistakes or negative outcomes should generally be stronger

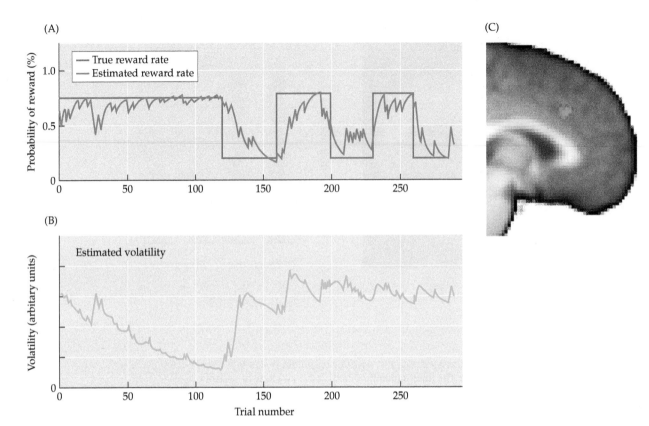

Figure 13.17 Activation in the dorsomedial prefrontal cortex tracks the volatility of the current environment Participants played a simple game in which they guessed which of two options—a blue box or a green box—would be followed by a monetary reward. (A) Over the first 120 trials of the experiment, the probability of reward was kept constant at 75 percent for the blue box and 25 percent for the green box. Then, over the next 170 trials, the reward probabilities (i.e., which item was most likely to lead to a reward) flipped back and forth between the two options, in blocks of about 30 trials. Shown are the true reward rate and the reward rate that would be estimated by a statistical algorithm that only monitored the reward outcomes. (B) The statistical algorithm also estimated the "volatility" of the environment. Low volatility means that the rules for reward are likely to be stable; high volatility means that the rules for reward are thought to be changing over time. (C) Activation in a region within dorsomedial prefrontal cortex was found to track the volatility in the decision environment, during the phase of the trial when participants were monitoring outcomes. (After Behrens et al. 2007.)

than signals about expected mistakes or positive outcomes, because the former are more important for future learning. This perspective can explain reward-learning tasks in which the dorsomedial prefrontal cortex exhibits increased activation under conditions of environmental **volatility**—that is, when the rules relating actions to outcomes are not stable over time (Figure 13.17).

Functional organization of dorsomedial prefrontal cortex

Whereas much effort has been expended in differentiating subregions within lateral prefrontal cortex, less research has focused on functional divisions in dorsomedial prefrontal cortex. An early review by cognitive neuroscientist Richard Ridderinkhof and colleagues showed that a variety of cognitive control processes were intercalated throughout dorsomedial prefrontal cortex, with no apparent organization. Evidence obtained in recent years indicates that particular subregions within dorsomedial prefrontal cortex may support distinct executive functions. An intriguing study by cognitive neuroscientists

Jean-Baptiste Pochon, Jonathan Cohen, and their colleagues demonstrated that a region along the cingulate sulcus showed increased activation in response to difficult judgments—specifically, which of two similar faces was more attractive—even when the task elicited no response conflict. This result suggests that this region may be important in resolving conflict at higher levels (i.e., "decision conflict") as opposed to competing motor actions.

Other studies have shown that increasingly complex sorts of control processes evoke activation in progressively more anterior regions within dorsomedial prefrontal cortex (Figure 13.18). Specifically, the incompatibility between potential responses (i.e., response-related control) evokes fMRI activation in the most posterior region, the difficulty of choosing between two options (i.e., decision-related control) evokes activation in a middle region, and deviations from an ongoing decision strategy in order to adopt a new decision strategy (i.e., strategy-related control) evoke activation in the most anterior region. Supporting this rough topography, a meta-analysis of work on the medial prefrontal cortex revealed a similar pattern: activation associated with decision-related control processes was systematically more anterior than that associated with response-related control processes. (The contributions of dorsomedial prefrontal cortex to higher-level decision making are revisited in Chapter 14.)

The topographical posterior-to-anterior gradient shown in Figure 13.18 has many similarities to that postulated for the lateral surface of the prefrontal cortex (see Figure 13.13). In both cases, relatively posterior regions support executive functions associated with selecting the appropriate motor action for a given behavioral context, while more anterior regions support functions related to implementing and modifying higher-order, abstract goals. A natural question is how the medial and lateral prefrontal cortices interact during executive functioning. Recent work on the connectivity between these brain regions provides converging evidence for such interrelations. Specifically, the more anterior regions of medial prefrontal cortex are preferentially connected to anterior but not posterior parts of lateral prefrontal cortex, as shown by fiber tracing in monkeys and diffusion tensor imaging in humans. A similar pattern has been demonstrated using fMRI functional connectivity both

Figure 13.18 Evidence for a topographical organization in dorsomedial prefrontal cortex (A) Participants in an fMRI experiment completed three different tasks with different control demands: a response-conflict task requiring inhibition of a potentiated motor response, a decision-conflict task comparing more difficult and less difficult decisions, and a strategy-conflict task involving occasional inhibition of a more common strategy for making a complex decision. Within dorsomedial prefrontal cortex, these three types of control evoked activation along a posterior-to-anterior gradient organized from least to most abstract. Squares indicate the centroids from a meta-analysis of the literature, for which the estimated activation maps are shown in (B). (After Venkatraman et al. 2009.)

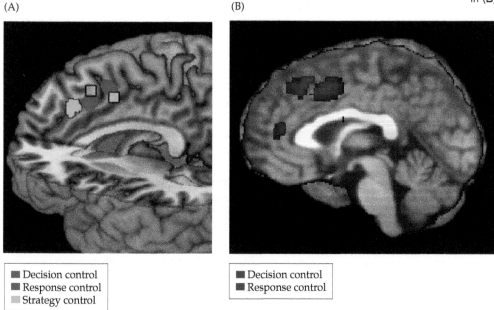

(A)

(B)

■ Decision control
■ Response control
■ Strategy control

■ Decision control
■ Response control

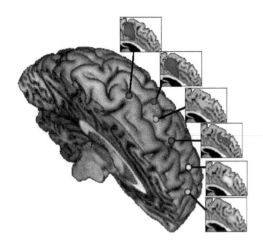

Figure 13.19 Evidence for topographical connections between medial and lateral prefrontal cortex Functional connectivity analyses were conducted on fMRI resting-state data (i.e., scans collected while participants were not performing an overt task). For seed regions in lateral prefrontal cortex, shown as colored dots, the analyses identified voxels in dorsomedial prefrontal cortex that had maximal functional connectivity (insets). The medial and lateral surfaces of the prefrontal cortex exhibited a consistent spatial pattern of connectivity—that is, posterior-to-posterior and anterior-to-anterior. This result suggests that the hierarchies shown in Figures 13.13 and 13.18 may be functionally interconnected. (From Taren et al. 2011.)

during performance of an executive processing task and within a nontask resting state (Figure 13.19). While much remains to be done to ascertain the functional relationships between the medial and lateral parts of the frontal lobe, it is clear that complex executive functions result not from the activity of single brain regions but from interactions among regions within larger networks.

Working Memory: Maintaining Information and Rules over Time

The executive functions introduced in the previous sections all facilitate the flexible and context-dependent control of behavior. In each case, these functions involve matching behavior to currently active goals. Left unaddressed, however, are the processes by which the brain keeps information online for effective executive processing. These processes, which collectively support what is often called **working memory**, involve the temporary maintenance and manipulation of information that is not currently available to the senses but that is necessary for successfully achieving short-term behavioral objectives. As the term implies, working memory is an active process that not only must maintain important information, but must inhibit irrelevant information to fit current behavioral goals.

A widely influential model of working memory was proposed by psychologist Alan Baddeley in the 1970s. In its more recent version, the **Baddeley model** consists of three capacity-limited *memory buffers* and a *control system* (Figure 13.20). Each memory buffer maintains a different kind of representation: a *phonological loop* holds sound-based representations, a *visuospatial sketchpad* holds visual object and spatial representations, and an *episodic buffer* contains integrated, multimodal representations. The control system in the model, which Baddeley called the *central executive*, is assumed to allocate processing resources to the memory buffers and to perform manipulations. Each memory buffer has two components: a *store* that holds information briefly, and a *rehearsal mechanism* that reactivates this information before it dissipates.

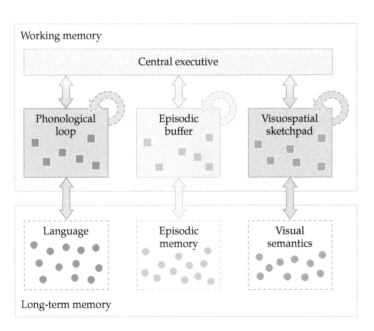

Figure 13.20 The Baddeley model of working memory Separate memory buffers hold phonological, visuospatial, and integrated multimodal information (the episodic buffer). The operation of the three buffers is taken to be controlled by a central executive. Dashed, curving arrows associated with each buffer represent rehearsal. (After Baddeley 2003.)

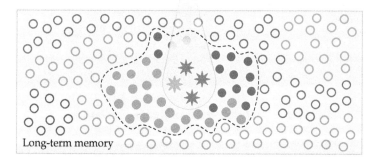

Figure 13.21 The Cowan model of working memory Different types of memory representations (open circles) are held within the same long-term memory store. Working memory consists of a subset of these representations in an activated state (filled circles). Only a few of these activated representations (stars) fall within the focus of attention (yellow "illuminated" area), which is controlled by the central executive. (After Cowan 1998.)

In the case of the phonological loop, these two components are respectively known as *phonological store* and *articulatory rehearsal*. Baddeley conceived of the articulatory rehearsal process as analogous to subvocal speech—that is, the "inner voice" we sometimes "hear" while reading or counting.

An alternative model, proposed by psychologist Nelson Cowan, contends that working memory is organized in two embedded levels (Figure 13.21). The first level of working memory consists of long-term memory representations in an "activated state." There is no fixed limit on the number of long-term memories that can be activated at one time, but activation decays rapidly unless it is rehearsed. In this model, unlike Baddeley's model, working memory representations for different types of information (verbal, visual, and so on) are all held in the same long-term memory store rather than in separate working memory stores. The second level of working memory in Cowan's model consists of activated representations that fall within the focus of executive control, which can hold up to four items at one time.

These two models of working memory have each been influential in psychological research for the past several decades. Notably, a few points of difference make testable cognitive neuroscience predictions. The Baddeley model suggests that the regions actively storing working memory representations are different from those storing long-term memories, whereas Cowan's model suggests that both regions are the same. Given that long-term memory representations of sensory information are stored in the sensory and association cortices pertinent to each type of stimulus information (see Chapter 8), Cowan's model suggests that working memory maintenance should be associated with sustained activity in these regions. The latter prediction is supported by current research. Another difference is that Baddeley's model suggests that the "store" and "rehearsal" components depend on different brain regions for each buffer, whereas Cowan's model does not. Moreover, although Baddeley's original model of working memory attributed the maintenance of visual object and spatial information to a single working memory component (the "visuospatial sketchpad"), it is now clear that object and spatial maintenance mechanisms can be dissociated at both the behavioral and neural levels. Thus, although both models have been used to explain a wide variety of behavioral phenomena, the Cowan model seems to be better supported by more recent research.

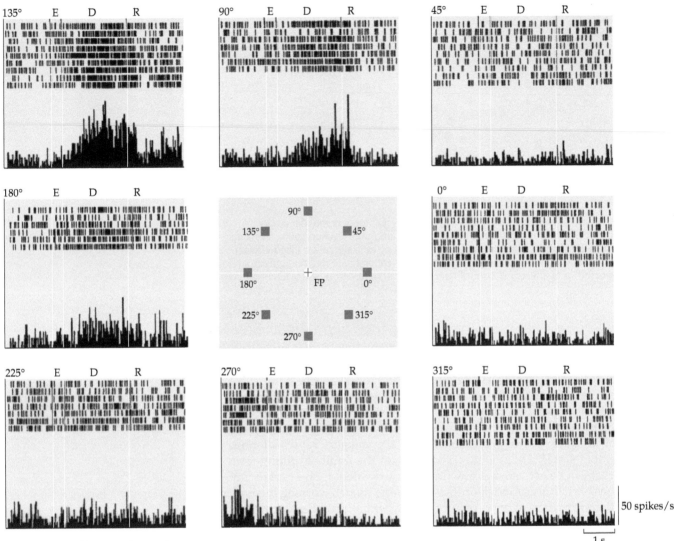

Figure 13.22 Neurons in monkey prefrontal cortex have a tuned "memory field" The neuron tuned to an orientation of 135 degrees showed delay-period activity to targets presented at this orientation, but not to targets at 270 degrees. E, encoding; FP, fixation point; D, delay; R, response. (After Funahashi et al. 1989.)

The following discussion builds on the Cowan model—that is, an executive process that transiently activates sensory representations—to consider how prefrontal cortex interacts with sensory cortices to support working memory.

Neural substrates of working memory

Studies of the neural basis for working memory have typically focused on what is called **delay-period activity**. The term *delay period* refers to the time between the initial activation of information in working memory and the use of that information to execute a particular action. Early and striking evidence for the role of dorsolateral prefrontal cortex neurons in working memory came from single-unit recordings in monkeys. When monkeys maintained a spatial location in working memory for a few seconds—to direct a later eye movement to that location—neurons in dorsolateral prefrontal cortex fired continuously during that delay period. A variety of studies by neurophysiologists Joaquin Fuster, Patricia Goldman-Rakic, and others showed that prefrontal neurons were selective for particular properties of the stimulus being maintained. As illustrated in Figure 13.22, a given prefrontal neuron might exhibit the greatest firing rate when a preferred spatial location was being held in memory (e.g., 135 degrees), but little to no firing when a nonpreferred spatial location was being remembered (e.g., 270 degrees). Prefrontal cortex neurons have since been shown to maintain information not only about spatial locations, but also about types of sensory stimuli, specific movements, or even the relative order of information within a sequence. Moreover, recordings from neurons in a number of other regions (e.g., parietal cortex, basal ganglia) have found delay-period activity, suggesting that such activity may be a general feature of information processing associated with the control of behavior and is instantiated broadly throughout the brain.

Subsequent functional neuroimaging studies built on this earlier work to elucidate the brain systems supporting working memory. Activation in lateral prefrontal cortex has been attributed to the active maintenance of information in working memory, on the basis of several findings:

1. Activation typically persists for the entire length of the delay period, whether a few seconds (as in the single-unit work) or 24 seconds or longer in some studies.

2. Activation generally increases as more information must be held in memory (e.g., maintaining five faces versus three faces), although the exact relationship between working memory load and activation amplitude differs across tasks.

3. Increased activation has been associated with better working memory performance, such that activation tends to be greater when the maintained information is used correctly at the end of the delay period.

4. Increased activation has been associated with resistance to the effects of distraction from a competing working memory task.

5. Activation tends to be greater when the task requires the *manipulation* of information in working memory (i.e., changing the content or order of information according to some rule), rather than simply *maintenance* of that information (Figure 13.23).

Together, these results uphold the conception that dorsolateral prefrontal cortex supports executive functions associated with selecting, maintaining, and rehearsing information held in working memory.

Conversely, substantial research indicates that the information held in working memory itself reflects information processing elsewhere in the brain, as would be consistent with the Cowan model. When attempting to remember phonological information, individuals with lesions in the left inferior parietal

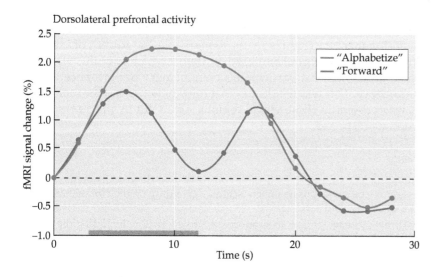

Figure 13.23 **Evidence that manipulation of information in working memory relies on dorsolateral prefrontal cortex** In an fMRI study, participants were presented with a series of letters to hold in working memory. Delay-period activation (gray bar) was found in both ventrolateral and dorsolateral prefrontal cortex regions, but dorsolateral prefrontal cortex activity was greater when the test condition involved manipulation ("alphabetize") than in a condition involving only maintenance ("forward"). (After D'Esposito et al. 2000.)

Figure 13.24 Using multivoxel pattern analysis (MVPA) to decode the contents of working memory (A) Participants viewed two spatial gratings and then were given a visual cue indicating which grating to maintain in memory during a delay interval. Then the participants saw a test grating and indicated whether that grating was rotated clockwise or counterclockwise compared to the grating being held in memory. (B) MVPA revealed that early visual regions (V1–V4) contained information that could be used to predict the orientation of the grating being held in memory (purple circles). The predictive power was similar to that obtained in a second, perceptual experiment (red circles) in which the stimuli were actually present on the visual display (i.e., not being held in memory), and the activation patterns found in the working memory experiment could be used to predict the orientation of stimuli in the perceptual experiment, and vice versa (green circles). (After Harrison and Tong 2009.)

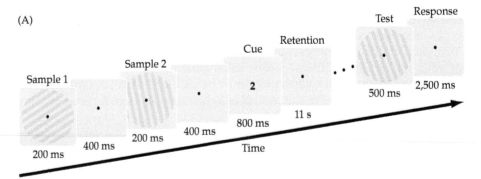

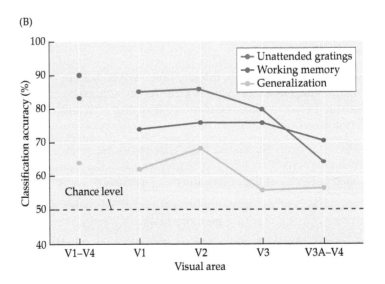

cortex have impaired working memory but normal long-term memory. And even though they have a normal capacity to articulate different letter sounds (e.g., for *P* or *V*), the working memory for those letters is not impaired by phonological similarity in these patients, unlike neurologically normal individuals, who rely on phonological representations for memory. In contrast, patients with damage to Broca's area show specific deficits in articulating letter sounds and words, which impair their ability to maintain this information in working memory.

Maintenance of simple visual information seems to involve sensory regions as well; features like color, motion direction, and spatial position all have been linked to the specific sensory regions (see Chapter 3) that process those object properties. In a recent example, multivoxel pattern analysis was used to decode the orientation directions of simple visual stimuli while they were held in working memory (Figure 13.24). Remarkably, the pattern of activation in regions of visual cortex could be used to predict which stimulus was being maintained, even when the participant's own memory performance was not better than chance. This result indicates that information about the maintained stimulus was present in these visual regions, albeit not in a form that led to the appropriate response.

Summary

1. Executive functions support the flexible control of goal-directed behavior. These processes may be conscious or nonconscious, depending on the circumstances in which they are evoked.

2. Several brain systems interact to support executive function, including the dorsolateral prefrontal cortex, ventromedial prefrontal cortex, posterior parietal cortex, anterior cingulate cortex, and basal ganglia.

3. The prefrontal cortex receives much of its input from the secondary sensory cortices and is richly interconnected with the parietal cortex. Projections from the prefrontal cortex extend primarily to the basal ganglia and the cortical motor systems, which together contribute to initiating and inhibiting actions.

4. In general, the lateral prefrontal cortex supports the initiating, inhibiting, shifting, and relating of novel rules for behavior. Its subregions are organized in a hierarchical fashion, such that the most posterior regions support the execution of relatively simple rules, while the most anterior implement and update higher-order goals that might be distant from immediate task demands.

5. In contrast, the ventral portions of the prefrontal cortex facilitate behavioral control in situations with well-established behavioral rules, as in social situations or in interactions with objects in the environment.

6. The dorsomedial prefrontal cortex monitors behavior and signals the need for increased allocation of executive control. Recent work indicates that dorsomedial prefrontal cortex may be organized along a posterior-to-anterior topography similar to that of dorsolateral prefrontal cortex.

7. Working memory refers to the maintenance and manipulation of information that is no longer directly available to the senses. Regions of the prefrontal cortex and parietal contribute to the successful engagement of working memory, through their influences on information processing in sensory regions.

8. Together, these executive control systems allow behavior to transcend simple stimulus-response associations, providing a foundation for many complex aspects of human activity.

> Go to the **COMPANION WEBSITE**
>
> sites.sinauer.com/cogneuro2e
> for quizzes, animations, flashcards, and other study resources.

Additional Reading

Reviews

BADDELEY, A. (2003) Working memory: Looking back and looking forward. *Nat. Rev. Neurosci.* 4: 829–839.

BADRE, D. AND M. D'ESPOSITO (2009) Is the rostro-caudal axis of the frontal lobe hierarchical? *Nat. Rev. Neurosci.* 10: 659–669.

BUSH, G., P. LUU AND M. I. POSNER (2000) Cognitive and emotional influences in anterior cingulate cortex. *Trends Cogn. Sci.* 4: 215–222.

COWAN, N. (1998) Visual and auditory working memory capacity. *Trends Cogn. Sci.* 2: 77.

MILLER, E. K. AND J. D. COHEN (2001) An integrative theory of prefrontal cortex function. *Annu. Rev. Neurosci.* 24: 167–202.

RIDDERINKHOF, K. R., M. ULLSPERGER, E. A. CRONE AND S. NIEUWENHUIS (2004) The role of the medial frontal cortex in cognitive control. *Science* 306: 443–447.

Important Original Papers

ALEXANDER, W. H. AND J. W. BROWN (2011) Medial prefrontal cortex as an action-outcome predictor. *Nat. Neurosci.* 14: 1338–1344.

ANDERSON, S. W., A. BECHARA, H. DAMASIO, D. TRANEL AND A. R. DAMASIO (1999) Impairment of social and moral behavior related to early damage in human prefrontal cortex. *Nat. Neurosci.* 2: 1032–1037.

BADRE, D. AND M. D'ESPOSITO (2007) Functional magnetic resonance imaging evidence for a hierarchical organization of the prefrontal cortex. *J. Cogn. Neurosci.* 19: 2082–2099.

BEHRENS, T. E., M. W. WOOLRICH, M. E. WALTON AND M. F. RUSHWORTH (2007) Learning the value of information in an uncertain world. *Nat. Neurosci.* 10: 1214–1221.

BOTVINICK, M., L. E. NYSTROM, K. FISSELL, C. S. CARTER AND J. D. COHEN (1999) Conflict monitoring versus selection-for-action in anterior cingulate cortex. *Nature* 402: 179–181.

BUSH, G., P. J. WHALEN, B. R. ROSEN, M. A. JENIKE, S. C. MCINERNEY AND S. L. RAUCH (1998) The counting Stroop: An interference task specialized for functional neuroimaging—Validation study with functional MRI. *Hum. Brain. Mapp.* 6: 270–282.

CHAO, L. L. AND R. T. KNIGHT (1995) Human prefrontal lesions increase distractibility to irrelevant sensory inputs. *NeuroReport* 6: 1605–1610.

COOLS, R., L. CLARK AND T. W. ROBBINS (2004) Differential responses in human striatum and prefrontal cortex to changes in object and rule relevance. *J. Neurosci.* 24: 1129–1135.

DAMASIO, H., T. GRABOWSKI, R. FRANK, A. M. GALABURDA AND A. R. DAMASIO (1994) The return of Phineas Gage: Clues about the brain from the skull of a famous patient. *Science* 264: 1102–1105.

FELLOWS, L. K. AND M. J. FARAH (2005) Is anterior cingulate cortex necessary for cognitive control? *Brain* 128: 788–796.

FUNAHASHI, S., C. J. BRUCE AND P. S. GOLDMAN-RAKIC (1989) Mnemonic coding of visual space in the monkey's dorsolateral prefrontal cortex. *J. Neurophysiol.* 61: 331–349.

GOLDMAN-RAKIC, P. S. AND L. J. PORRINO (1985) The primate mediodorsal (MD) nucleus and its projection to the frontal lobe. *J. Comp. Neurol.* 242: 535–560.

GOLDSTEIN, K. AND M. SCHEERER (1941) *Abstract and Concrete Behavior: An Experimental Study with Special Tests.* Psychological Monographs, Vol. 53, No. 2 (Whole No. 239). Evanston, IL: American Psychological Association.

HARRISON, S. A. AND F. TONG (2009) Decoding reveals the contents of visual working memory in early visual areas. *Nature* 458: 632–635.

HUETTEL S. A. AND G. MCCARTHY (2004) What is odd in the oddball task? Prefrontal cortex is activated by dynamic changes in response strategy. *Neuropsychologia* 42: 379–386.

KENNERLEY, S. W., M. E. WALTON, T. E. BEHRENS, M. J. BUCKLEY AND M. F. RUSHWORTH (2006) Optimal decision making and the anterior cingulate cortex. *Nat. Neurosci.* 9: 940–947.

KERNS, J. G., J. D. COHEN, A. W. MACDONALD III, R. Y. CHO, V. A. STENGER AND C. S. CARTER (2004) Anterior cingulate conflict monitoring and adjustments in control. *Science* 303: 1023–1026.

KOECHLIN, E. AND A. HYAFIL (2007) Anterior prefrontal function and the limits of human decision-making. *Science* 318: 594–598.

KOECHLIN, E., C. ODY AND F. KOUNEIHER (2003) The architecture of cognitive control in the human prefrontal cortex. *Science* 302: 1181–1185.

MCCARTHY, G., M. LUBY, J. GORE AND P. GOLDMAN-RAKIC (1997) Infrequent events transiently activate human prefrontal and parietal cortex as measured by functional MRI. *J. Neurophysiol.* 77: 1630–1634.

MILNER, B. (1963) Effects of different brain lesions on card sorting. *Arch. Neurol.* 9: 90–100.

MIYAKE, A., N. P. FRIEDMAN, M. J. EMERSON, A. H. WITZKI, A. HOWERTER AND T. D. WAGER (2000) The unity and diversity of executive functions and their contributions to complex "frontal lobe" tasks: A latent variable analysis. *Cogn. Psychol.* 41: 49–100.

POCHON, J. B., J. RIIS, A. G. SANFEY, L. E. NYSTROM AND J. D. COHEN (2008) Functional imaging of decision conflict. *J. Neurosci.* 28: 3468–3473.

SMITH, R., K. KERAMATIAN AND K. CHRISTOFF (2007) Localizing the rostrolateral prefrontal cortex at the individual level. *Neuroimage* 36: 1387–1396.

STROOP, J. R. (1935) Studies of interference in serial verbal reactions. *J. Exp. Psychol.* 18: 643–662.

TAREN, A. A., V. VENKATRAMAN AND S. A. HUETTEL (2011) A parallel functional topography between medial and lateral prefrontal cortex: Evidence and implications for cognitive control. *J. Neurosci.* 31: 5026–5031.

VALLENTIN, D., S. BONGARD AND A. NIEDER (2012) Numerical rule coding in the prefrontal, premotor, and posterior parietal cortices of macaques. *J. Neurosci.* 32: 6621–6630.

VENKATRAMAN, V., A. G. ROSATI, A. A. TAREN AND S. A. HUETTEL (2009) Resolving response, decision, and strategic control: Evidence for a functional topography in dorsomedial prefrontal cortex. *J. Neurosci.* 29: 13158–13164.

WALLIS, J. D., K. C. ANDERSON AND E. K. MILLER (2001) Single neurons in prefrontal cortex encode abstract rules. *Nature* 411: 953–956.

WILGUS, J. AND B. WILGUS (2009) Face to face with Phineas Gage. *J. Hist. Neurosci.* 18: 340–345.

Books

FINGER, S. (1994) *Origins of Neuroscience.* New York: Oxford University Press.

FUSTER, J. (2008) *The Prefrontal Cortex*, 4th Ed. London: Academic Press.

HUETTEL, S. A., A. W. SONG AND G. MCCARTHY (2004) *Functional Magnetic Resonance Imaging.* Sunderland, MA: Sinauer.

MACMILLAN, M. (2000) *An Odd Kind of Fame: Stories of Phineas Gage.* Cambridge, MA: MIT Press.

STUSS, D. T. AND R. T. KNIGHT (2002) *Principles of Frontal Lobe Function.* New York: Oxford University Press.

14

Decision Making

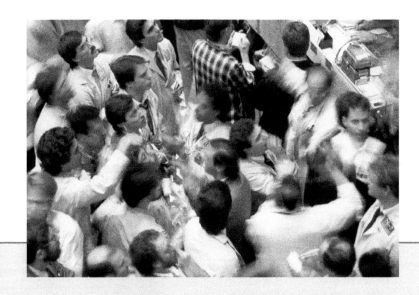

INTRODUCTION

Until recently, research on how people make decisions—whether large ones like choosing a college, or small ones like which brand of toothpaste to buy—has been conducted primarily within traditional economics. To understand decision processes, economists created **rational choice models**, which incorporate the different features of a decision into an algorithm that can evaluate and compare the different options (e.g., the prestige and cost of different colleges). Beginning in the 1970s, however, researchers in the nascent field of behavioral economics began to identify anomalies in the traditional rational choice models. People make choices—in both laboratory experiments and meaningful real-world situations—that could not be explained by those models. By the beginning of the present century, the integration of concepts from economics and neuroscience had led to the emergence of a new field called **neuroeconomics** or **decision neuroscience**, in hopes that the concepts and methods of neuroscience could help resolve issues in economics and related social sciences.

This chapter introduces some of the major behavioral phenomena and experimental methods that are central to decision-making research, and discusses how ongoing studies in cognitive neuroscience are shaping the way researchers think about decision making. It focuses on what is called *value-based decision making*, which means the selection of an option that leads to a preferred outcome (or set of outcomes). This approach extends the scope of decision making from the simpler situations considered in the previous chapter. For example, naming the ink color in a Stroop task requires executive functions for successful performance but does not involve personal value judgments in the same way as, say, the choice of a menu item at a restaurant.

■ INTRODUCTORY BOX ADDICTION TO GAMBLING

The 2003 World Series of Poker was the scene of an unusual championship match. One of the two finalists was Sam Farha, a professional poker player and veteran of hundreds of such tournaments. Sitting across the table was the improbably named Chris Moneymaker, an unknown who had never played in a face-to-face poker tournament before the series but was one of a new generation of online poker enthusiasts. Moneymaker bested more than 800 World Series entrants to reach the finals and, despite his inexperience at live tournament play, went on to defeat Farha and win a then-record $2.5 million. His victory signaled a turning point for the gambling industry. Within 2 years there were more than 2 million online poker players (both from the United States and from many other countries), and today more than 100,000 players are logged on and playing at any given time. Whereas high-stakes poker was once a game played by professionals in smoky back rooms, now anyone with a computer and some skill can win (or, far more likely, lose) substantial amounts of money online.

Online poker is simply the most visible example of a broader social problem. Taking into account all forms of gambling, estimates are that 1 to 2 percent of U.S. adults will at some time during their lifetime suffer from *pathological gambling disorder*, a serious condition that includes an inability to stop gambling despite significant negative consequences. (The more general term *problem gambling* is also used in the literature.)

Neuroimaging studies have shown that pathological gamblers have abnormal patterns of activation in brain regions critical for the evaluation of rewards. Deficits in reward processing might lead to maladaptive learning. For example, when people play a virtual slot machine while their brain is scanned using fMRI, activation of the ventral striatum observed in response to near misses (i.e., when the machine comes close to a winning combination but does not pay out any money) resembles the activation observed in response to actual winning plays (see figure). The magnitude of that activation is greater in individuals with gambling problems. Since the slot machine delivers rewards randomly, these gamblers should not learn from near misses. Yet their brains respond in a way that reinforces the problem behavior.

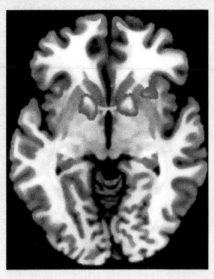
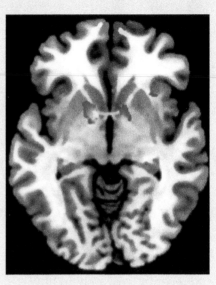

Wins > Losses   Near-miss loss > Full-miss loss

In a gambling paradigm, the reward system responds to near misses. Participants in an fMRI experiment played a simplified slot machine for real money. Reward-related brain regions, like the ventral striatum, showed greater activation on plays of the game in which they won money compared to plays in which they lost money (left panel). In some trials the slot machine stopped just before or just after a winning combination (a "near miss"); on other trials the slot machine stopped on a combination that was far from winning (a "full miss"). Notably, the near-miss trials evoked activation in the ventral striatum, even though the participant did not actually win any money (right panel). (From Clark et al. 2009.)

Pathological gambling affects some segments of the population much more than others. The rate of gambling problems is approximately three times higher in males aged 14 to 22 than in the population at large, and online gambling—with its easy access and cloak of privacy—represents a major source of abuse. Why adolescents and young adults are so susceptible to gambling is not clear. One possibility is the immaturity of executive control processes. Compared to other brain regions, the prefrontal cortex matures relatively late in development, with structural changes still observed in the late teens. Consistent with this delayed development, fMRI studies have frequently found differences between adolescents and adults in prefrontal cortex activation evoked by a variety of executive control paradigms. Impairments in executive control processes may limit adolescents' abilities to inhibit the attractive effects of rewards and to evaluate the future consequences of behavior.

Ironically, a second demographic group that is disproportionately afflicted

with pathological gambling is the elderly. For many older adults, gambling provides a much desired social opportunity, and retirees are frequent targets of casino marketing campaigns. As is the case for adolescents, multiple factors presumably contribute to the prevalence of gambling problems in the elderly. For example, older individuals are more likely than young adults to be impaired in decision-making tasks that rely on ventromedial prefrontal cortex.

Gambling problems can also be exacerbated by drugs that affect the brain's reward system. Parkinson's disease arises from the systematic degeneration of dopamine-synthesizing neurons in the midbrain, particularly within a region known as the substantia nigra. Loss of these neurons leads to a variety of symptoms that include the inability to control some types of motor movements. Treatment of **Parkinson's disease** often involves high doses of dopamine agonists, which ameliorate problems with motor control by mimicking the effects of dopamine and improve many patients'

■ **INTRODUCTORY BOX** *(continued)*

Pathological Gambling in Patients with Parkinson's Disease

BEFORE TREATMENT	ON DOPAMINE AGONIST	OFF DOPAMINE AGONIST
Patient A (age 54) gambled every few years.	Gambled almost daily; lost about $2,500.	Within a month, reported no interest in gambling.
Patient B (age 63) gambled every 3 months or so, without problems.	Reported "incredible compulsion" to gamble; gambled several times a week.	After a month, frequency of gambling was back to every few months.
Patient C (age 41) reported never having gambled.	Became "consumed" with gambling; lost $5,000 within a few months; exhibited compulsions for shopping and sex.	Two days after stopping treatment, reported no urge to gamble, and no other compulsions.
Patient D (age 50) had no history of gambling.	Gambled compulsively; remained at casinos for days at a time; exhibited hypersexuality and excessive drinking.	Within a month, reported no interest in gambling.

After Dodd et al. 2005.

quality of life. Yet after its use became widespread, this treatment was discovered to have an unexpected side effect: Parkinson's patients became much more likely to develop pathological gambling (about 5 to 7 percent), compared to individuals of similar age in the general population. In many Parkinson's cases under drug treatment, the development of pathological gambling has a sudden onset with uncontrollable compulsions, and it disappears soon after the patient stops treatment (see table). As reviewed later in the chapter, the neurotransmitter dopamine is important for reward-based learning, and it is the likely basis for these phenomena.

References

CLARK, L., A. J. LAWRENCE, F. ASTLEY-JONES AND N. GRAY (2009) Gambling near-misses enhance motivation to gamble and recruit win-related brain circuitry. *Neuron* 61: 481–490.

DODD, M. L., K. J. KLOS, J. H. BOWER, Y. E. GEDA, K. A. JOSEPHS AND J. E. AHLSKOG (2005) Pathological gambling caused by drugs used to treat Parkinson disease. *Arch. Neurol.* 62: 1377–1381.

DRIVER-DUNCKLEY, E., J. SAMANTA AND M. STACY (2003) Pathological gambling associated with dopamine agonist therapy in Parkinson's disease. *Neurology* 61: 422–423.

PAUS, T. (2005) Mapping brain maturation and cognitive development during adolescence. *Trends Cogn. Sci.* 9: 60–68.

The chapter begins by defining the core economic concepts of subjective value and uncertainty, and then progresses to more complex concepts from psychology, such as social context and decision rules (called *heuristics*). Applied examples are introduced throughout, from understanding consumer behavior to implications of decision-making research for clinical problems like addiction (see Introductory Box).

Decision Making: From Rational Choice to Behavioral Economics

Early theories of decision making were developed in response to largely practical concerns—for instance, how to make good bets in the context of gambling. The conception of probability as the likelihood of future events was first articulated in the seventeenth century by the French polymath Blaise Pascal. Pascal demonstrated that the relative probabilities of events could be determined by calculating the number of positive outcomes (e.g., winning rolls of dice) divided by the total number of possible outcomes (e.g., all potential rolls of dice). Pascal's insight soon led to the concept of **expected value**, derived by multiplying the probability of each possible outcome by its associated reward. For example, imagine being given the opportunity to roll a standard six-sided die, for which you would earn $1 multiplied by the number of spots rolled (e.g., 5 on the die

(A)

(B)

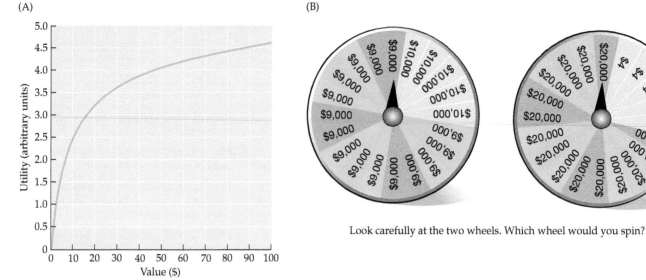

Look carefully at the two wheels. Which wheel would you spin?

Figure 14.1 The relation between objective value and subjective value (or utility) **(A)** Traditional economic models assume that the subjective value (also called *utility*) of money follows a concave function, according to the amount of wealth someone possesses. Doubling the amount of money, for example, results in less than a doubling of utility, as indicated in this schematic graph of utility plotted against monetary value. Note that utility is an abstract quantity that can be expressed only in arbitrary units. In addition, the specific shape of the utility curve differs across individuals. **(B)** People generally make decisions on the basis of expected utility, not expected value. If faced with a choice between the two options here, each presented as a "wheel of fortune," most people would choose the option on the left, even though it has a much lower expected value than the option on the right has.

means $5). The expected value of this gamble can be calculated to be $3.50, so it would seem wise to pay $3 to roll the die once, but unwise to pay $4. The simplest normative theory of decision making—that is, a theory of how people *should* make decisions—is to select the option with the highest expected value.

Expected value is an extraordinarily powerful concept, but it has clear limitations. Suppose a player in a coin-flipping game receives $2 if the coin comes up heads, but $0 for tails. A person who had to decide between playing the game once or receiving a sure $0.90 might do a quick expected-value calculation and choose to play. But what if the stakes were increased by a factor of 10,000? When considering a very similar problem, the eighteenth-century Swiss mathematician Daniel Bernoulli noted that most individuals would prefer the sure $9,000 (in his case in ducats, not dollars), although very rich individuals might consider a coin flip for $20,000 a reasonable investment.

Bernoulli explained this result by introducing the concept of **utility**, which reflects the *psychological* (as opposed to economic) value assigned to an outcome (Figure 14.1). He argued that the concept of expected value should be replaced by a new quantity: **expected utility**. Bernoulli pointed out that the utility of a small increase in wealth is inversely proportional to a person's current wealth. For example, the utility difference between having $0 and having $1,000 is much larger than the utility difference between $100,000 and $101,000—a phenomenon known as diminishing marginal utility.

Expected-utility theory and its variants have proved remarkably useful as a description of decision making, particularly in economic contexts, for more than two centuries. One result of this history is that the concept of **rationality** has come to dominate many accounts of decision making. Although there is no single agreed-upon definition of *rationality*, the term usually connotes consistency with some formal rules for decision making. Accordingly, rational decisions are characterized by preferences and decision rules that do not change in different contexts, and that are immune to whim or cognitive limitations. Rational decision makers also assume (by definition) that others will behave in a similarly rational manner; this assumption is important for understanding how people behave in interactive situations like bargaining, negotiating, and game playing.

Despite their intuitive attraction, rational choice models often fail to describe real-world behavior. For example, people pay to avoid risk when they buy insurance, but many of the same people pay to take on risk by buying lottery tickets that cost more than their expected value. The psychologists Daniel Kahneman

(A)

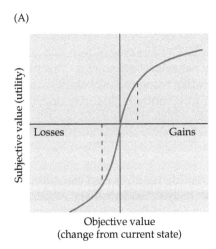

(B)

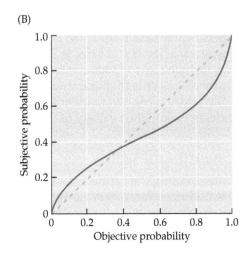

Figure 14.2 Reference dependence and probability weighting Prospect theory, which was developed by psychologists Daniel Kahneman and Amos Tversky, makes two primary assumptions about choice behavior. (A) Reference dependence. The subjective value of an outcome depends only on the change in objective value from an individual's current state. As shown in this schematic diagram, the slope of the subjective value function decreases with increasing magnitude (e.g., the subjective difference between $0 and $100 is greater than that between $1,000 and $1,100), and the slope is steeper for losses than for gains (e.g., the two dashed lines indicate losses and gains of similar objective magnitude). (B) Probability weighting. The subjective probability of an outcome (solid line) differs somewhat from its objective probability, such that low-probability events seem more likely than they really are, while high-probability events seem less likely than they really are. The dashed line shows the prediction of normative economic models; i.e., that subjective and objective probabilities should be matched. (After Tversky and Kahneman 1992.)

and Amos Tversky developed an approach to solving these behavioral puzzles that they called **prospect theory**. The term *prospect* refers to an option whose future rewards and probabilities are known or can be estimated. Prospect theory is an example of a descriptive theory of decision making in that it attempts to predict what people *will* choose; it is not a normative theory that describes what they *should* choose.

Prospect theory differs from expected-utility theory in two important ways. First, it assumes **reference dependence**: that people make decisions in terms of the anticipated gains and losses *compared to their current state*, largely ignoring how much wealth they actually have (Figure 14.2A). Thus, the current state serves as a reference point from which decision outcomes are evaluated. Both gains and losses are assumed to have diminishing marginal effects, as Bernoulli postulated, but the slope is steeper for losses (i.e., people want to avoid losses more than they want to seek gains). Though a novel concept for economics, reference dependence has a long history in psychology: it forms the core of the Weber-Fechner psychophysical model of sensory discrimination, as well as many adaptation effects (see Box 3B). Moreover, as will be considered later in the chapter, dopaminergic neurons in the midbrain change their firing rate in a reference-dependent manner.

Second, prospect theory proposes the idea of **probability weighting**, which means that people perceive probabilities in a highly subjective manner. People tend to overestimate the chances of low-probability events (e.g., winning the lottery) but underestimate the chances of high-probability events (Figure 14.2B). Again, this idea challenged core tenets of economic theory but was consistent with research in psychology. That humans (and other animals) showed biases in how they process infrequent events was well known to behavioral psychologists, who knew that training an animal using very infrequent rewards makes that training very resistant to extinction (i.e., weakening a learned association if rewards are no longer delivered). Similarly, studies of memory have shown that perceived frequency depends on how readily we can bring something to mind, and thus highly salient but rare events may be perceived as more common than they really are.

Prospect theory combined these two factors—reference dependence and probability weighting—to estimate the subjective utility of a decision outcome. It predicts a distinctive pattern of risk-averse and risk-seeking behavior. People should be risk-averse when faced with high-probability gains (e.g., preferring safe to risky investments), risk-seeking for low-probability gains (e.g., buying lottery tickets), risk-averse for low-probability losses (e.g., buying insurance), and risk-seeking for high-probability losses (e.g., keeping losing stocks in the hope that they recover). All of these diverse predictions are now supported by experimental data. Kahneman and Tversky's research—for which Kahneman was awarded the Nobel Prize in Economics in 2002 (Tversky was deceased, and thus ineligible)—supplied the foundation for **behavioral economics**. This new field seeks not only to characterize how factors like value and probability affect real-world choices, but to identify particular interventions that may improve decision making in a variety of contexts.

Reward and Utility

Understanding the neural basis of decision making requires first considering how the brain processes rewards that motivate choices. Rewards that have direct benefits for fitness, such as food, water, and sex, are called **primary reinforcers** (or *unconditioned reinforcers*). When decision-making experiments are conducted in non-human animals, the rewards are typically primary reinforcers that are valued even in the absence of training, such as drops of juice following successful performance of an experimental task. Many real-world decisions, at least for humans, do not involve primary reinforcers. Money, for example, has no intrinsic value but can be used to obtain other rewards; thus it is described as a **secondary reinforcer**. The removal of an aversive outcome following an action is called **negative reinforcement**, while the delivery of an aversive outcome is called **punishment**.

Two caveats are important to raise. First, the following sections will discuss learning and motivation specifically in the context of value-guided decision making. Other types of learning about positive and negative reinforcers (e.g., aversive responses to threatening stimuli, fear conditioning) involve brain circuitry important for affect and emotion, as was discussed in Chapter 10. Second, the brain regions and neurotransmitters discussed hereafter do not only contribute to decision making, but also have broader relevance for a wide range of adaptive behavior.

Dopamine: Pleasure or motivation?

For any animal to make behaviorally useful decisions, it must be able to predict the choices that lead to particular outcomes and to evaluate the reinforcement value of those outcomes, computing what economists refer to as subjective value or utility. Studies of the neural responses to rewards and their evaluation have generally implicated neural circuits that use the neurotransmitter **dopamine**. This important neurotransmitter contributes to many cognitive functions. As discussed in the Introductory Box, damage to dopamine neurons can lead to a difficulty in controlling motor movements, as evident in Parkinson's and Huntington's diseases. Dysfunction of the dopamine system has also been linked to a number of psychiatric conditions, including schizophrenia, depression, and attention deficit hyperactivity disorder. Conversely, other neurotransmitters also contribute to reward evaluation and decision making, as will be described later in this chapter. It is important, therefore, to understand the specific roles that dopamine neurons play in reward processing—while also recognizing that those roles are not always unique to dopamine or limited only to the processing of rewards.

Two important structures in the midbrain contain dopamine neurons: the substantia nigra and the **ventral tegmental area**, or **VTA** (Figure 14.3). Neurons in the substantia nigra contribute to motor control through their interconnections with the basal ganglia (see Chapter 5). Neurons in the VTA contribute to reward evaluation through their projections to the **nucleus accumbens** in the basal ganglia (sometimes referred to as the *ventral striatum*), the amygdala, and the hippocampus, as well as to cortical regions like the medial frontal lobe.

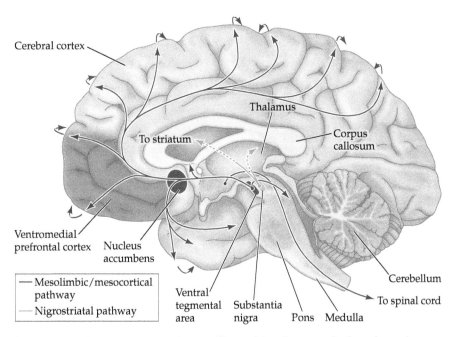

Cerebral cortex

Thalamus

To striatum

Corpus callosum

Ventromedial prefrontal cortex

Nucleus accumbens

Cerebellum

— Mesolimbic/mesocortical pathway
— Nigrostriatal pathway

Ventral tegmental area

Substantia nigra

Pons   Medulla

To spinal cord

Figure 14.3 Dopaminergic pathways The activity of neurons in the substantia nigra and ventral tegmental area of the midbrain is modulated by the neurotransmitter dopamine. These neurons project broadly throughout the brain, notably to the nucleus accumbens, other regions of the basal ganglia, and the ventral and medial parts of the prefrontal cortex.

Several lines of evidence have linked dopamine neurons in these circuits to reward processing. Particularly notable have been discoveries that essentially all drugs of abuse—with the possible exception of some psychedelic compounds like LSD—exert their addictive influence through alterations in the function of these dopamine neurons. Moreover, direct stimulation of dopamine neurons serves as a particularly potent reward. In the 1950s, neurophysiologists James Olds and Peter Milner implanted electrodes in the brains of rats along a white matter tract called the medial forebrain bundle. While this tract contains axons from a diverse array of brain regions, an important component comes from dopamine neurons in the brainstem that project onto the nucleus accumbens. If the rats were given a stimulating current from these electrodes each time they performed a particular behavior (e.g., sitting in a specific spot in their cage), they would perform that behavior repeatedly to the exclusion of everything else—neither eating or drinking, nor engaging in sex—potentially until death. On the basis of this intriguing evidence, dopamine came to be popularly known as the "pleasure chemical," a substance responsible for the feelings of liking and pleasure that accompany rewards as diverse as drugs, sex, and money.

This simple story—that dopamine signals pleasure—is incorrect. In a seminal study, psychologist Kent Berridge and his colleagues injected into the nucleus accumbens a chemical that was toxic for dopamine neurons, causing broad damage to the mesolimbic dopamine pathways. Without dopamine function, the rats became aphagic and would not eat even if starving. Yet these same rats exhibited normal reactions to pleasurable and aversive tastes (Figure 14.4). A sweet taste (sucrose solution delivered into the rats' mouths) generated tongue protrusions and licking, whereas a bitter taste (a quinine solution) led to mouth gaping and blocking the throat with the tongue. From these and similar results, Berridge argued that dopamine supported not liking, but *wanting*, or the motivation to pursue a reward. (This property has also been labeled *seeking*, to emphasize that dopamine pushes an organism into action.)

Figure 14.4 **Dopamine neurons are necessary for wanting, not liking** Rats treated with the neurotoxin 6-hydroxydopamine (6-OHDA) show dramatic decreases in the number of dopaminergic neurons within the striatum, compared to control animals. For example, in the experiment whose data are shown here, administration of 6-OHDA resulted in greater than 90 percent dopamine depletion in all rats (6-OHDA group), with subsamples showing greater than 98 percent depletion in the striatum (Ns) and greater than 99 percent depletion in the nucleus accumbens (Ac). These rats became aphagic, such that they would not seek out and eat food that was freely available in their cage. However, they showed normal hedonic or "liking" reactions (e.g., tongue protrusions and paw licking) to a sucrose solution delivered directly to their mouths (A). They also showed normal aversive reactions (e.g., gaping mouths, chin rubbing, and face washing) when that sugar water was made bitter by the addition of quinine (B). (After Berridge and Robinson 1998.)

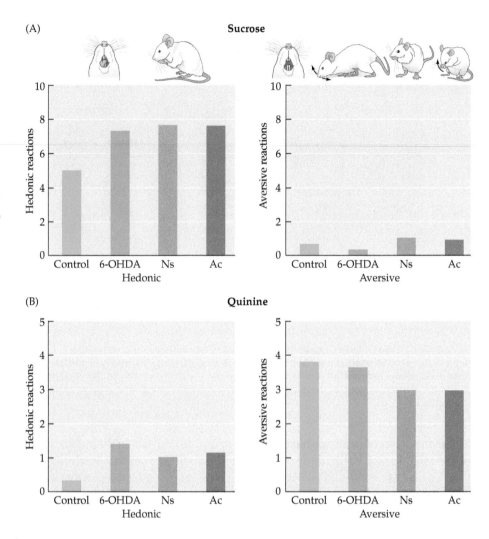

This perspective helped make sense of a counterintuitive feature of the stimulation research described earlier: even though the stimulation of this fiber tract seemed to evoke sensations of pleasure in the rat, dopamine release was not observed. Only when stimulation was randomly and unexpectedly delivered by the experimenters was dopamine release observed. It is now thought that sensations of pleasure accompany the activity of neurons sensitive to opioids and endocannabinoids, on the basis of evidence that direct delivery of those neurotransmitters to the ventral striatum (and other regions) increases the intensity of reactions associated with liking.

More recent work using functional neuroimaging has shown that activation in the nucleus accumbens is elicited by a wide range of motivationally relevant stimuli, including juice, money, social signals, donations to a favorite charity, and even the costly punishment of a noncooperative individual. Common to all of these cases is the reinforcement of a desirable association, whether learning about rewards or potentiating behavior. Conversely, any breakdown of motivation is accompanied by a diminishment of activation in the dopamine system.

In the phenomenon of reward undermining, an external reward actually reduces someone's engagement in a task. Participants in an fMRI study played a simple game in which they tried to stop a timer at exactly a target number. Subjects found this game rewarding and tried to perform well, even if they were receiving no explicit rewards—as shown by robust activation in the ventral

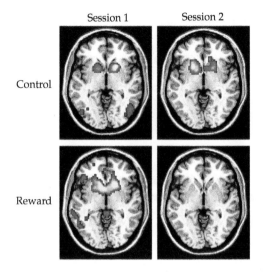

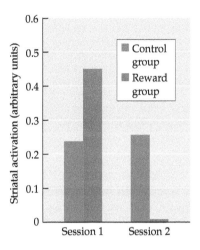

Figure 14.5 **Reward undermining** Economists have long recognized the possibility of reward undermining or "motivational crowding out," in which the delivery of a reward eliminates the intrinsic motivation to perform a task. In this fMRI experiment, two groups of participants played a simple stopwatch-timing game. The control group was not paid for playing the game, but successful plays in the game still evoked activation in the ventral striatum in each of two sessions. The reward group received monetary rewards for good performance in its first session of the game, during which time robust striatal activation was observed. The monetary rewards ceased in the second session, however, and the striatal activation was abolished. (After Murayama et al. 2010.)

striatum in a control group of unpaid participants across two sessions (**Figure 14.5**). Members of another experimental group were paid for their performance in the first session, and successful trials that resulted in payment led to activation in the ventral striatum. But when the experimental group was then told that there would be no monetary rewards in the second session, the activation in the ventral striatum disappeared. The participants still performed the task, but they now lacked any intrinsic motivation for performing well.

Reward prediction error

The previous section set forth the now-standard perspective that some midbrain dopamine neurons and their striatal targets support motivational processes, specifically links between actions and rewards. Left unanswered, however, is what information these dopamine neurons actually encode. Do they encode the value of the reward, the value of an action, or something else? Over the past 15 years, studies have converged to support a single and perhaps counterintuitive theory: phasic changes in the activity of dopamine neurons do not signal rewards themselves, but instead signal *changes in information*.

In a series of experiments, neurophysiologist Wolfram Schultz and his colleagues investigated how VTA neurons change their firing rate in response to rewarding stimuli. Monkeys with electrodes implanted in the VTA learned to press a lever when they saw a light, whereupon they would receive a squirt of juice (**Figure 14.6**). At the beginning of training, when the monkey was naïve about the experimental task, the delivery of the juice reward evoked a significant increase in VTA activity. As the monkey learned the task, however, the VTA neurons fired less and less to the juice reward and began firing more and more to the light. With learning,

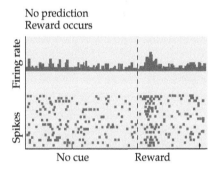

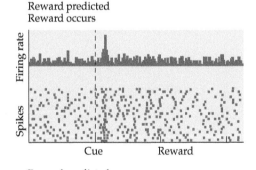

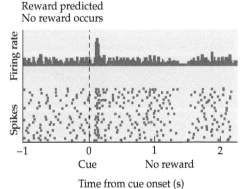

Figure 14.6 **Activity of midbrain dopaminergic neurons in response to expected and omitted rewards** Neurons in the ventral tegmental area (VTA) increase their firing rate in response either to unexpected rewards (top panel) or to cues that predict future rewards (middle panel), and show no change in response when a reward is delivered as expected (middle panel). However, they decrease their firing rates when a reward is expected but does not occur (bottom panel). (After Schultz et al. 1997.)

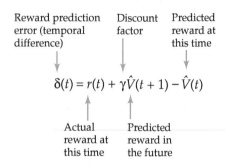

Figure 14.7 **Reward prediction error** Computational models of reward learning have been used to explain the signals carried by dopamine neurons. The most influential model contends that dopamine neurons carry a signal called *reward prediction error* (*RPE*), which combines three quantities: the actual reward received at a given point in time, new information gained about future rewards, and the reward that was predicted to be received. The RPE signal shares the essential properties of dopamine neurons (e.g., as shown in Figure 14.6), including increased firing to cues that provide new information about future rewards and no change in response to rewards that are fully predicted. (Equation from Schultz et al. 1997.)

therefore, the response of these particular dopamine neurons transferred from an unconditioned reinforcer to a conditioned stimulus that predicted that reinforcer. Moreover, if an expected reward did not occur, then the activity of the neurons decreased below baseline firing rates.

Subsequent studies by the same group suggested that the activation of VTA neurons is proportional both to the probability of reinforcement—with lower-probability rewards evoking greater activity—and to the magnitude of reinforcement. These results have since been replicated using functional neuroimaging studies in human participants, for whom activation in the ventral tegmental area (and its projection targets) increases in response to unpredictable rewards compared to predictable rewards.

Together, these studies indicate that dopamine neuron activity—at least in a subset of dopamine neurons—provides an index of **reward prediction error (RPE)**, which can be defined through a simple equation that combines two basic factors: (1) the difference between the reward that was received compared to what was expected, and (2) the change in information about future rewards. Note that the value of information depends on when a reward is expected (**Figure 14.7**). If a reward will not occur for a long time, then new information about that reward has less effect on midbrain dopamine neuron signals (for a similar phenomenon, see the discussion on temporal discounting later in the chapter). The reward prediction error signal can be used to guide behavior by means of **temporal difference learning**. The key idea in temporal difference learning is that successive states of the world (and, in turn, predictions about those states) are correlated over time.

As foreshadowed earlier in the chapter, the reward prediction error signal is substantially similar to the idea of reference dependence in prospect theory, in that both calculate subjective value in terms of transient changes from a current state, not absolute levels of reward. It is computationally efficient to track only unexpected changes in the world rather than the entire history of events over a long period of time. By taking advantage of the fast temporal resolution of EEG signals, very rapid brain responses can be identified that track unexpected reward outcomes (**Figure 14.8**). These rapid responses, which have been localized to the dorsomedial prefrontal cortex around the anterior cingulate gyrus, may in turn engage executive control processes to address ongoing task demands (see Chapter 13).

As described already, midbrain dopamine neurons project to many regions, most notably the basal ganglia (e.g., nucleus accumbens) and the ventromedial prefrontal cortex. An intriguing possibility is that information about rewards and punishments might modulate processing essentially everywhere in the brain, shaping all of the other cognitive functions considered in this textbook. Support for the idea of distributed reward processing comes from multivoxel pattern analysis (see Chapter 2) of fMRI data collected while human participants played a simple economic game (**Figure 14.9**). This analytic technique showed that classifiers that could distinguish winning and losing outcomes could be constructed from voxels in nearly all brain regions, including both primary

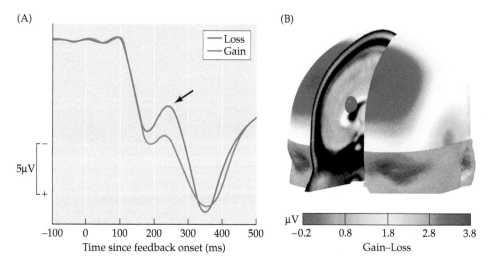

(A)

Loss
Gain

5μV

−100   0   100   200   300   400   500
Time since feedback onset (ms)

(B)

μV   −0.2   0.8   1.8   2.8   3.8
Gain–Loss

Figure 14.8   Rapid prefrontal cortex responses to monetary gains and losses
(A) By measuring brain functioning using EEG, cognitive neuroscientists can identify very rapid changes in brain activity associated with winning or losing money. Feedback about an unexpected monetary loss generates a negative-polarity ERP component within 200 milliseconds (black arrow in figure). (B) Source localization methods have linked this component to a dipole within the anterior cingulate gyrus, a region that contributes to the engagement of control systems within the brain, as introduced in Chapter 13. μV = microvolts. (After Gehring and Willoughby 2002.)

sensory regions and parts of prefrontal cortex. Similarly, studies using single-unit recording have revealed neurons sensitive to reward throughout much of the brain. While it seems clear that the midbrain dopamine system plays a critical role in the processing of reward, much remains to be understood about how other regions contribute to reward processing, especially in the context of decision making (Box 14A).

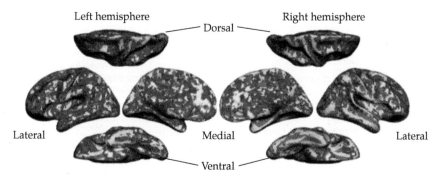

Left hemisphere   Right hemisphere
——— Dorsal ———

Lateral   Medial   Lateral

——— Ventral ———

Figure 14.9   Distributed influence of reward information throughout the brain
Researchers used multivoxel pattern analysis to identify brain regions where the local pattern of fMRI activation could predict whether a participant won or lost a simple competitive game (here, "matching pennies"). The reward outcome could be decoded from sets of voxels in nearly all regions, including both cortical and subcortical structures, suggesting that reward information modulates neuronal activity throughout the brain. Shown in the red-to-yellow color map are voxels contributing significant classification power (at a corrected $p < 0.001$). Of note, when the significance threshold was relaxed to a $p < 0.05$ threshold, more than 80 percent of the voxels in the brain passed significance testing. (After Vickery et al. 2011.)

■ BOX 14A LEARNING VALUES AND FORMING HABITS

Decision making is often considered to be an active, controlled process. When we think about the decisions that we have made in the past, the examples that leap most readily to mind typically involve conscious reflection about consequences and goals (e.g., selecting a college). Many of the examples used in this chapter do involve such goal-directed decisions; the fMRI activation shown in Figure 14.13, for example, represents the value associated with self-controlled choices of monetary rewards that may be delayed for several months before their receipt. Yet goal-directed choices represent only one facet of decision making. Many other important behaviors involve ongoing learning processes that relate value information to actions, often in the absence of reflection on our goals and desires.

Particularly relevant to day-to-day life are **habits**, or action tendencies that develop over time because of repeated reinforcement. Habits tend to involve relatively slow learning, but when established, they can be very resistant to change. Habits can be relatively innocuous, as when a student always sits in the same seat in the classroom. Or, in the case of a chronic drug abuser, they can be manifested in destructive, life-altering consequences. Two processes thought to be critical for reward learning and the development of habits are the ability to associate stimuli with rewards and the ability to choose motor actions that maximize future outcomes. Because of evidence implicating the basal ganglia both in stimulus-reward associations and in adaptive control of motor behavior, considerable research has been targeted at understanding how the basal ganglia's component regions may interact in reward learning and habit formation.

The basic features of reward learning can be seen in what are often called **actor-critic learning models**. Such models assume two brain systems: a *critic*

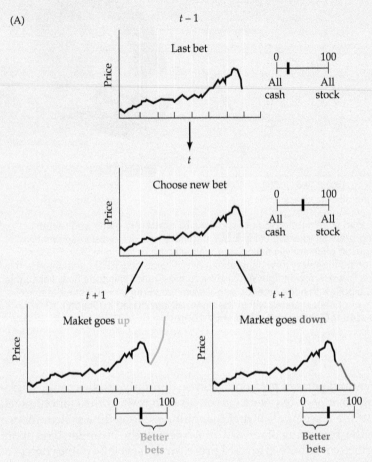

Real and fictive errors in a simple stock market game. (A) Participants in this fMRI experiment made a series of investment decisions within virtual stock markets. At each point in time (*t*), the participant could choose to allocate money in any proportion of stocks (i.e., betting that the market will go up) and cash (i.e., betting that the market will go down). This task generates two types of reward prediction errors: *real* RPEs based on the money invested in stocks, and *fictive* RPEs based on the money not so invested. For example, if all money was allocated to cash and then the market rose sharply, there would be a substantial positive fictive error. (After Lohrenz et al. 2007.)

that evaluates whether rewards are better or worse than expected, and an *actor* that updates the values of potential courses of behavior to increase the likelihood of future rewards. These two roles have been linked to separate components of the basal ganglia. Neurons in the ventral striatum (e.g., in the nucleus accumbens) provide critic signals associated with reward prediction error (RPE), via input

Responses to negative outcomes

To what degree, then, is the midbrain dopamine system specifically related to positive outcomes? Nearly all neuroeconomic experiments deliver or withhold some desirable outcome. In a typical task used with human subjects, winning money evokes an increase in fMRI activation in the nucleus accumbens, compared to not winning money. Similarly, tasks used with non-human primates show an increase in firing in response to the delivery of a juice reward

■ **BOX 14A** *(continued)*

(B)

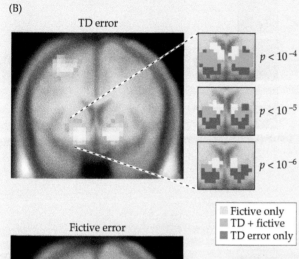

Fictive error

☐ Fictive only
☐ TD + fictive
■ TD error only

Activation in the striatum to real and fictive reward prediction errors. (B) RPEs associated with the money earned or lost by the participant on a given trial ("temporal difference" or "TD" error) are associated with activation in the ventral striatum. In contrast, activation associated with the money that could have been earned or lost—but was not actually won or lost, because the participant did not invest—was associated with more dorsal activation within the head of the caudate. The inset images are cropped to highlight the striatum and show the patterns of activation and overlap for these two error signals at different thresholds for significance. (After Lohrenz et al. 2007.)

from the VTA. In contrast, neurons in the dorsal striatum (e.g., in the head of the caudate) contribute to the creation and modification of plans for action, and thus have been linked to the actor role.

The separation between ventral and dorsal striatum also extends to other sorts of tasks. Activation of the ventral basal ganglia follows rewards in both classical conditioning (passive) and operant conditioning (active) tasks, whereas activation of the dorsal basal ganglia is observed only in operant conditioning (i.e., when rewards have implications for actions). In addition, research on executive function has linked the caudate to the establishment of mappings between specific stimuli and the required behavior.

It is important to recognize that actor-critic models update learning parameters in real time in response to each stimulus, action, and reward. This and similar approaches do not build inferences about the underlying structure of the environment or maintain a long history of rewards; as a result, they are simple and computationally efficient.

Even considering these constraints, such models can account for a wide array of decision-making behavior. Consider **fictive learning**, which refers to changes in behavior based on what might have been. As shown in Figure A, fictive learning is common within sequential decision processes like investing in the stock market. Even someone who does not own a particular stock might track the movements of that stock over time, trying to predict its future behavior to see how well a purchase of that stock might have paid off. A stock that rose unexpectedly, accordingly, would generate a *real* RPE signal in someone who owned it or a *fictive* RPE signal in someone who was merely watching it. Fictive error signals have been associated with activation in the caudate nucleus (Figure B), consistent with the potential contributions of such signals to learning the values of potential actions, as well as in the anterior cingulate cortex.

References

HAYDEN, B. Y., J. M. PEARSON AND M. L. PLATT (2009) Fictive reward signals in the anterior cingulate cortex. *Science* 324: 948–950.

LOHRENZ, T., K. McCABE, C. F. CAMERER AND P. R. MONTAGUE (2007) Neural signature of fictive learning signals in a sequential investment task. *Proc. Natl. Acad. Sci. USA* 104: 9493–9498.

O'DOHERTY, J. P., P. DAYAN, J. SCHULTZ, R. DEICHMANN, K. FRISTON AND R. J. DOLAN (2004) Dissociable roles of ventral and dorsal striatum in instrumental conditioning. *Science* 304: 452–454.

RANGEL, A., C. CAMERER AND P. R. MONTAGUE (2008) A framework for studying the neurobiology of value-based decision making. *Nat. Rev. Neurosci.* 9: 545–556.

compared to the unexpected omission of that reward. In contrast, almost no studies use truly negative outcomes. The challenge of using negative outcomes can be appreciated by thinking about how fMRI experiments are typically conducted: volunteer participants are recruited from the community, brought to the scanner to perform the task, and then paid some amount of money (e.g., $40) for their time. Even if the experimental task involves some winning trials and some losing trials, the participants know they will leave the experiment with money in their pocket. Thus, recent research has sought to understand

Figure 14.10 Identification of dopamine neurons that respond to both positive and aversive events Monkeys were trained that a set of cues predicted either fluid rewards (A) or aversive puffs of air to the face (B). CS, conditioned stimulus; ITI, intertrial interval; US, unconditioned stimulus. While many midbrain dopamine neurons exhibited a pattern of responses like that shown in Figure 14.6 (i.e., increased response to positive events, but decreased response to negative events), a subset of dopamine neurons showed increased responses to both positive and negative events. Shown in (C) are the responses of a single neuron to these cues. At the top of each subpanel are raster plots indicating the response of that neuron on individual trials, and at bottom are histograms showing the mean changes in firing rate of that neuron to a particular cue. (After Matsumoto and Hikosaka 2009.)

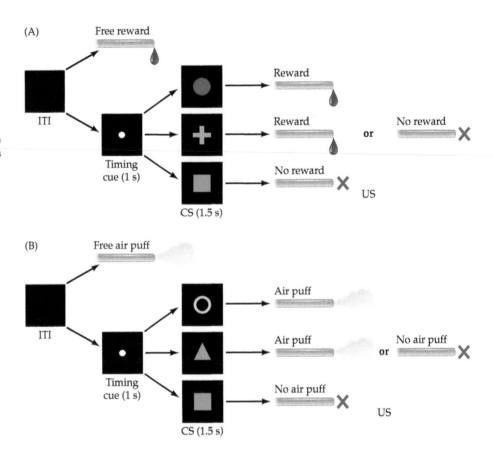

whether the dopamine signal might represent a factor other than the change in positive reinforcers.

An alternative theory posits that key reward-linked regions—notably the ventral striatum—respond not to rewards specifically, but instead to any stimulus that provides information important for future behavior. Such stimuli, which are sometimes called *salient events*, would include positive reinforcers (e.g., squirts of juice) as well as negative reinforcers (e.g., electric shocks) and even the unexpected absence of a predicted reward. Unexpected and distracting events have been shown to evoke activation in the basal ganglia, especially in ventral regions like the nucleus accumbens. In a typical experiment, fMRI participants perform a simple executive function task, such as judging whether each of a series of visually presented numbers is odd or even, while irrelevant auditory sounds are simultaneously presented. When an alerting sound like a dog bark or siren occurs, activation in the ventral striatum increases, and the magnitude of that activation is proportional to how much response time slows on the executive function task. It is not known to what extent similar effects occur in other parts of the brain's reward circuitry. Some studies have suggested that the appearance of an unexpected stimulus, but perhaps not other forms of arousal, modulates activation of the substantia nigra and VTA in the midbrain.

Salience-based explanations have difficulty, however, in answering the question of why dopamine neuron activity decreases when rewards are unexpectedly absent. The dopamine neuron whose data is shown in Figure 14.6, for example, evinces a clear difference between the delivery and omission of rewards: the unexpected delivery of a reward leads to an increase in its activity, while the unexpected omission of a reward leads to a decrease in its activity. If this neuron were responding to salient events, one might expect to observe increases in its activity in both cases.

(C)

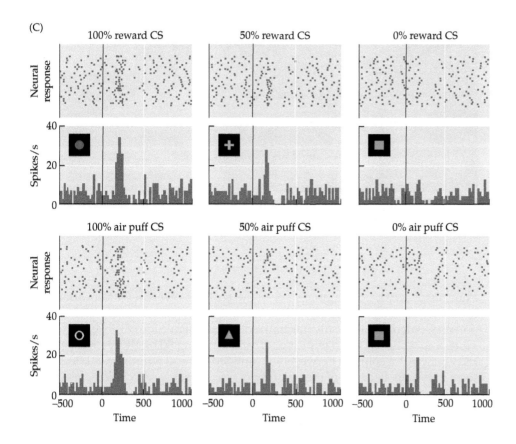

Studies by neurophysiologist Okihide Hikosaka and his colleagues suggested a way of reconciling the contradictory evidence for salience-related activity in the dopamine system. These researchers modified the basic paradigm of Schultz and colleagues so that monkeys worked to avoid punishments, specifically irritating puffs of air to the eye (Figure 14.10). When recording single-unit activity from neurons in the midbrain, they found that some neurons exhibited increased activity not only to fluid rewards but also to the aversive air puffs. This result suggests that there may be heterogeneity in the population of dopamine neurons, with the activity of some neurons tracking positive reinforcers and others tracking punishments. Both sorts of neurons may contribute to the identification of behaviorally relevant events, perhaps through projections to different targets in the cerebral cortex and basal ganglia.

Uncertainty: Risk, Ambiguity, and Delay

Neuroeconomic research on decision making is also concerned with how people deal with uncertainty. The term *uncertainty* means different things in different settings, but it can be thought of as the psychological state of having limited information, as often occurs in the making of real-world decisions. Research in neuroeconomics has investigated two main sorts of uncertainty: uncertainty about *what* outcome will occur, and uncertainty about *when* an outcome will occur. The former typically leads to what is often called **risk aversion** (with the related concept of **ambiguity aversion**); the latter leads to **delay discounting**. These concepts will be considered in more detail in the following sections.

Risk and ambiguity

A decision involves risk if it has multiple potential outcomes with known or estimable probabilities. Betting on red or black in roulette is a prototypical

Figure 14.11 Brain regions associated with risk Meta-analysis of a large number of fMRI studies indicated several brain regions consistently associated with both the anticipation of probabilistic rewards and decisions about probabilistic outcomes. Key regions identified include the anterior insula (aINS), the dorsomedial prefrontal cortex (dmPFC), and the posterior parietal cortex (not shown here). (From Mohr et al. 2010.)

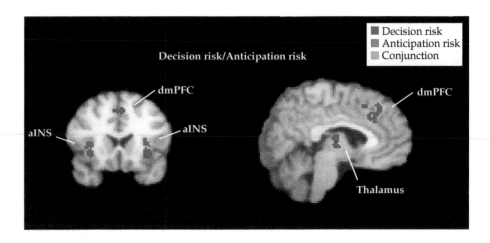

example of a risky decision, as are many sorts of investment allocations or consumer choices. Risk is often defined roughly as the estimated variance in potential outcomes, typically normalized by the magnitude of those outcomes. Thus, a coin flip between winning $20 and winning $0 might seem relatively risky, whereas a coin flip between winning $10,020 and winning $10,000 might seem very safe. Because of the ubiquity of risk in real-world choices, researchers studying the neural basis of risky decisions have used a diverse range of paradigms, leading to a broad array of brain regions being implicated in different aspects of risk processing.

Meta-analytic techniques (see Box 1A) can be used to identify brain regions whose activation tends to track the degree of risk present in a situation, in the absence of other confounding economic variables (e.g., intertemporal delay, social context). Four cortical regions have been identified as significantly associated with the risk of a decision: dorsolateral prefrontal cortex, dorsomedial prefrontal cortex, posterior parietal cortex, and the anterior insula (Figure 14.11). The first three of these reflect a subset of the regions discussed in Chapter 13 as critical for executive functions; that is, to deal with a risky choice, people may consistently engage particular executive functions that are not specific to risk itself. The anterior insula, however, is less often considered within the context of executive control, and more often discussed because of its contributions to emotional processing (see Chapter 10). Yet it has been consistently linked to risk not only in standard economic decisions, but also for the anticipation of probabilistic losses and gains. This result, and those of individual studies specifically implicating the anterior insula in decision making, suggests that the anterior insula is associated with the monitoring of aversive signals (e.g., interoceptive states) that push behavior away from risky options and toward greater certainty.

Within the other regions identified by this meta-analysis, some additional differentiation is possible. In executive function tasks that do not involve economic decision making, the psychological state of uncertainty leads to increased activation in the dorsomedial prefrontal cortex. Only particular types of uncertain decision making activate this region, however. When uncertainty reflects limited information about what decisions should be made in response to a stimulus, then the magnitude of dorsomedial prefrontal activation is proportional to the amount of uncertainty about the decision. But when the uncertainty of an outcome reflects a distribution of potential probabilistic outcomes (e.g., when rolling dice) but not different decisions, then activation does not increase with increasing risk. This dissociation is consistent with the perspective in

(A)   Lateral orbitofrontal cortex

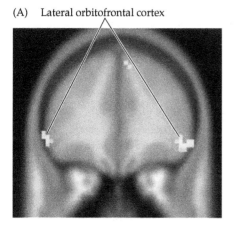

(B)   Lateral prefrontal cortex

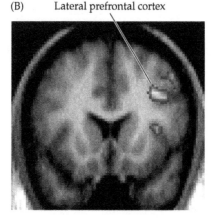

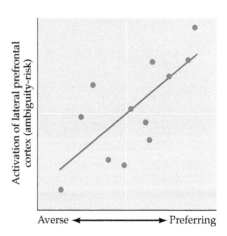

Activation of lateral prefrontal cortex (ambiguity–risk)

Averse ◄──────► Preferring

Figure 14.12   Decision making in the face of economic ambiguity Many people are averse to ambiguity, which is defined by economists as a situation in which one must make a decision without knowing the probabilities of the possible outcomes. (A) Compared to risk in decision making, ambiguity in decision making evokes increased activation in the orbitofrontal cortex, perhaps because of its aversiveness. (B) Ambiguity also evokes increased activation in lateral prefrontal cortex, which may reflect the need to think about the possible probabilities and to construct a decision rule. Supporting this latter interpretation, the magnitude of activation in the lateral prefrontal cortex during decision making under ambiguous circumstances depends on whether the subject prefers or is averse to ambiguity. (A from Hsu et al. 2005; B after Huettel et al. 2006.)

Chapter 13 that dorsomedial prefrontal cortex sends signals indicating that the surrounding environment has changed from what was expected, not simply that several outcomes could occur.

In contrast to risk, a decision involves ambiguity if the probabilities of its outcomes cannot be known. In typical laboratory tasks, ambiguity is evoked by eliminating people's ability to estimate probabilities. For example, someone completely unfamiliar with the game of cricket would not know which team to bet on, or even know how to think about the relevant factors. Many economic theorists consider risk and ambiguity to involve similar processes for subjective assessment of probability; others argue for a distinction between these categories. If clear differences were to emerge between the patterns of brain activation evoked by risk and by ambiguity—especially within regions critical for decision making—then cognitive neuroscience data could provide insight into new directions for research in economics. Research now indicates that this is indeed the case. In particular, ambiguity evokes increased activation in a region of posterior ventrolateral prefrontal cortex that had been previously associated with setting up rules for performing complex tasks (Figure 14.12).

Delay: Discounting future rewards

How strongly a person wants something often depends on the length of the delay until it can be obtained. In general, people judge rewards to be less valuable the farther in the future they will occur, and must overcome this **temporal discounting** tendency when saving for the future or avoiding impulse purchases. A paradox raised by temporal discounting is the development of time-inconsistent preferences. Most people prefer smaller immediate rewards to slightly larger delayed rewards. For example, people tend to prefer receiving $100 now (we'll call this Option A) compared to $110 a week from now (Option B). On the other hand, given the option of receiving $100 in 52 weeks (C) or $110 in 53 weeks (D), most people choose Option D. Preferring A over B but D over C reflects an inconsistency in choices; after 52 weeks, the second decision would

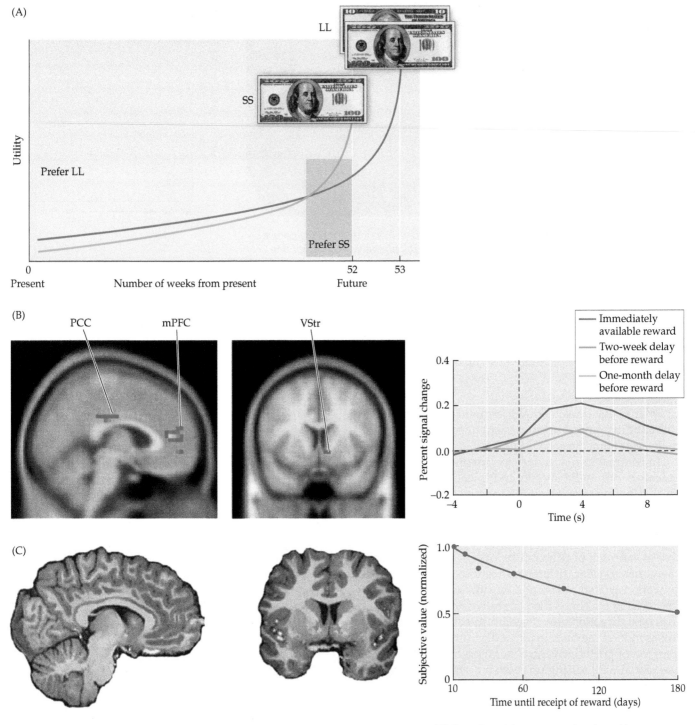

Figure 14.13 **Temporal discounting** (A) Data from laboratory and real-world experiments indicate that people's discount rate for money follows a hyperbolic function, with a very rapid increase in valuation for immediately available rewards. This function explains some paradoxes in choice behavior, including potential reversals from preferring larger, later (LL) rewards to preferring smaller, sooner (SS) rewards as those rewards become more immediate. (B) Analysis of decisions involving immediately available rewards revealed greater activation of reward-related regions, such as the ventral striatum (VStr), compared to decisions involving future rewards. mPFC, medial prefrontal cortex; PCC, posterior cingulate cortex. (C) A study using a different analysis method revealed that activation of the same regions tracked the subjective value of rewards, regardless of the time until delivery. (B after McClure et al. 2004; C after Kable and Glimcher 2007.)

become exactly the same situation as the first, so anyone who chooses A should also choose C. Behavioral anomalies of this sort have led to the development of models of hyperbolic discounting (Figure 14.13A), such that rewards are discounted very steeply over short time intervals, but more slowly over long time intervals. Cognitive neuroscientists, similarly, have investigated whether temporal discounting reflects the competitive interaction of two distinct neural processes (a **dual-system model**) or just a single neural process.

Dual-system models have a long history in psychology and economics. The most general form of such models—as advocated by Daniel Kahneman—posits two types of decision processes. System 1 is fast, parallel, automatic, and context-dependent. Emotionally guided decisions, as when people are tempted by an immediately available reward, are often linked to System 1. System 2 is slower, serial, controlled, and evidence-based. Decisions involving deliberation or cost-benefit analysis are often linked to System 2.

Whether a dual-system model is consistent with neural processing during intertemporal choice was investigated by functional brain imaging (Figure 14.13B). Choices that involved an immediate reward (i.e., money that could be received today) activated the ventral striatum and the medial and ventral prefrontal cortex, consistent with the postulated response of System 1. In contrast, lateral prefrontal cortex and other executive function regions were similarly active regardless of the delay until reward, as would be expected of System 2. This dissociation was interpreted to indicate that choices of short- or long-term rewards depend on the interaction between two systems, which were linked in this study to the dopaminergic reward system and lateral prefrontal cortex, respectively.

Subsequent studies, however, argued against the dual-process model of temporal discounting. An fMRI experiment using a similar design but different sorts of analyses showed that the magnitude of activation within reward-related regions tracked the subjective value of a reward regardless of its delay (Figure 14.13C). That is, the activation in those regions followed a function similar to hyperbolic discounting, with a very rapid decrease in people whose behavioral data indicated that they were very averse to waiting, but minimal decline in people who were very patient. This result supported a single-process model in which the reward system tracks the value of all potential outcomes, not just those available immediately.

As discussed later, in the section on integration, current cognitive research largely supports this second, single-process model, even though substantial evidence from behavioral economics and psychology exists for dual-process models (see Kahneman's engaging book, *Thinking, Fast and Slow*, cited in this chapter's Additional Reading section.) How could this discrepancy be reconciled? A useful perspective comes from the discussion of executive function introduced at the outset of Chapter 13. The hallmark of an executive function is that it modulates processes occurring elsewhere in the brain. Similarly, within temporal discounting, the role of the lateral prefrontal cortex (and other regions) may not be to compete with value-related regions, but to modulate activity within those regions. As one supporting example, repetitive TMS delivered to the lateral prefrontal cortex leads to a decrease in choices of a delayed option in an intertemporal choice task.

Social Context

Most of the decisions discussed so far involve the judgments and preferences of individuals acting in isolation. Many decisions, however, depend on information about other people. Consider, for example, a poker player who is dealt a good hand. Betting too much might scare potential opponents out of the game, and betting too little would minimize the potential winnings. To make good decisions, therefore, a player must evaluate not only his or her hand, but the effects of potential actions on the decisions of others. The following sections build on social cognitive functions introduced in Chapter 11 to consider how social information contributes to decisions across a range of contexts, from serving as highly motivating rewards to engendering future cooperation in interactive games.

Social rewards

It may seem self-evident that social stimuli reinforce a wide range of behaviors. Flip through almost any magazine, and you see smiling attractive faces and bodies in most advertisements. Marketers know that including appealing social images, even of unknown faces, increases interest in their products. Our daily interactions with others are shaped by social cues like smiles, glances, and gestures. The viability of charitable and nonprofit organizations, moreover, depends on our prosocial attitudes: many people show a remarkable willingness to donate money and time for the benefit of others, even individuals whom they will never meet.

Given these common experiences, it may seem unsurprising that social stimuli such as attractive faces robustly evoke activation in reward-related regions like the ventral striatum and ventromedial prefrontal cortex. Such responses are not merely associated with physical features, however, like those associated with attractiveness. Information about social relationships also contributes, often in complex ways. When monkeys are trained in a simple "pay-per-view" task that involves trade-offs between juice rewards (e.g., larger and smaller quantities) and social rewards (e.g., photographs of different monkeys in their social group), they are willing to forgo appreciable amounts of juice to view important social images (Figure 14.14).

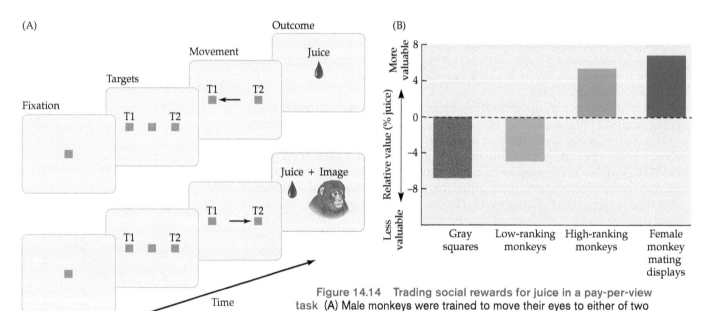

Figure 14.14 Trading social rewards for juice in a pay-per-view task (A) Male monkeys were trained to move their eyes to either of two targets. Movements to one target (T1) led to a juice reward; movements to the other target (T2) led to a juice reward and the opportunity to view an image of the face of another monkey in the same social group, of a female monkey mating display, or of a neutral gray square. The amount of juice associated with each movement was varied across blocks, so that the researchers could calculate the relative value (in juice) associated with each sort of image. (B) Monkeys were willing to give up substantial amounts of juice to view the female monkey mating displays or high-ranking male monkeys, but required additional juice payments to view low-ranking male monkeys or the gray square. (After Deaner et al. 2005.)

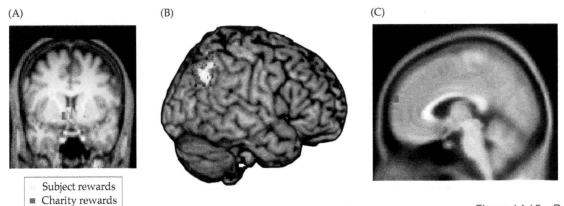

(A)
(B)
(C)

Subject rewards
Charity rewards
Overlap

Figure 14.15 Brain regions associated with prosocial behavior (A) Activation of the ventral striatum is evoked both when fMRI participants receive money for themselves and when money is allocated to a respected charitable cause. (B) Activation of the lateral parietal cortex increases when people engage in social cognition tasks: identifying other people, tracking actions of other agents in the environment, or simulate the thoughts of others. The magnitude of lateral parietal cortex activation in a simple social cognition task predicts individual differences in self-reported altruism. (C) The medial prefrontal cortex (mPFC) has been implicated in a variety of processes related to mentalizing, or thinking about others' mental states. Activation in the mPFC during charitable giving tasks predicts the altruistic donation of money or time helping others. (A from Harbaugh et al. 2007; B from Tankersley et al. 2007; C from Waytz et al. 2012.)

Rewards experienced by others also constitute an important class of social stimuli. Such rewards can have striking influences on behavior, as when people donate money to a charity that delivers food or medicine to a distant foreign country—even though the donors may never visit that country, much less meet the specific recipients of their gifts. Broadly considered, two, nonexclusive theories have been proposed to explain prosocial behavior of this sort—both now supported by cognitive neuroscience data.

The first theory proposes that charitable giving is motivated by internal reward signals—sometimes called the "warm glow" of giving—that reinforce that behavior, despite its cost. Several studies now link activation of the ventral striatum, in particular, to giving to a desirable charity (Figure 14.15A). The second theory contends that prosocial behavior requires social cognition processes that recognize another individual's needs, as a prerequisite for actions to help that individual (Figure 14.15B,C). Research now shows that several brain regions associated with social cognition (see Chapter 11), including the lateral parietal cortex and medial frontal cortex, predict the degree to which an individual will engage in altruistic behavior toward others.

Social cooperation

Decision making can quickly become complex when multiple individuals are involved, each with limited information and different preferences. The branch of decision science that studies how decisions are made in such circumstances is known as **game theory**, in part because many of its concepts can be easily expressed as simple interpersonal games (Figure 14.16). Most games can be formalized in terms of a payoff matrix that plots the possible choices of each player along its axes and the outcomes for each player in its cells. Such games provide a natural framework for studying cooperative behavior.

When the game known as the *prisoner's dilemma* (see Figure 14.16A) is repeated over many trials, consistent cooperation by the two players yields the best mutual outcome. Although defection makes more money for a player on any given trial, it often causes the opponent to defect as well, lowering the total amount earned. Functional neuroimaging studies of the prisoner's dilemma game have suggested that cooperation itself evokes activation in the nucleus accumbens, among other reward-related regions. An intuitive explanation of this result is that repeated cooperation is experienced as rewarding by research participants. Yet, as discussed earlier in the chapter, activity of the neurons in the nucleus accumbens (and other reward-related regions) tends to be more associated with *information* about future rewards than with the experience of current rewards.

(A) Prisoner's dilemma

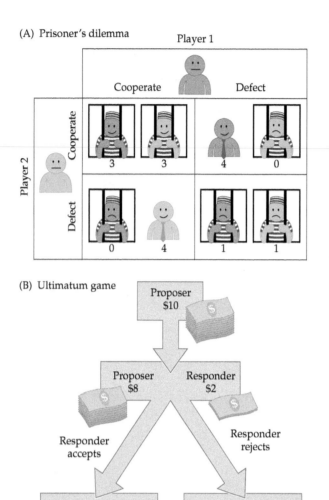

(B) Ultimatum game

(C) Trust game

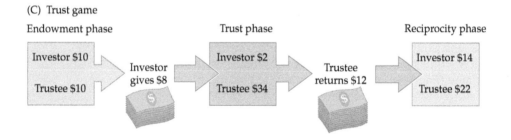

Figure 14.16 **Some commonly studied games** (A) The prisoner's dilemma. The terms *cooperate* and *defect*, typically used in descriptions of this game situation, refer, respectively, to cooperating with the partner by remaining quiet or defecting to the police by confessing. The numbers below each person indicate the personal utility of that outcome, from 4 ("going free") to 0 ("longest sentence"). (B) The ultimatum game. One player (the proposer) is given a sum of money (e.g., $10) that he may divide between himself and another player (the responder). The responder then decides to accept the division or reject it. If the division is rejected, neither player receives anything at all. (C) The trust game. The two players start the game with equal sums of money. The investor can keep the money or give any fraction of it to the trustee, whereupon the money is multiplied by some factor (e.g., tripling in value). The trustee then decides how much of the total amount to return to the investor.

Cooperation, instead, may predict increased reward on future trials, through the development of trust. An intriguing approach to studying cooperative behavior has been the simultaneous recording of fMRI data from individuals in two scanners who are playing a game against each other. This approach, called **hyperscanning** (Figure 14.17A), allows behavioral and brain changes in one individual to be predicted from the behavioral and brain changes in another individual. Data from a multiple-round *trust game* (see Figure 14.16C) show that activation in the caudate (dorsal striatum) seems to signal an intention to subsequently trust one's opponent (Figure 14.17B–D). In early rounds of the game, activation of the trustee's caudate increases after the trustee's opponent invests money; that is, the brain responses occur following a cooperative action. Once trust has been established in later rounds, however, the caudate is activated earlier in the trial; it now anticipates the later cooperation.

This change from reactive to anticipatory activity in the caudate has been interpreted as the building of a model about the opponent, which then can be used to decide whether to trust that person. A hyperscanning approach has been used subsequently to demonstrate that the pattern of activation within the cingulate gyrus, which is linked to evaluations of the need for cognitive

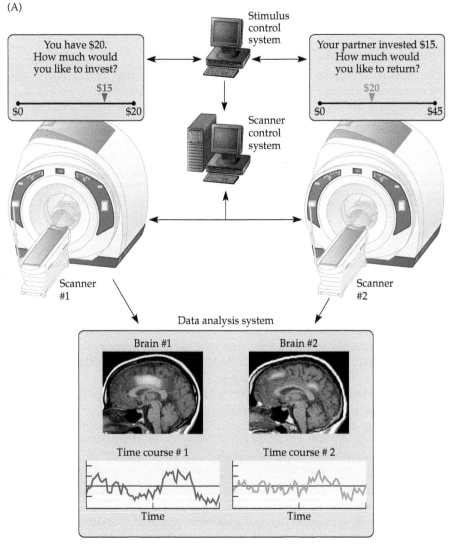

(A)

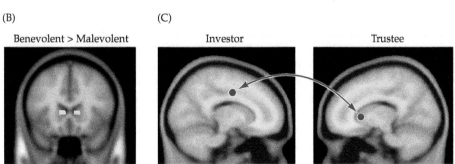

(B) Benevolent > Malevolent

(C) Investor   Trustee

Figure 14.17 **The neural correlates of trust in decision making** (A) By recording fMRI data simultaneously from two individuals playing a competitive game—an approach called *hyperscanning*—researchers can use brain signals observed in one individual to predict similar signals observed in another individual. (B) A variety of socially rewarding actions activate the basal ganglia, specifically in the head of the caudate nucleus. Shown here are voxels that exhibited greater fMRI activation to benevolent, cooperative actions than to malevolent, selfish actions in an investment game. (C) The researchers recorded fMRI data from the investor and the trustee simultaneously, examining the relations between fMRI activation in the cingulate cortex of the investor and in the caudate of the trustee. (D) On early trials, activation in the trustee lagged activation in the investor by about 16 to 18 seconds, which corresponds to the delay between the investor's decision and the trustee's decision. But after the two people had played the game six times, the trustee's brain shifted earlier in time (arrows indicate the time lag with maximal correlation). The authors interpreted this change as reflecting the developing intention to trust, based on an expectation of fair behavior by the opponent. (B–D after King-Casas et al. 2005.)

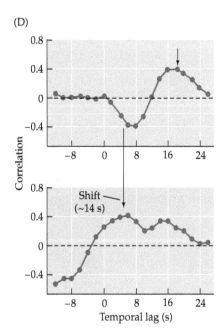

(D)

control, differs between evaluation of one's own decisions and presentation of the opponent's decisions.

Whether to cooperate depends on how well one can predict another person's goals. In several neuroimaging studies, subjects played the same game against human and computer opponents. When playing against computer opponents—and knowing that their opponents are computers—subjects are much less likely to evaluate the reasoning behind an opponent's actions or to retaliate against unfair behavior. Consistent with these behavioral effects, decision making in games against computers is often accompanied by reduced activation in brain regions associated with reward or social cognition. Decision making does not depend simply on the available choices and potential outcomes, but on how one interprets others' actions and uses that information to guide one's own decisions.

Social punishment

A key contributor to social cohesion comes from censuring people who violate social norms—a phenomenon known as **altruistic punishment**. Suppose that you anonymously observe two people playing an interactive game, like the trust game described in the previous section; you can watch them, but they do not know anything about you. After cooperating well for some time, the trustee suddenly decides to take all of the money for that trial, leaving the investor with nothing. The rules of the game give you the option to punish the trustee; if you give up $5 of your own money, you will reduce the trustee's earnings by $20. Do you sacrifice your money to punish another person—even if you will never interact with that person again in the future? In an fMRI study of this sort of game, increased activation is observed in the ventral striatum when subjects can altruistically punish their opponents, and that activation increases in subjects who are willing to spend more money to exert greater punishment.

In another class of games that has been particularly well studied, resources are allocated by one decision maker and accepted by another. A classic example is the *ultimatum game* (see Figure 14.16B), in which one player proposes a division of a pot of money, and the other player responds to that division by accepting the offer (in which case the money is split accordingly) or rejecting it (in which case no one gets any money). A purely rational responder would accept any offer, no matter how small, because rejecting it results in no money at all. Yet many studies have shown that responders tend to reject offers that they deem unfair, even when relatively large stakes are involved (e.g., being offered $40 out of a total of $200). Rejecting unfair offers has been interpreted as a way of censuring antisocial behavior—and the risk of rejection pushes people toward making more fair offers in the first place.

Unfair offers in the ultimatum game have been linked to activation in the insular cortex. Moreover, insular activation increases with the perceived amount of unfairness in the offer, and it is greater for offers that will be rejected later. In contrast, activation in the dorsolateral prefrontal cortex was relatively consistent across conditions in one study, regardless of whether an offer was rejected. These results were initially interpreted as supporting the dual-system framework introduced earlier in the chapter: the insular activation provides an emotional signal that can override a more rational evaluation of the outcomes in dorsolateral prefrontal cortex. That the insular cortex supports processing of the affective components of complex decisions has indeed been supported by a range of other work, both on risky decision making (see Figure 14.11) and on emotional processing more generally (see Chapter 10). However, other work challenges the idea that dorsolateral prefrontal cortex supports the rational evaluation of outcomes. Application of TMS to lateral prefrontal cortex caused acceptance rates to increase; that is, when this region was disrupted, participants' choice became more consistent with rational economic models

(A)

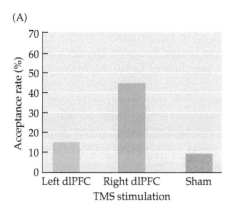

(B)

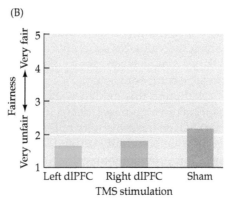

Figure 14.18 Disruption of processing in dorsolateral prefrontal cortex (DLPFC) increases acceptance of unfair offers in the ultimatum game Participants played an ultimatum game while receiving transcranial magnetic stimulation (TMS) to either the left dlPFC or the right dlPFC, or a sham TMS session that simulated the experience of TMS without delivering magnetic fields. (A) When participants were offered an unfair division of money (i.e., they would receive 4 Swiss Francs, while their partner would receive 16), they tended to reject those offers following sham stimulation or stimulation of left dlPFC. Following stimulation of right dlPFC, however, they were much more likely to accept those unfair offers. (B) TMS did not alter the participants' judgments of fairness; those offers were still seen as very unfair, regardless of stimulation condition. (After Knoch et al. 2006.)

(Figure 14.18). Such results led to the different conclusion that lateral prefrontal cortex supports not economic rationality, but self-control (see Chapter 13).

Integration: Combining and Comparing Information to Reach a Decision

Some of the most difficult kinds of decisions arise when we must compare very different sorts of outcomes. How do we decide which is more valuable: the experience of having dinner with friends at a nice restaurant or the money we would save by eating at home alone? Which would be a better use of an unexpected windfall: buying a new car or going on a long-awaited vacation? Decisions of this sort are much more complex than the simple financial choices described earlier. They involve not only rewards, risk, and social components, but also some sort of comparison across categories, as when we consider the relative value of an experience (e.g., a vacation) versus a practical and physical good (e.g., a car). Such cross-category decisions are especially challenging, as evident in the common lament about "comparing apples and oranges" or in the Latin maxim *de gustibus non est disputandum* ("tastes are not disputable").

Despite the many practical and experimental challenges, there has been substantial progress in understanding how different contributors to subjective value are integrated into a decision. Initial research focused on integration within simple perceptual tasks; more recent studies have examined more complex tasks involving economic choice. In both sorts of tasks, key advances came from the identification of neurons whose activity tracked the subjective value of a stimulus, independently of the specific factors that contributed to that value. Such a general response to value has become known as a *common currency signal* used by the brain.

Perceptual decision making

Early research showed that different contributors to the value of an action—such as the probability that it would be rewarded or the magnitude of potential rewards—were integrated into a common representation of value within regions of the brain associated with action selection. The first single-unit recording study of the effects of value on decision making was conducted in monkeys by neurobiologists Michael Platt and Paul Glimcher. As introduced in Chapter 5, they chose to record in a region of the parietal lobes called the **lateral intraparietal area** (**LIP**) because that region had been theorized to represent a nexus between low-level attentional signals and high-level motor outputs. Expected value had a marked effect on neurons in this region (see Figure 5.16). The firing rate increased to stimuli associated with larger or more probable rewards, especially early in the trials, before the monkey could execute a particular motor plan. Subsequent work from these and other investigators has now elucidated some of the functions of this region. When monkeys are placed in a simulated foraging task, in which the values of different responses change dynamically, the activation of LIP neurons also changes dynamically as a function of the relative value of the possible courses of action.

Although this evidence shows that area LIP is important in at least some aspects of value-based decision making, its specific contributions are not yet clear. Given the sensitivity of this region to visuospatial input and to eye movements, one possibility is that LIP activation is specific to that particular motor system (i.e., oculomotor control). Some evidence for this idea is provided by the observation that manipulating the probability of reward in an eye-movement task also influences the activity of neurons within the superior colliculus, a structure directly concerned with the control of eye movements. More generally, LIP activity might reflect the transformation of value to action, consistent with demonstrations that LIP neurons track short-term fluctuations in the value of different response options. This latter perspective is consistent with neuroimaging studies showing that the parietal cortex supports the generation and modification of rules for action (see Chapter 13). Subsequent work has indicated that multiple areas within both prefrontal and parietal cortex support the integration of sensory and value information in advance of a decision.

The integration of information relevant to a decision has been harder to study with functional neuroimaging because of the spatial coarseness of the relevant data. However, researchers have had some success using perceptual categories that elicit significantly different regional activations, such as in the different object category regions within the ventral temporal lobe. Photographs of faces and houses provide a natural pair of categories; and if sufficient noise is introduced, they can be made difficult to discriminate. When subjects make decisions about whether a given stimulus is a face or a house, activation in the ventral temporal lobe increases in the stimulus-appropriate regions proportional to the clarity of the stimulus. However, concurrent activation is observed along the superior frontal sulcus in the dorsolateral prefrontal cortex that is independent of stimulus category, and greatest for simple discriminations (Figure 14.19). In contrast, regions supporting processes related to attentional or cognitive control are more active for difficult discriminations.

A major catalyst for research on perceptual decision making has been the development of **drift-diffusion models** (also called *diffusion decision models*). As the name implies, these models assume that the decision process is a random-walk process (*drift*) from a neutral state toward thresholds for action. Such models can

Figure 14.19 The prefrontal cortex integrates information in perceptual decisions When subjects make decisions about whether a given stimulus is a face or a house, activation increases in the stimulus-appropriate regions. (A) Activation of a region of the left dorsolateral prefrontal cortex (dlPFC) was correlated with activation of a face-selective region in the fusiform gyrus and a place-selective region in the parahippocampal gyrus. (B) When activity increased in the relevant region of the dlPFC, subjects tended to be correct in their decisions. When activity was reduced, subjects were often incorrect. These results suggest that this region is important for integrating perceptual information to reach a useful decision. (After Heekeren et al. 2004.)

(A)

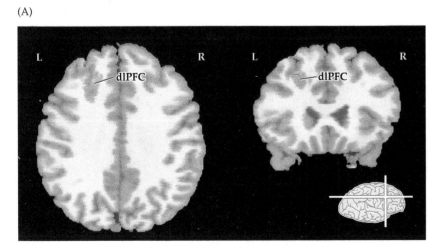

(B)

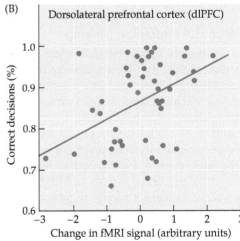

quantitatively separate several contributors to information integration: the rate of information accumulation, the confidence needed to reach a decision, and the relative bias toward one option or another. Though originally developed to explain features of response time distributions found in psychological research, these models have now been applied with great success to both single-unit and fMRI data (**Box 14B**).

Value-based decision making

The challenge in understanding value integration comes into sharper focus when considering a simple consumer purchase like putting a few coins into a vending machine to buy a soda. Within that single transaction are two very different sorts of rewards. Monetary rewards are abstract, highly portable, able to be aggregated or divided arbitrarily, storable for long periods, and have value only through trades for other goods and services. A can of soda has tangible biological value through the calories and fluid it provides, has a limited life span, cannot be aggregated or divided, and generates a range of sensory and affective states when consumed. Yet despite these differences, we have no trouble deciding whether to sacrifice a given amount of money for a given amount of soda. Current models of value-based decision making posit that the brain compares rewards with very different properties by encoding information about each reward into abstracted value signals that can then be compared computationally. Some evidence now supports the idea that neuronal circuitry coding for reward value independent of modality (i.e., a common currency for reward) is located within the ventral prefrontal cortex.

Damage to the ventral prefrontal cortex has been long recognized to impair self-control (see Chapter 13). In the early 1990s, however, research by neuroscientists Antoine Bechara, Antonio Damasio, and their colleagues showed that patients with ventromedial prefrontal damage were relatively insensitive to negative feedback in economic decision making. When performing the **Iowa Gambling Task** (**Figure 14.20A**), for instance, these patients persistently select the decks with a negative expected value, despite their accumulating monetary losses. In addition, when selecting the bad decks, unlike normal individuals these patients exhibit no anticipatory skin conductance response (see Chapter 10 for discussion of the somatic marker hypothesis). The researchers interpreted these results to mean that damage to the ventromedial prefrontal cortex makes patients insensitive to bodily signals about the risk or safety of upcoming choices; thus, patients' behavior is driven by the frequent large gains, whereas neurologically normal individuals learn from the infrequent losses.

Supporting this conclusion, subsequent studies showed that these patients failed to demonstrate regret following losses in gambling tasks. In one striking example (**Figure 14.20B**), patients with damage to ventromedial prefrontal cortex actually performed much better than did neurologically normal controls in a probabilistic investment task; unlike control subjects, who tended to become conservative after losses, the patients were just as willing to take risks following losses

Figure 14.20 Changes in decision-making behavior following brain lesions (A) The Iowa Gambling Task was developed by Antoine Bechara, Antonio Damasio, and their colleagues to characterize deficits in decision making shown by some clinical patients. Participants in this task are presented with four decks of cards. Decks A and B have large hypothetical rewards (e.g., $100) on every card, but also infrequent very large losses—leading to a negative expected value. Decks C and D are associated with small rewards (e.g., $50) on every card but only small losses on some of the cards—leading to a positive expected value. Neurologically normal adults learn over time to choose primarily from the good decks, while patients with damage to ventromedial prefrontal cortex (VM patients) do not. (B) In a simple betting game, neurologically normal individuals tended to become more risk-averse over time, particularly following losing bets. Patients with damage to ventromedial prefrontal cortex, insular cortex, and related regions (target patients) did not show this pattern, remaining relatively risk-neutral over the course of the experiment. Such patients, but not control patients with damage in other regions, tended to earn more money in the game than did individuals without brain damage. (A after Bechara et al. 2000; B after Shiv et al. 2005.)

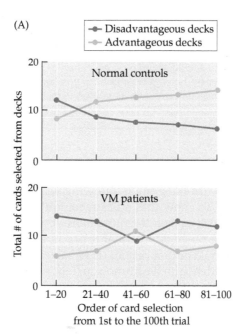

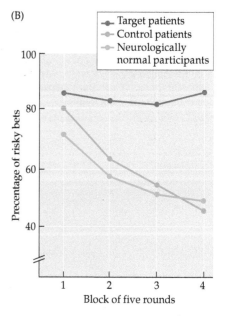

■ BOX 14B MODELING SIMPLE DECISIONS

Imagine walking up to the counter in a coffee shop. You order your regular espresso and then look down and see two pastries, one chocolate and the other fruit-filled. You pause, your eyes flit back and forth between them, and after a few seconds you select one of the two options. This seems like such a simple decision, in that it has only two options and takes only a short time to complete. But that surface simplicity belies a surprisingly complex decision process. From the outset, you might have a particular bias toward one option. As the decision process unfolds, your brain accumulates information in favor of each option, drawing upon both the current sensory experience and your memories for past events. In addition, you have to balance the competing goals of choosing the best option and making the decision quickly. Researchers studying simple decisions of this sort have sought answers to two sorts of questions: What does the decision maker choose? And how long does it take to make that choice? The answers to these two questions turn out, perhaps surprisingly, to be interrelated.

The coffee shop decision described here shares many features with the simple perceptual-motor decisions introduced in Chapter 5 (see Box 5C). In the perceptual-motor task, the participant—typically, a monkey undergoing single-unit recording—watches a display containing a number of flashing dots. On test trials, a small fraction of the dots will move coherently to either the left or right. If the monkey moves its eyes in the corresponding direction, it receives a small juice reward. While the monkey is watching the dot motion, the activity of neurons in the motion-sensitive region MT is greater for highly coherent displays than it is for less coherent displays.

(A)

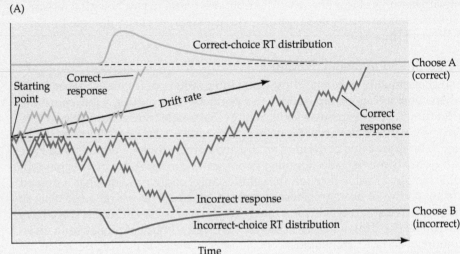

Drift-diffusion modeling. (A) In the drift-diffusion model, information integration is simulated by a random-walk process that begins at a starting point (center line) and then drifts toward one of two thresholds. Here, the upper threshold corresponds to a correct choice (e.g., in the dot motion paradigm, choosing "left" when the dots are moving to the left), and the lower threshold corresponds to an incorrect choice. Even though sensory information tends to be biased toward the upper, correct threshold (based on the drift rate), the noise in processing may lead to drift to the lower, incorrect threshold on some trials. RT, response time. (After Ratcliff and McKoon 2008.)

How might information from sensory regions (e.g., MT) be integrated to facilitate a decision? The drift-diffusion modeling mentioned in the text provides an elegant explanation for several aspects of simple two-option decisions. The core assumption of the drift-diffusion model is that, during a decision, information continually accumulates from a neutral starting point toward either of two response thresholds (Figure A). As the model name implies, the information accumulation process consists of a noisy, random-walk drift. Information consistent with one alternative (e.g., dots moving to the right) biases the drift toward the associated threshold, with the rate of drift proportional to the quality of the evidence (e.g., faster drift for more coherent dot motion). If a decision maker becomes more cautious (i.e., requires more evidence before making a decision), then the thresholds move farther from the starting point, thereby predicting that decisions will have slower response times but also be more accurate. This model can explain core properties of decision behavior, such as how probability and stimulus similarity affect both choices and response time distributions.

A strong prediction of the drift-diffusion approach is that decisions are made—

as they were following wins. Taken together, these studies suggest a deficit in reward integration following ventral prefrontal damage.

To show that a brain region actually codes a common currency signal, however, would require more specific evidence: its neurons should be sensitive to a range of potential rewards, and the relative firing rate to a given reward should be proportional to its subjective value. The brain region with the strongest evidence for a common currency signal is the orbitofrontal cortex, particularly within its ventromedial aspect. Neurons in this region respond to a range of

■ BOX 14B (continued)

and a motor action executed—when the amount of accumulated information passes a particular threshold. For an oculomotor decision like moving the eyes in response to the coherence of moving dots, the activity of neurons in the brain region LIP is consistent with that prediction. Beginning with the onset of dot motion, there is a gradual increase in the activity

of LIP neurons if the stimulus information indicates a movement toward a location in the cells' receptive field, with more rapid increases in firing rate when the motion is more coherent (Figure B, left panel). If the same responses from the same neurons are now aligned to the onset of the movement (Figure B, right panel), then a striking consistency is revealed: as soon as the

firing rate passes a threshold of about 65 spikes per second, the monkey initiates the eye movement.

While the temporal resolution of fMRI is too coarse for tracking the dynamic changes in brain response during the information integration process, that technique can identify regions whose overall activation on a trial is consistent with the predictions of a drift-diffusion model. Using such a model-based approach implicates the posterior parietal cortex (including a region that may correspond to LIP) and the dorsomedial prefrontal cortex as particularly important in integration during simple decision making. Combining fMRI with high-temporal resolution approaches, like MEG or EEG, has shown promise for elucidating the specific contributions of parietal and prefrontal cortices to the choice process.

A firing-rate threshold in area LIP neurons predicts the initiation of decisions. (B) The data here come from single-unit recording in monkeys during the dot motion paradigm introduced in Chapter 5. Each line represents the average activity of LIP neurons to moving dots of a given coherence, with solid lines indicating movements into the neurons' receptive fields and dashed lines indicating movements away. The neurons' firing rate tends to increase more rapidly when the dot motion is more coherent (left panel). If the same data are now time-locked to the motor movement (right panel), all of the curves overlap immediately before the movement, such that the movement is initiated when the firing rate reaches a particular threshold. This consistency supports the idea that LIP neurons integrate signals about motion coherence—from area MT and other visual regions—in order to accumulate evidence in favor of specific motor movements. (After Roitman and Shadlen 2002.)

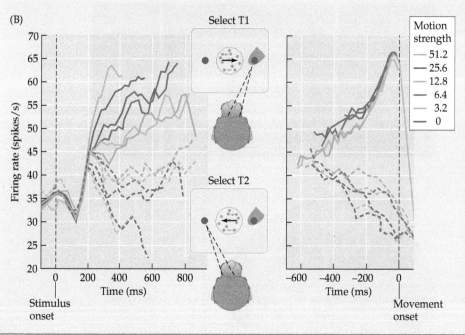

References

HARE, T. A., W. SCHULTZ, C. F. CAM-ERER, J. P. O'DOHERTY AND A. RANGEL (2011) Transformation of stimulus value signals into motor commands during simple choice. *Proc. Natl. Acad. Sci. USA* 108: 18120–18125.

HUNT, L. T., N. KOLLING, A. SOLTANI, M. W. WOOLRICH, M. F. S. RUSHWORTH AND T. E. J. BEHRENS (2012) Mechanisms underlying cortical activity during value-guided choice. *Nat. Neurosci.* 15: 470–476.

RATCLIFF, R. AND G. MCKOON (2008) The diffusion decision model: Theory and data for two-choice decision tasks. *Neural Comput.* 20: 873–922.

ROITMAN, J. D. AND M. N. SHADLEN (2002) Response of neurons in the lateral intraparietal area during a combined visual discrimination reaction time task. *J. Neurosci.* 22: 9475–9489.

rewards, such as typical fluid rewards for monkeys, like juices, water, milk, or tea. Moreover, the firing rate of those neurons tracks the subjective value of a chosen option in simple decision making (**Figure 14.21**).

More recent research using fMRI in humans has dramatically expanded the range of paradigms that can be used to test the common currency hypothesis. A number of studies by neuroeconomist Antonio Rangel and his colleagues have shown that ventral prefrontal activation tracks the subjective value of decision options. A typical paradigm in these studies presents a large number

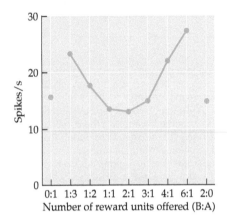

Figure 14.21   Responses of orbitofrontal cortex neurons to the value of fluid rewards Monkeys were given a series of choices between cues that predicted well-learned rewards. For example, Cue A might predict grape juice while Cue B might predict water. Behavioral testing was used to quantify the relative value of each reward type, such that a monkey might prefer grape juice over water if their quantities were equal, but prefer to get two units of water instead of one unit of grape juice. Single-unit recordings revealed that the activity of neurons in the orbitofrontal cortex tracked the relative value of rewards, not the rewards themselves. (After Padoa-Schioppa and Assad 2006.)

of consumer goods (e.g., inexpensive snacks like candy bars) and asks the participants to indicate how much money they would be willing to pay for each good. Following the experiment, one or more of those goods are selected randomly for potential sale to the participant, based on the reported subjective value (i.e., their "willingness to pay" for the good). Activation in a specific region of posterior ventromedial prefrontal cortex increases with increased subjective value, for a range of goods and experiences (Figure 14.22A), even when goods are being passively viewed without an overt decision (Figure 14.22B).

(A)

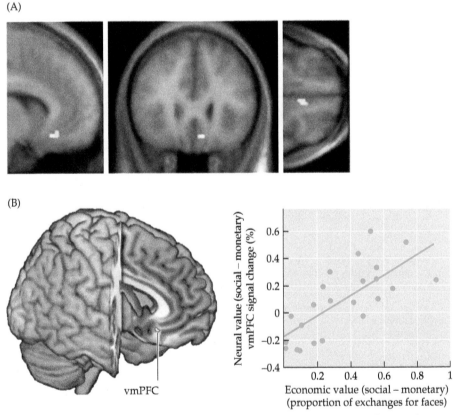

(B)

Figure 14.22   Activation in posterior ventromedial prefrontal cortex (vmPFC) is associated with willingness to pay (A) A number of studies have implicated the posterior part of the ventromedial prefrontal cortex in decision value. Specifically, when people make simple consumer choices—here, what to pay for candy bars and other snack items—activation in the posterior vmPFC tracks the amount of money people are willing to pay for a given item. (B) This property extends to non–consumer goods as well. When individuals passively viewed a series of faces and passively received monetary rewards, their relative brain responses to those social and monetary rewards predicted their later decisions about trading one type of reward for another. (A from Plassmann et al. 2007; B after Smith et al. 2010.)

Heuristics in Decision Making

As already noted, decision makers do not always approach choices with a rational weighing of costs and benefits. Many decisions are made by following rules, referred to as **heuristics**, that allow people to simplify a complex decision situation into something more tractable. Suppose that you are traveling to a city for the first time and you need to find a place to eat dinner. There are two nearby restaurants, about which you know nothing—save that you've heard of one but not the other. Which restaurant do you choose? In situations analogous to this one, most people choose the familiar option. Doing so turns out to be a relatively fast and efficient approach to decision making, because familiarity tends to be correlated with popularity and other positive qualities. But, using a familiarity heuristic will not work in all situations: some well-known restaurants might be of low quality, while newer or less well-known restaurants might serve much better food. As this example illustrates, we use heuristics because they tend to work well in many situations, although they can be misleading in others.

The idea that heuristics play an important role in decision making was first popularized by economist and psychologist Herbert Simon in the 1950s. Simon recognized that organisms have finite computational resources—what he called **bounded rationality**—and must often make decisions under time constraints, rendering rational consideration impractical or even impossible. An example is shopping for food at a grocery store. A typical shopper does not analyze the advantages and disadvantages of all possible options, but instead adopts a much simpler strategy that identifies an important feature such as price, selects a few candidate items to examine secondary features, and then buys the item that is most acceptable. Such decisions involve determination not of the optimal choice, but of a choice that is simply "good enough." Simon called this heuristic **satisficing**, a neologism that combines *satisfy* and *suffice*.

Some heuristics are linked to the concepts of reward evaluation introduced earlier. The **anchoring heuristic** refers to the tendency of reference points to bias subsequent value judgments. If people are asked to estimate an unknown quantity (e.g., "How many countries from the continent of Africa are in the United Nations?"), their estimates are lower when they are given a low value as a reference point (e.g., "Is it more or less than 10? Estimate how many.") compared to when they are given a high value as a reference. Marketers rely on this effect when pricing luxury goods, which are often labeled with inflated "suggested retail prices" that are then discounted within a store. Accordingly, telling people that the wine they are drinking is expensive increases activation in ventromedial prefrontal cortex, compared to labeling the same wine as inexpensive. Moreover, the magnitude of the anchoring effect for a given person is predicted by the difference in activation between the two labeled values.

In the related **endowment effect**, people require more money when they are selling something they own than they would be willing to spend to buy an identical good. For example, participants in a laboratory experiment who were handed coffee mugs might state that they would sell the mugs for only $7; but other participants (chosen randomly) might state that they would pay only $4 for such mugs. The magnitude of the endowment effect across individuals has been shown to co-vary with how well the ventral striatum tracks price discrepancies. These and similar heuristics are consistent with the perspective that key reward-related brain regions respond to changes in reward from a reference point, not absolute values of reward.

Other heuristics involve strategies for setting up and evaluating a decision problem, and in many ways they are similar to concepts introduced in Chapter 13. People tend to be relatively risk-averse when cued to think about what could

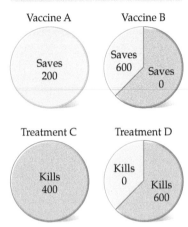

You are trying to halt the spread of a disease in a village of 600 people.

Vaccine A — Saves 200

Vaccine B — Saves 600 / Saves 0

Treatment C — Kills 400

Treatment D — Kills 0 / Kills 600

Figure 14.23 **Framing effects in decision making** (A) Framing effects. Suppose you are a physician trying to halt the spread of a fatal disease with two vaccines: a proven one that will save 200 of 600 villagers (Vaccine A), and an untested one that has a 33 percent chance of saving all 600 and a 67 percent chance of saving none (Vaccine B). Which do you choose? Now suppose instead that you have two therapeutic options for the disease: a known treatment that definitely will kill 67 percent of the villagers (Treatment C), and an untested one that has a 33 percent chance of killing none and a 67 percent chance of killing them all (Treatment D). Again, which do you choose? Most people choose the vaccine that will save 200 people for sure (Vaccine A) and the therapeutic intervention that has a chance of killing no one (Treatment D). Note, however, that the two decision situations are identical, with Vaccine A equivalent to Treatment C, and Vaccine B equivalent to Treatment D; the only difference is that one is framed in terms of saving and the other in terms of killing.

be gained from an action, but relatively risk-seeking when cued to think about what could be lost (Figure 14.23). This **framing effect** occurs even when the actual outcomes are kept constant. For instance, people shift their planned retirement date by as much as several years depending on whether the instructions frame waiting as a loss (i.e., forgone benefits for a number of years) or as a gain (i.e., higher annual income). Simple changes in the instructions can shift financial choices that involve many thousands of dollars. Because of the potential power of framing effects for shaping real-world behavior, there has been substantial interest in the computational algorithms that generate framing effects, as well as in the brain systems involved.

Decisions inconsistent with the framing effect have been shown to evoke increased activation in dorsomedial prefrontal cortex and the amygdala (Figure 14.24). Specifically, activation in these regions is highest when people are cued to think about monetary gains but are still risk-seeking, or when people are cued to think about monetary losses but are still risk-averse. An initial interpretation of these results is that emotional processes can occasionally intervene in risky decisions, leading to irrational biases like framing.

This interpretation—at least with regard to the dorsomedial prefrontal cortex—has been called into question by subsequent work on other heuristics. If a decision option could lead to a complex set of monetary gains and losses (e.g., equal chances of $80, $27, $10, –$40, or –$90), some people use a rational analytic approach like calculating the expected utility of each option by multiplying each outcome by its probability. Others, however, tend to use a heuristic, simplifying outcomes as either "good" or "bad" compared to a particular aspiration level (in this example, for instance, three outcomes are good and two are bad). For

Figure 14.24 **Activation in dorsomedial prefrontal cortex (dmPFC) associated with counterframe choices** (A) Within an economic version of a framing task, activation in the dmPFC increases when people make choices that run opposite of the normal framing effect. (B) There is increased activation when people choose risky options for decisions that are described in terms of monetary gains. But when the same decisions are instead described in terms of monetary losses, activation in the dmPFC is greater when people make safer choices. (After De Martino et al. 2006.)

(A)

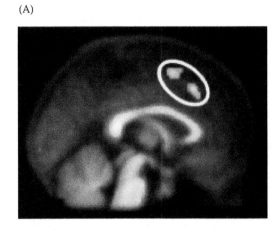

(B)

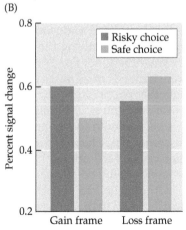

both sorts of people, activation in dorsomedial prefrontal cortex is observed when they use a decision strategy different from their usual tendency. This result suggests that the dorsomedial prefrontal cortex contributes not to any particular heuristic, but to executive processes associated with changing from one heuristic to another.

In summary, we and many other animals make decisions in many real-world situations by using heuristics rather than by making more reflective, calculated choices. Heuristics usually work to our advantage because they are statistically valid across a wide range of situations; but for the same reason, they often lead to wrong choices, as seen in the examples illustrated.

Future Directions

To create satisfactory models of decision making will require the synthesis of concepts from economics, psychology, and neuroscience. Popular accounts, however, often gloss over the limitations and difficulties associated with integrating these diverse fields, proffering breathless headlines such as "Researchers Discover Why Some People Seek Out Risks," or "Scientists Find the Part of the Brain That Makes People Cooperate" (Figure 14.25). These sorts of reports are at best a mixed blessing; they promote new and exciting research but encourage the fallacy of **neurorealism**, which is the tendency to regard brain measurements associated with conclusions about behavior as more real and convincing than they are. Neuroscience will not supplant other approaches for

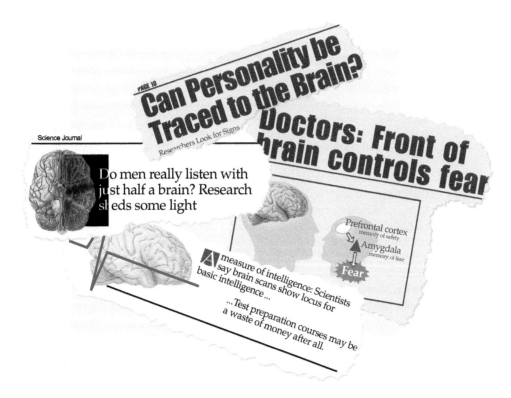

Figure 14.25 Studies of cognitive functions picked up by the popular media often lead to sensationalism Because the intended audience knows neither the anatomy nor the jargon used to describe it, sweeping simplifications are commonplace (e.g., treating the frontal lobe as a unitary structure). Moreover, complex concepts like personality, intelligence, or emotion are falsely linked to specific areas, and erroneous inferences are drawn about behavior—for example, how one can become a better parent or investor in the stock market. (All headlines are taken from actual news reports from CNN or ABC.)

■ BOX 14C NEUROMARKETING

Most applications of cognitive neuroscience have been within the medical domain. Research on the neuroscience of decision making, however, has become increasingly relevant for applications to real-world consumers, leading to the emergence of **neuromarketing**. Applied research in neuromarketing seeks to develop algorithms that can use neuroscience data from a small group of individuals—in a sense, a focus group consisting of human brains—to predict consumer choices for real-world products. This may seem like an unnecessary expense, in that marketers do not need to measure brain activity to determine whether a particular advertisement causes more people to buy their product; they can simply measure purchasing behavior, as has been done for decades. Yet there has been an explosion of interest in neuromarketing research, and many companies have used it for product development and marketing. If neuroscience simply duplicates basic measurements of behavior—at greater apparent expense—then why has neuromarketing grown so rapidly?

To understand why neuromarketing has attracted such attention, consider the key goals of commercial marketing, which extend well beyond measuring purchas-

Activation in the ventromedial prefrontal cortex tracks subjective preferences. Functional MRI activation in the ventromedial prefrontal cortex (top) was different in subjects anticipating a squirt of Coke or Pepsi bottom, *y*-axis), depending on whether the subject tended to prefer Coke or Pepsi in a prior taste test (bottom, *x*-axis). (After McClure et al. 2004.)

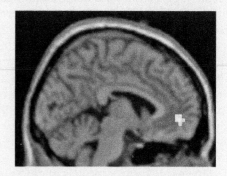

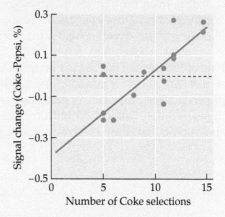

ing behavior. Modern marketing research attempts to improve all aspects of the consumer product cycle: developing new products and advertisements, assessing the factors that shape consumer preferences (e.g., understanding how a given brand influences choices), and getting the right messages to the right consumers through market segmentation. Neuroscience methods have been applied in each of these areas.

Think about an advertisement for a consumer good (e.g., clothing) on television. A typical 15-second commercial contains about 10 separate video segments, each with multiple images, all targeted toward a single message. Traditional methods for assessing and optimizing advertisements involve showing the commercial to potential consumers and

studying decision making; it will be a useful tool for many applications, but it will not replace traditional methods for economic or psychological analysis. Thus, a key challenge for cognitive neuroscientists who study decision making lies in building productive links between neuroscience and other disciplines.

Moreover, like other complex cognitive functions, decision making does not exist in isolation. Real-world choices rely on the processes of attention, memory, and emotion described in other chapters. People rarely, for example, make decisions of the sort studied in typical laboratory paradigms, such as choices between monetary gambles with known probability and fixed outcomes. Most decisions involve more tangible and meaningful outcomes, for which we often have substantial prior knowledge. As decision-making paradigms become increasingly realistic, researchers will need to incorporate these other cognitive functions in their models.

Even with these caveats, however, research on the cognitive neuroscience of decision making can serve as a bridge between basic decision science and some real-world applications (Box 14C). For instance, economists are increasingly interested in populations whose decision making is systematically maladaptive, such as addicts, habitual criminals, sociopaths, and others with behavioral pathologies. Because different neural deficits characterize each group, a policy of intervention that might be appropriate for one group would not necessarily be appropriate for others. Maladaptive decision making is especially evident in drug addiction. Addicts make repeated poor decisions that contribute to

■ **BOX 14C** *(continued)*

then soliciting evaluative data afterward (e.g., intent to purchase). Because such methods are retrospective and based on the commercial as a whole, they do not provide information about the individual segments or images within the commercial. To optimize the design of commercials, neuromarketing firms record physiological signals during commercial viewing using EEG, fMRI, skin conductance, eye tracking, or another technique. Such approaches hold promise for gaining real-time information about consumer attitudes that would normally be unobtainable using standard interview techniques. Similar approaches have been applied to optimizing print advertisements and product packaging, such as in the redesign of the labels for Campbell's Soup products.

Neuroscience may also contribute to an improved understanding of how different factors are integrated into consumer preferences. In some cases, findings from specific research studies may point to targets for neuromarketing applications. An engaging example comes from an fMRI study that examined preferences between two major soft drinks, Coke and Pepsi. When participants awaited delivery of small squirts of those drinks, activation in the ventromedial prefrontal cortex was correlated with subjects' behavioral pref-

erences. Subjects who were more likely to choose Coke in a taste test showed greater activation when Coke was presented, and the reverse was observed for those who were more likely to choose Pepsi (see figure).

This observation suggested that activity within a brain region known to be important for value integration also tracks preferences between well-known consumer products. Furthermore, when subjects who preferred Coke were cued with an image of a Coke can before the squirt, activation in the hippocampus and in the dorsolateral prefrontal cortex increased, whereas no such change was observed for Pepsi cues. One interpretation of this result is that mnemonic associations, learned over years of exposure to advertising, are activated by hippocampal and prefrontal systems, thus modulating subjective preferences.

Evidence of this sort can also be an important tool for market segmentation, the process of grouping consumers so that advertising and product development can be targeted to specific types of individuals. Most market segmentation is based on demographic factors like age, gender, and household income. Those factors are good predictors of the sorts of products that might inter-

est certain consumers (e.g., people with below-average household income would rarely purchase luxury cars). They are less useful, however, in predicting the biases or preferences (e.g., risk aversion) that a consumer might bring to the decision process. As cognitive neuroscience research develops more reliable indicators of individual differences in brain function, those indicators may become useful for segmenting populations of consumers according to different decision processes, which would complement the current focus on economic and social indicators.

References

ARIELY, D. AND G. S. BERNS (2010) Neuromarketing: The hope and hype of neuroimaging in business. *Nat. Rev. Neurosci.* 11: 284–292.

MCCLURE, S. M., J. LI, D. TOMLIN, K. S. CYPERT, L. M. MONTAGUE AND P. R. MONTAGUE (2004) Neural correlates of behavioral preference for culturally familiar drinks. *Neuron* 44: 379–387.

VENKATRAMAN, V., J. A. CLITHERO, G. J. FITZSIMONS AND S. A. HUETTEL (2012) New scanner data for brand marketers: How neuroscience can help better understand differences in brand preferences. *J. Consum. Psychol.* 22: 143–153.

addiction, placing themselves in situations that offer the potential for relapse and engaging in self-destructive behavior, despite experience with its long-term consequences.

Economists have encapsulated these decision processes within models that can seek to predict the course and consequences of addiction under the assumption that addictive decisions will be understood only when they are considered in the context of the brain systems responsible for reward evaluation and decision making. Collaborations of economists, neuroscientists, and clinicians are beginning to tackle these difficult problems.

Summary

1. Concepts derived from cognitive neuroscience and behavioral economics interact usefully in the emerging discipline of neuroeconomics.

2. In decision making, one option is selected from a set on the basis of prior knowledge, expectations about outcomes, and preferences about potential rewards.

3. Early research in economics combined ideas about expected value and probability weighting to create expected-utility models of rational decision makers. More recent economic research incorporates ideas from psychology about heuristics and biases, in recognition that many real-world decisions show systematic deviations from rational choice models.

4. Information about the risk associated with a decision modulates activation in control regions within prefrontal and parietal cortices, as well as in the insular cortex.

5. Single-unit recording studies from dopaminergic midbrain neurons and their projection targets in the basal ganglia and cortex indicate that many such neurons show increases in activity to unexpected positive reinforcers, and to cues that predict future reinforcers. These changes in activity have been described as signaling a reward prediction error that reflects information about rewards, but not necessarily rewards themselves.

6. The key challenge in decision making comes from the integration of diverse information (e.g., different reward types, risk, social context) into a common currency for decision making. Research now indicates that the ventromedial prefrontal cortex plays an important role in the reward integration process.

Additional Reading

Reviews

CLITHERO, J. A., D. TANKERSLEY AND S. A. HUETTEL (2008) Foundations of neuroeconomics: From philosophy to practice. *PLoS Biol.* 6: e298.

GLIMCHER, P. W. AND A. RUSTICHINI (2004) Neuroeconomics: The consilience of brain and decision. *Science* 306: 447–452.

PLATT, M. L. AND S. A. HUETTEL (2008) Risky business: The neuroeconomics of decision making under uncertainty. *Nat. Neurosci.* 11: 398–403.

RANGEL, A., C. CAMERER AND P. R. MONTAGUE (2008) A framework for studying the neurobiology of value-based decision making. *Nat. Rev. Neurosci.* 9: 545–556.

TVERSKY, A. AND D. KAHNEMAN (1974) Judgment under uncertainty: Heuristics and biases. *Science* 185: 1124–1131.

Important Original Papers

BACH, D. R., B. SEYMOUR AND R. J. DOLAN (2009) Neural activity associated with the passive prediction of ambiguity and risk for aversive events. *J. Neurosci.* 29: 1648–1656.

BECHARA, A., H. DAMASIO AND A. R. DAMASIO (2000) Emotion, decision making and the orbitofrontal cortex. *Cereb. Cortex* 10: 295–307.

BECHARA, A., H. DAMASIO, D. TRANEL AND A. R. DAMASIO (1997) Deciding advantageously before knowing the advantageous strategy. *Science* 275: 1293–1295.

BERRIDGE, K. C. AND T. E. ROBINSON (1998) What is the role of dopamine in reward: Hedonic impact, reward learning, or incentive salience? *Brain Res. Rev.* 28: 309–369.

DEANER, R. O., A. V. KHERA AND M. L. PLATT (2005) Monkeys pay per view: Adaptive valuation of social images by rhesus macaques. *Curr. Biol.* 15: 543–548.

DE MARTINO, B., D. KUMARAN, B. HOLT AND R. J. DOLAN (2009) The neurobiology of reference-dependent value computation. *J. Neurosci.* 29: 3833–3842.

DE MARTINO, B., D. KUMARAN, B. SEYMOUR AND R. J. DOLAN (2006) Frames, biases, and rational decision-making in the human brain. *Science* 313: 684–687.

DE QUERVAIN, D. J. AND 6 OTHERS (2004) The neural basis of altruistic punishment. *Science* 305: 1254–1258.

FIGNER, B. AND 6 OTHERS (2010) Lateral prefrontal cortex and self-control in intertemporal choice. *Nat. Neurosci.* 13: 538–539.

FLAGEL, S. B. AND 9 OTHERS (2011) A selective role for dopamine in stimulus-reward learning. *Nature* 469: 53–57.

GEHRING, W. J. AND A. R. WILLOUGHBY (2002) The medial frontal cortex and the rapid processing of monetary gains and losses. *Science* 295: 2279–2282.

HARBAUGH, W. T., U. MAYR AND D. R. BURGHART (2007) Neural responses to taxation and voluntary giving reveal motives for charitable donations. *Science* 316: 1622–1625.

HUETTEL, S. A., C. J. STOWE, E. M. GORDON, B. T. WARNER AND M. L. PLATT (2006) Neural signatures of economic preferences for risk and ambiguity. *Neuron* 49: 765–775.

KABLE, J. W. AND P. W. GLIMCHER (2007) The neural correlates of subjective value during intertemporal choice. *Nat. Neurosci.* 10: 1625–1633.

KAHNEMAN, D. AND A. TVERSKY (1979) Prospect theory: An analysis of decision under risk. *Econometrica* 47: 263–291.

KING-CASAS, B., D. TOMLIN, C. ANEN, C. F. CAMERER, S. R. QUARTZ AND P. R. MONTAGUE (2005) Getting to know you: Reputation and trust in a two-person economic exchange. *Science* 308: 78–83.

KNOCH, D., A. PASCUAL-LEONE, K. MEYER, V. TREYER AND E. FEHR (2006) Diminishing reciprocal fairness by disrupting the right prefrontal cortex. *Science* 314: 829–832.

KNUTSON, B., G. W. FONG, C. M. ADAMS, J. L. VARNER AND D. HOMMER (2001) Dissociation of reward anticipation and outcome with event-related fMRI. *Neuroreport* 12: 3683–3687.

LAMMEL, S., D. I. ION, J. ROEPER AND R. C. MALENKA (2011) Projection-specific modulation of dopamine neuron synapses by aversive and rewarding stimuli. *Neuron* 70: 855–862.

MATSUMOTO, M. AND O. HIKOSAKA (2009) Two types of dopamine neuron distinctly convey positive and negative motivational signals. *Nature* 459: 837–841.

McCLURE, S. M., D. I. LAIBSON, G. LOEWENSTEIN AND J. D. COHEN (2004) Separate neural systems value immediate and delayed monetary rewards. *Science* 306: 503–507.

MOHR, P. N., G. BIELE AND H. R. HEEKEREN (2010) Neural processing of risk. *J. Neurosci.* 30: 6613–6619.

MURAYAMA, K., M. MATSUMOTO, K. IZUMA AND K. MATSUMOTO (2010) Neural basis of the undermining effect of monetary reward on intrinsic motivation. *Proc. Natl. Acad. Sci. USA* 107: 20911–20916.

PADOA-SCHIOPPA, C. AND J. A. ASSAD (2006) Neurons in the orbitofrontal cortex encode economic value. *Nature* 441: 223–226.

PLASSMANN, H., J. O'DOHERTY AND A. RANGEL (2007) Orbitofrontal cortex encodes willingness to pay in everyday economic transactions. *J. Neurosci.* 27: 9984–9988.

PLATT, M. L. AND P. W. GLIMCHER (1999) Neural correlates of decision variables in parietal cortex. *Nature* 400: 233–238.

RACINE, E., O. BAR-ILAN AND J. ILLES (2005) fMRI in the public eye. *Nat. Rev. Neurosci.* 6: 159–164.

SANFEY, A. G., J. K. RILLING, J. A. ARONSON, L. E. NYSTROM AND J. D. COHEN (2003) The neural basis of economic decision-making in the Ultimatum Game. *Science* 300: 1755–1758.

SCHULTZ, W., P. DAYAN AND P. R. MONTAGUE (1997) A neural substrate of prediction and reward. *Science* 275: 1593–1599.

SHIV, B., G. LOEWENSTEIN, A. BECHARA, H. DAMASIO AND A. R. DAMASIO (2005) Investment behavior and the negative side of emotion. *Psychol. Sci.* 16: 435–439.

SMITH, D. V., B. Y. HAYDEN, T.-K. TRUONG, A. W. SONG, M. L. PLATT AND S. A. HUETTEL (2010) Distinct value signals in anterior and posterior ventromedial prefrontal cortex. *J. Neurosci.* 30: 2490–2495.

TANKERSLEY, D., C. J. STOWE AND S. A. HUETTEL (2007) Altruism is associated with an increased neural response to agency. *Nat. Neurosci.* 10: 150–151.

TVERSKY, A. AND D. KAHNEMAN (1992) Advances in prospect theory: Cumulative representation of uncertainty. *J. Risk Uncertain.* 5: 297–323.

VENKATRAMAN, V., J. W. PAYNE, J. R. BETTMAN, M. F. LUCE AND S. A. HUETTEL (2009) Separate neural mechanisms underlie choices and strategic preferences in risky decision making. *Neuron* 62: 593–602.

VICKERY, T. J., M. M. CHUN AND D. LEE (2011) Ubiquity and specificity of reinforcement signals throughout the human brain. *Neuron* 72: 166–177.

WAYTZ, A., J. ZAKI AND J. P. MITCHELL (2012) Response of dorsomedial prefrontal cortex predicts altruistic behavior. *J. Neurosci.* 32: 7646–7650.

ZINK, C. F., G. PAGNONI, M. E. MARTIN-SKURSKI, J. C. CHAPPELOW AND G. S. BERNS (2004) Human striatal responses to monetary reward depend on saliency. *Neuron* 42: 509–517.

Books

CAMERER, C. (2003) *Behavioral Game Theory: Experiments in Strategic Interaction.* Princeton, NJ: Princeton University Press.

GIGERENZER, G., P. M. TODD AND THE ABC RESEARCH GROUP (1999) *Simple Heuristics That Make Us Smart.* New York: Oxford University Press.

GLIMCHER, P. W., C. F. CAMERER, E. FEHR AND R. A. POLDRACK (2009) *Neuroeconomics: Decision Making and the Brain.* London: Academic Press.

HASTIE, R. AND R. M. DAWES (2001) *Rational Choice in an Uncertain World: The Psychology of Judgment and Decision Making.* Thousand Oaks, CA: Sage.

KAHNEMAN, D. (2011) *Thinking, Fast and Slow.* New York: Farrar, Straus and Giroux.

MEYER, J. S. AND L. F. QUENZER (2005) *Psychopharmacology: Drugs, the Brain, and Behavior.* Sunderland, MA: Sinauer.

15

Evolution and Development of Brain and Cognition

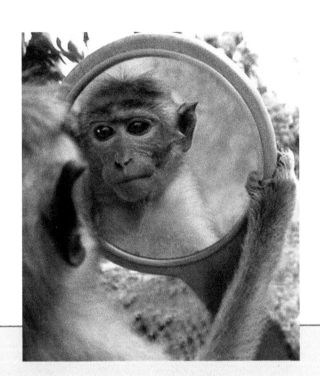

INTRODUCTION

As the pioneering geneticist Theodosius Dobzhansky famously said, "Nothing in biology makes sense save in the light of evolution." Important and often overlooked issues in cognitive neuroscience are how and why cognitive abilities have evolved in many (although certainly not all) animals, and why cognitive abilities are so highly developed in humans compared to other species.

These questions can be considered from two related perspectives: the evolution of cognitive abilities over the eons (a process called phylogeny); and the development of cognitive abilities during the maturation of an individual member of a species (ontogeny). Like all other biological features of an organism, an individual's cognitive abilities are determined in part by intrinsic developmental programs whose rules are inherited and are often referred to as the contribution of "nature." In addition, the experience of each maturing human shapes the development and maintenance of the neural circuitry underpinning cognitive abilities; this aspect is often referred to as the contribution of "nurture." Another broad, if anthropocentric, question underlying these evolutionary and developmental concerns is the extent to which the cognitive abilities of humans set us apart from other species, if indeed they do. Reasonable answers to these questions provide a basis for beginning to understand what it means to be human.

Any description of the present status of this effort must include the influence of evolutionary and developmental processes on the organization of cognitive functions and the neural circuits that mediate them; indeed, the pressures of natural selection have presumably been the driving force for the emergence of all cognitive processes and their neural underpinnings during development, as well as in the adult. Just as the evolution of other morphological structures has enabled organisms to adapt to particular environmental challenges, brain evolution has shaped the ability of animals to respond successfully to specific

■ INTRODUCTORY BOX SAVANT SYNDROME

A fascinating developmental anomaly of human cognition is exhibited by rare individuals who until recently were referred to as *idiots savants*; the current literature tends to use the less pejorative phrase *savant syndrome* to describe the condition. Savants are people who, for a variety of poorly understood reasons (typically brain damage in the perinatal period), are severely restricted in most mental activities but extraordinarily competent and mnemonically capacious in one particular domain (different individuals excel in different areas). The grossly disproportionate skill compared to the rest of their limited mental life can be striking. Indeed, these individuals—whose special talent may be in calculation, history, art, language, or music—are usually diagnosed as severely retarded.

A good example of someone with savant syndrome was given the fictitious name "Christopher" in a detailed study carried out by psychologists Neil Smith and Ianthi-Maria Tsimpli. Christopher was discovered to have severe brain damage at just a few weeks of age (perhaps as the result of rubella during his mother's pregnancy, or anoxia during birth; the record is uncertain on this question). He had been institutionalized since childhood because he was unable to care for himself. He could not find his way around, had poor hand-eye coordination, and exhibited a variety of other deficiencies. Tests on standard IQ scales were low, consistent with his general inability to cope with daily life. Scores on the Wechsler Scale, a more comprehensive intelligence test with separate assessments for verbal comprehension, working memory, arithmetic, and so on, were, on different occasions, 42, 67, and 52—well below the level generally considered to reflect mental retardation.

Despite his severe mental incapacitation, Christopher took an intense interest in books from the age of about 3, particularly those providing factual information

and lists such as telephone directories and dictionaries. At about age 6 or 7, Christopher began to read technical papers that his sister sometimes brought home from work, and he showed a surprising proficiency in foreign languages. His special talent in the acquisition and use of language (an area in which savants are often particularly limited) grew rapidly. As an early teenager, Christopher could translate from—and communicate in—a variety of languages, in which his skills were described as ranging from rudimentary to fluent; these included Danish, Dutch, Finnish, French, German, modern Greek, Hindi, Italian, Norwegian, Polish, Portuguese, Russian, Spanish, Swedish, Turkish, and Welsh. This extraordinary level of linguistic accomplishment is all the more remarkable because he had no formal training in language even at the elementary school level, and he could not play tic-tac-toe or checkers because he was unable to grasp the rules needed to make moves in these games.

The neurobiological basis for such extraordinary capacities is not well understood. Notably, the co-occurrence of savant syndrome and autism is particularly high; one in 10 individuals with autism qualifies as having extraordinary abilities in some domain, and roughly 50 percent of individuals with savant syndrome also have autism. It has been suggested that the lack of interest in other individuals and concomitant deficits in the development of social skills exhibited by people with autism may permit the rededication of information-processing circuits from social interaction to other interests, such as memorizing the phone book or learning dozens of languages. Savants clearly spend a great deal of their mental time and energy practicing the skills that they find rewarding. Such investment could, in theory, result in the rededication of neural circuits in a fashion similar to changes in brain function that occur in blind individuals who develop acute sensory aware-

ness in hearing and touch. The result is that the relevant associations savants make become especially rich, as Christopher's case demonstrates.

From an evolutionary point of view, savant syndrome is a puzzle, since there is no convincing evidence of truly extraordinary individuals within any particular non-human animal species. Yet some species have grossly exaggerated cognitive abilities in some domains. For example, Clark's nutcrackers store pine seeds to retrieve and eat over the long winter in the mountains of the western United States. These birds can apparently remember the locations of upwards of 20,000 seeds stored in random places, avoid the caches they have already eaten, and update their memories when they observe their stores pilfered by others. Having knowledge of the specialized abilities of animals like the nutcracker may offer unique potential for understanding the extraordinary cognitive abilities of human savants and their underlying neural bases.

References

Howe, M. J. A. (1989) *Fragments of Genius: The Strange Feats of Idiots Savants*. New York: Routledge.

Miller, L. K. (1989) *Musical Savants: Exceptional Skill in the Mentally Retarded*. Hillsdale, NJ: Erlbaum.

Smith, N. and I.-M. Tsimpli (1995) *The Mind of a Savant: Language Learning and Modularity*. Oxford: Basil Blackwell.

Smith, S. B. (1983) *The Great Mental Calculators: The Psychology, Methods, and Lives of Calculating Prodigies, Past and Present*. New York: Columbia University Press.

Treffert, D. A. (2009) The savant syndrome: An extraordinary condition. A synopsis: past, present, future. *Philos. Trans. R. Soc. Lond. B* 364: 1351–1357. doi: 10.1098/rstb.2008.0326.PMC2677584.

information-processing challenges confronted in nature throughout development and adulthood. The evolution of any new functional capacity builds on preexisting traits, and similar solutions to similar problems are often achieved in unrelated species. Further, the time course of cognitive and neural milestones over development often retraces the evolutionary trajectory of changes in cognition and behavior.

Understanding the organization of cognitive systems in the adult human brain thus profits from comparative studies of the brains and behaviors of both other animals and human infants and children, as well as examination of the fossil and archaeological records of changes in brains and behavior over millennia. Such observations suggest that the increasing size and complexity of the neocortex was a key factor in the emergence of the increasingly sophisticated cognitive abilities in humans compared with other primates, and in adults compared with infants and children. The evidence reviewed in this chapter indicates that adult human cognition comprises a mosaic of abilities that are shared with infants and children, as well as with other primates. For example, cognitive processes mediating social interaction, quantitative estimation, and memory show similar behavioral signatures in human infants, non-human primates, and adults, and they appear to rely on the same neural circuits.

This convergence of structure and function hints at a shared history of adaptation to similar environmental and social problems confronted by our ancestors and those of our closest primate relatives. Viewed through the lens of comparative biology, such homologies in brain and cognition appear to reflect specialized adaptations to the demands of navigating complex social environments and foraging for hard-to-find foods, which profit from enhanced capacities for social perception, numerical estimation, and memory. Despite these shared cognitive and neural traits, some abilities, including language and the capacity for symbolic culture, find full expression only in the human adult. The fossil and archaeological records, as well as the record of biological change preserved in the human genome, provide a tantalizing glimpse into the prehistory of human cognition.

Early Thinking about the Evolution and Development of Cognition

Charles Darwin's monumental work *On the Origin of Species*, published in 1859, recognized and carefully documented the now generally accepted idea that each organism's morphological features represent an amalgam of traits broadly shared with other animals because of the descent of different species from a common ancestor. In proposing descent by natural selection, however, Darwin emphasized that common traits become more specialized to adapt a given species to survival and reproduction in a particular ecological niche. Thus, morphological evolution can be viewed, in Darwin's words, as "descent with modification," which thereby increases the "fitness" of any plant or animal to its local environment. Although subsequent empirical and theoretical work in biology and genetics has modified this scheme by recognizing the importance of genetic drift, developmental constraints, and other factors, the process of **adaptation** to specific features of the local environment remains the dominant theme in understanding the forces that shape any biological feature, including the human brain.

While Darwin generally avoided discussing the evolution of behavior in his initial treatise, he was nonetheless convinced that his ideas about the body should apply equally to mental traits and abilities. For example, in his "Notebook M," Darwin wrote: "Evolution of man now proved. Metaphysics must flourish. He who understands baboon would do more toward metaphysics than Locke." In his subsequent book *The Expression of the Emotions in Man and Animals*, published in 1872, Darwin endeavored to show that basic behavioral reactions to emotions such as anger, joy, and disgust are conserved across a variety of animals, including humans (**Figure 15.1**). Although his views about the evolution of human cognitive traits were radical at the time, Darwin provided

Figure 15.1 Conserved behavioral reactions In *The Expression of the Emotions in Man and Animals*, Darwin endeavored to show that behavioral reactions to many basic emotions are similar (conserved) across different species. These drawings from the book compare the aggressive (A) and submissive (B) poses of a dog and a cat. (From Darwin 1871.)

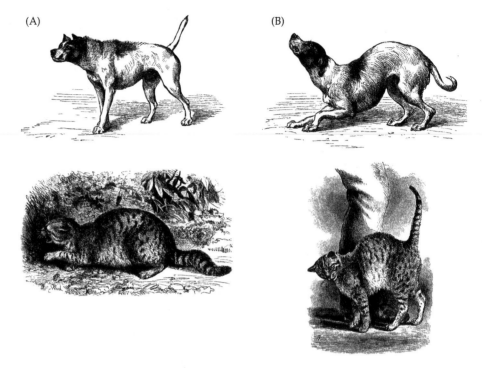

a biological framework for thinking about the relationship between brain and behavior that informs cognitive neuroscience today (Box 15A).

The other side of the coin with regard to what makes us what we are is our own individual experience and development. Early ideas about human cognitive development derived principally from the work of the Swiss developmental psychologist Jean Piaget, working in the 1940s and 1950s. Even though many "baby diaries" in which parents and keen observers like Charles Darwin provided detailed accounts of their infants' behavioral development had been published, it was Piaget who initiated the scientific study of infant cognition.

Piaget believed that children actively construct an understanding of the world as they adapt to their environment, through processes he called **assimilation** and **accommodation**. In some circumstances, children assimilate new people, events, and objects into their preexisting schemes of thought. In other situations, children might react to a new person, event, or object by changing or modifying their scheme of thought through *accommodation*. In Piaget's view, children move through a series of stages, each of which is characterized by cognitive limitations. For example, he believed that children in the first sensory-motor period lacked object permanence, rendering them incapable of representing objects that were out of view.

The ideas of Darwin and Piaget set the stage for subsequent work aimed at understanding the evolution and development of cognition in biological and, ultimately, neurobiological terms. Although some of their ideas have been discredited by subsequent work in cognitive neuroscience, the broad outlines of their programs continue to influence thinking about the development and evolution of brain and cognition.

One important thread running through both Piaget's and Darwin's writings is the biological dictum that ontogeny (development) recapitulates phylogeny (evolutionary history)—an idea advanced by the embryologist Ernst Haeckel in the nineteenth century. This hypothesis holds that the morphological, behavioral, or cognitive stages an organism passes through during development parallel changes in these same features during the course of evolution, and that more basic features appear before more advanced ones. Endorsing this notion,

■ BOX 15A DARWIN AND THE BRAIN

The impact of Darwin's work on biology was revolutionary (see figure), and his prescient and wide-ranging scientific viewpoint is as applicable to the organization of the brain as to the body.

Before Darwin published his great trilogy (*On the Origin of Species*; *The Descent of Man, and Selection in Relation to Sex*; and *The Expression of the Emotions in Man and Animals*), most anatomical studies of the brain were undertaken to support a special role for man in the universe, an enterprise called *natural theology*. The anatomist Richard Owen, for example, concluded that humans are not primates, but are a taxonomically unique group of mammals based on the greater development of the cerebral cortex in comparison to apes and other animals. Similarly, Sir Charles Bell, a physician and theologian now remembered chiefly for his contributions to understanding the facial paralysis known as Bell's palsy, argued that humans possessed muscles of facial expression without counterpart in the animal kingdom. Bell declared that the corrugator supercilii muscle, which knits the brow in concern or sadness, was designed by the Creator precisely to convey the presence of a mind.

One of Darwin's main goals was to combat this naïve thinking by demonstrating continuity in morphology and behavior among humans and other animals. Thus, *The Expression of the Emotions in Man and Animals* reads as a detailed catalog of similar facial expressions in humans and other animals, implying similar underlying emotional states and brain processes. Darwin's writings on brain and cognition, however, studiously avoided explaining such things in terms of adaptation, which was otherwise a central part of Darwin's evolutionary theory. As the modern psychologist Paul Ekman notes, this omission probably reflected Darwin's need to emphasize continuity over adaptive diversity in debates with creationists—debates that were often played out then, as now, under intense public scrutiny.

Another reason for Darwin's reluctance to apply the principle of adaptation to the study of the brain was the difficulty of explaining how gradual changes in form could improve function enough to enhance reproductive fitness. Indeed, Darwin acknowledged this problem head-on in his explanation for the evolution of the vertebrate eye on page 190 of *On the Origin of Species*:

To suppose that the eye, with all its inimitable contrivances for adjusting the focus to different distances, for admitting different amounts of light, and for the correction of spherical and chromatic aberration, could have been formed by natural selection, seems, I freely confess, absurd in the highest possible degree. Yet reason tells me, that if numerous gradations from a perfect and complex eye to one very imperfect and simple, each grade being useful to its possessor, can be shown to exist; and if further, the eye does vary ever so slightly; and if any of the variations be inherited; and if any of the variations be ever useful to an animal under changing conditions of life, then the difficulty of believing that a perfect and complex eye could be formed by natural selection, though insuperable by our imagination, can hardly be considered real.

No doubt Darwin felt similarly about the brain, emotions, and other cognitive processes. Of course, Darwin and his contemporaries had no knowledge of the existence of genes per se—although Darwin's grasp of the nature of the hereditary mechanism was both presciently accurate and fundamental to the ideas he put forth. However, he could not have foreseen the discovery of regulatory genes and their wide-ranging role in creating evolutionary novelty, any more than he could have foreseen the technologies of functional neuroimaging.

References

BELL, C. (1824) *Essays on the Anatomy and Philosophy of Expression*. London: Murray.

DARWIN, C. (1872) *The Expression of the Emotions in Man and Animals*. London: Murray.

OWEN, R. (1866) *On the Anatomy of Vertebrates*. London: Longmans, Green.

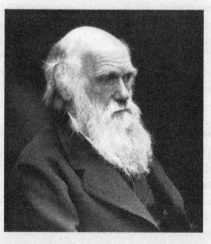 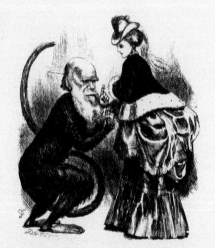

The debate over evolution, particularly as applied to human emotions and cognition, evoked strong reactions. Darwin was often depicted as part monkey to lampoon his argument that humans and non-human primates shared a common ancestor.

a central discovery of developmental and comparative research in cognitive neuroscience is that the cognitive traits that humans share with other animals tend to emerge early in human development.

Despite this similarity, however, the simplistic notion that development faithfully retraces the evolutionary trajectory of a species has been fully discredited. Instead, cognitive neuroscientists, like other biologists, now recognize that evolution acts on early developmental stages, as well as on adults, to adapt brain and cognition to the behavioral demands facing the organism, subject to the constraints imposed by the processes of physical and cognitive maturation.

Early Brain Development

The first challenge in developmental and evolutionary studies of brain and cognition is to understand how these two biological features are related. Since the outcome of development (an animal's phenotype, which is shaped by both its genotype and experience) provides the raw material for both the expression of cognition in behavior and its subsequent modification by evolution, understanding the ontogeny of the brain provides a useful starting point.

Somewhere around the twentieth day of human embryogenesis, the nervous system begins to develop. At this time the neural tube emerges, eventually giving rise to the brain and spinal cord. The cells of the neural tube are undifferentiated stem cells known as **neural precursor cells**. The anterior end of the neural tube soon begins to develop the components that can be recognized as those of the adult brain by generating three distinct vesicles that will eventually give rise to the forebrain, midbrain, and hindbrain (Figure 15.2). The locus of cell division is at the inner surface of the neural tube, a region called the *ventricular zone*. The neuronal precursor cells migrate outward (toward the surface of the neural tube), where they eventually differentiate into neurons. Those neurons in the emerging brain and spinal cord that are the last to be generated migrate to the most superficial layers of the gray matter (see the Appendix), whereas neurons generated earlier in development remain in the deepest layers of the brain. In general, the development of the nervous system progresses from head to tail, as is apparent in Figure 15.2.

In humans, on the order of 20 to 100 billion neurons (depending on the method of cell counting) and several times that many glial cells are generated from these neural precursor cells, most between the sixth and eighth weeks of gestation and nearly all before the end of the second trimester. Thus, virtually all the neurons in the neocortex on which cognition will ultimately depend are present in the late-stage human embryo. With a few exceptions, no new neurons are generated after birth—an important fact that must be taken into account in any theory of cognitive development.

Neuronal differentiation and myelination

After reaching their destination in a given region of the brain or spinal cord, neural precursor cells differentiate to form distinct cell types. In differentiation, transcription factors turn off some genes and turn on others. This modulatory process is determined by both the lineage of the neuron and local signals arising from its position in the developing brain. The result is the remarkable regional diversity of cell types that populate the adult brain, a diversity that is already evident at birth. The key features that distinguish neuronal types are the signaling properties of the action potentials they generate, the transmitter agents they employ, the receptor molecules they incorporate at postsynaptic sites, and the morphology of their axons and dendrites, all of which reflect their ultimate connectivity and thus function.

In parallel with neuronal differentiation, glial cells differentiate and begin to perform their myriad functions. Particularly important is the differentiation of the glial class called **oligodendrocytes**, which elaborate the myelin that ensheathes many varieties of neuronal axons in the nervous system. **Myelination** increases the speed of action potential conduction and thus improves the efficiency of neuronal signaling and processing generally. On the basis of this

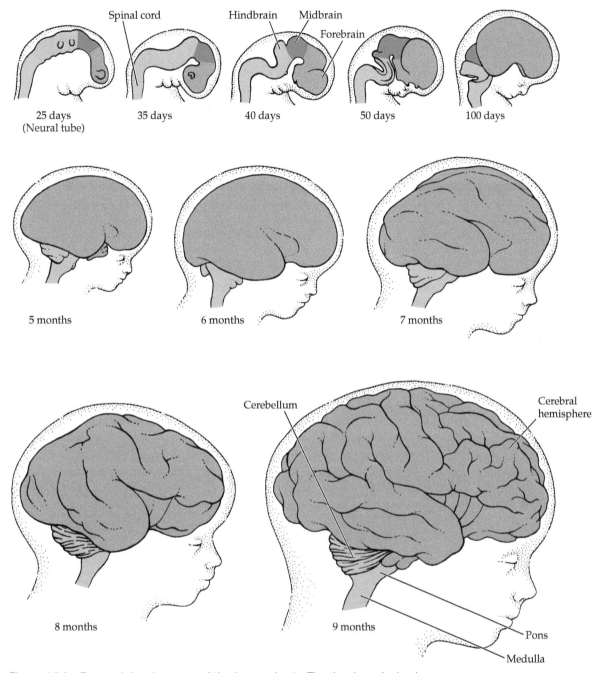

Figure 15.2 Prenatal development of the human brain The drawings depict the development of the brain from the neural tube over the course of human gestation. Note the exceptional growth of the forebrain, which gives rise to the cerebral hemispheres. (After Cowan 1979.)

fact and correlative evidence, it is widely assumed that myelination is important in the emergence of cognitive functions in both evolution and individual development. Myelination begins relatively late in human gestation (at about 29 weeks), and many major tracts are not fully myelinated until adolescence. Indeed, some white matter tracts, such as the arcuate fasciculus that links Broca's and Wernicke's language areas, continue to become myelinated into the third decade of life. As shown in Figure 15.3A, myelination more or less parallels the emergence of complex cognitive functions in a number of brain regions.

(A) Time course of myelination

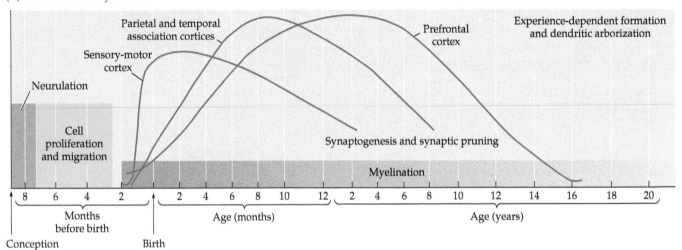

Figure 15.3 Progression of two key developmental processes (A) Myelination in the human brain. (B) Synaptogenesis. The density of synaptic contacts is plotted here as a function of time, pooled across all cortical layers in a rhesus monkey. (A after Casey et al. 2005; B after Bourgeois and Rakic 1993.)

(B) Synaptic prevalence in rhesus development

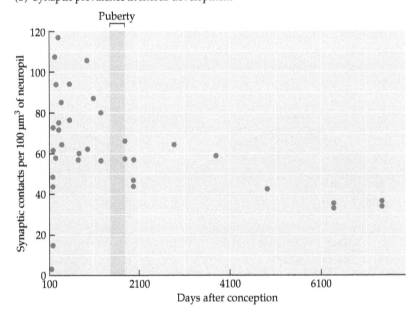

The development of neural connections

Once precursor cells have migrated to their destinations and differentiated into neurons, they send out axons to contact other cells, and dendrites to transmit and receive the information that determines their ultimate function. The emerging axons are guided to their targets by molecular cues in the local environment. Having reached the target cells (which can be other neurons, muscle cells, or gland cells) the axon endings form synapses (see the Appendix). A great deal of cellular and molecular work has shown that synapse formation is determined primarily by surface and secreted molecules that are specific to each target.

Synaptogenesis, the formation of synapses, begins early in gestation and peaks at different times in different brain regions. Two quite different factors affect the assessment of synaptogenesis in the brain: its rate in a given brain region, and the maximum number of synapses per unit volume in a given region at different times over the human life span. The latter value is presumably a measure of the complexity of neural processing in the region of interest. The rate of synaptogenesis is straightforward in principle, but the number of synapses counted at any point in life in a given brain is subject to many factors, of which the rate of synapse formation is only one. Another obvious factor is synapse loss, which is evident throughout development and the rest of the human life span as synaptic contacts turn over and change under the influence of experience.

Thus, the relationship between synaptogenesis and overall synaptic numbers in relation to cognitive functions is controversial. Extraordinarily careful electron microscopic studies of developing rhesus monkey brains carried out by neuroanatomist Pasko Rakic and his colleagues indicate that in primates, the overall number of synapses increases progressively until adolescence, and it falls thereafter (Figure 15.3B).

The processes of synaptic production and synaptic change vary from region to region. Synaptogenesis tends to proceed earlier in brain regions whose functions are important early in life compared to regions whose functions depend more on postnatal experience, which develop more slowly and remain plastic longer. It is now known, mainly through in vivo imaging studies, that synaptogenesis is always accompanied by synapse loss and rearrangement, a pruning process that presumably reflects the adjustment of the numbers of synapses to the needs of the target cells. For similar reasons, some neuronal populations are overproduced and die in early development, although this phenomenon seems limited largely to the death of neurons in the spinal cord and plays relatively little part in the developing brain. Taken all together, these variations are likely to influence cognitive development, as well as differences between species wrought by evolution. As described in Chapters 8 and 9, synaptic change is ongoing throughout life and forms a basis for learning and memory.

Another general aspect of cortical development is the importance of connectivity as a determinant of function. Since the general organization of neocortex is broadly similar across all regions of the brain (see the Appendix), the question arises whether neurons in one region might work just as well if transplanted to another region. In fact, considerable evidence suggests that this is indeed the case. For example, in experimental animals auditory cortex has been observed to process visual information after surgical rewiring of thalamic inputs. Similarly, when a region of embryonic visual cortex is transplanted into the somatosensory cortex, the transplanted tissue becomes similar to that of the recipient somatosensory cortex.

Although cortical neurons are certainly not all the same, evidence of this sort implies that all neural processing across the neocortex must have much in common, and that what particular neurons end up doing depends greatly on their inputs and the areas that they in turn innervate. More generally, the plasticity of neuronal function is greatest early in cortical development, and many transplantation experiments indicate that the ability of cortical progenitor cells to produce neurons of different phenotypes declines over time. Whereas early progenitor cells can assume multiple potential forms and functions, later progenitors become progressively restricted in their potential fates.

Linking Brain and Cognitive Development

By 2 years of age, a child's brain has reached about 80 percent of its adult weight, and by 5 years it is, on average, about 90 percent of adult size. However, longitudinal MRI studies have shown that some remodeling of gray and white matter in the cortex continues throughout life; indeed, average brain weight changes continually, peaking in the late teenage years and declining thereafter (Figure 15.4A). A series of large-scale longitudinal MRI studies in which children's brains were visualized anatomically every 2 years showed changes in gray and white matter volume through adolescence. Specifically, total cerebral volume reaches a peak at approximately 11.5 years in females and 14.5 years in males,

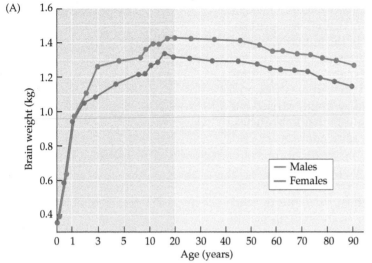

(A)

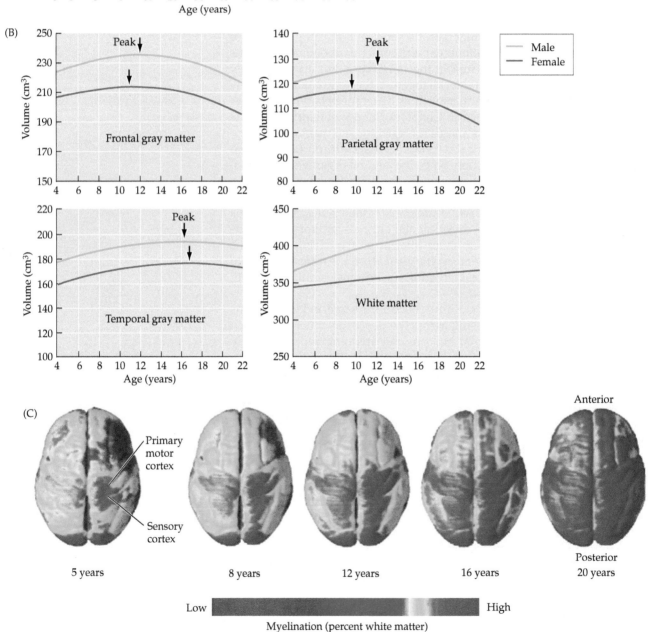

Figure 15.4 **Anatomical measures of human brain development** (A) The average weight of the human brain over the life span. The brain continues to grow in mass for about two decades; then brain weight gradually declines, presumably representing a loss of neural circuitry in the aging brain. (B) The change in volume of frontal, parietal, and temporal gray matter, as well as white matter, between ages 2 and 22 years. The data reflect 243 scans from 145 subjects scanned at 2-year intervals. (C) Dorsal view of the dynamic changes as gray matter matures over the cortical surface. The color changes here are an amalgam and represent units of gray matter volume for 13 different subjects, each scanned four times at approximately 2-year intervals. (A after Dekaban and Sadowsky 1978; B,C after Lenroot and Giedd 2006; images in C courtesy of N. Gogtay.)

(B)

Frontal gray matter

Parietal gray matter

Temporal gray matter

White matter

— Male
— Female

(C)

Primary motor cortex

Sensory cortex

5 years   8 years   12 years   16 years   20 years

Anterior

Posterior

Low ———————————————— High

Myelination (percent white matter)

and the rate of brain growth differs for different brain regions (Figure 15.4B). For example, regions that control primary functions, such as motor and sensory systems, develop first, followed by the temporal and parietal cortices associated with language and spatial attention (Figure 15.4C). Importantly, the last brain regions to mature are the prefrontal and lateral temporal cortices involved in the integration of sensory-motor processes, the modulation of attention and language, and critical aspects of decision making. These latter cognitive functions are also the latest to develop in behavioral studies.

Whereas white matter volume increases steadily throughout the brain during childhood, adolescence, and into adulthood, gray matter volume follows an inverted U-shaped trajectory that peaks at somewhat different times in adolescence for different brain regions. The loss of gray matter in some brain regions in late adolescence and early adult life probably reflects the elimination of some neuronal connections, in keeping with evidence in monkeys that the overall number of synapses in the neocortex increases through adolescence and then begins to decline slowly. This eventual decline also accords with average brain weight over the human life span, which decreases steadily during the adult years.

Individual variability in the development of a given brain region is sometimes correlated with differences in cognition as well. A longitudinal study comprising multiple structural brain scans from over 300 neurologically normal children demonstrated that the dynamics of brain development provide a better prediction of individual differences in cognition than does mere brain size alone. In that study, the rate of change in the thickness of cortical gray matter was more predictive of IQ than were absolute differences in cortical thickness (Figure 15.5).

In addition to brain structure, patterns of brain function accompany changes in cognition over development. This is particularly clear for developmental changes in executive function. In one study, children (7 to 12 years old) and

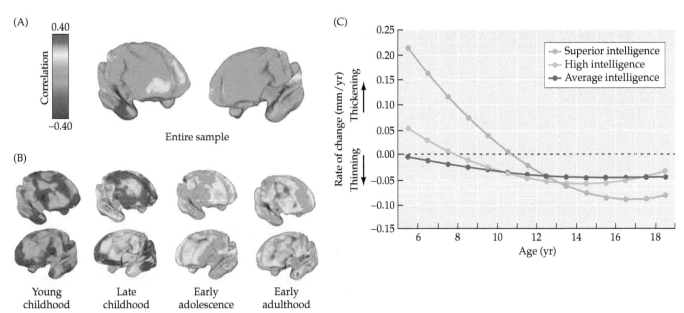

Figure 15.5 Correlations between IQ and cortical thickness (A) Correlations were positive but modest for all areas except the anterior temporal cortex, which showed a negative correlation. (B) Correlations in different age groups. The youngest children showed negative correlations with higher IQ associated with thinner cortex in temporal and frontal regions. The relationship reversed by late childhood. (C) Children with superior intelligence showed the highest rate of change in cortical thickness in the right superior and medial frontal gyrus. Positive values indicate increasing cortical thickness. (After Shaw et al. 2006.)

young adults (21 to 24 years old) were scanned with fMRI during a simple task in which they were required to press a button in response to all letters except the letter *X*. This task shows clear developmental improvement, with adults making fewer erroneous button presses. When erroneous responses to *X*s were successfully inhibited, activation was seen in several regions of the prefrontal cortex, including the anterior cingulate, orbitofrontal cortex, and inferior and middle frontal gyri in both children and adults. Compared to adults, children showed significantly greater activation in the dorsolateral prefrontal cortex and anterior cingulate cortex. By contrast, adults showed more activity in orbitofrontal cortex than did children. Across all ages, individuals with higher orbitofrontal activation and lower dorsolateral prefrontal activation performed better on the task. These findings suggest that changes in prefrontal cortex function throughout development shape changes in executive function.

Brain size and the evolution of cognition

Given the relationship between brain maturation and cognition observed during development, it seems reasonable to suppose that differences in cognitive abilities between species are in some broad way dependent on differences in brain structure and function. Since most studies of cognitive evolution focus on complex, flexible, goal-directed behavior, a global metric such as brain size would seem a simple and reasonable starting point to test this idea.

Among vertebrates, mammals and birds generally have larger brains (and certainly larger volumes of cerebral cortex; see the next section) than do fishes, amphibians, or reptiles, and no one would dispute the fact that these differences in brain volume are somehow related to differences in the apparent cognitive abilities of these various taxonomic groups. Among mammals, moreover, rats have smaller brains than cats or monkeys, which in turn have smaller brains than dolphins and humans, seemingly confirming the general tendency of cognitive abilities and brain size to track together. Collectively, these observations suggest that brain size is indeed an important determinant of behavioral complexity and flexibility. This conclusion makes good sense because as the number of neurons in the brain increases, the number and complexity of functions that the brain can perform are likewise expected to increase.

A closer look at the relationship between absolute brain size and cognition, however, raises the troubling observation that some seemingly intelligent animals have smaller brains than other animals not known for their cognitive prowess (Figure 15.6). This observation implies that the relationship between absolute brain size and cognition is not so simple (see Box 15B).

The resolution of this puzzle is in part answered by the relation of brain size and body size: it makes little sense to consider the size of an animal's brain

(A) Macaque

(B) Cow

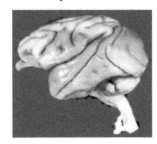
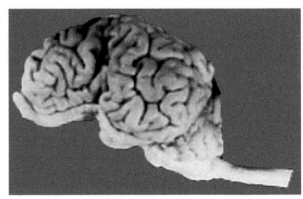

Figure 15.6   Brain size does not correlate absolutely with cognitive ability Lateral views of the brains of a macaque monkey (A) and a cow (B), shown to scale. Even though the macaque's cognitive abilities are superior to those of the cow, its brain is significantly smaller, as well as less folded. (Courtesy of the University of Wisconsin and Michigan State University Comparative Mammalian Brains Collection.)

without adjusting this metric for the size of the animal's body, since—cognitive abilities aside—the brain would presumably need to be somewhat larger simply to organize the behavior of larger bodies. The differential measurement of individual body parts in relation to the whole to is known as allometry (the prefix *allo* means "other" in Greek), and the general proportionality of brain and body size reflects the fact that as the body grows larger, more neurons are needed to process sensory inputs, motor outputs, and their central interactions.

The allometric relationship of brain and body size is highly variable among species. Thus, the line that fits to the scatter of brain size plotted against body size in **Figure 15.7A** makes it obvious that some animals have brains that are larger than body size alone would suggest, whereas others do not. For instance, humans, dolphins, and crows have larger brains than expected for their average body size, whereas opossums, ostriches, and some other animals have smaller brains than one might expect. Moreover, birds and mammals have larger brains for their body size than do reptiles and fishes. These deviations from allometrically predicted brain size, often referred to as *residual brain size*, correspond more closely to relative cognitive ability than does brain size alone. Within any particular group of vertebrates, relative brain size is also correlated, at least roughly, with apparent cognitive capacity (**Figure 15.7B**). Whether or not relative brain sizes of individuals within a species scale with their specific cognitive abilities, however, remains hotly debated (**Box 15B**).

Figure 15.7 Importance of brain size relative to body size Note that the scale is logarithmic in all cases. (A) Brain weight as a function of body weight. Red lines indicate the allometric scaling relationship between brain size and body size, determined by linear regression. The blue and green areas indicate minimal polygons enclosing the data points for mammals (blue) and for fishes and a reptiles (green). (B) Allometric relationship of brain size and body size for placental (modern) mammals. Note that primates (black dots) have much larger brains given their body sizes than do rodents and rabbits (Glires; red dots) or deer, antelope, and the like (artiodactyls; blue dots)–animals not known for their cognitive skills. (A after Jerison 1977; B after Striedter 2005.)

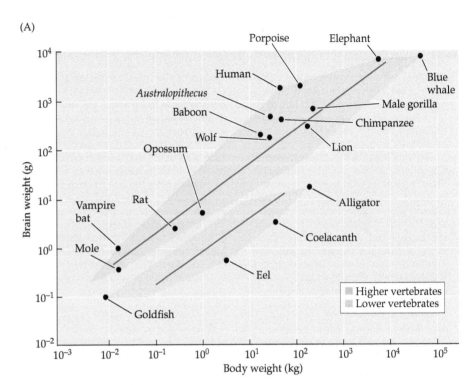

(A)

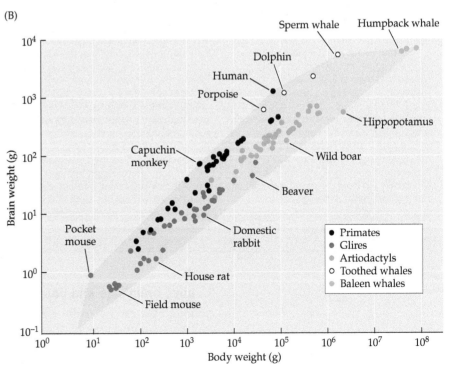

(B)

■ BOX 15B BRAIN DIFFERENCES IN MODERN HUMANS: IMPLICATIONS FOR COGNITION

A wealth of neuroanatomical, physiological, and behavioral data support the hypothesis that brain size and complexity predict cognitive abilities across a wide diversity of species. However, whether differences in brain size *within* a species are associated with differences in cognition remains a subject of debate. The debate is especially heated when differences in brain size and cognitive behavior in humans are being considered. Historically, scientists have often tried to link overall brain size to differences in performance by using global measures of cognitive performance such as IQ tests.

Several prominent nineteenth-century scientists—including the statistician Francis Galton (who, incidentally, was Darwin's cousin), the American physician Samuel Morton, and the French neuroanatomist Paul Broca (who determined that the left frontal lobe is responsible for articulate speech; see Chapter 12)—argued that individual differences in brain size (often estimated by a method no more scientific than simply measuring the head) accurately predicted a person's intelligence. Unfortunately, this approach was used to support, either implicitly or explicitly, notions of racial and gender superiority that buttressed Western conventional wisdom of the time, which asserted that white European males had larger brains—and consequently greater intelligence—than everyone else in the world.

Careful reanalysis revealed much of this original research to be badly flawed. For example, evolutionary biologist Stephen Jay Gould demonstrated that Morton's measurements of cranial capacity (an index of brain size based on measuring the interior volume of the skull) in specimens of different races were inaccurate and highly biased toward finding larger brain sizes for European males. Moreover, it is now clear that it is difficult to measure general intelligence in individuals with different cultural, educational, and socioeconomic backgrounds. Despite recognition of these methodological problems, the legacy of this nineteenth-century mind-set has continued to bedevil psychology, neuroscience, and society right into the twenty-first century.

Individual human beings clearly vary in cognitive ability, as well as in brain size. But such differences among human groups are small and often difficult to interpret, not least because the brain is a mosaic of interrelated modules and systems serving distinct behavioral functions. It thus makes more sense to consider more specifically whether variation in the size, physiology, cell structure, and molecular biology of such components corresponds to the efficiency or complexity of the behavioral functions they enable.

For example, the size of each of the various components of the visual system, including the optic tracts, lateral geniculate nucleus, and primary visual cortex, is intimately related within an individual; across subjects, however, these elements vary substantially in size. As described in Chapter 3, visual acuity corresponds closely to the cortical space allocated to each part of the visual field, suggesting (along with much other evidence) that the quality of cortical processing is a function of the amount of cortical space given over to that function. Structural differences of this sort may also underlie gender differences in cognitive abilities such as language and spatial navigation. It has long been known, for example, that women are much less likely than men to suffer a debilitating loss of language (aphasia) following strokes involving cortical language areas in the left hemisphere. This gender difference suggests that women process language more bilaterally than men do—a hypothesis supported by recent neuroimaging studies demonstrating stronger lateralization of language processing in males than in females.

Stronger lateralization in males also extends to visuospatial information processing, as revealed by both lesion and functional neuroimaging studies. These observed sex differences in brain organization could be related to differences in cognitive performance, specifically to the superior verbal abilities of females, on average, and to the superior visuospatial navigation abilities in males revealed by standardized tests. Note, however, that such tests are subject to the same criticisms as the IQ tests described earlier.

These and other differences in brain structure and cognitive performance in men and women seem likely to derive from the interplay of sex hormones and experience during development. Gender differences in the spatial navigation ability of experimental animals, for example, have been linked to differences in the size of the hippocampus in male and female voles and rats, which is known to be determined by the action of sex hormones during development.

These observations notwithstanding, the links among gender, hormones, experience, brain structure, and cognition in humans remain hotly debated. Given the enormous cultural, political, and educational implications of these kinds of findings, much more work will be required to understand the biological mechanisms that contribute to the wide range of differences in cognitive performance seen across groups and across individuals within groups.

References

ANDREWS, T. J., S. D. HALPERN AND D. PURVES (1997) Correlated size variations in human visual cortex, lateral geniculate nucleus, and optic tract. *J. Neurosci.* 17: 2859–2868.

BOYNTON, G. M. AND R. O. DUNCAN (2002) Visual acuity correlates with cortical magnification factors in human V1 [Abstract]. *J. Vision* 2(10): 11a.

GOULD, S. J. (1981) *The Mismeasure of Man.* New York: Norton.

KIMURA, D. (1996) Sex, sexual orientation, and sex hormones influence human cognitive function. *Curr. Opin. Neurobiol.* 6: 259–263.

Relative brain size and cerebral complexity

Although the ratio of brain size to body size predicts cognitive abilities fairly well across a wide range of animals, this observation does not explain why or how this correlation exists. One argument is that the scaling relationship between brain size and body size in Figure 15.7 reflects the average amount of neural processing "machinery" necessary for maintaining a body of a particular size. According to this view, positive deviations in brain size from expectations based on body size would afford the animal extra neural processing capacity for additional abilities that transcend the usual housekeeping functions (**Box 15C**). The extra capacity could then be devoted to cognitive functions that are particularly advantageous for behavioral success in some ecological niches.

A second, not mutually exclusive, possibility is that changes in the relationship of brain and body size are associated with concomitant changes in the *structure* of the brain, as well as in its size. For example, the six-layered neocortex is the most recently evolved part of the forebrain, is found only in mammals, and is widely agreed to be the seat of many advanced cognitive functions. Allometric analyses indicate that the size of the neocortex scales positively with the size of the rest of the brain: as the brain gets larger, the neocortex gets larger.

This proportionality, however, varies among different animal groups. That is, the allometric relationship relating neocortex size to brain size has the same slope, but different intercepts in different species. For example, simian primates (monkeys and apes) have proportionately larger neocortices given the size of the rest of their brains than do prosimian primates (lemurs and lorises; **Figure 15.8**), which in turn have proportionately larger neocortices than would be expected compared to insectivores (e.g., hedgehogs and shrews). Thus, as the size of the brain relative to body size increases, the relative size of the neocortex also increases. In at least this respect, the differential scaling of brain structures is important in the evolution of cognitive capacities.

(A)

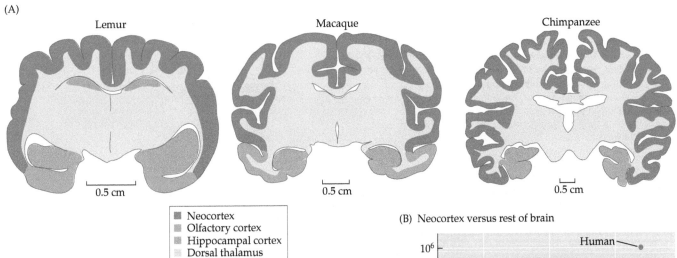

Neocortex
Olfactory cortex
Hippocampal cortex
Dorsal thalamus

Figure 15.8 Neocortex size as a function of brain size
(A) Diagrammatic coronal sections through lemur, macaque, and chimpanzee brains (note the different scales). Increasing brain size is associated with a disproportionate increase in the size and complexity of the neocortex, at the expense of the hippocampus, olfactory cortex, and thalamus. (B) Neocortex size as a function of the size of the rest of the brain in primates. The dashed line indicates proportional scaling. The slope of the function is greater than 1 in this double logarithmic plot, indicating that in primates neocortex size becomes disproportionately larger as brain size increases. (A after University of Wisconsin Brain Collection; B after Stephan et al. 1981.)

(B) Neocortex versus rest of brain

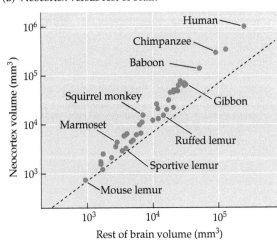

■ BOX 15C EVOLUTION OF HUMAN BRAIN AND COGNITION EVIDENT IN THE FOSSIL RECORD

In many respects, human neural and cognitive evolution has simply elaborated on trends that are well established in non-human primates; in other respects, however, human brain evolution has been marked by distinctive deviations from other primates. For example, like other primates, the human brain represents a larger fraction of body size than in other mammals. Nonetheless, the trajectory of brain evolution relative to body size has been steeper within the lineage leading to modern humans compared to the lineage of non-human primates (Figure A).

The fossil (i.e., skeletal and other organismal remains) and archaeological (i.e., artifacts of human activity) records provide clues about the coevolution of brain structure and cognition in humans. The primate lineage leading to humans first diverged from the great apes between 5 and 8 million years ago. Somewhat surprisingly, this divergence was not characterized by major neurological changes. The first adaptive change distinguishing ancestral humans, or **hominids**, from apes was not neurological, but morphological, entailing upright bipedal walking. The first human ancestors, known as **australopithecines** and found in eastern and southern African fossil beds dated to 3 to 4 million years ago, had brains about the same size as modern-day chimpanzees (see Figure A). However, the human evolutionary career thereafter (Figure B) is characterized by both gradual, progressive changes and relatively rapid advancements in brain size and cognition.

The first member of the genus **Homo**, the group to which modern humans belong, diverged from an australopithecine ancestor around 2.5 million years ago (see Figure B). This species, dubbed *Homo habilis* ("handy man"), had a brain that was about 50 percent larger than those of its ancestors, and it was the first human ancestor to produce crude stone tools (Figure C). About 800,000 years later, *Homo erectus* ("erect man") diverged from an earlier *Homo* species. Again, this evolutionary event was characterized by major advancements in brain size and cognition. Early *Homo erectus* fossils reveal brains that were about a third larger than the brains of early *Homo habilis*. Moreover, *Homo erectus* made stone tools of greater complexity and symmetry than those made by earlier humans (see Figure C) and also began to use fire, presumably reflecting greater cognitive capacity.

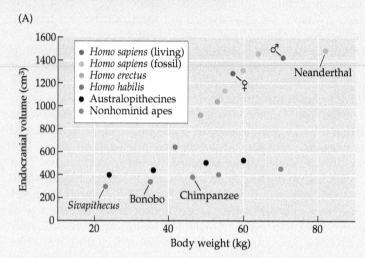

(A)

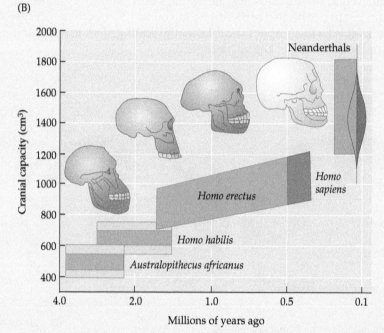

(B)

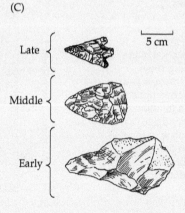

(C)

(A) Brain size is disproportionately large in relation to body size in humans and their immediate ancestors (hominids) compared to apes. (B) Brain size has increased in sudden jumps, as well as gradual changes, during hominid evolution. Shaded regions indicate the range of variation in brain size. (C) The sophistication of the stone tools produced by hominids increased in parallel with increasing brain size over the course of evolutionary time. Bottom: Early Paleolithic tools associated with *Homo habilis* and early *Homo erectus*. Middle: Middle Paleolithic tools associated with late *Homo erectus* and early *Homo sapiens*. Top: Upper Paleolithic tools found with the skeletal remains of anatomically modern humans. (A after Hofman 1983; C after Tattersall et al. 1988.)

■ **BOX 15C** *(continued)*

(D)

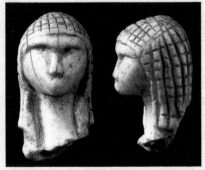

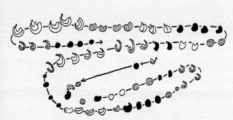

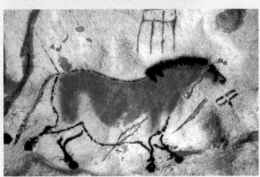

(D) Anatomically modern humans in Ice Age Europe began to produce symbolic art indicative of greatly enhanced cognitive abilities. Shown here are a carved woman's head from Brassempouy, in southern France, about 23,000 years old; lunar phases incised on a piece of bone, 30,000 to 40,000 years old; and a cave painting of a horse from Lascaux, France, approximately 15,000 years old.

possessed an extremely sophisticated arsenal of stone tools, including long blades and hafted spear points (i.e., points with handles, which make much more effective weapons than a simple pointed implement with no handle). These were also the first humans to produce symbolic representations and art (Figure D). In addition, they buried their dead with jewelry and other items, indicating that they apparently had religious beliefs of some type.

Together, the size and morphology of the brain, and archaeological traces of ancient behavior, suggest that adult human cognitive capacities have changed little in the past 200,000 years. Although some evidence suggests that certain aspects of human biology continued to evolve (e.g., the sickle-cell trait and malarial resistance in sub-Saharan Africans; adult lactose-tolerance in northern European dairying cultures), the technological and intellectual achievements of today's humans largely reflect the accumulation and storage of knowledge by purely cultural means—and often outside the brain, in books and computers. These feats highlight the remarkable capacity of the human brain to rapidly adapt to new physical and social contexts, and to use information in new ways unanticipated by evolution.

Homo erectus was an extremely successful species, persisting for about 2 million years and colonizing what are now Africa, Europe, and Asia. During that time, hominid brain size increased gradually, and the stone tools produced by *Homo erectus* progressed in sophistication. These advances in brain and cognitive ability apparently permitted *Homo erectus* to survive in a wide variety of climates, utilize a variety of resources, and even navigate open oceans to reach Australia. Throughout the Old World, *Homo erectus* continued to evolve and adapt to local conditions until the late Pleistocene era, from 200,000 to about 50,000 years ago. In what is today western Europe and the Middle East, *Homo erectus* evolved into **Neanderthals**, who,

rather surprisingly, had brains that were even larger than those of modern humans (although it should be noted that their bodies were slightly heavier as well); in this instance, overall brain size does not align very well with the relatively primitive material culture of Neanderthals.

Modern humans, *Homo sapiens* (meaning, for better or worse, "wise man") evidently arose on the African continent about 200,000 years ago and rapidly spread throughout the world, in some cases driving other hominid populations, including Neanderthals, to extinction, and in other cases interbreeding with them. The competitive advantage of anatomically modern humans was almost certainly due, at least in part, to their superior cognitive abilities. Early *Homo sapiens*

References

CHASE, P. G. AND H. L. DIBBLE (1987) Middle Palaeolithic symbolism: A review of current evidence and interpretations. *J. Anthropol. Archaeol.* 6: 263–296.

HOFMAN, M. A. (1983) Evolution of brain size in neonatal and adult placental mammals: A theoretical approach. *J. Theor. Biol.* 105: 317–332.

TATTERSALL, I., E. DELSON AND J. VAN COUVERING, EDS. (1988) *Encyclopedia of Human Evolution and Prehistory.* New York: Garland.

WYNN, T. (2002) Archaeology and cognitive evolution. *Behav. Brain Sci.* 25: 389–438.

In addition to changes in the size of the brain itself and the relative size and complexity of structures like the neocortex, there is evidence that the complexity of neuronal circuitry has increased during evolution. A family tree (properly called a *cladogram*) plotting the number of distinct neuronal cell types found in several vertebrate taxonomic group indicates that, as brain-to-body-weight ratios increased over evolutionary time, so did forebrain complexity (**Figure 15.9**). If the number of neuronal cell types found within a brain underlies the number and complexity of the computations that the brain can perform, then

Figure 15.9 Forebrain complexity In this cladogram, each bar indicates the number of different cell groups found in representative species of each major vertebrate group. Colored dots indicate when forebrain complexity is likely to have increased (orange) or decreased (green). (After Striedter 2005.)

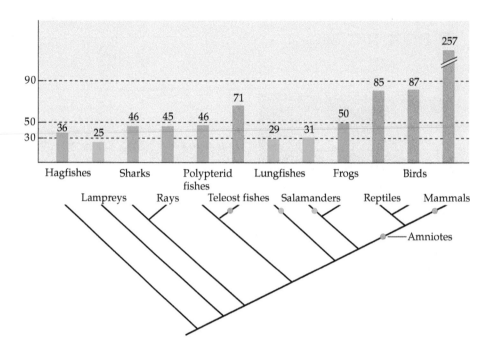

the impact of brain size on cognitive capacity may be due in part to increases in the complexity of neuronal circuitry.

Evolution of Brain Development

The overall size, regional complexity, and histological diversity of the brain would seem to reflect both prior adaptations of ancestral species and contemporary responses to adaptive pressures favoring the evolution of particular behavioral capacities. An important question raised by these observations is how these changes in brain size and structure are generated during development. The question becomes particularly intriguing when one considers the relatively small number of coding sequences available in animal genomes for specifying the size and structure of the brain (keeping in mind that the entire human genome contains fewer than 30,000 genes).

In fact, recent genetic discoveries revealed a family of genes that seem to play a role in controlling brain size development. Evolutionary changes in cognitive ability appear to be strongly related to the way brain size scales with body size across species, suggesting that relatively small changes in the genetic programs controlling brain size could result in profound changes in cognition. This argument is endorsed by the recent finding that genes involved in determining brain size in humans have evolved rapidly within the primate lineages leading to humans (Figure 15.10). Genes such as *microcephalin-1* (*MCPH1*) appear, in part, to underlie the growth and differentiation of neurons. Mutations in the *microcephalin* gene family lead to severe reductions in head and brain size, resulting in adults with brains about the size of chimpanzee brains; not surprisingly, such individuals have severe mental retardation. Relatively small changes in such genes could, in principle, provide a mechanism for scaling brain size across primates, at the same time providing the wherewithal for enhanced cognitive function.

Just how such a small number of genes might actually generate the diversity of brain size and complexity in different animals is not known. One model, developed by neurobiologist Barbara Finlay and her collaborators, suggests that changes in the timing of neurogenesis during brain development can account

(A)

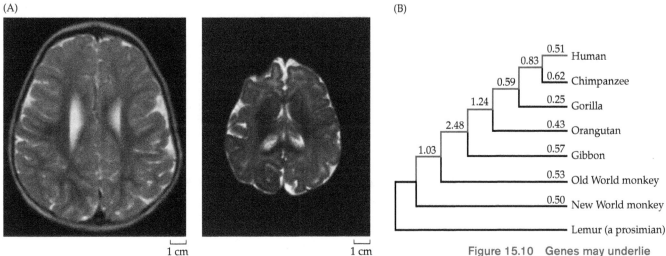

(B)

Figure 15.10 **Genes may underlie evolutionary changes in brain size** (A) Brains of a normal 8-month-old child (left) and an 8-month-old child with microcephaly (right). (B) Cladogram based on the nucleotide substitution rate for the *microcephalin-1* (*MCPH1*) gene in primates. Higher proportions indicate more nonsynonymous mutations (i.e., mutations specifying a different amino acid than was originally present). The lineage leading to humans (red) shows the fastest substitution rate, suggesting accelerated adaptive evolution. (From Gilbert et al. 2005.)

for regional diversity. To understand the merits of this model, it is useful to compare rats and macaque monkeys in terms of the developmental time at which neurons cease to be generated in different brain regions (Figure 15.11A). The sequence of neurogenesis in various brain structures follows the same pattern in both species, with, for example, brainstem neurons (locus coeruleus) being born first, then limbic neurons (septal nucleus), and finally neocortical neurons. In macaques, however, the neocortex develops later, relative to the rat, than the brainstem. This differential timing might explain the large expansion of the neocortex in macaques and other primates compared to rodents (Figure 15.11B). Therefore, merely stretching out the period of development of a particular brain area could, in principle, increase the number of neurons generated—and thus the size of a given brain area.

(A)

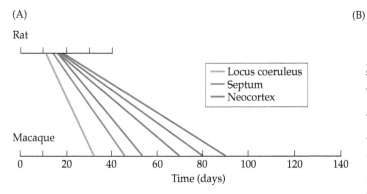

(B)

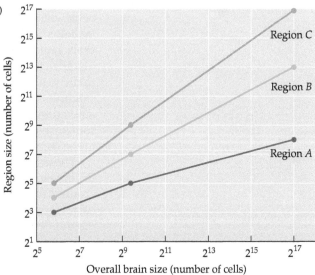

Figure 15.11 **Developmental timing may explain differences in brain structure size** (A) Timing of the end of neuronal generation in different brain structures is compared here for rats and macaques. While the locus coeruleus develops at about the same time in both species, the neocortex takes much longer to mature in macaques. (B) Finlay and Darlington's "late equals large" model of timing effects on brain region size. Three different brain regions contain cells generated at different times (*A* first, *C* last) in three species with small, medium, and large brains. Region *C* is disproportionately large in the largest species as a result of having had more time for neuronal proliferation and maturation. (A after Clancy et al. 2001; B after Finlay and Darlington 1995.)

Evolutionary Specializations of Brain and Behavior

The discussion so far has focused on the evolution and development of overall cognitive capacities inferred from behavioral flexibility and concomitant changes in total brain size and the size of some component structures. Just as important, however, are the specialized cognitive and behavioral mechanisms that have evolved to solve specific information-processing problems encountered in the natural environment. Adaptive specializations for particular types of behavior and cognitive functions have, until recently, received less attention than have questions concerning the evolution of more general characteristics of the brain shared by many different species.

In the 1960s, one of the first indications that animals might preferentially process certain types of information at the expense of others was the observation that rats readily associate the taste of lithium chloride with the nausea induced by its ingestion, but they have much greater trouble learning that bright lights predict nausea. In contrast, rats learn to associate bright lights with electric shock far more quickly than they learn to associate a specific taste with a shock. These findings challenged the then-dominant behaviorist notion that all behavior can be explained through simple associative learning, and suggested that, at the very least, animals are predisposed to learning particular types of stimulus-response relationships that are more likely to occur in their ecological niche.

Later studies in birds further supported the idea that the adaptation of behavior to specific environmental and social contexts is a driving force behind brain evolution. For example, male songbirds produce a repertoire of species-specific songs during development, and adult males sing these songs to attract mates and defend territory (see Chapter 12). Different songbird species show striking differences in the number of songs they can learn to produce. Even within a single species of songbirds, some individuals learn many more songs than do others, and the number of songs a male produces affects his eventual reproductive success.

Such behavioral differences among species or individuals could be realized through changes in overall brain size, as described in the previous section, or through specific adaptations of the neural circuits involved in producing the behavior. Such specializations are sometimes referred to as **functional neural modules**, and the differential elaboration of modular regions is termed **mosaic brain evolution**. Functional and neuroanatomical studies indicate that neural modules can become exquisitely specialized for processing information vital to the ways in which a particular species interacts with its environment. For example, rats and mice navigate their environments at night by touch, and autoradiographic, histological, and electrophysiological studies of the primary somatosensory cortex show that mice and rats overrepresent tactile sensibility in the corresponding sensory cortex.

These rodents possess an array of facial whiskers that is highly specialized to convey information about the size, shape, texture, and motion of objects around the head and face. A corresponding module of cortex called a whisker barrel represents each whisker, and the overall representation of the whiskers is disproportionately large relative to the rest of the body surface (Figure 15.12A). A similarly precise overrepresentation of the fingers and lips is apparent in the human somatosensory cortex and underlies the fine sensory discrimination abilities of these structures (Figure 15.12B). Similarly, the overrepresentation of the fingers in the primary motor cortex contributes to the ability to move them with high precision (see Chapter 5). Modularity is also a feature of the visual system, as described in Chapter 3.

(A)

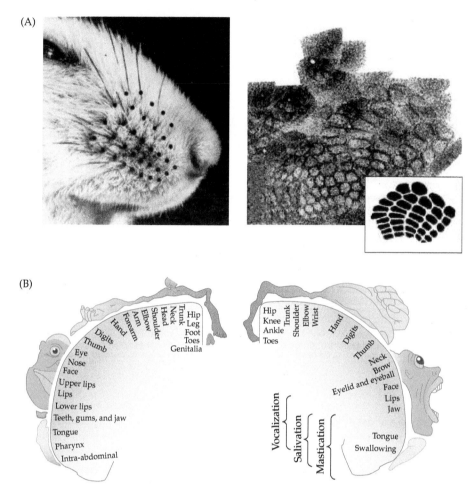

(B)

Figure 15.12   Overrepresentation of critical body parts in sensory and motor maps (A) Barrels in mouse somatosensory cortex (right) contain a precise, but disproportionately large, representation of the whiskers, the source of much sensory information in these animals. (B) Distorted topographical maps of the body surface in human somatosensory (left) and motor (right) cortices. (A from Woolsey and Van der Loos 1970; B after Penfield and Boldrey 1937.)

Evolution and development of learning and memory

The evolution and development of specialized brain regions that deal with the special processing needs of a given species are well documented, and many of these structural specializations are clearly related to cognitive abilities. The neural systems supporting learning and memory offer a particularly compelling example of specialization during evolution and development.

In non-human animals, even closely related species can differ substantially in their ability to learn and remember information, and these differences appear to be related to underlying differences in brain size and structure. For instance, members of the corvid (crow) family vary in the degree of their reliance on stored food, as well as on structural specializations of the mouth and throat for carrying food during storing (Figure 15.13A). Similar variation is seen among chickadees and titmice, in which some species store food while others do not. In general, species that rely on stored food show greater capacity to remember the location and contents of food caches for long periods. These differences

(A)

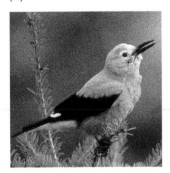

Clark's nutcracker

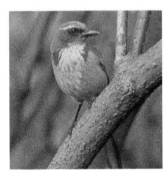

Scrub jay

(B) Absolute hippocampus size

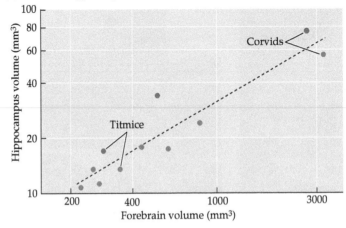

Figure 15.13 The size of some brain structures correlates with behavior The hippocampus is specialized for remembering the location of stored food in birds, and its size varies accordingly. (A) Two members of the crow (corvid) family. Clark's nutcracker (top) displays highly specialized behavior for storing and retrieving food. In contrast, the western scrub jay (bottom), a feeding generalist, is relatively unspecialized for food caching. (B) Hippocampal volume plotted against forebrain volume for two families of birds: corvids and parids (titmice). Food-storing species (red) tend to have larger hippocampal formations than the size of the forebrain as a whole would suggest. (After Krebs et al. 1989.)

in memory are associated with differences in the size of the hippocampus, a structure important for encoding information in memory that is pertinent to navigation in many animals and to declarative memory in humans (**Figure 15.13B**). By the same token, species that do not store food have a disproportionately smaller hippocampus. These observations strongly support the conclusion that neural structures become highly specialized for solving the specific information-processing problems faced by a species.

Primate brains also show specializations for learning and memory. Such variation among species may reflect the demands of foraging for widely dispersed and ephemeral food sources. Endorsing this idea, the relationship between brain size and body size differs in primates that forage for different types of foods. Primates whose diet is high in ripe fruit tend to have larger brains for their body size than do primates that eat mostly leaves or insects (**Figure 15.14A**). Enhanced brain size in fruit-eating primates compared with leaf- or insect-eating primates could represent an adaptation to the complex spatial and temporal distribution of ripe fruits. In the tropics, fruit tends to ripen in a piecemeal fashion, and on trees dispersed over long distances throughout the forest. A diet rich in ripe fruit thus requires the ability to learn and remember both the temporal and spatial distribution of resources across a wide area. Leaf eaters, however, typically possess digestive specializations permitting them to extract energy from the abundant leaf matter located more or less anywhere in the forest. Insect eaters tend to forage opportunistically, but they typically have small enough bodies that they can satisfy their nutritional needs within a relatively small area.

This framework predicts that fruit-eating primates should possess better spatial learning and memory abilities than should otherwise similar primates that forage on leaves, insects, or even tree sap. Testing this model experimentally showed that fruit-eating tamarin monkeys remember the locations of food sources for much longer periods than do sap-eating marmosets, even though the two species have a similar body size and possess the same cooperative social

(A)

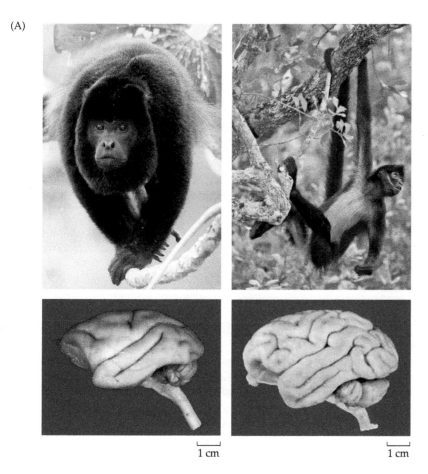

1 cm   1 cm

Figure 15.14 The foraging hypothesis
This concept posits that the demands of "specialized" feeding on widely dispersed and/or ephemeral food sources favor the evolution of enhanced cognition. (A) The brains of a howler monkey (a leaf-eating generalist feeder; left) and a spider monkey (a fruit-feeding specialist; right) are shown at the same scale. Note the spider monkey's appreciably larger brain and greater number of gyri. (B) Allometric plot of brain weight versus body weight for bats. Bat species feeding on fruit, flowers, or blood are plotted in red; insectivorous bats are plotted in black. The more generalist insectivorous bats have smaller brains for their body size than do bats specialized for feeding on fruit, flowers, or blood. (A brain images courtesy of University of Wisconsin and Michigan State University Comparative Mammalian Brain Collections; B after Stephen et al. 1981.)

(B)

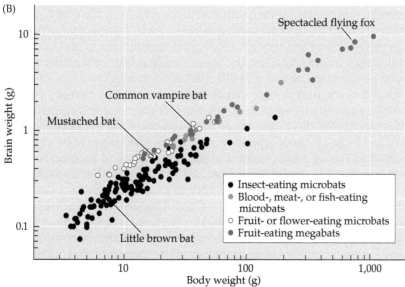

system. The foraging model is further supported by the observation that bats that eat fruit, flowers, or blood—all of which are difficult to obtain—have larger brains for their body size than do insect-eating bats (**Figure 15.14B**).

Learning and memory differ not only across species, but also over development. A paradox of early memory is that although infants clearly learn and store an enormous amount of information during the first few years of life (acquisition of language and motor skills, increasingly acceptable social behavior, and

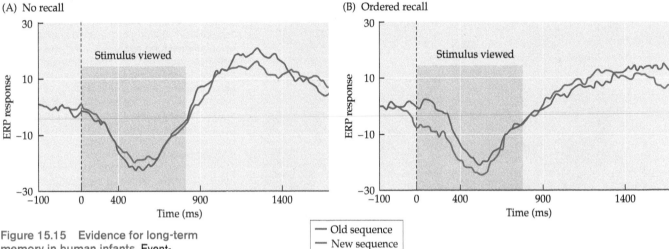

(A) No recall

(B) Ordered recall

— Old sequence
— New sequence

Figure 15.15 Evidence for long-term memory in human infants Event-related potential waveforms at a frontal electrode site recorded as infants viewed static images of an experimenter performing a two-step sequence with props. These data were collected 1 week after the infants viewed a live demonstration of the experimenter acting out the sequence. Data plotted in (A) reflect the subset of infants who later showed no recall for the two-step sequence. In contrast, data plotted in (B) reflect the subset of infants who later showed evidence of ordered recall. (After Bauer et al. 2003.)

so on), adults have very little explicit memory of this period—a phenomenon termed **childhood amnesia**.

Despite our apparent inability to recall events from early childhood, abundant experimental evidence suggests that children do in fact form memories of events they experience in the first few years of life. For example, infants can be cued to imitate action sequences from memory. Infants as young as 9 months can reliably recall ordered action sequences, and the robustness of such long-term recall increases with age. Infants as young as 13 months can remember two- and three-step sequences for as long as 8 months under the appropriate conditions. Importantly, the same factors that influence adult declarative memory—such as the number of experiences with an event, the nature of the event, and the availability of cues that support event retrieval—also influence children's ability to recall events. Thus, even though adults do not remember experiences from early childhood, infants form robust memories that last for months and are influenced by the same factors that affect adult memories.

At the end of the first year of life, changes in long-term memory (such as being able to successfully emulate a two-step action sequence) coincide with major changes in the development of circuits within the hippocampus. As discussed in Chapter 9, these hippocampal circuits are thought to be important for the temporal order of information stored as declarative memories, which may in turn support the emergence of episodic memory as it is understood in adults. Consistent with this idea, variability in an ERP component associated with novelty detection recorded from the scalp of 9-month-old infants predicts their long-term memory for ordered sequences (Figure 15.15). Only those infants whose brain waves registered a difference between old and new sequences 1 week after first seeing them showed subsequent memory for the sequences one month later when they were given an opportunity to manipulate the objects they originally saw. Brain indices of memory retention after 1 week predicted infants' behavioral reactions to objects several weeks later, thus demonstrating a form of long-term memory.

Evolution and development of quantitative cognition

Many forms of number use in humans depend on explicit symbols, making a great deal of cognitive processing necessary for solving even simple addition problems. However, humans also possess an ability to represent number that appears to have evolved well before language or human cultures existed. This

approximate number system (ANS) provides a rough estimate of the number of items seen, heard, or remembered. Much the same way that perceptual systems discriminate stimulus qualities based on the ratio of their intensities—an effect known as the **Weber-Fechner law**—the ANS discriminates numbers of stimuli by their ratios, as described in Box 12C. Remarkably, the same ratio dependence has been shown to characterize the numerical judgments made by a variety of non-human animals, human babies, and even human adults.

Although only an adult human with number words and concepts can represent large quantities with precision, precursors of human mathematical abilities are present in human infants and non-human animals. The value of such skills is not hard to imagine, since a change in number is often biologically relevant. However, sorting out the importance of number from other variables can be experimentally challenging. For example, 10 seeds are more numerous than 5 seeds, but they also weigh more and have greater surface area. Three alarm calls emitted in sequence are more numerous than two, but they are also longer in overall duration and cumulatively contain more sound energy. Nevertheless, it is possible to show that many non-human animals represent number independently of other physical dimensions and that animals can use these abstract numerical representations to make approximate computations. The remarkable overlap in reaction time and accuracy between monkeys and humans when comparing two arrays differing in number implies a common nonverbal representational scheme (Figure 15.16).

Preverbal infants in the first year of life are also sensitive to the abstract numerical properties of their environments. A variety of clever procedures that rely on measuring the location and duration of an infant's gaze demonstrate that babies can differentiate visual and auditory arrays on the basis of number and independently of alternative variables that, in nature, are correlated with number. Furthermore, discrimination in infancy follows Weber's law. For example, Figure 15.17 illustrates that, when shown two streams of changing visual arrays, infants prefer to look at the stream that alternates between two numerical values (e.g., 8 dots–16 dots–8 dots–…) compared to a constant numerical stream (e.g., 8 dots–8 dots–8 dots–…). Even more impressive, the magnitude of

(A)

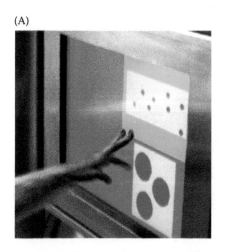

(B)

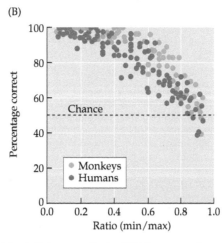

(C)

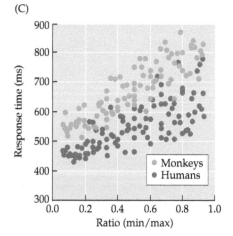

Figure 15.16 **Human and monkey numerical distance effects** (A) Here a monkey is engaging in a numerical ordering task using a touch screen. (B) Monkey and human performance in the numerical ordering task are plotted as a function of the ratio between the two numerical values being compared. (C) Response time is plotted here as a function of the ratio between the two numerical values being compared for monkeys and human college students. (After Cantlon and Brannon 2006.)

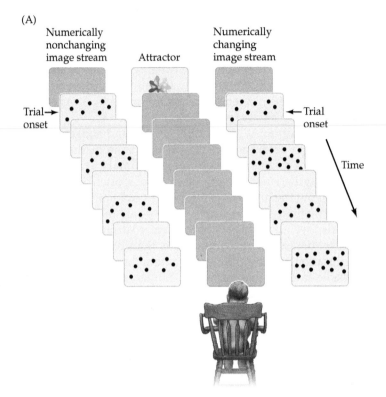

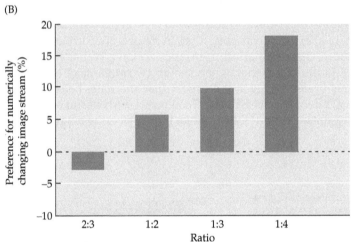

Figure 15.17 Behavioral evidence for an approximate number sense in human infants (A) A numerical change detection paradigm. During each trial, infants were presented with two image streams simultaneously on two peripheral screens. The amount of time the infants looked at each of the two streams was measured. The numerically changing image stream showed images with two different numerosities in alternation; the numerically nonchanging image stream showed images with the same numerosity. (B) Six-month-old infants showed significant preference scores for numerically changing image streams when the values in the changing stream differed by a 1:2, 1:3, or 1:4 ratio, but not when they differed by a 2:3 ratio. (After Libertus and Brannon 2010.)

a baby's preference for the numerically changing stream depends on the ratio between the two alternating values.

Convergent evidence from studies of people with brain damage and from neuroimaging studies implicate parietal cortex, principally near the intra-parietal sulcus (IPS), in numerical processing in adult humans. Importantly

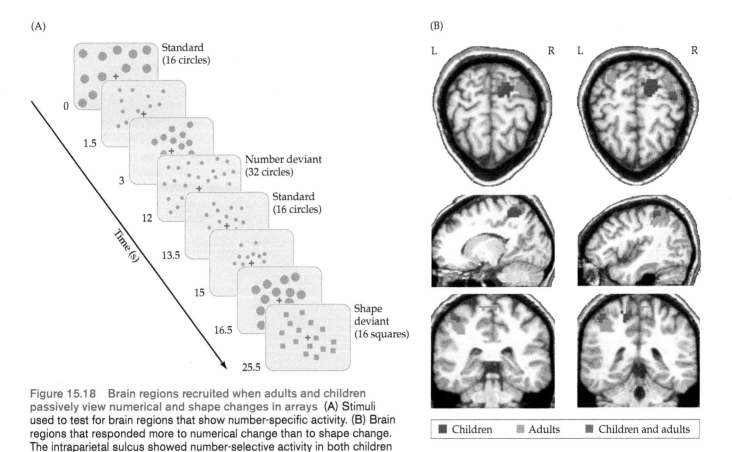

Figure 15.18 Brain regions recruited when adults and children passively view numerical and shape changes in arrays (A) Stimuli used to test for brain regions that show number-specific activity. (B) Brain regions that responded more to numerical change than to shape change. The intraparietal sulcus showed number-selective activity in both children and adults. (After Cantlon et al. 2006.)

the same brain region appears to be recruited when infants and very young children perform numerical tasks. For example, a study with infants using near-infrared spectroscopy (NIRS) showed that the IPS in the right hemisphere responds selectively to changes in the number of elements compared to changes in shape of a visual stimulus. Similarly, both 4-year-old children and adults show selective recovery of fMRI BOLD responses to changes in the number of stimuli but not changes in the shape of stimuli within the same IPS region (Figure 15.18). In rhesus macaques, cells in the prefrontal and parietal cortices respond selectively to specific numerical values (Figure 15.19). The sensitivity of individual neurons to number is broader for larger numbers, consistent with encoding number on a ratio scale.

Collectively, these findings strongly implicate the IPS as a critical component, if not the physical embodiment, of the ANS. One implication of this conclusion is that the ubiquitous problem of quantifying things in the world selectively favored the evolution of a homologous brain circuit supporting approximate number judgments early in primate evolution, and this circuit is operational early in human infancy. These ideas raise the question of how the brains of other animals, as diverse as birds, bees, and spiders, make numerical judgments in a way similar to those made by the ANS in monkeys and humans.

Evolution and development of social cognition

Most primates, including humans, live in relatively large social groups structured around kinship, dominance hierarchies, and cooperative alliances. Managing these social relationships relies on individual recognition, status assessment,

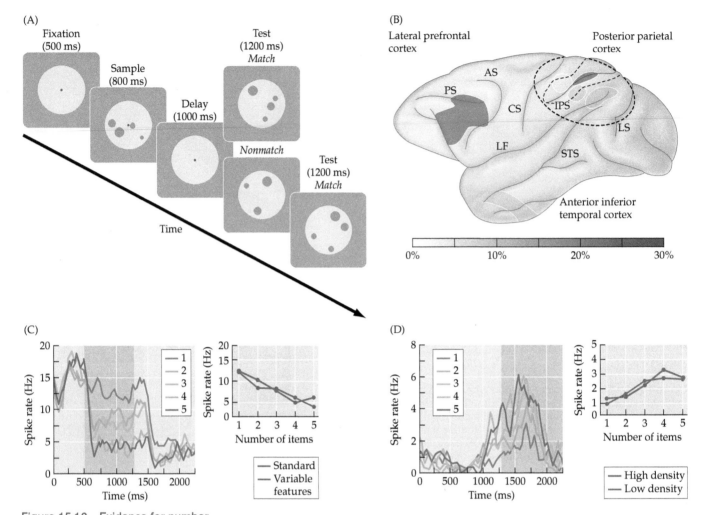

Figure 15.19   Evidence for number cells in the parietal cortex of the monkey brain (A) Stimuli like these were used in the task structure illustrated here to test macaques during electrophysiological recording. Monkeys viewed sample arrays and after a short delay were required to release a bar when the test array matched the sample array in number. (B) This lateral view of a monkey brain shows recording sites. Color coding indicates the relative proportion of number-selective cells. AS, arcuate sulcus; CS, central sulcus; IPS, intraparietal sulcus; LF, lateral fissure; LS, lunate sulcus; PS, principal sulcus; STS, superior temporal sulcus. (C) Firing rate is plotted as a function of sample numerosity during the sample period (darker shaded region) for a neuron that was maximally responsive to one item, the numeral 1. (D) Here, firing rate is plotted as a function of sample numerosity during the delay period (darker shaded region) for a neuron that was maximally responsive to four items. (After Nieder and Miller 2004.)

and long-term memory for prior interactions. Furthermore, it would be adaptive for primates to be able to infer the intentions of other individuals from their expressions and state of attention, as well as to be able to deceive others. Such socially sophisticated behavior implies an ability to infer the internal mental state of other individuals (see Chapter 11). This hypothesis of socially driven brain evolution is often referred to as the *Machiavellian intelligence hypothesis*, after the notorious political theorist of the Italian Renaissance.

The suggestion that the more highly evolved cognitive abilities of primates in general and humans in particular have been socially driven is supported by several observations. First, primate societies are arguably among the most complex in the animal kingdom, and primates as a group possess relatively large forebrains. Moreover, other animals that live in complex social groups, such as dolphins and killer whales, also have relatively large brains. Second, various measures of advanced brain development among primates correlate with measures of social complexity such as deception rate, number of grooming partners, and frequency of social learning and innovation (**Figure 15.20**). Third, the primate brain also shows specializations for processing social information. Both human and non-human primates, for example, possess neurons in the temporal and occipital cortex selective for the identity and direction of gaze in a viewed face (**Figure 15.21A**; see also Figure 3.27A). Moreover, electrical stimulation of areas containing such face-selective neurons in monkeys can induce them to report seeing a face; stimulation of the temporal cortex and

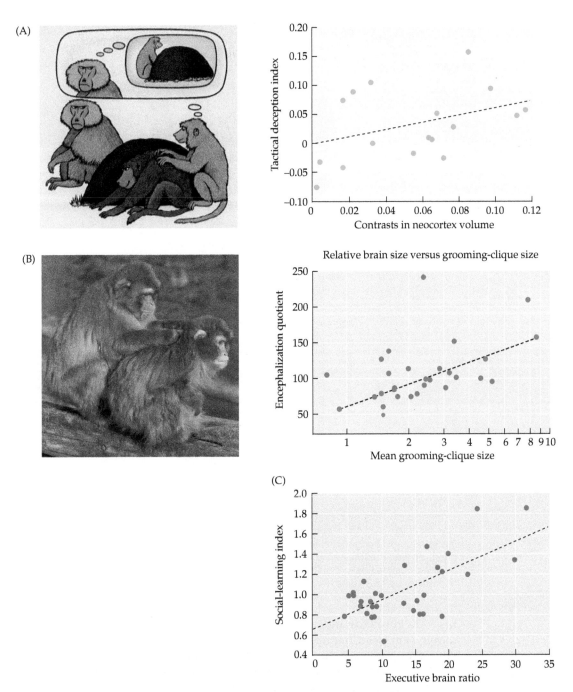

Figure 15.20 The social, or Machiavellian, intelligence hypothesis Most primates live in groups that favor the evolution of sophisticated social skills, including the ability to infer the emotions and intentions of others. Such skills would favor the evolution of advanced cognition in primates. (A) The sort of tactical deceptive abilities illustrated in the cartoon on the left tend to be greater in primates with larger neocortices. (B) Encephalization quotient, a measure of brain size to body size, scales positively with grooming-clique size, which is the typical number of animals that an individual spends time grooming. (C) Social-learning frequency scales positively with executive brain ratio, a measure of the elaboration of advanced brain structures, including the prefrontal cortex. (A after Byrne and Corp 2004; B after Kudo and Dunbar 2001; C after Reader and Laland 2002.)

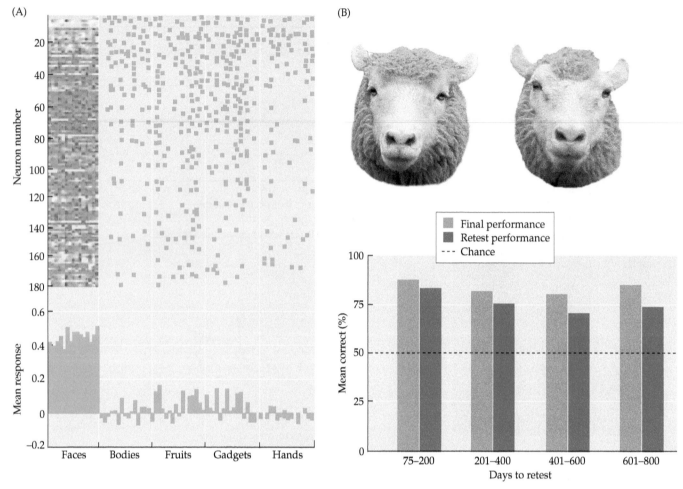

Figure 15.21 Social recognition (A) Neurons in a face "patch" in the monkey temporal lobe identified by fMRI respond selectively to faces. Each tick (upper portion of panel) marks neuronal firing to a stimulus by the individual neurons displayed in each row in the graph. Average responses across all neurons were robust for faces but weak for other complex objects (lower portion of panel). (B) Sheep can remember the faces of their cohorts for up to 3 years. (A after Tsao et al. 2006; B after Kendrick et al. 2001.)

fusiform gyrus can induce transient prosopagnosia—a specific deficit in face recognition (see Chapter 3) in human surgical patients. Such specializations are not unique to primates, however; sheep have similar face-selective neurons in their temporal cortices and, despite their simple social system, are adept at recognizing and remembering social identities (Figure 15.21B).

Remarkably, the neural circuits implicated in identifying individuals, attending to the face and body cues that communicate their intentions, and acting on this information not only are well developed in human and non-human primates but are shaped by social conditions even during adulthood. A recent study experimentally manipulated group size, from one to six individuals, in a colony of rhesus macaques. The monkeys' brains were subsequently scanned while they were anesthetized. Structural MRI scans showed that the gray matter in the superior temporal sulcus region of cortex—an area known to contain neurons selective for faces—was thicker in monkeys with larger social networks (Figure 15.22). Furthermore, there was stronger functional coupling between this region and a region of prefrontal cortex implicated in planning and decision making. Finally, these relationships were more pronounced in monkeys with higher status. Together, these observations endorse the idea that

(A)

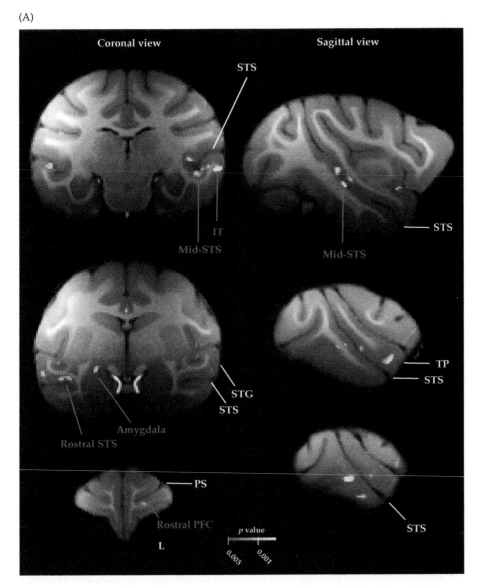

(B)

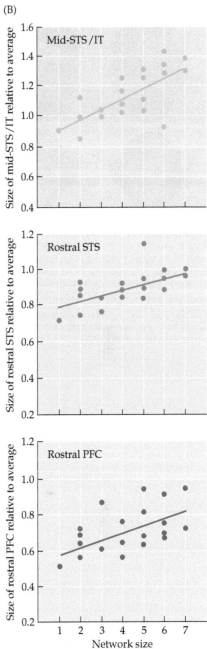

Figure 15.22 Social networks and the brain (A) Rhesus macaques were assigned to groups of one to seven individuals, and over 1 year later their brains were scanned for anatomical differences with MRI. Gray matter thickness positively correlated ($p < 0.005$, cluster size > 5 cubic millimeters) with social group size in the temporal lobe and rostral prefrontal cortex (rostral PFC). Red leaders and text indicate regions where network size effects were observed. White leaders and text indicate anatomical landmarks. IT, inferotemporal cortex; L, left; PS, principal sulcus; STG, superior temporal gyrus; STS, superior temporal sulcus; TP temporal pole. (B) The relationship between social network size and a measure of the size of the mid-STS/IT, rostral STS, and rostral PFC, relative to the overall average. Measures greater than 1 indicate that voxels in an individual's MRI scan must be compressed to match the group average. (After Sallet et al. 2011.)

individual experience can shape the structure and function of neural circuits supporting specialized types of cognition, and they hint at the remarkably interplay of development, experience, and evolution in adapting individuals and species to specific information-processing problems presented by the physical or social environment.

Supporting the importance of social interaction in the evolution of human cognition, developmental studies suggest that specializations for processing

(A)

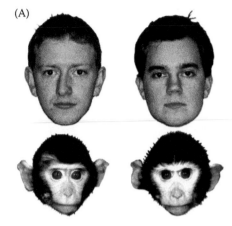

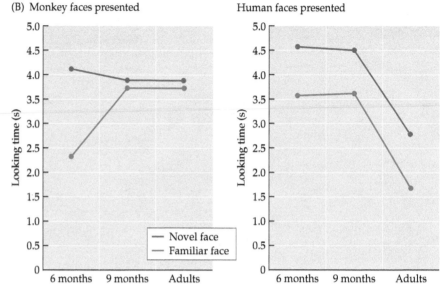

Figure 15.23   The "own species" effect (A) Sample stimuli. (B) Six-month-old infants show longer looking times when presented with both novel monkey (left graph) and human (right graph) faces. In contrast, 9-month old infants (and adults) differentiate novel faces from familiar faces only in humans. (After Pascalis et al. 2002.)

social information appear early in human ontogeny and become refined with the development of social expertise, and that their dysfunction in conditions like autism can have devastating consequences. Infants enter the world with a bias to attend to faces, and even in the first few months of life they differentiate novel individuals from each other. Much like adults, infants only a few days old show superior discrimination for upright faces compared to inverted faces. Further, the P100 and P400 ERPs recorded from 3-month-old infants differentiate upright and inverted faces as well.

Building on this initial face-processing bias, face perception in infancy is also shaped by experience. For example, 6-month-old infants show similar recognition memory for both monkey faces and human faces. By 9 months, however, infants, like adults, are better able to recognize human faces compared to monkey faces (Figure 15.23). Increasing specialization for own-species faces mirrors the phenomenon of perceptual narrowing seen in speech perception, in which infants initially perceive phonemes of all languages but gradually lose the ability to perceive phonemes not present in the language they are exposed to (see Chapter 12).

As might be expected, given the highly social nature of our species, failure to develop normal social cognition can have devastating consequences. Autism, for example, is a disorder that affects about three to six in every 1,000 children and, as described in Chapter 11, involves many social deficits. Individuals with autism tend to avoid both physical and eye contact with others. They show heightened interest in the inanimate world, often fixating on particular objects. In addition, children with autism tend to fail theory-of-mind tasks and generally show reduced interest in other people. In contrast to typically developing children and adults, people with autism spend significantly less time examining people's eyes and instead focus on the mouth or body when shown images of people.

By contrast, children with Williams syndrome—a neurodevelopmental disorder characterized by high verbal abilities but otherwise low IQ and excessive sociability—show relatively normal social cognition, orienting to faces and successfully passing theory-of-mind tests. The contrast between children with Williams syndrome, who are typically social and talkative, and children with autism, who are typically antisocial and reticent, has been interpreted by some as evidence that social cognition depends on a dedicated brain system that can be disturbed during development. However, research by developmental psychologist Annette Karmiloff-Smith and her colleagues suggests some caution in the interpretation of this contrast. For example, children with Down syndrome show impaired face processing but nonetheless pass theory-of-mind tests. Karmiloff-Smith argues that segregation of social cognition may occur postnatally, through experience with normal social and speech input. In any event, developmental disorders of this sort are clearly complicated and are more likely to depend on a cascade of developmental events that has gone awry than on the loss of a specific regional function.

Evolution and development of language

As introduced in Chapter 12, two brain regions in the left hemisphere appear to be major substrates for language processing in humans. Broca's area in the frontal cortex plays a critical role in language production, and lesions in this area produce an aphasia characterized by halting, inarticulate speech. Wernicke's area in the temporal lobe contributes to language comprehension, and lesions in this area result in deficits in producing meaningful utterances.

Although it was initially thought that Broca's and Wernicke's areas were unique to humans, it now appears that they represent elaborations of brain areas present in non-human primates (Figure 15.24). Field playback experiments of species-specific vocalizations in macaques have shown a right-ear

(A) Macaque

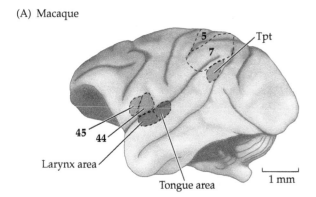

(B) Human

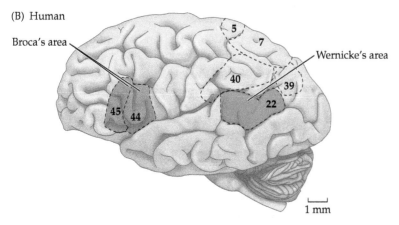

Figure 15.24 Vocal communication–related cortical areas in macaques and humans Areas 44 and 45 in the macaque (A) correspond to Broca's area in humans (B), whereas the temporal parietal junction (Tpt) in macaques has apparently been elaborated as Wernicke's area in humans. Areas 39 and 40 in the human parietal lobe have no homologue in macaques, although some investigators contend that lateral area 7 in the macaque is homologous with these areas. (A after Preuss and Goldman-Rakic 1991; B after Petrides et al. 2005.)

Figure 15.25 Language areas in the brains of non-human primates? The figure shows PET activation in three different rhesus monkeys in response to the vocalizations that these animals use in social communication. The areas activated are arguably similar to the major language areas in the human brain. Whether this activity is comparable to the activity elicited by speech in the human brain remains a matter of active investigation and some dispute. (The letters A, B, and C in the inset identify the levels of brain sections shown.) (From Gil-da-Costa et al. 2006.)

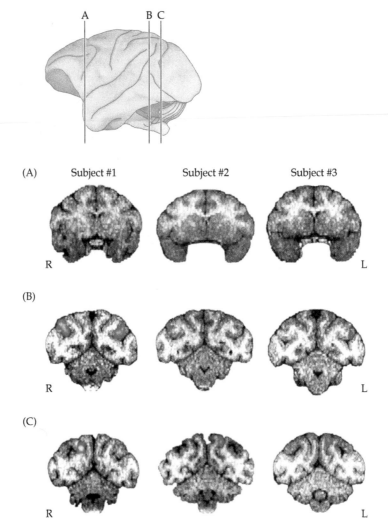

response advantage (and thus a left-hemisphere processing bias) similar to the left-hemisphere lateralization of language in humans. Furthermore, the left temporoparietal area in macaques (roughly corresponding to Wernicke's area in humans) is larger in the left hemisphere than the right. Similarly, the ventrolateral frontal cortex of the macaque (roughly corresponding to Broca's area in humans) is specialized for fine control of the orofacial musculature and has a cellular structure generally similar to that found in Broca's area in humans. Recent PET studies also revealed the homologue of Wernicke's area in rhesus monkeys to be activated when the monkeys hear species-specific vocalizations (Figure 15.25). Together, these observations support the idea that specialized features of human speech are built on adaptations for social and perhaps vocal communication already present in non-human primates.

Despite these shared brain areas associated with vocal communication, human language is both qualitatively and quantitatively distinct from animal communication (see Chapter 12). The linguistic complexity and cultural capacity of humans remains even more enigmatic when considered in light of the fact that most of the basic brain structures contributing to language and other cognitive abilities in humans are shared with other primates. These observations suggest that the neurobiological source of human language and culture might lie in other unique structural or functional characteristics of the brain, as well as morphological features outside the brain (such as the vocal tract).

Developmental studies indicate that the left hemisphere shows early specialization for speech processing in young human infants. For example, behavioral studies have shown that infants show better speech discrimination when sounds are presented to the right ear (and thus preferentially processed by the left hemisphere). Functional MRI studies have confirmed that the left hemisphere is indeed predominant in speech processing in early infancy. Infrared optical imaging has also shown that there is greater left-hemisphere activation in newborns for normal speech compared to speech played backward. Although the complete network of brain regions needed for adult language processing described in Chapter 12 is not fully apparent in the infant brain, a subset of these regions is clearly active early in development. This evidence, together with the fact that newborns are responsive to speech and capable of learning the full range of phonemes in the world's languages, argues strongly for language circuitry arising from developmental programs that precede experience.

Despite this evidence, it is obvious that the relevant brain regions are influenced by language experience; after all, we learn a native or other languages during the early years of life and beyond, and do so more effectively before the end of a critical period that ends late in childhood (see also the review of language deprivation studies in children in Chapter 12).

ERP studies in children and adults further support this conclusion. Studies of language processing in adults show that posterior temporoparietal ERPs generated by the left hemisphere differentiate "open-class" words (nouns and verbs) from "closed-class" words that convey grammatical relationships (prepositions, determiners, and conjunctions). At 20 months of age, infants understand the meaning of open- and closed-class words but do not exhibit distinct ERP responses to the two classes. By 28 to 30 months, however—the point at which most children are beginning to speak in short sentences—ERPs differentiate open- and closed-class words. By 3 years of age, children are speaking in complete sentences and employing closed-class words correctly, and ERPs show the mature pattern of left-hemisphere asymmetry to closed-class words. These results suggest that brain systems for aspects of language become more specialized over development as the child masters increasingly complex linguistic challenges.

Another approach to these questions has been to study language development in patients with brain injuries, left- versus right-brain injuries in particular. Surprisingly, these studies reveal that language development is not much different for children with left- compared to right-hemisphere trauma when the damage occurs very early in life. Thus, although behavioral and neuroimaging data demonstrate that laterality for speech processing emerges early in infancy and continues to develop with linguistic experience, other brain regions appear to take on language functions when the brain is injured early in development.

Summary

1. Understanding how changes in brain structure and function lead to changing cognitive abilities that are apparent during the course of infancy, childhood, and adolescence, as well as across species, remains an important goal for cognitive neuroscience.

2. A great deal of brain development takes place prenatally, driven by intrinsic genetic and epigenetic programs that lay the foundation for adult cognitive skills. These programs specify the development of neural systems that vary among species in ways reflecting inheritance from a common ancestor, as well as adaptation to local conditions.

3. The brain continues to develop and organize its connectivity postnatally, in a process that continues through adolescence and, to a diminished degree, throughout adult life. This plasticity is particularly important for the emergence of uniquely human faculties, like reading and writing.

4. Different brain regions mature at different rates, and this variation appears to explain many of the changes evident in cognitive behavior during development. Such changes in the timing of critical events in the emergence of brain structures that underlie cognition may explain differences in brain and behavior that characterize different species.

5. Social complexity may have been a particularly important selective factor in the evolution of cognition and its neural mechanisms in human and non-human primates. Consequently, disorders attended by social impairments, such as autism, are particularly devastating.

Additional Reading

Reviews

BUNGE, S. A. AND P. D. ZELAZO (2006) A brain-based account of the development of rule use in childhood. *Curr. Dir. Psychol. Sci.* 15: 118–121.

CASEY, B. J., N. TOTTENHAM, C. LISTON AND S. DURSTON (2005) Imaging the developing brain: What have we learned about cognitive development? *Trends Cogn. Sci.* 9: 104–110.

CLAYTON, N. S. AND J. R. KREBS (1995) Memory in food-storing birds: From behaviour to brain. *Curr. Opin. Neurobiol.* 5: 149–154.

GILBERT, S. L., W. B. DOBYNS AND B. T. LAHN (2005) Genetic links between brain development and brain evolution. *Nat. Rev. Genetics* 6: 581.

JOHNSON, M. H. (2001) Functional and brain development in humans. *Nat. Rev. Neurosci.* 2: 475–483.

LENROOT, R. K. AND J. N. GIEDD (2006) Brain development in children and adolescents: Insights from anatomical brain magnetic resonance imaging. *Neurosci. Behav. Rev.* 30: 718–729.

NELSON, C. (2001) The development and neural bases of face recognition. *Infant Child Devel.* 10: 3–18.

NEVILLE, H. J. AND D. BAVELIER (2002) Specificity and plasticity in neurocognitive development in humans. In *Brain Development and Cognition: A Reader*, 2nd ed. M. H. Johnson, Y. Munakata and R. O. Gilmore (eds.). Malden, MA: Blackwell, pp. 251–271.

PELPHREY, K. A. AND E. J. CARTER (2007) Brain mechanisms underlying social perception deficits in autism. In *Human Behavior and the Developing Brain*, 2nd Ed., D. Coch, G. Dawson and K. Fischer (eds.). New York: Guilford.

VAN PRAAG, H., G. KEMPERMANN AND F. H. GAGE (2000) Neural consequences of environmental enrichment. *Nat. Neurosci.* 1: 191–198.

Important Original Papers

BAILLARGEON, R. (1987) Object permanence in 3.5- to 4.5-month-old infants. *Devel. Psychol.* 23: 665–664.

BOURGEOIS, J. AND P. RAKIC (1993) Changes of synaptic density in the primary visual cortex of the macaque monkey from fetal to adult stage. *J. Neurosci.* 13: 2801–2820.

CLUTTON-BROCK, T. H. AND P. H. HARVEY (1980) Primates, brains, and ecology. *J. Zool. Soc. London* 190: 309–323.

DEHAENE-LAMBERTZ, G., S. DEHAENE AND K. HERTZ-PANNIER (2002) Functional neuroimaging of speech perception in infants. *Science* 298: 2013–2015.

DUNBAR, R. I. M. (1993) Coevolution of neocortical size, group size and language in humans (with commentary). *Behav. Brain Sci.* 16: 681–735.

FINLAY, B. L. AND R. B. DARLINGTON (1995) Linked regularities in the development and evolution of mammalian brains. *Science* 268: 1578–1584.

JOLLY, A. (1966) Lemur social behavior and primate intelligence. *Science* 153: 501–506.

MILLS, D. L., C. PRAT, R. ZANGL, C. L. STAGER, H. J. NEVILLE AND J. F. WERKER (2004) Language experience and the organization of brain activity to phonetically similar words: ERP evidence from 14- and 20-month-olds. *J. Cogn. Neurosci.* 16: 1452–1464.

MISCHEL, W. (1981) Metacognition and the rules of delay. In *Social Cognitive Development*, J. H. Flavell and L. Ross (eds.). Cambridge: Cambridge University Press, pp. 240–271.

PLATT, M. L., E. M. BRANNON, T. BRIESE AND J. A. FRENCH (1996) Differences in feeding ecology predict differences in memory between lion tamarins (*Leontopithecus rosalia*) and marmosets (*Callithrix kuhli*). *Anim. Learn. Behav.* 24: 384–393.

RAKIC, P. (1974) Neurons in rhesus monkey visual cortex: Systematic relation between time of origin and eventual disposition. *Science* 183: 425–427.

SALLET, J. AND 9 OTHERS (2011) Social network size affects neural circuits in macaques. *Science* 334: 697–700.

SAWAGUCHI, T. (1989) Relationships between cerebral indices for "extra" cortical parts and ecological categories in anthropoids. *Brain Behav. Evol.* 43: 281–293.

WIMMER, H. AND J. PERNER (1983) Beliefs about beliefs: Representation and constraining function of wrong beliefs in young children's understanding of deception. *Cognition* 13: 41–68.

WYNN, K. (1992) Addition and subtraction by human infants. *Nature* 358: 749–750.

Books

ALLMAN, J. (2000) *Evolving Brains.* New York: Freeman.

DE HAAN, M. AND M. H. JOHNSON (2003) *The Cognitive Neuroscience of Development.* London: Psychology Press.

JERISON, H. (1973) *Evolution of the Brain and Intelligence.* New York: Academic Press.

JOHNSON, M. H. (2005) *Developmental Cognitive Neuroscience.* Malden, MA: Blackwell.

NELSON, C. A. AND M. LUCIANA (2001) *Handbook of Developmental Cognitive Neuroscience.* Cambridge, MA: MIT Press.

PLATT, M. L. AND A. A. GHAZANFAR, EDS. (2012) *Primate Neuroethology.* New York: Oxford University Press.

PURVES, D. (1988) *Body and Brain.* Cambridge, MA: Harvard University Press.

RUFF, H. A. AND M. K. ROTHBART (1996) *Attention in Early Development.* Oxford: Oxford University Press.

STRIEDTER, G. F. (2005) *Principles of Brain Evolution.* Sunderland, MA: Sinauer.

APPENDIX

The Human Nervous System

This Appendix briefly reviews human nervous system structure and function. It is intended as a convenient guide to basic aspects of physiology and anatomy.

Cellular Components of the Nervous System

The fact that **cells** are the elements that make up all animal tissues was recognized early in the nineteenth century. Not until the twentieth century, however, did neuroscientists finally agree that the nervous system, like all other organ systems, comprises these fundamental units, and that the cells of the nervous system are exceptional in only some details. Pioneering histological studies led to the further consensus that the cells of the nervous system can be divided into two broad categories:

- **Nerve cells**, or **neurons**, are specialized to generate and propagate electrical signals. Information transmitted in the form of these electrical signals is the basis of sensation, behavior, and physiological processes in all animals; it is also the source of the cognitive abilities that reach their most complex expression in human beings. Our current understanding of this signaling process represents one of the more dramatic success stories in modern biology.

- **Neuroglial cells** comprise a variety of cell types that support and hold together nervous tissue; they are frequently referred to simply as **glia**— the Greek word for "glue"—and they play a variety of important roles in neural function. In contrast to neurons, neuroglial cells are not capable of electrical signaling, but some types (notably the *Schwann cells*, discussed a little later) have a crucial effect on the speed at which a neuron's electrical signals travel.

Like other cells, each nerve cell has a **cell body** containing a nucleus and **organelles** (endoplasmic reticulum, ribosomes, Golgi apparatus, mitochondria, and others) that are essential to the function of all cells (Figure A.1). The distinguishing features of nerve cells arise from their specialization for *intercellular communication*. Neurons are characterized by a single, often quite long extension from the cell body called an **axon**, and by shorter branches called **dendrites** (also called *dendritic branches* or *dendritic processes*). The axon's purpose is to convey information, usually in the form of electrical impulses, over distances that range from millimeters to meters (the latter representing axons that extend

Figure A.1 **Major features of nerve cells (neurons)** The drawing on the left shows a typical neuron, identifying the cell body (soma), its dendritic arborization, and the initial part of its axon. The blowup of the vicinity of the nerve cell body shows the variety of organelles that neurons share with other cell types, as well as the axonal, dendritic, and synaptic specializations that make nerve cells unique.

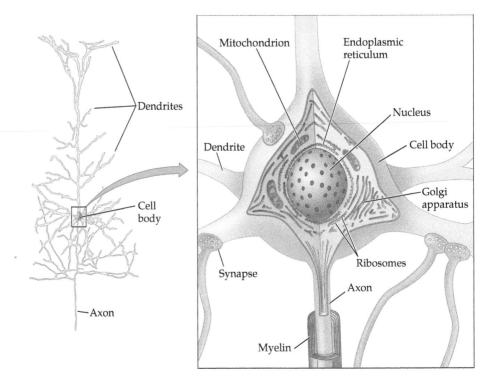

from the spinal cord to the arms and legs). Dendrites receive information from the axonal endings arising from other nerve cells.

Neurons in humans and other mammals are unusual in their extraordinary numbers; the human brain alone is estimated to contain some 100 billion neurons and several times as many neuroglial supporting cells. The neurons that make up the human nervous system also display a much greater range of distinct cell types than do the cells of other organ systems, whether this judgment is made on the basis of neuronal morphology or the variety of their physiological properties. This structural and functional diversity, and the rich interconnection of nerve cells to form intricate signaling ensembles called **neural circuits**, is the foundation on which all cognitive functions are built.

Nerve Cells and Their Signaling Functions

The transfer of information from one neuron to another is typically mediated by a variety of **neurotransmitters**. These molecules are released from **synapses** and change the electrical potential across the membrane of the neuron they contact. As a rule, many nerve cells converge on a single target neuron, and the terminal axon branches of each neuron typically diverge to contact a number of other target neurons. The convergent input onto a neuron at any moment is integrated at the point of origin of the axon from the cell body—a region called the **axon hillock**—to determine whether the neuron will carry the signal forward to its own target cells.

The mechanism that carries signals to additional target cells is called the **action potential**, a self-regenerating wave of electrical activity that begins at the axon hillock and propagates to the synaptic endings at the axon's terminus. Specialization for signal conduction is reflected in many aspects of axons, including a variety of proteins present in axonal membranes—**ion channels** and **ion pumps**—that support action potential propagation. The energy that ion pumps expend maintaining ionic gradients in the face of signaling is the

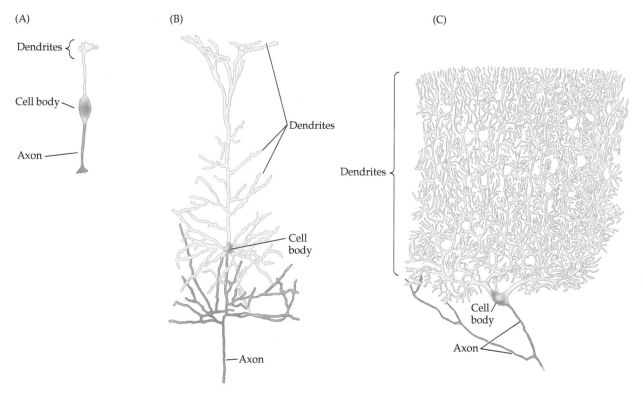

(A)

Dendrites {

Cell body

Axon

(B)

Dendrites

Cell body

Axon

(C)

Dendrites {

Cell body

Axon

Figure A.2 Dendritic "trees" Examples of the variety in the shape and extent of dendrites in the human nervous system. (A) Retinal bipolar neuron. (B) Cortical pyramidal neuron. (C) Cerebellar Purkinje neuron. In each example, the axon of the neuron continues well beyond the region of the cell body shown.

primary reason that neurons are so metabolically costly. In addition to other nerve cells in the brain and the rest of the central nervous system, the target cells contacted by axonal endings include the autonomic ganglion cells, muscle cells, and glandular cells throughout the body.

In addition to the axon, the other salient morphological features of most nerve cells are the number and arrangement of their dendrites. Dendritic geometries range from a complete lack of dendrites (in a very small minority of neurons) to elaborate *dendritic arborizations* (**Figure A.2**). Dendrites, together with the cell body, provide the major site for the synaptic contacts from other nerve cells.

An important functional feature enabled by the morphological diversity of neuronal dendritic geometries is that the number of inputs that a particular neuron receives is generally proportional to the complexity of its dendritic arborization: nerve cells that lack dendrites are innervated by just one or a few other nerve cells, whereas those with increasingly elaborate dendrites are contacted by a commensurately larger number of other neurons. The number of inputs received by a single human neuron varies from 1 to about 100,000. This range reflects a fundamental purpose of the different nerve cell types—namely, to integrate information from other neurons. The number of inputs to a given neuron is therefore an important determinant of its function.

As already mentioned, the endings of neuronal axons are specialized to transfer information onto the dendrites and cell bodies of the neurons they contact via the release of neurotransmitter substances. When an action potential arrives at these axon terminals, the associated change in the membrane potential of the terminal causes the secretion of neurotransmitter molecules. Typically, the *presynaptic terminal* of the axon (also called a *synaptic bouton*) is immediately adjacent to an elaborate complementary *postsynaptic specialization* of the dendrite or cell body of the contacted cell. There is, however, no physical continuity between the pre- and postsynaptic elements at such **chemical synapses** (Figure A.3; see also Figure A.1). In the brain, and elsewhere in the nervous system, a small minority of the neural contacts are *electrical synapses* that operate quite differently from chemical synapses.

Synaptic communication between two neurons is accomplished by the diffusion of neurotransmitter molecules from the presynaptic terminal across an intervening space, called the **synaptic cleft**, where the molecules bind to **neurotransmitter receptors**, which are proteins embedded in the membrane of the postsynaptic specialization. The synaptic contacts on dendrites and cell bodies are actually a special elaboration of the secretory apparatus found in many types of non-neural cells, such as the cells of the pancreas that secrete insulin or the cells of the gut that secrete digestive enzymes. The secretory organelles

Figure A.3   A chemical synapse This schematic diagram details the sequence of events initiated when an action potential arrives at the presynaptic axon terminal. The subsequent transfer of information to the postsynaptic specialization is accomplished by a variety of neurotransmitter molecules that cross the synaptic cleft and bind to receptor molecules embedded in the membrane of the postsynaptic cell.

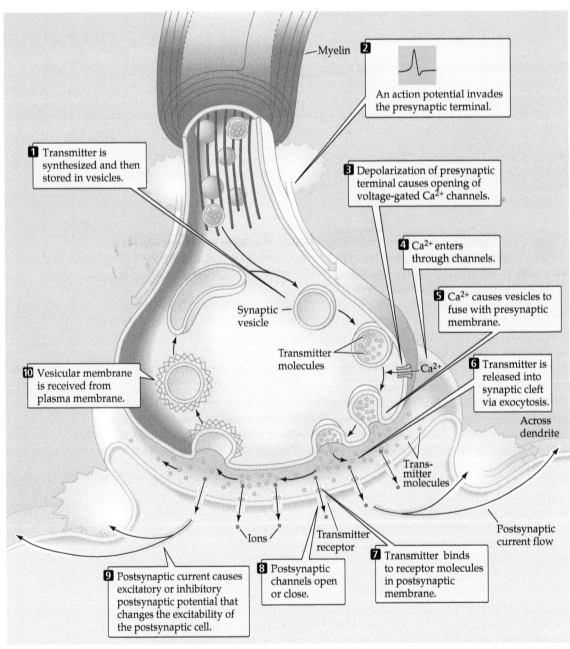

Myelin

2 An action potential invades the presynaptic terminal.

1 Transmitter is synthesized and then stored in vesicles.

3 Depolarization of presynaptic terminal causes opening of voltage-gated Ca^{2+} channels.

4 Ca^{2+} enters through channels.

5 Ca^{2+} causes vesicles to fuse with presynaptic membrane.

Synaptic vesicle

Transmitter molecules

Ca^{2+}

6 Transmitter is released into synaptic cleft via exocytosis.

10 Vesicular membrane is received from plasma membrane.

Across dendrite

Transmitter molecules

Postsynaptic current flow

Ions

Transmitter receptor

7 Transmitter binds to receptor molecules in postsynaptic membrane.

9 Postsynaptic current causes excitatory or inhibitory postsynaptic potential that changes the excitability of the postsynaptic cell.

8 Postsynaptic channels open or close.

in the presynaptic terminal of chemical synapses are called **synaptic vesicles**, and each one is filled with several thousand neurotransmitter molecules (see Figure A.3).

The binding of neurotransmitters to receptors opens or closes ion channels in the postsynaptic membrane, which, as noted, changes the postsynaptic membrane potential; these potential changes are, in the aggregate, the information that is read out at the axon hillock, determining whether the contacted cell fires an action potential or remains silent. This process underlies signaling throughout the nervous system.

Functional Organization of the Human Nervous System

Although the cellular level provides a logical starting point in thinking about the nervous system, neural function depends on interactions of nerve cells in circuits and systems.

Neural circuits

As already mentioned, all cognitive functions depend on the operation of groups of interconnected neurons called neural circuits. Although the arrangement of neural circuits varies greatly according to the function of the different components of the nervous system, certain features and the relevant terminology are common to all neural circuitry.

A first step in understanding neural circuitry is to learn the nomenclature. Nerve cells that carry information *centrally*—that is, toward the central nervous system (the brain or spinal cord) or, more generally, toward any neural processing structure—are called **afferent neurons**. Nerve cells that carry information *peripherally*—away from the central nervous system (or away from the structure in question)—are called **efferent neurons**. These terms are used mainly in describing the inputs and outputs of the brain; within the brain itself, and within the cerebral cortex in particular, the question of whether signals are traveling centrally or peripherally is largely moot.

Nerve cells that participate only in the local aspects of a circuit, as in many components of the brain, are called **interneurons** (or, alternatively, *local circuit neurons*). These three classes—afferent neurons, efferent neurons, and interneurons—are the basic constituents of all neural circuits.

A simple example of a neural circuit is the **spinal reflex arc**, the most familiar of which is the "knee-jerk" response (Figure A.4A). The afferent limb of the reflex arc comprises bipolar **sensory neurons** whose cell bodies are located in dorsal root ganglia of the spinal cord (discussed later) and whose peripheral axons terminate in special sensory receptors in the relevant muscles. (As described in Chapters 3 and 4, each of the five senses employs different, highly specialized receptors that *transduce* energy in the environment into neural signals.) The processes of these bipolar afferent neurons run centrally to contact target nerve cells in the spinal cord. The primary targets are **motor neurons** in the spinal cord, which in turn give rise to the axons that form the efferent portion of the reflex arc. One group of these efferent motor neurons projects to flexor muscles in the limb, and the other to extensor muscles.

In addition to sensory neurons and motor neurons, the interneurons of the spinal cord make up the third element of the spinal reflex circuit. The interneurons serve a *modulatory function*—as do the local neurons in many neural circuits. The interneurons of this knee-jerk circuit receive synaptic contacts from the afferent sensory neurons and make synapses on the efferent motor neurons that project to the flexor muscles (i.e., muscles that cause the limb to fold up—bending the leg at the knee as in this case, or the arm at the elbow). The

Figure A.4 **A simple neural circuit** (A) The elements of the myotatic stretch reflex (the knee-jerk reflex). (B) Diagram showing the ability to record electro-physiological responses from each element during the execution of the reflex in an experimental animal, thus revealing the detailed function of its constituent neurons.

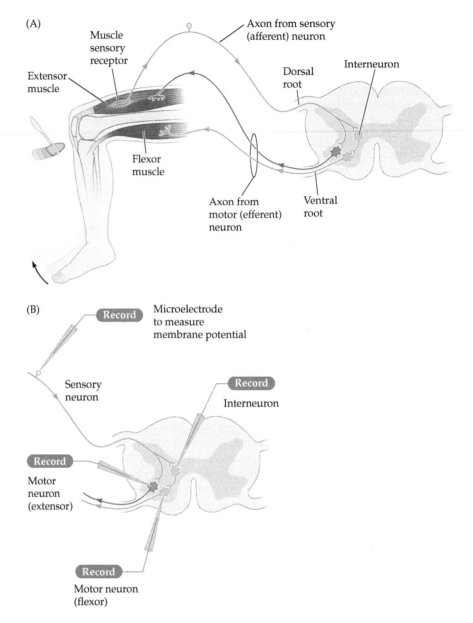

synaptic connections between the sensory afferents and the extensor efferents are **excitatory**, causing the extensor muscles to contract and thus extend the leg; conversely, the interneurons activated by the afferents are **inhibitory**, and their activation by the afferent axons diminishes electrical activity in motor neurons, causing the flexor muscles to become less active. The result is a complementary activation of the synergist muscles and inactivation of the antagonist muscles that control the position of the leg. The net outcome is that when the muscles connected to the patellar tendon are briefly stretched by the tap of the reflex hammer, the leg extends. A more detailed picture of the events underlying a stretch reflex or any other neural circuit can be obtained by electrophysiological recording (Figure A.4B).

Electrophysiological recording has been and continues to be a mainstay of modern neuroscience, including cognitive neuroscience (Box A1; see also Chapter 2). There are two basic approaches to measuring electrical activity at the cellular level: extracellular recording, in which an electrode is placed *near* the nerve cell of interest to detect action potential activity; and intracellular recording, in which the electrode is placed *inside* the cell and records changes in membrane potential, as seen in Box A1. Extracellular recordings detect only action potentials; such recordings are widely used in studies of cognitive functions in non-human primates and, to a limited extent, in humans during neurosurgery. Intracellular recordings are more revealing because they detect the graded **synaptic potentials** that trigger action potentials, but they are difficult to do in living animals. Synaptic potentials also arise at sensory receptors in the periphery, where they are called **receptor potentials**. The changes in membrane potential that together are the basis of neural signaling can thus be measured from each element of the circuit before, during, and after a stimulus occurs. By comparing the onset, duration, and frequency of receptor, synaptic, and action potential activity in each cell, a detailed functional picture of any circuit can be established (see Figure A.4B and Box A1 for an example).

Neural systems

Neural circuits are typically grouped together to form neural systems that serve broad functional purposes (Figure A.5). The most obvious of these systems are:

- The **sensory systems** (visual, auditory, mechanosensory, and chemosensory) that acquire and process information from the environment.
- The **motor systems** that allow an animal to respond to sensory and stored information by activating **effectors**—muscles or glands. The motor neurons that activate the skeletal muscles to generate body movement make up the **somatic motor system**, whereas those that govern cardiac muscle, the smooth muscles of the gut and other organs, and the glands constitute the **visceral** or **autonomic motor system**.

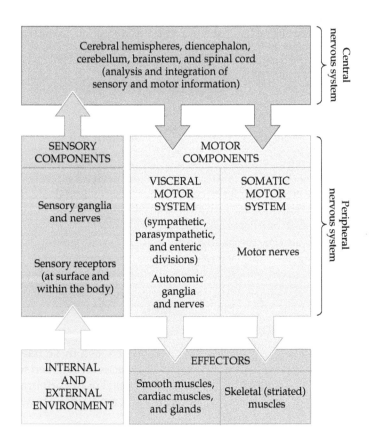

Figure A.5 **Organization of the human nervous system** This schematic diagram illustrates the flow of information through the central and peripheral components of the human nervous system. Stimuli from the environment send signals to the brain and spinal cord (the *central nervous system*) via the *sensory* components of the *peripheral nervous system*. Processing circuits in the central nervous system interpret the significance of this sensory input and in turn send signals via the *motor* components of the peripheral nervous system. These signals result in a large array of actions, both voluntary and involuntary, which are carried out by effectors, the body's muscles and glands.

■ BOX A1 INTRACELLULAR RECORDING FROM NERVE CELLS

All neural signaling depends on changes in the permeability of nerve cell membranes to different ions. Such changes in ion permeability alter the distribution of electrical charges across the neuronal membrane, thus changing the *membrane potential* of the affected neurons. The most informative—but not always the most feasible—way to observe the events underlying neural signaling is to insert a microelectrode into the cell that directly measures the electrical potential across the neuronal membrane. A typical microelectrode used in such intracellular recording is a piece of glass tubing pulled to a fine point with an opening of less than 1 micrometer (micron) in diameter; the electrode is then filled with a good electrical conductor. This conductive core can then be connected to a voltmeter (an oscilloscope) that records the transmembrane voltage of the nerve cell over time.

When a microelectrode is inserted through the membrane of a neuron, it records a negative potential, indicating that the cell has a means of generating a constant voltage across its membrane when it is at rest. This voltage, called the *resting membrane potential*, depends on the type of neuron being examined, but it is always a small fraction of a volt (typically −50 to −100 millivolts).

An electrical current can be injected by inserting a second microelectrode into the same neuron and connecting that electrode to a battery. (In the natural course of events, such a stimulating current would emanate from the action of neurotransmitter molecules on postsynaptic neurons, or from sensory receptor activation; Figure A.) If the polarity of the current delivered in this way makes the membrane potential more negative (called **hyperpolarization**), nothing dramatic happens. The membrane potential simply changes in proportion to the magnitude of the injected current. Such hyperpolarizing responses do not engage the action potential mechanism and are therefore called *passive electrical responses*.

The membrane potential changes that are apparent with intracellular recording from neurons, as might be obtained from the arrangement shown in Figure A.4B. Such changes, which are shown as they would be recorded on an oscilloscope, are the basis of all neuronal signaling. (A) An action potential. (B,C) Dashed lines indicate the onset of the action potential that would normally be elicited by these excitatory synaptic potentials. (D) An inhibitory synaptic potential. mV = millivolts.

A much different phenomenon is seen if current of the opposite polarity is delivered, so that the membrane potential of the nerve cell becomes more positive than the resting potential (called **depolarization**). In this case, at a certain level of membrane potential called the **threshold potential**, an action potential occurs (see Figure A). The action potential is an active response generated by the membrane properties of neurons. It appears on an oscilloscope as a brief change (1–5 milliseconds long) from negative to positive in the transmembrane potential. Importantly, the amplitude ("height") of the action potential is independent of the magnitude of the current used to evoke it; that is, larger currents do not elicit larger action potentials. The action potentials of a given neuron are therefore said to be *all or none*, because they occur either fully or not at all. However, if the amplitude or duration of the stimulus current is increased sufficiently, multiple action potentials occur. Thus, the intensity of a stimulus is encoded in the *frequency* of action potentials rather than in their amplitude.

Intracellular electrodes, as noted in the text, can record synaptic potentials and receptor potentials when the electrode is near synapses or sensory receptors, respectively. A chemical synapse that releases a transmitter molecule whose interaction with postsynaptic receptors brings the membrane potential of the contacted neuron closer to

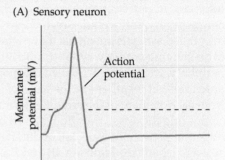

(A) Sensory neuron

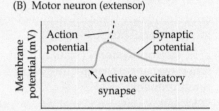

(B) Motor neuron (extensor)

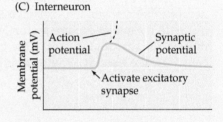

(C) Interneuron

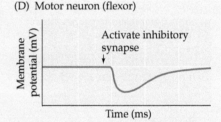

(D) Motor neuron (flexor)

the threshold of action potential initiation by depolarization is called an *excitatory synapse* (producing an *excitatory postsynaptic potential*, or *EPSP*; Figures B and C), whereas a transmitter that acts to hyperpolarize the postsynaptic membrane (or simply stabilizes it at the resting level) is called an *inhibitory synapse* (Figure D).

The majority of neurons and neural circuits, however, lie between these relatively well-defined input and output systems. These are collectively referred to as associational systems. The associational systems at the level of the cerebral cortex, together with their subcortical components, are what mediate the functions of greatest interest to cognitive neuroscience.

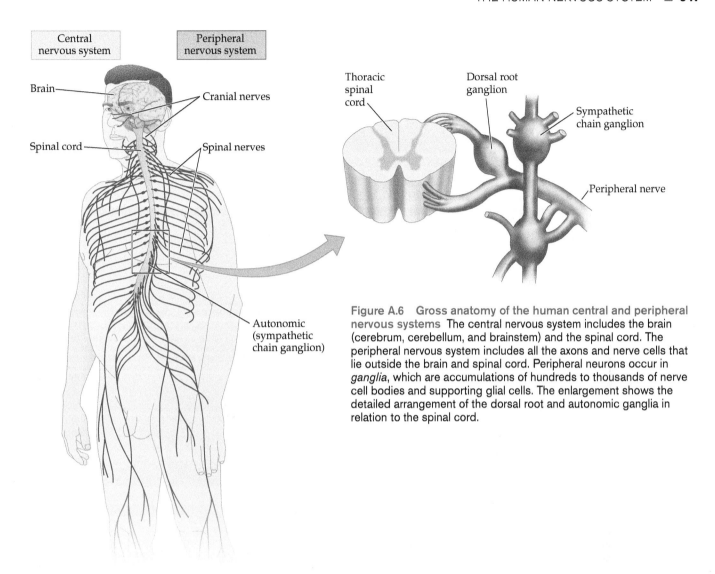

Figure A.6 Gross anatomy of the human central and peripheral nervous systems The central nervous system includes the brain (cerebrum, cerebellum, and brainstem) and the spinal cord. The peripheral nervous system includes all the axons and nerve cells that lie outside the brain and spinal cord. Peripheral neurons occur in *ganglia*, which are accumulations of hundreds to thousands of nerve cell bodies and supporting glial cells. The enlargement shows the detailed arrangement of the dorsal root and autonomic ganglia in relation to the spinal cord.

Structural Organization of the Human Nervous System

In addition to the broad functional distinctions described in the previous section, the nervous system of humans and other vertebrates is conventionally divided anatomically into central and peripheral components (Figure A.6). The **central nervous system** includes the brain (cerebrum, cerebellum, and brainstem) and the spinal cord. The **peripheral nervous system** comprises all the axons and nerve cells that lie outside the brain and spinal cord. Even in humans, rather surprisingly, there may be about as many neurons in the peripheral nervous system (mostly in the gut) as in the brain. These peripheral neurons are located in ganglia, which are local accumulations (hundreds to thousands) of nerve cell bodies and supporting glial cells. The axons of the peripheral nervous system are gathered into nerves (bundles of axons and supporting cells); nerves can arise from the brainstem, spinal cord, or sensory and autonomic ganglia.

Within the central nervous system, nerve cells are arranged in two general configurations (Figure A.7A). **Nuclei** are relatively compact accumulations of neurons that have functionally related inputs and outputs; these collections range from a few hundred to millions of nerve cell bodies and their connections throughout the brain and spinal cord. In general, nuclei define the functional

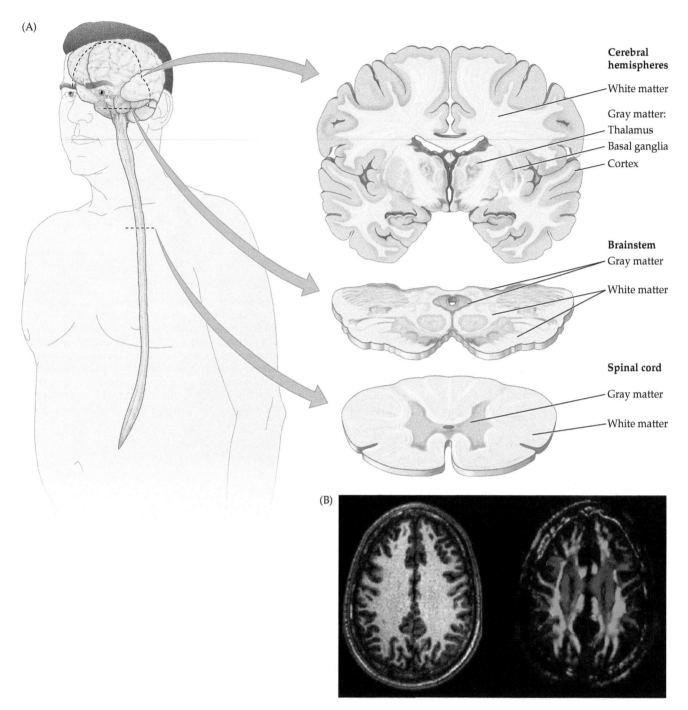

Figure A.7 Some key structural features of the central nervous system
(A) Distinctions between gray matter and white matter in the brain and spinal cord. The coronal section through the cerebral hemispheres indicates the cerebral cortex and some of the major subcortical nuclei (the basal ganglia) that are of particular interest in the text. (B) The major white matter tracts of the cerebrum are seen in a horizontal magnetic resonance imaging section (left); various tracts can be functionally distinguished (by different colors) using a method called diffusion tensor imaging (right). (Magnetic resonance imaging [MRI] techniques are explained in Chapter 2.) (B courtesy of the Johns Hopkins Medical Institute, Laboratory of Brain Anatomical MRI.)

organization of the central nervous system at the **subcortical** level (i.e., the components of the brain that lie beneath the cerebral cortex). In contrast, the *cerebral cortex* is the sheetlike, folded array of billions of nerve cells that covers the surfaces of the cerebral hemispheres and cerebellum. (The term *cortex*—plural, *cortices*—is from the Latin for "bark" and refers to the outer layer of a structure.)

Axons in the central nervous system are gathered into **tracts** (Figure A.7B), which are in this sense equivalent to peripheral nerves. Within a tract, glial cells of the central nervous system, called *oligodendrocytes*, envelop the central axons. In much the same way, glial cells of another type, known as *Schwann cells*, wrap the peripheral nerves. The envelopment of axons by oligodendrocytes and Schwann cells gives rise to a multilayered, membranous coating called **myelin** (see Figure A.1) that surrounds many central and peripheral axons. Myelin exerts important effects on the transmission of neural signals, by increasing the speed at which action potentials are conducted along axons.

Two other key histological terms are used to distinguish nuclei and cortices from axon tracts: **gray matter** refers to the nuclei and/or cortices, which are rich in neuronal cell bodies and synapses; **white matter** refers to axon tracts (see Figure A.7A). These names arose from the color of the respective regions in the postmortem brain. The relative whiteness of the axon tracts arises from the predominance of myelinated axons in the major central nervous system pathways.

A final feature of the overall organization of the human nervous system concerns the various types of ganglia in the peripheral nervous system. **Sensory ganglia** (singular, *ganglion*) lie adjacent to either the spinal cord (where they are referred to as **dorsal root ganglia**; see Figure A.6) or the brainstem (where they are called **cranial nerve ganglia**; see Figure A.9A). As mentioned already, the nerve cells in sensory ganglia send axons to the periphery that end in (or on) specialized receptors that transduce information about a wide variety of stimuli.

The organization of **autonomic ganglia** in the visceral, or autonomic, motor division of the peripheral nervous system is a bit more complicated. Visceral motor neurons in the brainstem and spinal cord form synapses with peripheral motor neurons that lie in these ganglia. In the **sympathetic division** of the autonomic motor system, the ganglia are along or in front of the vertebral column (see Figure A.6) and send axons to a variety of peripheral targets (blood vessels, piloerector muscles, heart, lungs, and many more). In the **parasympathetic division**, the ganglia are found within the organs they innervate, which generally receive input from the sympathetic division as well. Broadly speaking, *sympathetic activity* prepares the organism for the expenditure of metabolic energy, whereas *parasympathetic activity* initiates processes that conserve or store energy.

One major component of the visceral motor system is the **enteric division** (some neuroscientists prefer to think of it as a more or less separate system) made up of numerous small ganglia scattered throughout the wall of the gut. The ganglia of the enteric division modulate processes specifically concerned with digestion.

Major Subdivisions of the Central Nervous System

The central nervous system is considered to have seven basic parts: the spinal cord, medulla, pons, midbrain, cerebellum, diencephalon, and the two cerebral hemispheres (the *cerebrum*; Figure A.8). The medulla, pons, and midbrain are collectively called the **brainstem**; the diencephalon and cerebral hemispheres are collectively called the **forebrain**.

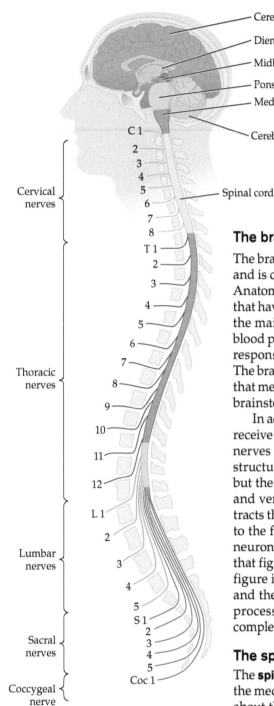

Cerebrum ⎱ Forebrain
Diencephalon ⎰

Midbrain ⎫
Pons ⎬ Brainstem
Medulla ⎭

Cerebellum

C 1
2
3
4
5
6
7
8
T 1
2
3
4
5
6
7
8
9
10
11
12
L 1
2
3
4
5
S 1
2
3
4
5
Coc 1

Cervical nerves

Thoracic nerves

Lumbar nerves

Sacral nerves

Coccygeal nerve

Spinal cord

Figure A.8   Subdivisions of the human central nervous system This lateral view indicates the seven major components of the central nervous system (right) and the five different segmental levels of the vertebral column that encase the spinal cord (left). Spinal (or segmental) nerves from the spinal cord pass through foramina (openings) in the spinal column to innervate much of the body.

The brainstem

The brainstem lies between the forebrain and the upper end of the spinal cord and is conventionally divided into **midbrain, pons**, and **medulla** (Figure A.9A). Anatomically, it is a highly complex structure that houses many of the nuclei that have immediate control of the reflex functions that are most important for the maintenance of life. These include the reflexes that determine heart rate, blood pressure, breathing rate, the coughing and vomiting responses, digestive responses, level of consciousness, and basic aspects of reward and pleasure. The brainstem's internal structure is characterized by the presence of the nuclei that mediate these functions. Many of these nuclei are located in the core of the brainstem, called the reticular formation (Figure A.9B).

In addition, the brainstem houses the nuclei of the **cranial nerves** that either receive input from cranial sensory ganglia via their respective cranial sensory nerves or give rise to axons that form the cranial motor nerves. (The overall structure is thus basically the same as that of the spinal cord, described next, but the gray matter is no longer so clearly collected into dorsal, intermediate, and ventral regions.) In addition, the brainstem is the conduit for the major tracts that either relay sensory information from the spinal cord and brainstem to the forebrain, or relay motor commands from the forebrain back to motor neurons in the brainstem and spinal cord. Other structures in the brainstem that figure importantly in the text are the **superior** and **inferior colliculi**, which figure in the control of eye movements and auditory processing, respectively; and the **substantia nigra** and **ventral tegmental area**, which are important in processing *reward* (i.e., feedback associated with a desired stimulus or the completion of a goal).

The spinal cord

The **spinal cord** extends caudally (tailward) from the brainstem, running from the medullary-spinal junction at about the level of the first cervical vertebra to about the level of the twelfth thoracic vertebra (see Figure A.8). The vertebral column—and the spinal cord contained within it—is divided into cervical, thoracic, lumbar, sacral, and coccygeal regions. Each of these segments gives rise to peripheral nerves called the spinal (or segmental) nerves that innervate much of the body. Sensory information carried by the afferent axons in the spinal nerves enters the cord via the dorsal roots, and motor commands carried by the efferent axons leave the cord via the ventral roots (see Figure A.4A). Once the dorsal and ventral roots join, sensory and motor axons (with some exceptions) travel together in the spinal nerves.

The interior of the cord is formed by gray matter, which is surrounded by white matter (see Figure A.7). In transverse sections, the gray matter is conventionally divided into dorsal (posterior), lateral, and ventral (anterior) "horns"

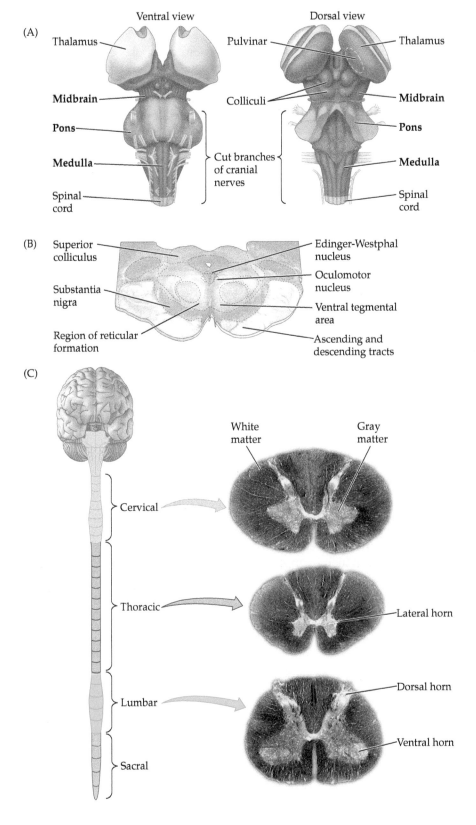

(A) Ventral view / Dorsal view

Ventral view labels: Thalamus, Midbrain, Pons, Medulla, Spinal cord, Cut branches of cranial nerves

Dorsal view labels: Pulvinar, Colliculi, Thalamus, Midbrain, Pons, Medulla, Spinal cord

(B) Superior colliculus, Substantia nigra, Region of reticular formation, Edinger-Westphal nucleus, Oculomotor nucleus, Ventral tegmental area, Ascending and descending tracts

(C) Cervical, Thoracic, Lumbar, Sacral, White matter, Gray matter, Lateral horn, Dorsal horn, Ventral horn

Figure A.9 Human brainstem and spinal cord (A) Ventral and dorsal views showing the three major divisions of the brainstem: medulla, pons, and midbrain. The structure rostral to the midbrain is the diencephalon. (B) Cross section of the brainstem at the level of the midbrain, indicating the reticular formation, the cranial nerve nuclei visible at this level (Edinger-Westphal and oculomotor), the major ascending and descending tracts, and other structures of special importance for cognitive issues. (C) Organization of the spinal cord, indicating the major subdivisions of the spinal cord gray matter and the major ascending and descending tracts.

(Figure A.9C). The neurons of the **dorsal horns** receive sensory information that enters the spinal cord via the dorsal roots of the spinal nerves. The **lateral horns** are present primarily in the thoracic region and contain the visceral motor neurons that project to the sympathetic ganglia. The **ventral horns** contain the cell bodies of motor neurons that send axons via the ventral roots of the spinal nerves to terminate in striated (skeletal) muscles.

The white matter of the spinal cord represents a complex collection of axon tracts related to specific functions. Some of these tracts carry ascending (i.e., going toward the brain) sensory information from the body's mechanoreceptors, while others include axons that travel from the cerebral cortex and brainstem to contact spinal motor neurons and interneurons. Still others carry information locally between spinal cord levels to better coordinate motor actions.

Surface features of the brain

Many key features of the human brain are apparent simply from examining its surface. The major structures visible in this way are the cerebral hemispheres, the cerebellum, and the medullary (caudal) portion of the brainstem. The **cerebral hemispheres** are notable for their large size—they account for about 85 percent of the brain by weight—and their highly folded surface (Figure A.10A). Neuroanatomists and evolutionary biologists have argued for at least a century about the significance of cerebral convolutions, without reaching any clear resolution. All agree, however, that the infolding of the cerebral hemispheres allows a great deal more cortical surface area (about 0.6 square meters on average) to exist within the confines of the cranium than would otherwise be possible.

The convex convolutions of the brain are known as **gyri** (singular, *gyrus*), and the concavities between the gyri are called **sulci** (singular, *sulcus*) or, if they are especially deep, **fissures**. The brain's sulci and gyri figure heavily in the description of cognitive functions. The most important of the gyri are shown in Figure A.10B; although this figure may seem overly detailed, it is especially helpful in discussions of particular brain regions.

Despite its convolutions, the surface of the cerebral hemispheres is a continuous sheet of neurons and supporting cells about 2 millimeters thick called the **cerebral cortex** (recall that the term *cortex* is Latin for "bark"). The sheet is layered in a manner that varies from one region to another, and although they remain poorly understood, these differences are functionally important. Some of these differences and the generic organization of cortical circuitry (which is central to all cognitive functions) are described in Box A2.

The lateral surface view of the human brain in Figure A.10 is also the best perspective from which to appreciate the **lobes** of the cerebral hemispheres, which are again essential descriptors in discussing cognitive functions. Each

Figure A.10 Surface views of the human brain (A) The left cerebral hemisphere in lateral view (the front of the brain is to the left). **(B)** Approximate location of some of the major gyri and other features of the brain surface that are important landmarks in several chapters of this book.

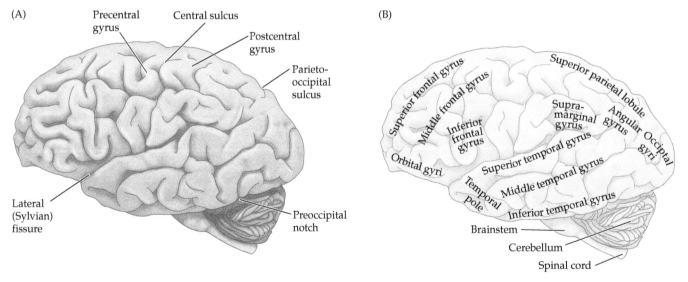

(A) Precentral gyrus · Central sulcus · Postcentral gyrus · Parieto-occipital sulcus · Lateral (Sylvian) fissure · Preoccipital notch

(B) Superior frontal gyrus · Middle frontal gyrus · Inferior frontal gyrus · Orbital gyri · Superior parietal lobule · Supramarginal gyrus · Angular gyrus · Occipital gyri · Superior temporal gyrus · Middle temporal gyrus · Inferior temporal gyrus · Temporal pole · Brainstem · Cerebellum · Spinal cord

■ BOX A2 ORGANIZATION OF THE CEREBRAL CORTEX

ecause cognitive functions are so closely tied to the cerebral cortex, a general understanding of cortical structure and the organization of its canonical circuitry is especially important. Most of the cortex that covers the cerebral hemispheres is *neocortex*, defined as cortex that has six cellular layers, or *laminae* (singular, *lamina*).

Each layer comprises populations of cells that are distinguished by their different densities, sizes, shapes, inputs, and outputs. The layers are designated by numerals 1 to 6 (or, alternatively, Roman numerals I to VI), with letters for laminar subdivisions (e.g., layers 4a, 4b, and 4c in the primary visual cortex).

Nerve cell bodies are rich in elements such as the cell nucleus and ribosomes, which tend to stain darkly with chemically basic nerve cell stains such as cresyl violet acetate. These so-called *Nissl stains* (named after Franz Nissl, who first described this technique when he was a medical student in nineteenth-century Germany) provide a dramatic picture of brain structure at the histological (microscopic) level. The most striking feature revealed in this way is the distinctive cortical lamination evident in humans and other mammals (Figure A).

Neocortex has six layers, but other brain regions have fewer. The infolded cortex of the hippocampus, for example, has only four laminae. The hippocampal cortex is regarded as evolutionarily more primitive and is therefore called *archicortex* to distinguish it from the six-layered neocortex. (All mammals have a well-developed hippocampus, but many have relatively rudimentary neocortex.) Another type of cortex, *paleocortex*, generally has three layers and is found on the ventral surface of the cerebral hemispheres and along the parahippocampal gyrus in the medial temporal lobe. The functional significance of different numbers of laminae in neocortex, archicortex, and paleocortex is not known, although it seems likely that the greater number of layers in neocortex means that more complex processing takes place there than in archicortex or paleocortex.

To a considerable degree, cortical lamination corresponds to the predominance of different neuronal types, and generally different input/output characteristics. For example, neocortical layer 4 is typically rich in *stellate neurons*, which have locally ramifying axons; and in the primary sensory cortices, these neurons receive input from the thalamus, the major sensory relay from the peripheral nervous system. Layer 5, and to a lesser degree layer 6, contains large *pyramidal neurons* whose axons typically leave the cortex. The generally smaller pyramidal neurons in layers 2 and 3 (which are not as distinct as their differing numeral assignments suggest) have

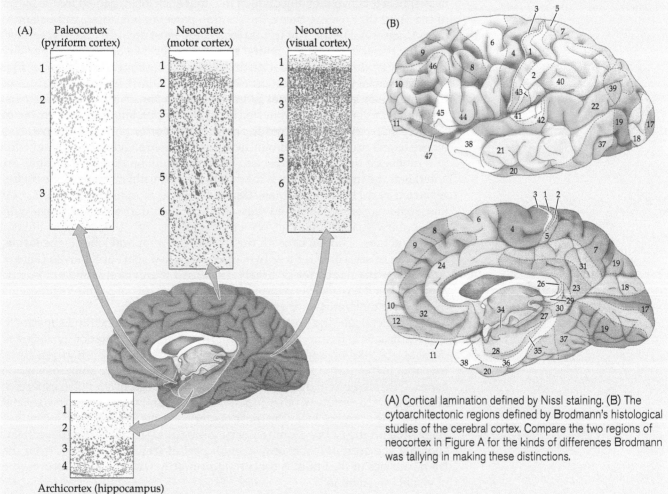*(Continued on next page)*

(A) Cortical lamination defined by Nissl staining. (B) The cytoarchitectonic regions defined by Brodmann's histological studies of the cerebral cortex. Compare the two regions of neocortex in Figure A for the kinds of differences Brodmann was tallying in making these distinctions.

■ BOX A2 *(continued)*

primarily connections to and from other cortical regions (called *corticocortical connections*), and layer 1 contains mainly axons and dendrites, with few nerve cell bodies present.

Despite the overall uniformity of neocortical lamination, regional differences based on laminar features have long been apparent, allowing investigators to identify anatomically distinct subdivisions of the cerebral cortex (Figure B). Early in the twentieth century, the German neurologist Korbinian Brodmann described about 50 such distinct regions, which he called *cytoarchitectonic areas*; today they are more commonly referred to as *Brodmann areas* (the phrase *cytoarchitectonic area* is simply jargon for a cortical region defined by a specific distribution of neurons as revealed with Nissl stains). Brodmann

defined these regions with little or no knowledge of their functional significance. Eventually, however, studies of patients in whom one or more cortical areas had been damaged, along with much other evidence, showed that many of the regions neuroanatomists had identified on histological grounds are also functionally distinct. Although useful in a number of contexts, designating Brodmann areas is not particularly helpful in an introductory textbook like this.

These variations notwithstanding, the circuitry of all cortical regions has common features. First, each cortical layer has a primary source of inputs and a primary output target. Second, each area has connections in the vertical axis (called *columnar* or *radial* connections), as well as connections in the horizontal

axis (*lateral* connections). Third, cells with similar functions tend to be arrayed in vertically aligned groups that span all of the cortical layers and receive inputs that are often segregated into radial or columnar bands. Finally, interneurons within specific cortical layers give rise to extensive local axons that extend horizontally in the cortex, often linking functionally similar groups of cells. The circuitry of any particular cortical region tends to be a variation on this canonical pattern of inputs, outputs, and vertical and horizontal patterns of connectivity. The similarity of neocortical structure and circuit organization across the entire cerebrum suggests that there must be a common denominator of cortical operation, although no one has yet deciphered what it is.

---

hemisphere is conventionally divided into four such lobes, named for the bones of the skull that overlie them: the frontal, parietal, temporal, and occipital lobes (**Figure A.11A,B**). The frontal lobe is the most anterior and is separated from the parietal lobe by the **central sulcus**. The central sulcus is an especially important landmark because it distinguishes the motor cortices anterior to it from the sensory cortices posterior to it. A particularly important feature of the frontal lobe is the **precentral gyrus**. (The prefix *pre-*, in anatomical contexts, refers to a structure that is anterior to, or in front of, another.) The cortex of the precentral gyrus is referred to as the **motor cortex** and contains neurons whose axons project to the motor neurons in the brainstem and spinal cord that innervate the skeletal muscles. The temporal lobe extends almost as far anterior as the frontal lobe but is inferior to (underneath) it, the two lobes being separated by the **lateral** (or **Sylvian**) **fissure**. The uppermost region of the temporal lobe contains cortex concerned with audition; the inferior portions deal with high-order visual information, object recognition, and categorization, among other functions. Hidden beneath the frontal and temporal lobes is the **insula**, which can be seen only if these two lobes are pulled apart or removed (**Figure A.11C**). The insular cortex is largely concerned with visceral and autonomic function, but it has also been implicated in a wide array of cognitive functions that involve motivational or emotional states.

The parietal lobe lies posterior to (behind) the central sulcus and superior to (above) the lateral fissure. The **postcentral gyrus**, the most anterior gyrus in the parietal lobe, harbors cortex that is concerned with somatic (bodily) sensation; this area is therefore referred to as the **somatic sensory** (or **somatosensory**) **cortex**. Other regions of the parietal lobe mediate aspects of attention, aspects of language, and a variety of other functions. The boundary between the parietal lobe and the occipital lobe (the most posterior of the hemispheric lobes) is a somewhat arbitrary line from the parieto-occipital sulcus to the preoccipital "notch." The occipital lobe, only a small part of which is apparent from the lateral surface of the brain, is concerned primarily with the initial processing of visual information.

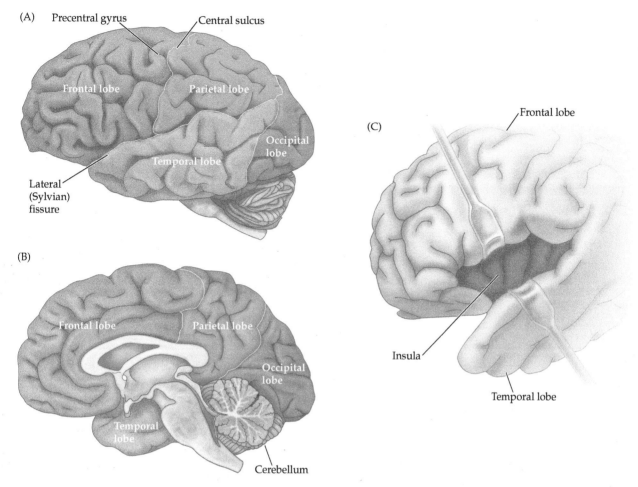

Figure A.11 Four lobes of the human brain (A) The lobes as seen from the lateral surface of the left hemisphere. (B) The lobes as seen from the medial surface. (C) Location of the insula.

Other surface features of the brain are best seen from a ventral perspective (**Figure A.12**). Extending along the inferior (lower) surface of the frontal lobe near the midline are the **olfactory tracts**, which arise from enlargements at their anterior ends called the **olfactory bulbs**. The olfactory bulbs receive input from neurons in the epithelial lining of the nasal cavity; the axons from these neurons make up the **olfactory nerve**. On the ventromedial surface of the temporal lobe, the **parahippocampal gyrus** conceals the **hippocampus**, a highly convoluted cortical structure that figures importantly in certain kinds of memory. Medial to the parahippocampal gyrus is the **uncus**, a protrusion that includes the **pyriform cortex**. The pyriform cortex is the target of the olfactory tract and processes olfactory information.

In the central region of the ventral surface of the forebrain is the **optic chiasm**; immediately posterior to it lies the ventral surface of the **hypothalamus**, including the base of the **pituitary gland** (the infundibular stalk in figure A.12) and the **mammillary bodies**. Posterior to the hypothalamus are two large tracts, oriented roughly rostral–caudally, the **cerebral peduncles**. These tracts contain axons from the cerebral hemispheres that project to the motor neurons in the brainstem and into the lateral and ventral columns of the spinal cord, as well as axons traveling to forebrain structures. Finally, the ventral surfaces of the

Figure A.12   Ventral view of the human brain Some brain structures, including the olfactory tract and the optic chiasm, are best seen from this ventral ("bottom-up") perspective.

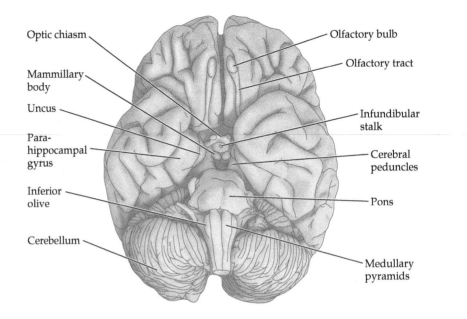

Optic chiasm

Mammillary body

Uncus

Para-hippocampal gyrus

Inferior olive

Cerebellum

Olfactory bulb

Olfactory tract

Infundibular stalk

Cerebral peduncles

Pons

Medullary pyramids

pons, medulla, and cerebellar hemispheres are all readily apparent on the ventral surface of the brain.

When the two cerebral hemispheres of the brain are pulled apart and the underlying brainstem is divided by cutting in the midline, all of the brain's major subdivisions plus a number of additional structures are visible on the medial surface of the hemispheres (Figure A.13A,B; see also Figure A.11B). In this view, the frontal lobe extends forward from the central sulcus, the medial end of which can just be seen. The **parieto-occipital sulcus**, running from the superior to the inferior aspect of the hemisphere, separates the parietal and occipital lobes. The **calcarine sulcus** marks the location of the primary visual cortex on the medial surface of the occipital lobe, running at very nearly a right angle from the parieto-occipital sulcus. A long, roughly horizontal sulcus, the **cingulate sulcus**, stretches across the medial surface of the frontal lobe, extending into the anterior parietal lobe. The prominent gyrus below it, the **cingulate gyrus**, figures prominently in discussions of emotion and social cognition. These structures are also important in the regulation of visceral motor activity, which is closely tied to emotional expression. Finally, ventral to the cingulate gyrus is the midsagittal surface of the **corpus callosum**, a massive white matter tract that is the major route for the transfer of information between the two cerebral hemispheres.

Although parts of the diencephalon, brainstem, and cerebellum are visible on the ventral surface of the brain, their overall structure is especially clear in views of the medial surface. From this perspective, the **diencephalon** can be seen to consist of two parts (Figure A.13C). The **thalamus**, the largest component of the diencephalon, comprises a number of nuclear subdivisions, all of which relay information to the cerebral cortex from other parts of the brain; the most posterior part of the thalamus is called the **pulvinar** (see Figure A.9A), which is important in visual attention. The hypothalamus, a small but crucial part of the diencephalon, is devoted to the control of homeostatic (stability-maintaining) and reproductive functions, often over natural cycles such as days or months. The hypothalamus is intimately related, both structurally and functionally, to the pituitary gland, an endocrine organ whose posterior part is attached to the hypothalamus by the pituitary stalk.

Figure A.13 View of the brain surface after separating the hemispheres at the midline (A) An overview of the major features visible after bisecting the brain in the midsagittal plane (see Box A3). (B) The major gyri, sulci, and other features visible in this view after removal of the brainstem. (C) Blowup of a region of the diencephalon, indicating the thalamus and some of the major landmarks that are important in the text.

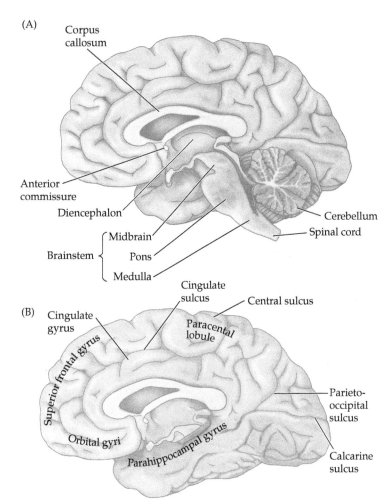

(A)

Corpus callosum

Anterior commissure

Diencephalon

Brainstem {
Midbrain
Pons
Medulla
}

Cerebellum

Spinal cord

The midbrain, which can be seen only in this medial view, lies caudal to the thalamus; as noted, the superior and inferior colliculi define the midbrain's dorsal (back-facing) surface, or *tectum* (meaning "roof"). Several midbrain nuclei, including the substantia nigra, lie in the ventral portion, or **tegmentum** ("covering") of the midbrain. The pons ("bridge") lies caudal to the midbrain along the midsagittal surface, and the **cerebellum** lies over the pons, just beneath the occipital lobe of the cerebral hemispheres; in fact the pons is largely a collection of nerve cell axons and nuclei related to the cerebellum. The cerebellum's major function is coordination of motor activity, posture, and equilibrium, although it is implicated in some cognitive functions as well. From the midsagittal surface, the most visible feature of the cerebellum is the **cerebellar cortex**, a continuous, layered sheet of cells folded into ridges and valleys called **folia** (singular, *folium*).

Finally, the most caudal structure seen from the midsagittal surface of the brain is the medulla, which merges into the spinal cord.

Internal features of the brain

Many structures are not visible from any brain surface but are apparent when the organ is cut in sections and examined grossly (i.e., with the unaided eye) or, as is commonly done, stained with one of a variety of chemical agents that highlight different structures, such as the stains for myelin that accentuate the brain's white matter tracts. Understanding this sectional anatomy is especially pertinent to cognitive neuroscience because internal structures can be seen quite easily in the sections routinely generated by the noninvasive brain imaging techniques that are described in detail in Chapter 2. Modern brain imaging methods are used far more widely today than is the examination of postmortem brain sections in the pathology laboratory (see Figure A.7B). Thus, a major challenge—and a basic requirement in cognitive neuroscience—is learning to move easily from surface neuroanatomy to recognizing the brain's internal structures. Box A3 provides a brief overview of some anatomical terminology needed for understanding the brain as a whole and in histological or MRI sections.

(B)

Cingulate gyrus

Cingulate sulcus

Central sulcus

Paracentral lobule

Superior frontal gyrus

Orbital gyri

Parahippocampal gyrus

Parieto-occipital sulcus

Calcarine sulcus

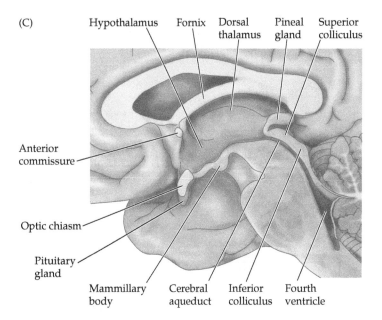

(C)

Hypothalamus   Fornix   Dorsal thalamus   Pineal gland   Superior colliculus

Anterior commissure

Optic chiasm

Pituitary gland

Mammillary body   Cerebral aqueduct   Inferior colliculus   Fourth ventricle

■ BOX A3 ANATOMICAL TERMINOLOGY

An obstacle to understanding the internal structure of the brain is the sometimes confusing nomenclature used to specify anatomical locations. Although many of the terms used to describe spatial orientation in the brain are the same as those used for anatomical descriptions of the rest of the body, the meanings of some of the terms differ. For the body, the anatomical terms in common use refer to the long axis, which is more or less straight. The long axis of the central nervous system, however, has a bend in it. Thus, in describing the brain the simplest terms are *anterior* and *posterior*, which indicate the direction of the front (face) and back of the head, respectively. However, the somewhat more difficult terms *rostral* and *caudal* are also used for some descriptions; *rostral* indicates the direction toward the nose (Latin *rostrum* means "beak") and caudal toward the "tail" (*caudum*), which refers to the base of the skull. When applied to the long axis of the body, the distinctions anterior–posterior and rostral–caudal are synonymous, both indicating "top to tail"; but because of the bend in the axis of the nervous system, they have somewhat different meanings in brain anatomy, as indicated in Figure A. This discrepancy is not a major problem but is important to be aware of.

The terms *dorsal* and *ventral* present a similar case. When speaking of the body or spinal cord axes, *dorsal* refers to the back (Latin *dorsum*) and *ventral* to the front, or belly (Latin *ventrum*). When referring to the brain, however, *dorsal* refers to the upper and *ventral* to the lower surface (see Figure A). Other spatial descriptions apply in the same way to the brain and the body. These include *medial* and *lateral*, toward the midline (center) or to the side (left or right), respectively; and *inferior* and *superior*, above and below.

More significant for cognitive neuroscience is the terminology applied to *sections* (i.e., slices) of the brain—either those made by a knife in the neuropa-thology lab, or the sections that are now routinely visualized by noninvasive brain imaging techniques (see Chapter 2). By convention, sections of the brain that are parallel to the rostral–caudal axis are referred to as *horizontal* or *axial*, sections taken in the plane that divides the brain's two hemispheres are called *sagittal*, and sections in the plane of the face are called *frontal* or *coronal* (Figure B).

The sectional terminology for the spinal cord, though it does not figure significantly in this book, is based on the terms used in considering sections of the body as a whole. Thus, the plane of section perpendicular to the long axis of the body or spinal cord is called a *transverse* (or "cross") section, and sections parallel to the long axis of the body or spinal cord are called *longitudinal*. In a transverse section through the spinal cord, the terms *dorsal–ventral axis* and *anterior–posterior axis* indicate the same direction.

(A) A bend in the long axis of the nervous system arose as humans evolved upright posture, leading to an angle of about 120 degrees between the long axis of the brainstem and that of the rest of the brain. As explained here, this evolutionary fact introduces some special considerations in describing anatomical location in the brain. (B) The major planes of section used in cutting or imaging the brain.

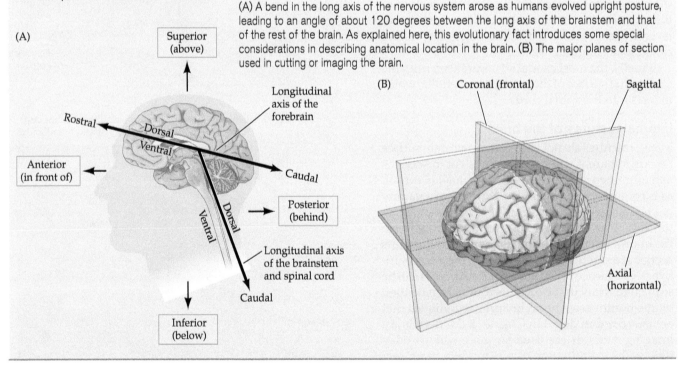

In any plane of section, the cerebral cortex is evident as a thin layer of neural tissue that covers the entire cerebrum. The largest structures embedded within the cerebral hemispheres are two nuclei called the **caudate** and **putamen** (together these nuclei are referred to as the **striatum**), which are closely associated with another nucleus, called the **globus pallidus** (Figure A.14A,B). Because of the related location and function of these three nuclei, they are referred to collectively as the **basal ganglia** (the use of the term *ganglia* in this case is an exception to the usual usage of this word described earlier in its application to collections of peripheral nerve cells; this idiosyncratic use is historical and refers to a collection of related nuclear structures). As Figure A.14C suggests, the basal ganglia are visible in horizontal sections through the mid-dorsal to mid-ventral portion of the forebrain, in frontal sections from just rostral to the uncus to the level of the diencephalon, and in all paramedian sagittal sections.

The neurons in the large nuclear complexes of the basal ganglia receive input from the cerebral cortex and participate in the organization and guidance of complex motor functions, as well as many other cortical feedback loops, many of which are relevant to a range of cognitive functions. In the base of the forebrain, ventral to the basal ganglia, are several smaller clusters of nerve cells known as the **septal**, or **basal, forebrain nuclei**. The function of these latter nuclei is not well understood, but they are of particular interest because of their involvement in the early signs and symptoms of Alzheimer's disease.

The other clearly discernible structure visible in coronal sections through the cerebral hemispheres at the level shown in Figure A.14A is the **amygdala**, a collection of nuclei that lies in front of the hippocampus in the anterior pole of the temporal lobe. Some nuclei of the amygdala are especially important in emotional processing.

In addition to these cortical and nuclear structures, the internal anatomy of the brain shows the major axon tracts mentioned earlier. As already mentioned, the two cerebral hemispheres are interconnected by the corpus callosum, which is apparent in the majority of coronal sections; in some anterior sections, the much smaller **anterior commissure**, another interhemispheric tract, can also be seen (as in Figure A.14A). Another tract that is pertinent in the text is the **fornix**, which connects the hippocampus and the hypothalamus (see Figure A.14B). Finally, axons descending from and ascending to the cerebral cortex assemble into another very large and extensive tract called the **internal capsule**. The internal capsule lies just lateral to the thalamus (which is how it gets its name, since it forms a sort of

Figure A.14 Internal brain structures seen in coronal sections These coronal views reveal important structures in the deep gray matter of the brain. (A) This section passes through the basal ganglia (caudate, putamen, and globus pallidus) and the amygdala. (B) This more posterior coronal section includes the thalamus. All of these structures are of major significance in cognitive studies. (C) This "transparent" lateral view shows the approximate locations of the sections in (A) and (B).

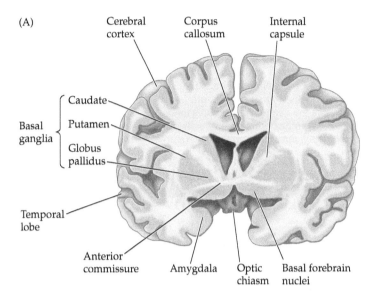

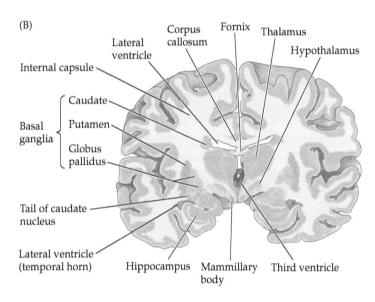

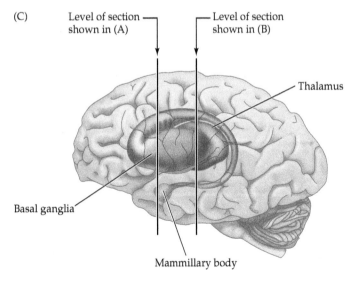

Figure A.15 The ventricular system
The ventricles are a series of interconnected spaces deep in the forebrain
and brainstem. These spaces are filled
with cerebrospinal fluid. (A) Lateral
view showing the main features of the
system. (B) This "transparent" lateral
view shows the ventricular system as a
whole. (C) Another "transparent" view of
the ventricles, this one from the brain's
dorsal surface, looking downward.

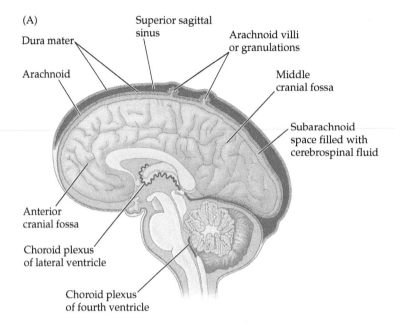

(A)

Dura mater

Arachnoid

Superior sagittal
sinus

Arachnoid villi
or granulations

Middle
cranial fossa

Subarachnoid
space filled with
cerebrospinal fluid

Anterior
cranial fossa

Choroid plexus
of lateral ventricle

Choroid plexus
of fourth ventricle

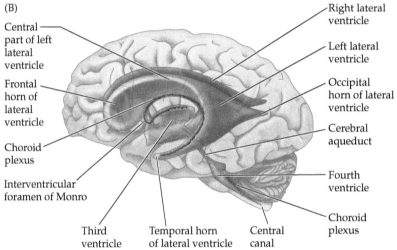

(B)

Central
part of left
lateral
ventricle

Frontal
horn of
lateral
ventricle

Choroid
plexus

Interventricular
foramen of Monro

Third
ventricle

Temporal horn
of lateral ventricle

Central
canal

Right lateral
ventricle

Left lateral
ventricle

Occipital
horn of lateral
ventricle

Cerebral
aqueduct

Fourth
ventricle

Choroid
plexus

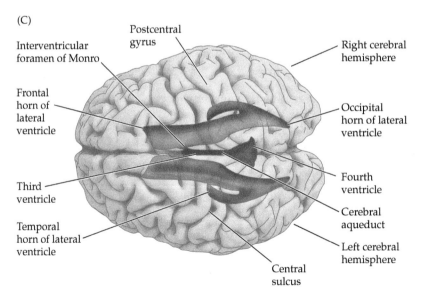

(C)

Interventricular
foramen of Monro

Postcentral
gyrus

Frontal
horn of
lateral
ventricle

Third
ventricle

Temporal
horn of lateral
ventricle

Central
sulcus

Right cerebral
hemisphere

Occipital
horn of lateral
ventricle

Fourth
ventricle

Cerebral
aqueduct

Left cerebral
hemisphere

"capsule" around the thalamus), and many internal capsule axons arise from or terminate in the dorsal thalamus. As might be expected from its location, the internal capsule is most obvious in frontal sections through the middle third of the rostral–caudal extent of forebrain, or in horizontal sections through the level of the thalamus. The axons of the internal capsule enter the cerebral peduncles that connect the cerebral hemispheres to the brainstem. Thus, the internal capsule is the major pathway linking the cerebral cortex to the rest of the brain and spinal cord.

The ventricular system

It is important to be familiar with another feature of the internal anatomy of the brain: the ventricular system (**Figure A.15**), the location of which is particularly helpful in interpreting noninvasive brain images. The ventricles of the brain are a series of interconnected, fluid-filled spaces that lie deep in the forebrain and brainstem. Ventricles are the adult reflection of the open space (the *lumen*) of the embryonic neural tube, around which the central nervous system initially develops (see Chapter 15). The largest of these spaces are the **lateral ventricles** (one within each of the cerebral hemispheres). The lateral ventricles are best seen in frontal sections, where their ventral surface is defined by the basal ganglia, their dorsal surface by the corpus callosum, and their medial surface by the septum pellucidum, a membranous tissue sheet that forms part of the midline sagittal surface of the cerebral hemispheres.

The **third ventricle** forms a narrow midline space between the right and left thalamus, and it communicates with the lateral ventricles through a small opening (the *interventricular foramen*) at the anterior end of the third ventricle. The third ventricle is continuous caudally with the **cerebral aqueduct**, which runs through the midbrain. At its caudal end, the aqueduct opens into the **fourth ventricle**, a larger space in the dorsal pons and medulla. The fourth ventricle narrows caudally to form the central canal of the spinal cord.

The ventricles are filled with **cerebrospinal fluid**, and the lateral, third, and fourth ventricles are the sites of the **choroid plexus**, which produces this fluid. Cerebrospinal fluid percolates through the ventricular system and flows into the subarachnoid space through perforations in the thin covering of the fourth ventricle; the fluid is eventually absorbed by specialized structures called arachnoid villi, and is thus returned to the venous circulation. Although the ventricles have no obvious function other than serving as conduits for the circulation of cerebrospinal fluid, their locations provide excellent landmarks for deciphering brain sections.

The Brain's Blood Supply

As is apparent in various chapters of this text, much insight into cognitive functions has come from the clinical consequences of **stroke**, a generic term that refers to the clinical and neuropathological results of interrupting the blood supply to one or another region of the brain. Such interruptions can be caused by the obstruction of an artery or by hemorrhage (bleeding) from a blood vessel that ruptures. The resulting damage is referred to as a **brain lesion**, a term that also refers to damage from other causes, including trauma and tumors.

The blood supply of the brain is particularly significant because neurons are more sensitive to oxygen deprivation than are other kinds of cells, which generally have lower rates of metabolism. Brain tissue deprived of oxygen and glucose as a result of compromised blood supply is especially likely to sustain transient or permanent damage. Even a brief loss of blood supply (a few minutes), referred to as **ischemia**, can cause cellular changes that, if not quickly reversed, lead to cell death.

Figure A.16 **Major arteries of the brain** The primary features of the vessels that supply blood to the brain are seen here from the ventral perspective. The enlargement shows the circle of Willis, a ring of arteries at the base of the brain.

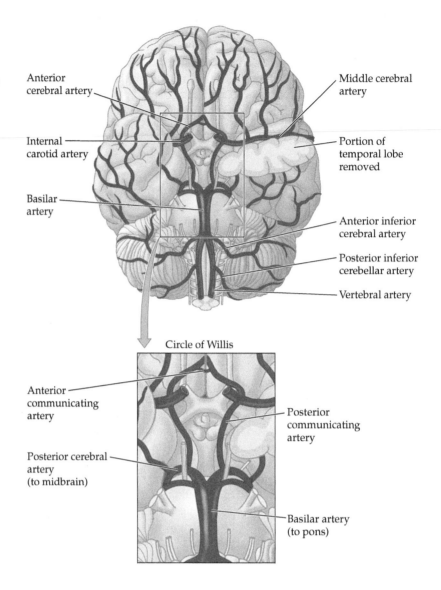

Anterior cerebral artery

Internal carotid artery

Basilar artery

Middle cerebral artery

Portion of temporal lobe removed

Anterior inferior cerebral artery

Posterior inferior cerebellar artery

Vertebral artery

Circle of Willis

Anterior communicating artery

Posterior cerebral artery (to midbrain)

Posterior communicating artery

Basilar artery (to pons)

The human brain receives blood from two sources: the internal carotid arteries, which arise at the point in the neck where the common carotid arteries bifurcate (diverge); and the vertebral arteries (**Figure A.16**). The internal carotid arteries branch to form two major cerebral arteries: the anterior and middle cerebral arteries. The right and left vertebral arteries come together at the level of the pons on the ventral surface of the brainstem to form the midline basilar artery. The basilar artery in turn joins the blood supply originating from the internal carotids in an arterial ring at the base of the brain called the **circle of Willis** (see the enlargement in Figure A.16). The posterior cerebral arteries arise at this confluence, as do two small bridging arteries: the anterior and posterior communicating arteries. Conjoining the two major sources of cerebral vascular supply via the circle of Willis presumably improves the chances that at least some regions of the brain will continue to receive blood if one of the major arteries becomes occluded.

The anterior and middle cerebral arteries form what is referred to clinically as the anterior circulation of the forebrain. Each of these arteries gives rise to branches that supply the cortex and to branches that penetrate the basal surface of the brain and supply deep structures such as the basal ganglia, thalamus, and internal capsule. The posterior circulation of the brain comprises the posterior cerebral, basilar, and vertebral arteries, which supply the posterior cerebral cortex, midbrain, and brainstem.

Although these and many other details of brain vasculature are important primarily in clinical practice, some knowledge of the brain's blood supply is helpful for understanding a variety of issues in cognitive neuroscience. Historically, the functional consequences of compromised blood supply provided a great deal of information about the location of various cognitive functions in the human brain, and today neurological patients continue to be a valuable source of information about brain functions pertinent to cognitive neuroscience.

Go to the **COMPANION WEBSITE**

sites.sinauer.com/cogneuro2e
for quizzes, animations, flashcards,
and other study resources.

Glossary

A1 See *primary auditory cortex*.

A2 See *secondary auditory cortex*.

abulia A symptom of brain damage, often to the frontal lobes, that manifests as flat affect, limited willpower, and reduced motivation. [13]

accommodation A stage of child development in which children learn to react to novel entities by modifying their schemes of thought. Compare *assimilation*. [15]

acquired sociopathy A personality change, often following focal damage to the frontal lobes, in which a person's behavior becomes sociopathic. [13]

acquisition In conditioning, the gradual learning of a conditioned response. Compare *extinction*. [8]

action potential The electrical signal conducted along neuronal axons by which information is conveyed from one place to another in the nervous system. [1, Appendix]

actor-critic learning model A framework for learning that posits two independent elements: a critic that learns rules mapping actions to rewards, and an actor that learns the optimal policy for selecting actions. [14]

acuity The ability of a sensory system to accurately discriminate spatial detail; usually tested by the ability to spatially discriminate two points, as in the Snellen eye chart exam for vision. Applies to all the sensory systems, but most obviously to vision and somatic sensation. [3]

adaptation The process by which organisms come to achieve a better fit to their environment, typically through the process of natural selection. [15]

ADHD See *attention deficit hyperactivity disorder*.

affective neuroscience The study of the neurobiological basis of emotions. [10]

afferent neuron An axon that conducts action potentials from the periphery to more central parts of the nervous system. Compare *efferent neuron*. [Appendix]

agonist A neuropharmacological agent that mimics the action of a neurotransmitter. Compare *antagonist*. [2]

altruistic punishment An action taken to harm another individual, at personal cost, in order to enforce a social norm (e.g., sacrificing one's own money in order to punish someone who cheats in a game). [14]

ambiguity aversion The tendency to prefer choice options whose outcome probabilities are known over options with unknown probabilities (i.e., that have ambiguity). [14]

amnesia The pathological inability to remember or to establish memories. See also *anterograde amnesia* and *retrograde amnesia*. [8]

amygdala A collection of nuclei in the temporal lobe that forms part of the limbic system; its major functions concern autonomic, emotional, and sexual behavior. [10, Appendix]

anchoring heuristic A bias in decision making in which judgments are influenced by a number that serves as a reference point, or anchor, for further deliberations. [14]

anhedonia Reduced experience of positive affect; often accompanies depression. [10]

anosognosia Lack of awareness of one's own disability. [5]

ANS See *approximate number system*.

antagonist A neuropharmacological agent that opposes or interferes with the action of a neurotransmitter. Compare *agonist*. [2]

anterior cingulate cortex The portion of the midline frontal lobe comprising the anterior extent of the cingulate gyrus and adjacent cortex; its dorsal regions are associated with executive functions. [13]

anterior commissure A small midline fiber tract that lies at the anterior end of the corpus callosum; like the callosum, it connects the two hemispheres. [Appendix]

anterograde amnesia The inability to lay down new memories. Compare *retrograde amnesia*. [8]

aperture problem The challenge of determining the speed and direction of a moving line when its ends are obscured by an opening such as a circular hole or a vertical rectangle. [3]

aphasia A language deficit that arises from damage to one of the cortical language areas, typically in the left hemisphere. [12]

apparent motion The sensation of motion elicited by presentation of a stimulus in two successive positions over a brief interval. [3]

approximate number system (ANS) A neural circuit or set of circuits providing a non-symbolic, fuzzy sense of the quantity of objects or events perceived, shared by human adults, preverbal infants, and animals. [15]

aprosodia   The inability to inflect speech with the usual emotional color that the right hemisphere typically contributes to language. Characterized by a monotonic or "robotic" speech pattern. [12]

area 6   See *supplementary motor cortex*.

area LIP   See *lateral intraparietal area*.

arousal   1. A global state of the brain (or the body) reflecting an overall level of responsiveness. Compare *attention*. [6] 2. The degree of intensity of an emotion. [10]

assimilation   A stage of child development in which young children deal with novel entities by encompassing them in their preexisting thought schemes (e.g., assuming any woman who seems to be the child's mother's age is also a mother). Compare *accommodation*. [15]

association cortices   See *cortical association areas*.

associativity   In long-term potentiation, the enhancement of a weakly activated group of synapses when a nearby group is strongly activated. [8]

attention   The marshalling of cognitive processing resources on a particular aspect of the external or internal environment, or on internal processes such as thoughts or memories. Compare *arousal*. [6]

attention deficit hyperactivity disorder (ADHD)   A childhood disorder of unknown cause characterized by impulsiveness, short attention span, and continual activity. [13]

attentional blink   A cognitive phenomenon, typically observed in a rapidly presented stream of stimuli, in which the ability to successfully report a second target stimulus occurring within 150 to 450 milliseconds of a successfully reported first target in the stream is decreased. [6]

attentional stream paradigm   A paradigm used in attention research in which two or more segregated series of stimuli are presented in parallel and subjects selectively attend to one of the series to perform a task. [6]

auditory brainstem response (ABR)   See *brainstem evoked response*.

auditory N1   The first major negative ERP wave elicited by an auditory stimulus, arising mainly from secondary auditory cortex and peaking at about 100 milliseconds after the stimulus; can be strongly modulated by auditory spatial attention. [6]

auditory scene   The overall perception of the auditory environment at any point in time. Analogous to the perception of a visual scene. [4]

australopithecines   Human-like primate species that lived in the Plio-Pleistocene era (5 to 1.5 million years ago) which were bipedal and dentally similar to humans, but had a brain size not much larger than modern apes. Which of these species gave eventual rise to humans remains a topic of debate amongst anthropologists. [15]

autism spectrum disorder   A childhood disorder of unknown cause, characterized by social disengagement that varies greatly in severity. [10]

autobiographical memory   Memory of one's personal experience. [9]

autonomic ganglia   Collections of autonomic motor neurons outside the central nervous system that innervate visceral smooth muscles, cardiac muscle, and glands. [Appendix]

autonomic motor system   Also called *visceral motor system*. The very large component of the nervous system that is dedicated to proper functioning of the viscera (all the organs that maintain the well-being of the body and brain). [Appendix]

awareness   A cognitive/perceptual state in which an individual both shows knowledge of an event or stimulus and can report the subjective experience of having that knowledge. Compare *self-awareness*. [7]

axon   The extension of a neuron that carries the action potential from the nerve cell body to a target. Compare *dendrite*. [Appendix]

axon hillock   The initial portion of an axon, closest to the cell body; the point where action potentials are typically initiated. [Appendix]

Baddeley model   A model, proposed by Alan Baddeley, positing that working memory consists of three memory buffers (the phonological loop, the visuospatial sketchpad, and the episodic buffer) that briefly maintain information, as well as a central executive that allocates attentional resources to the buffers. [13]

Balint's syndrome   A neurological syndrome, caused by bilateral damage to the posterior parietal and lateral occipital cortex, that has three hallmark symptoms: (1) *simultanagnosia*, the inability to attend to and/or perceive more than one visual object at a time; (2) *optic ataxia*, the impaired ability to reach for or point to an object in space under visual guidance; and (3) *oculomotor apraxia*, difficulty voluntarily directing the eye gaze toward objects in the visual field with a saccade. Simultanagnosia is the sign most closely associated with the syndrome, and the one most studied from a cognitive neuroscience standpoint. [7]

basal forebrain nuclei   Also called *septal forebrain nuclei*. A complex of primarily cholinergic nuclei that lies between the hypothalamus in the diencephalon and the orbital cortex of the frontal lobes; concerned with alertness and memory, among other functions. [Appendix]

basal ganglia   A group of nuclei lying deep in the subcortical white matter of the frontal lobes that organize motor behavior. The caudate, putamen, and globus pallidus are major components of the basal ganglia; the subthalamic nucleus and substantia nigra are often included. [5,13,Appendix]

basic emotion   An emotion that is innate, pan-cultural, evolutionarily old, shared with other species, and expressed by a particular physiological pattern and facial configuration. Compare *complex emotion*. [10]

basilar membrane   The membranous sheet in the cochlea of the inner ear that contains the receptor cells (hair cells) that initiate audition. [4]

behavioral economics   A new social science discipline that combines elements of traditional economics and psychology to explain real-world decisions, including observed biases in choice. [14]

behavioral LTP   A change in synaptic efficacy similar to long-term potentiation (LTP) that follows an actual learning experience. [8]

behaviorism   A perspective in cognitive psychology that holds that only directly observable behavior, and not internal mental states, can be studied scientifically. [1]

belt areas   See *secondary auditory cortex*.

BER   See *brainstem evoked response*.

biased competition   a theory of attention that proposes that stimulus inputs compete in a mutually inhibitory fashion for neural processing priority and that a key role of attention is to bias the processing towards those items that are attended. [6]

binding problem   The neural and cognitive processing problem by which the multiple features of an object (e.g., its color, shape, orientation) are integrated together to yield a single perceptual object. Tends to be called a "problem" because is it still mostly unclear how this is accomplished in the brain. [7]

binocular   Pertaining to both eyes. Compare *monocular*. [3]

binocular rivalry   The bi-stable visual experience that occurs when the right and left eyes are presented with incompatible or conflicting images and visual perception alternates between the two images every few seconds. [3,7]

blindsight   The ability of people who are blind, usually because of damage to portions of their visual cortex, to identify the properties of simple visual stimuli when forced to guess. [7]

blocked design   A task design used in PET studies and sometimes in fMRI studies where multiple trials of the same type are grouped together in blocks. The brain activity is then analyzed by comparing neural activity across the entire block against blocks containing another type of trials, or with a different cognitive condition. Compare *event-related design*. [2]

blood oxygenation level–dependent (BOLD) contrast
A measurement of brain activity using fMRI that is based on the local variations in deoxygenated hemoglobin that result from the changes in blood flow induced by neural activity. [2]

BOLD   See *blood oxygenation level–dependent contrast*.

bounded rationality   The idea that biological limitations on cognitive processing prevent people from making decisions or from reasoning in a fully rational manner. [14]

brain lesion   A localized region of brain damage. [Appendix]

brainstem   The portion of the brain that lies between the diencephalon and the spinal cord; comprises the midbrain, pons, and medulla. [Appendix]

brainstem evoked response (BER)   Also called *auditory brainstem response* (*ABR*). A series of small electrical brain waves that are elicited during the first 10 milliseconds after onset of a brief auditory stimulus and that can be detected at the scalp. BERs reflect activity in the auditory brainstem nuclei as the sound stimulus information reaches them in sequence via the auditory afferent pathways. [6]

brightness   Technically, the apparent intensity of a source of light; more generally, a sense of the effective overall intensity of a light stimulus. Compare *lightness*. [3]

Broca's aphasia   Also called *motor aphasia* or *production aphasia*. A language deficit arising from damage to Broca's area in the frontal lobe and characterized by difficulty in the production of speech. Compare *Wernicke's aphasia*. [12]

Broca's area   An area in the ventral posterior region of the left frontal lobe that helps mediate language expression; named after the nineteenth-century anatomist and neurologist Paul Broca. Compare *Wernicke's area*. [12]

calcarine sulcus   The major sulcus on the medial aspect of the human occipital lobe; the primary visual cortex lies largely within this sulcus. [Appendix]

Cannon-Bard theory   Also called *diencephalic theory*. A theory of emotion, developed by Walter Cannon and Philip Bard in the 1920's, emphasizing the role of the hypothalamus and related parallel processing routes for emotional expression and emotional experience. [10]

caudate   One of the three major nuclei that make up the basal ganglia in the cerebral hemispheres; together with the putamen, serves as the input structure for the globus pallidus. Damage to the caudate nucleus leads to hyperkinetic movement disorders such as Huntington's disease. [Appendix]

cell   The basic biological unit of life, defined by a membrane or wall that encloses cytoplasm and, in eukaryote organisms (including all plants and animals), a nucleus. [Appendix]

cell body   Also called *soma*. The portion of a neuron that houses the cell's nucleus; axons and dendrites typically extend from the neuronal cell body. [Appendix]

central nervous system   The brain and spinal cord of vertebrates (by analogy, the central nerve cord and ganglia of invertebrates). Compare *peripheral nervous system*. [Appendix]

central sulcus   A major sulcus on the lateral aspect of the cerebral hemispheres that forms the boundary between the frontal and parietal lobes. Its anterior bank contains the primary motor cortex; the posterior bank contains the primary sensory cortex. [Appendix]

cerebellar cortex   The superficial gray matter of the cerebral hemispheres. [Appendix]

cerebellum   The prominent hindbrain structure that is concerned with motor coordination, posture, balance, and some cognitive processes; composed of a three-layered cortex and deep nuclei, and attached to the brainstem by the cerebellar peduncles. [5,Appendix]

cerebral achromatopsia   Loss of color vision as a result of damage to the visual cortex. [3]

cerebral aqueduct   The portion of the ventricular system that connects the third and fourth ventricles. [Appendix]

cerebral cortex   The superficial gray matter of the cerebellum. [1,Appendix]

cerebral hemispheres   Also called *cerebrum*. The two halves of the forebrain. [Appendix]

cerebral peduncles   The major fiber bundles that connect the brainstem to the cerebral hemispheres. [Appendix]

cerebrospinal fluid   A normally clear and cell-free fluid that fills the ventricular system of the central nervous system; produced by the choroid plexus in the lateral ventricles. [Appendix]

chemical synapse   A synapse that uses a chemical transmitter agent; the most common type of synapse in the mammalian brain. [Appendix]

childhood amnesia   Also called *pediatric amnesia*. In adults, the inability to remember the early years of childhood. [8,15]

choreiform movement   Uncontrollable, dancelike ("choreiform") writhing or twisting associated with damage to the basal ganglia, as occurs in disorders such as Huntington's disease. [5]

choroid plexus   Specialized epithelium in the ventricular system that produces cerebrospinal fluid. [Appendix]

cingulate gyrus   The gyrus that surrounds the corpus callosum. [Appendix]

cingulate sulcus   A sulcus on the medial aspect of the cerebral hemispheres defined by the cingulate gyrus. [Appendix]

circle of Willis   A ring of arteries at the base of the midbrain; connects the posterior and anterior cerebral circulation. [Appendix]

circumplex model   A way to graphically represent the relationships among emotions by ordering them along the circumference of a circle formed by intersecting two orthogonal axes of valence and arousal at the circle's center. Compare *vector model*. [10]

classical conditioning   Also called *conditioned reflex*. The modification of an innate reflex by associating its normal triggering stimulus with an unrelated stimulus. The unrelated stimulus comes to trigger the original response by virtue of this repeated association. Compare *operant conditioning*. [8]

coactivation   Two areas of the brain are said to be coactivated if they both show higher activity in a specific task. Statistically, coactivation is reflected by a positive correlation of activity between two areas. [2]

cochlea   The portion of the inner ear specialized for transducing sound energy into neural signals. [4]

cocktail party effect   An attentional phenomenon in which an individual can selectively focus attention on one particular speaker while tuning out other simultaneously occurring conversations. [6]

cognition   "Higher-order" mental processes. [1]

cognitive functions   The set of processes that allow humans and many other animals to perceive external stimuli, to extract key information and hold it in memory, and ultimately to generate thoughts and actions that help reach desired goals. [1]

cognitive map theory   A theory positing that the hippocampus mediates memory for spatial relations among objects in the environment. Compare *episodic memory theory* and *relational memory theory*. [9]

cognitive model   A explanatory framework that invokes unobserved internal states to predict how stimuli lead to actions. [1]

cognitive neuroscience   A scientific discipline that seeks to create models that explain the interrelations between brain function and cognitive functions. [1]

cognitive reappraisal   A form of emotion regulation in which individuals use cognitive resources to alter the meaning of a situation in order to reduce or change its emotional impact. [10]

cognitive science   A scientific discipline that seeks to understand and model the information processing associated with cognitive functions. [1]

coincidence detector   A neuron that detects simultaneous events, as in sound localization. [4]

color   The subjective sensations elicited in humans (and presumably many other animals) by different spectral distributions of light. [3]

color constancy   The similar color appearance of surfaces, despite different spectral returns from them; usually applied to the similar appearance of objects under different illuminants. Compare *color contrast*. [3]

color contrast   The different color appearance of surfaces despite similar spectral returns from them. Compare *color constancy*. [3]

color space   The depiction of human color experience in diagrammatic form by a space with three axes representing the perceptual attributes of hue, saturation, and color brightness. [3]

coma   A pathological state of profound and persistent unconsciousness. [7]

complementarity   The combination of data across multiple methods for measuring brain function, often to improve inferences about the nature of the generative neural processes. [1]

complex emotion   An emotion that is learned, socially and culturally shaped, evolutionarily new, and typically expressed by a combination of the response patterns that characterize basic emotions. Compare *basic emotion*. [10]

computerized tomography (CT)   An imaging method in which X-rays acquired at multiple angles are used to build a three-dimensional structural image of biological tissue. [2]

conceptual priming   A form of direct priming in which the test cue and the target are semantically related. Compare *perceptual priming* and *semantic priming*. [8]

conditioned reflex   See *classical conditioning*.

conditioned response (CR)   In classical conditioning, the reflex (normally innate in response to a particular unconditioned stimulus) that is triggered by a novel stimulus by virtue of repeated association. Compare *unconditioned response*. [8]

conditioned stimulus (CS)   In classical conditioning, the novel stimulus that eventually comes to trigger the innate reflex by virtue of repeated association. Compare *unconditioned stimulus*. [8]

conditioning   The generation of a novel response that is gradually elicited by repeated pairing of a novel stimulus (the conditioned stimulus) with a stimulus that normally elicits the response being studied (the unconditioned stimulus). Compare *priming* and *skill learning*. [8]

confabulation   In patients with memory disorders, the generation of false memories for complex autobiographical events. [9,13]

conjunction target   A target in a visual search task that is characterized by having a unique combination of two visual features. Because the time taken to find a conjunction target increases linearly with the number of distracters, its detection is thought to require serial focused attention to each item till the specified target is found. Compare *pop-out stimulus*. [7]

connectionist   Pertaining to the connectivity of neural networks whose connection weights vary according to experience. [12]

consciousness   An intriguing but puzzling concept that includes the ideas of wakefulness, awareness of the world, and awareness of the self as an actor in the world. [7]

consolidation   The strengthening of memory traces following encoding. [9]

consonant   Typically an unvoiced (atonal) element of speech that begins and/or ends syllables. [12]

context memory test   See *source memory test*. [9]

contextual fear conditioning   A form of emotional learning in which fear responses are acquired in response to environments that predict the presence of an aversive stimulus. [10]

convergence   The combination of results across multiple experimental paradigms, often to support inferences about an unobservable internal state. [1]

corpus callosum   The large midline fiber bundle that connects the cortices of the two cerebral hemispheres. [Appendix]

correct rejection In recognition memory test, correctly classifying an new item as "new." Compare *false alarm, hit,* and *miss.* [9]

cortical association areas Also called *association cortices.* The regions of cerebral neocortex that are not involved in primary sensory or motor processing. [3]

cortical columns See *cortical modules.*

cortical magnification The disproportionate representation of cortical space according to peripheral receptor density (such as occurs for the central representation of the fovea of the human eye). [3]

cortical modules Also called *cortical columns.* Vertically organized groups of cortical neurons that process the same or similar information; examples are ocular dominance columns and orientation columns in the primary visual cortex. [3]

cortisol A steroid hormone released by the adrenal gland that is involved in the stress response. Called *corticosterone* in rodents. [10]

covert attention The focusing of visual attention toward a location or item in the visual field without shifting the direction of gaze. Can apply to other sensory modalities or to attentional paradigms. Compare *overt attention.* [6]

CR See *conditioned response.*

cranial nerve ganglia The sensory or motor ganglia associated with the 12 cranial nerves. Compare *dorsal root ganglia.* [Appendix]

cranial nerves Nerves projecting from the cranial motor nuclei to sense organs or muscles, mostly of the face, head, eyes, or neck. [Appendix]

CS See *conditioned stimulus.*

CT See *computerized tomography.*

cyclopean fusion The normal sense, when looking at the world with both eyes, that we see it as if with a single eye. [3]

decision neuroscience See *neuroeconomics.*

declarative memory Also called *explicit memory.* Memory available to consciousness that can be expressed by language. Compare *nondeclarative memory.* [8]

default mode Brain processes that occur in the absence of active executive control; a pattern of brain activation reflecting a set of cognitive processes that are typically more engaged during passive experience. [11]

default-mode network A network of the brain that includes the posterior cingulate cortex, the ventral anterior cingulate cortex, and the medial inferior prefrontal cortex and that has been proposed to be engaged when the brain is either "idling," not engaged in any specific cognitive task, or directing attention inwardly. [7]

delay conditioning A form of classical conditioning in which the conditioned stimulus is still ongoing when the unconditioned stimulus starts, and they both terminate at the same time. Compare *trace conditioning.* [8]

delay discounting See *temporal discounting.*

delay line The time delay generated by axons of different lengths; a mechanism important in coincidence detection. [4]

delay-period activity In cognitive neuroscience studies of working memory, the observation of neural signals that persist while the research subject maintains information over time. [13]

dendrite Also called *dendritic branch* or *dendritic process.* The extension of a neuron that receives synaptic input; usually branches near the cell body. Compare *axon.* [Appendix]

dendritic field potential An electrical potential induced in the dendritic tree of a neuron by input from the axons of other neurons; this electrical activity can often also be detected at the scalp as an EEG or ERP response. Compare *local field potential.* [2]

dendritic spine A small extension from the surface of a dendrite that receives synapses. [8]

depolarization Changing the membrane potential of a neuron in the positive direction, which initiates an action potential if threshold is reached. Compare *hyperpolarization.* [Appendix]

depth In vision the perception of distance from the observer. [3]

diaschisis A disruption of the function of one brain area caused by focal damage to another, distant part of the brain. Often, the proper functioning of a brain area relies upon receiving input and stimulation from other, distant areas, so that if a distant area is damaged, the "down-stream" area can be affected as well. [2]

dichromat A color-deficient human (and the majority of mammals) whose color vision depends on only two cone types. Compare *trichromat.* [3]

diencephalic theory See *Cannon-Bard theory.*

diencephalon The portion of the brain that lies just rostral to the brainstem; comprises the thalamus and hypothalamus. [Appendix]

diffusion decision model See *drift-diffusion model.*

diffusion tensor imaging (DTI) A method of MRI that can show the preferred directions of diffusion within tissue; useful for the imaging of fiber tracts of the brain. [2]

digit-span task A working memory test in which the subject is asked to immediately recall a random string of numbers, which is gradually increased until recall fails. [8]

direct priming Also called *repetition priming.* The facilitation of recall in which the prime and the target are identical or have the same name. Compare *indirect priming.* [8]

disinhibition syndrome Also called *frontal disinhibition syndrome.* A collection of behavioral signs and symptoms, typically caused by damage to the ventral prefrontal cortex; manifested by a loss of control, inappropriate outbursts, and a lack of inhibition in social settings. Compare *dysexecutive syndrome.* [13]

dissociative identity disorder A clinical condition characterized by at least two distinct and relatively enduring personalities that alternately control a person's behavior. [11]

domain-specific theory Theory which postulates that semantic memory is organized by semantic categories, such as living vs. nonliving things. Compare *sensory/functional theory.* [9]

dopamine A catecholamine neurotransmitter involved in learning and reward evaluation, among other roles in the nervous system of humans and other animals. [14]

dopamine system refers to the circuits in the brain that include neurons that release the neurotransmitter dopamine. The dopaminergic neurons, which are mostly located in the ventral tegmental area of the midbrain, the substantia nigra pars compacta, and the hypothalamus, have been particularly associated with reward. [2]

dorsal horn The dorsal portion of the spinal cord gray matter, which contains neurons that process sensory information. Compare *lateral horn* and *ventral horn*. [Appendix]

dorsal root ganglia The segmental sensory ganglia of the spinal cord that contain the first-order sensory neurons whose axons project centrally. Compare *cranial nerve ganglia*. [Appendix]

dorsal stream A partially segregated visual processing pathway passing from primary visual cortex through extrastriate areas to the higher-order association cortices of the parietal cortex; thought to be concerned primarily with spatial aspects of visual processing. Compare *ventral stream*. [3]

dorsolateral prefrontal cortex A functional division of the prefrontal cortex roughly corresponding to the middle and superior frontal gyri, as located anterior to motor cortex and the frontal eye fields. Compare *ventrolateral prefrontal cortex*. [13]

dorsomedial prefrontal cortex A functional division of the prefrontal cortex roughly corresponding to the medial surface dorsal to the corpus callosum. Compare *ventromedial prefrontal cortex*. [13]

double dissociation A functional relationship in which one area of the brain is experimentally shown to be associated with a particular task or cognitive function and not with another task or function, whereas another area is shown to be involved in the second task or function but not the first. This demonstration thus distinguishes the cognitive roles of different regions in a more rigorous way than does simply showing that the two regions in question respond differently. [2]

drift-diffusion model A mathematical description of decision-making behavior in terms of competing processes that drift in a random-walk fashion toward boundaries. Also called *diffusion decision model*. [14]

DTI See *diffusion tensor imaging*.

dual-system model A framework for decision making that posits the existence of two independent systems—typically, a fast emotional system and a slower cognitive system—whose interactions over time predict choices. [14]

dynamic causal modeling A successor to structural equation modeling which tests *directional* models of functional connectivity against brain data to determine the relative likelihood of the activity in one area of the brain causing the activity in others. [2]

dysexecutive syndrome Also called *frontal dysexecutive syndrome*. A collection of behavioral signs and symptoms, typically caused by damage to the dorsolateral prefrontal cortex; manifested by an inability to change behavior willfully and flexibly according to context. Compare *disinhibition syndrome*. [13]

eardrum See *tympanic membrane*.

early selection A model of attention postulating that attentional mechanisms can selectively filter out or attenuate irrelevant sensory input at an early processing stage, before the completion of sensory and perceptual analysis. Compare *late selection*. [6]

effector A muscle or gland that provides the output of neural processing. [Appendix]

efferent neuron An axon that conducts information away from the central nervous system. Compare *afferent neuron*. [Appendix]

electrophysiological recording Any of various methods of recording electrical activity in the nervous system. [Appendix]

embodiment A sense of physical location of the self within one's own body. [11]

emotion A set of physiological responses, action tendencies, and subjective feelings that adaptively engage humans and other animals to react to events of biological and/or individual significance. [10]

emotion regulation The voluntary or involuntary deployment of resources to gain control over emotional responses. [10]

emotional perseveration The continuation of an emotional response to a stimulus after the emotional significance of the stimulus has changed and the response is no longer appropriate. [10]

empathy The ability to share the same feelings expressed by another individual. Compare *sympathy*. [11]

encoding Also called *learning*. The incorporation of new information into a memory store, which requires the modification or creation of memory traces. Compare *retrieval*. [8]

endogenous attention A form of attention in which processing resources are directed voluntarily to specific aspects of the environment; typically prompted by experimental instructions or, more normally, by an individual's goals, expectations, and/or knowledge. Compare *exogenous attention*. [6]

endowment effect A bias in decision making in which people will pay less to buy something than they would accept to sell the same thing, if they already possessed it. [14]

engram Also called *memory trace*. The physical basis of a stored memory. [8]

enteric division The division of the autonomic motor system that is specifically concerned with regulating the behavior of the gut. [Appendix]

epinephrine A catecholaminergic neurotransmitter and hormone involved in many body functions, including the fight-or-flight response coordinated by the autonomic nervous system. [10]

episodic memory Declarative memory that refers to memory for personally experienced past events. Compare *semantic memory*. [9]

episodic memory theory A theory positing that the hippocampus is critical for episodic memory but not for semantic memory. Compare *cognitive map theory* and *relational memory theory*. [9]

ERN See *error-related negativity*.

EROS See *event-related optical signals*.

ERP See *event-related potential*.

error-related negativity (ERN) An electrophysiological marker that occurs when participants make errors in cognitive tasks. [11,13]

event-related design A task design used in fMRI studies in which trials or events of different types may follow one another in randomized order and the neural responses from the different events can be extracted from the measured signals. Analogous to the extraction of event-related potentials (ERPs) from ongoing EEG and to the construction of peristimulus histograms from single-neuron recordings. Compare *blocked design*. [2]

event-related optical signals (EROS) A noninvasive optical imaging approach based on the fact that when brain tissue is illuminated, even through the skull, the amount of transmitted versus scattered light varies as a function of whether the neuronal tissue is electrically active. [2]

event-related potential (ERP) Voltage fluctuations in an ongoing brain EEG that are triggered by sensory and/or cognitive events; the changes reflect the summed electrical activity of neuronal populations specifically responding to those events and are extracted from the ongoing EEG by time-locked averaging. [2]

excitatory Pertaining to a synaptic effect that brings the membrane of the postsynaptic cell closer to threshold, thereby making firing of the postsynaptic cell more likely. Compare *inhibitory*. [Appendix]

executive function The cognitive functions that allow flexible and goal-directed control of thought and behavior. [13]

exogenous attention Also called *reflexive attention*. A form of attention in which processing resources are directed to specific aspects of the environment in response to a sudden stimulus change, such as a loud noise or sudden movement, that attracts attention automatically. Compare *endogenous attention*. [6]

expected utility The personal value (i.e., utility) placed on the potential outcome of a decision, as derived from the combination of the value and probability of its potential outcomes. Compare *expected value*. [14]

expected value The average value in a particular currency (e.g., dollars) of the potential outcome of a decision as weighted by the relative probabilities of those outcomes. Compare *expected utility*. [14]

explicit memory See *declarative memory*.

external ear The cartilaginous elements of the visible ear (the pinna and concha). [4]

extinction The gradual disappearance of a conditioned response that is no longer being rewarded. [8]

extracellular recording Recording the electrical potentials in the extracellular space near active neurons. Compare *intracellular recording*. [2]

extrastriate visual cortical areas Regions of the visual cortex that lie outside the *primary* (striate) *visual cortex*; includes higher-order visual processing areas such as V4, MT, and MST. [3]

eyeblink conditioning A paradigm in which a puff of air is repeatedly paired with a tone until the tone by itself elicits blinking. [8]

FA See *fractional anisotropy*.

false alarm In recognition memory test, incorrectly classifying a new item as "old." Compare *correct rejection*, *hit*, and *miss*. [9]

familiarity The feeling of having experienced an event at some point in the past, even though no specific associations or contextual detail come to mind. Compare *recollection*. [9]

fear conditioning A form of emotional learning in which fear responses are acquired to cues that predict the occurrence of an aversive stimulus. See also *contextual fear conditioning*. Compare *fear extinction*. [10]

fear extinction A form of emotional learning in which fear responses are reduced by repeated presentation of a feared stimulus without any unpleasant consequences. Compare *fear conditioning*. [10]

feature integration theory A model of attention postulating that the visual perceptual system is organized as a set of feature maps, each providing information about the location(s) in the visual field of a particular feature. The model also proposes that attention is required to integrate the feature information from these separate maps into a perceptual whole. [7]

feature similarity gain model A model in which the attentional modulation of the amplitude (gain) of a sensory neuron's response depends on the similarity of the features of the currently relevant target and the feature preferences of that neuron. [6]

FFA See *fusiform face area*.

fiber tract Bundles of axons in the brain that carry neuronal signals between brain areas. [2]

fictive learning The adjustment of rules for behavior based on reward outcomes that were observed, but not received directly. [14]

fissure A deep cleft in the surface of the brain; can be either between two lobes (e.g., the lateral fissure between the frontal and temporal lobes) or an especially deep *sulcus* (e.g., the calcarine fissure in the occipital lobe). [Appendix]

flashbulb memory The concept that traumatic memories are vividly and accurately represented in the brain as though the event were recorded through the flash of a camera. [10]

fMRI adaptation One way of using repetition suppression within an fMRI paradigm that uses pairs of similar stimuli. If the second stimulus induces less activity than the first stimulus (or prime) in a particular brain area, then it can be inferred that the region in some way supports a process common to the two stimuli. [2]

fMRI See *functional magnetic resonance imaging*.

folia (sing. folium) The ridges and valleys that are apparent in the cerebellar cortex. [Appendix]

forebrain The anterior portion of the brain that includes the cerebral hemispheres (the telencephalon and diencephalon). [Appendix]

form The perception of object geometry or shape; one of the major visual perceptual qualities. [3]

formant One of several frequencies that represent the natural resonances of different components of the vocal tract. [12]

fornix (pl. fornices) An axon tract, best seen from the medial surface of the divided brain, that interconnects the hypothalamus and hippocampus. [Appendix]

fourth ventricle The ventricular space that lies between the pons and the cerebellum. Compare *third ventricle* and *lateral ventricles*. [Appendix]

fovea The area of the human retina specialized for high acuity; contains a high density of cones and few rods. Most mammals do not have a well-defined fovea, although many have an area of central vision (called the *area centralis*) in which acuity is higher than in more eccentric retinal regions. [3]

fractional anisotropy (FA) The degree to which water diffuses in a preferred direction within tissue. Higher levels of fractional anisotropy are thought to reflect greater amounts of white-matter (i.e., fiber tract) integrity. [2]

framing effect   A mode of representing a decision-making scenario that changes the decisions people make, even though the basic structure of the problem is left unchanged. [14]

frequency band   A specific frequency range within a spectrum, usually referring to oscillatory electrical brain activity. [2]

frontal disinhibition syndrome   See *disinhibition syndrome*.

frontal dysexecutive syndrome   See *dysexecutive syndrome*.

frontal eye fields   A region of the prefrontal cortex in human and non-human primates, often associated with area 8a, that plays a key role in voluntary visual orienting movements. [5]

frontopolar cortex   The most anterior part of the prefrontal cortex. [13]

fugue state   Transient states of confusion in which self-relevant knowledge is temporarily unavailable to consciousness. [11]

functional connectivity   How the activity of one brain region varies with the activity in other brain regions. [2]

functional magnetic resonance imaging (fMRI)   A non-invasive method for imaging brain activity that uses imaging pulse sequences generated by a magnetic resonance scanner; the signal measured is caused by hemoglobin-based changes in blood oxygenation and blood flow that are induced by local neural activity. [2]

functional neural module   A specialized, encapsulated neural circuit that has evolved to process specific types of information relevant to solving the problems a particular species confronts in its natural environment. [15]

fundamental frequency   The first vibratory mode in the harmonic series evident in the sound spectra generated by a vibrating string or column of air. [4]

fusiform face area (FFA)   A region of the fusiform gyrus that shows enhanced responses to faces relative to other objects. [3,11]

game theory   A subfield of behavioral economics that investigates how people make decisions in simple, well-controlled games. [14]

ganglion (pl. ganglia)   A structurally and functionally discrete collection of neurons (individually referred to as *ganglion cells*) in the periphery (i.e. outside the central nervous system). Not to be confused with the *basal ganglia*, a group of structures that lie within the brain. Compare *nucleus*. [Appendix]

gating   Allowing or permitting. The basal ganglia, for example, gate movement initiation. Channels through the neuronal membrane are often gated, allowing the access of certain ions under certain conditions. [5]

glia   See *neuroglial cells*.

globus pallidus   One of the three major nuclei that make up the basal ganglia in the cerebral hemispheres; relays information from the caudate and putamen to the thalamus. [Appendix]

glomerulus (pl. glomeruli)   Any of the characteristic collections of neurons in the olfactory bulb that are formed by dendrites of mitral cells and terminals of olfactory receptor cells, as well as the axons and dendrites of local interneurons. [4]

grammar   The system of rules implicit in a language. [12]

gray matter   Regions of the central nervous system that are rich in neuronal cell bodies; includes the cerebral and cerebellar cortices, the nuclei of the brain, and the central portion of the spinal cord. Compare *white matter*. [Appendix]

guided search   A cognitive model positing that there are two basic components that determine the allocation of attention during visual search : a component driven by stimulus (bottom-up) information and one driven by top-down influences based on high-level factors and behavioral goals. [7]

gustatory system   Also called *taste system*. The peripheral and central components of the nervous system dedicated to processing and perceiving taste stimuli. [4]

gyrus (pl. gyri)   Any of the ridges in the folded cerebral cortex. Compare *sulcus*. [Appendix]

habit   A well-established pattern of thought or behavior. [14]

habituation   The process by which a behavioral response to the same stimulus decreases in intensity, frequency, or duration when that stimulus is repeated over and over. Compare *sensitization*. [8]

hair cell   The receptor cell in the inner ear for transducing sound stimuli (or other mechanical stimuli in the case of vestibular hair cells) into neural signals. [4]

harmonic series   The series of vibratory modes evident in the spectra produced by resonating objects. [4]

Hebbian learning   The idea, proposed by Donald Hebb in the late 1940s, that when presynaptic and postsynaptic neurons fire action potentials together, the strength of the synaptic connections between them is enhanced. Hebb's rule is often state as "cells that fire together wire together." [8]

hemiballismus   A neurological disorder resulting from unilateral damage to the basal ganglia; manifested by flinging movements of the limbs contralateral to the lesion. [5]

hemispatial neglect   A deficit in the ability to attend to the left side of space, and often to the left side of objects, typically caused by damage to the right parietal lobe. Occasionally damage to the left parietal lobe can cause corresponding deficits for attending to the right side of space, but much more rarely. [7]

heuristic   A rule or procedure derived from past experience that can be used to solve a problem (e.g., in decision making, perception, or some other aspect of cognition). [14]

hippocampus (pl. hippocampi)   A specialized cortical structure located in the medial portion of the temporal lobe; in humans, concerned with declarative memory, among many other functions. [10,Appendix]

hit   In recognition memory test, correctly classifying an old item as "old." Compare *correct rejection*, *false alarm*, and *miss*. [9]

hominids   The family of primates that includes humans and their bipedal ancestors but not great apes (although some taxonomists include all African apes, humans, and human ancestors in this family). [15]

Homo   The genus of humans and their ancestors characterized by upright walking, a relatively large brain, certain advanced dental features, and toolmaking. [15]

homunculus (pl. homunculi)   Literally "little man" (Greek), often used in referring to the shape of a primary sensory or motor cortical map. Also used to refer (often negatively) to the dualist notion of a non-neurally based "self." [2,4]

HPA axis   See *hypothalamic-pituitary-adrenal axis*.

Huntington's disease   An autosomal dominant genetic disorder in which a single gene mutation results in damage to the basal ganglia that causes personality changes, progressive loss of the control of voluntary movement, and eventually death. [5]

hyperpolarization   Changing the membrane potential of a neuron in the negative direction, driving it away from threshold and making it less likely to initiate an action potential. Compare *depolarization*. [Appendix]

hyperscanning   An fMRI technique in which data are collected simultaneously across more than one MRI scanner, often while individuals are playing a multiplayer game. [14]

hypothalamic-pituitary-adrenal (HPA) axis   The primary information-processing pathway for stress responses; connects the hypothalamus, pituitary gland, and adrenal gland. [10]

hypothalamus   A collection of small but critical nuclei in the diencephalon that lies just inferior to the thalamus; governs reproductive, homeostatic, and circadian functions. [10,Appendix]

illumination   The light that falls on a scene or surface. [3]

illusory conjunction   A perceptual process in which sensory features from different objects in a scene are falsely perceived as being part of the same object. [7]

imaging genomics   See *neuroimaging genomics*.

implicit memory   See *nondeclarative memory*.

indirect priming   The facilitation of recall by an item (the prime) that is not directly related to that item. For example, the word *winter* may indirectly prime both *summer* and *snow*. Compare *direct priming*. [8]

individual difference   Variation in a cognitive function or other trait across people, often as can be related to a particular biological predictor. [1,10]

inferior colliculi (sing. inferior colliculus)   Paired structures on the dorsal surface of the midbrain; concerned with auditory processing. Compare *superior colliculi*. [4,Appendix]

inhibition of return   A phenomenon in an exogenously cued spatial attention paradigm that is apparent as a slower behavioral response to a target stimulus presented at the (validly) cued location later than 300 milliseconds after the cue. [6]

inhibitory   Pertaining to a synaptic effect that makes the firing of the postsynaptic cell less likely. Compare *excitatory*. [Appendix]

instrumental learning   See *operant conditioning*.

insula   Literally "island" (in Latin). The portion of the cerebral cortex that is buried within the depths of the Sylvian fissure (lateral sulcus). [4,Appendix]

intention tremor   A tremor that occurs during performance of a voluntary motor act. Characteristic of cerebellar pathology. [5]

intentional stance   The assumption that others are agents motivated to behave in a way that is consistent with their current mental state. [11]

interaural intensity difference   The difference in the intensity of a sound stimulus at the two ears; contributes to sound localization. Compare *interaural time difference*. [4]

interaural time difference   The difference in the time of arrival of a sound stimulus at the two ears; contributes to sound localization. Compare *interaural intensity difference*. [4]

internal capsule   A large white matter tract that lies between the diencephalon and the basal ganglia; contains, among others, sensory axons that run from the thalamus to the cortex and motor axons that run from the cortex to the brainstem and spinal cord. [Appendix]

interneuron   Also called *local circuit neuron*. Literally, a neuron in a circuit that lies between primary sensory and primary effector neurons; more generally, a neuron that branches locally to innervate other neurons. [Appendix]

interoception   The sense of the internal state of the organism. [11]

intracellular recording   Recording the potential between the inside and outside of a neuron with a microelectrode. Compare *extracellular recording*. [2]

inverse optics problem   The impossibility of knowing the world directly by means of light stimuli; arises because of the ambiguity of light patterns projected onto the retina. [3]

ion channel   A membrane protein that uses the passive energy of concentration gradients (created by *ion pumps*) to allow the passage of ions across the cell membrane. [Appendix]

ion pump   A membrane protein that uses metabolic energy to create ion concentration gradients across neuronal membranes. Compare *ion channel*. [Appendix]

Iowa Gambling Task   An experimental paradigm, developed by Antonio Damasio and colleagues at the University of Iowa, that tests subjects' sensitivity to risk and reward; the test reveals that patients with damage to the inferior prefrontal cortex tend to make risk-seeking choices. [14]

ischemia   A paucity or complete lack of blood supply; a common cause of stroke. [Appendix]

item recognition test   Memory test that measure memory for the occurrence of items independently of their contexts. [9]

James-Lange theory   A theory, developed by William James and Carl Lange in the 1880's, positing that emotions are determined by the pattern of feedback from the body periphery to the cerebral cortex. [10]

joint attention   The sharing of a common focus of attention across at least two individuals. [11]

Klüver-Bucy syndrome   A rare behavioral syndrome following damage to the anterior temporal lobe that includes a lack of appreciation for the motivational significance of objects in the environment, hyperorality, and altered sexual behavior; named after Heinrich Klüver and Paul Bucy. [10]

larynx   The portion of the upper respiratory tract that lies between the trachea and the pharynx. [12]

late selection   A theory of attention postulating that all stimuli are processed through the completion of sensory and perceptual analysis before any selection or influence of attention occurs. Compare *early selection*. [6]

lateral fissure   Also called *Sylvian fissure*. The cleft on the lateral surface of the human brain that separates the temporal and frontal lobes. [Appendix]

lateral geniculate nucleus   The thalamic nucleus that relays information from the retina to the cerebral cortex. Compare *medial geniculate nucleus*. [3]

lateral horn   The lateral portion of the spinal cord gray matter, which mediates sympathetic motor responses. Compare *dorsal horn* and *ventral horn*. [Appendix]

lateral intraparietal area (LIP)   Also called *area LIP*. A part of the inferior parietal lobule that plays a key role in orienting attention and the eyes to a location in space. [14]

lateral prefrontal cortex   The portion of the frontal lobes that lies along the lateral surface of the cerebral cortex, usually restricted to regions anterior to motor cortex. [13]

lateral ventricles   The major ventricle in each of the two cerebral hemispheres. Compare *third ventricle* and *fourth ventricle*. [Appendix]

learning   1. See *encoding*. 2. The combined effect of all encoding, storage, and retrieval in gradually enhancing the performance of a particular task. [8]

left parietal effect   In ERP studies of recognition memory, the phenomenon, occurring at about 400 to 800 milliseconds after the stimulus, whereby old items elicit greater positivity over left parietal regions than do new items. Compare *right frontal effect*. [9]

levels of processing   Declarative memory encoding is usually better when information is processed at a semantic (deep) level rather than at a perceptual (shallow) level. [8]

LFP   See *local field potential*.

lightness   In vision, the apparent reflectance of a surface. Compare *brightness*. [3]

limbic system theory   The theory, developed by Paul MacLean in the 1940's, positing that structures of the limbic forebrain constitute a system that generates emotions. [10]

LIP   See *lateral intraparietal area*.

lobes   The four major regions of the cerebral cortex: the frontal, parietal, occipital, and temporal lobes. [Appendix]

local circuit neuron   Also called *interneuron*. A neuron whose local connections contribute to processing circuitry. [5]

local field potential (LFP)   A *dendritic field potential* that is recorded intracranially close to the dendritic source (i.e., locally). [2]

localization of function   The idea that the brain may have distinct regions that support particular cognitive functions. [1]

locus coeruleus   A small adrenergic nucleus in the rostral brainstem that projects widely in the brain; it plays a role in the sleep-waking cycle, mediating alertness, and attention. [7]

long-term depression (LTD)   A long-lasting diminishment of synaptic strength as a result of repetitive activity. Compare *long-term potentiation*. [8]

long-term potentiation (LTP)   A long-lasting enhancement of synaptic strength as a result of repetitive activity. Compare *long-term depression*. [8]

loudness   The sensory quality elicited by the intensity of sound stimuli. [4]

lower motor neuron   Also called *primary motor neuron*. A motor neuron that directly innervates muscle. Compare *upper motor neuron*. [5]

LTD   See *long-term depression*.

LTP   See *long-term potentiation*.

luminance   The physical measure of light intensity. [3]

magnetic resonance imaging (MRI)   A noninvasive imaging method based on the behavior of atomic nuclei (particularly hydrogen) within a strong magnetic field; provides excellent soft-tissue contrast of brain anatomy, and can also be used to measure functional brain activity noninvasively. See also *functional magnetic resonance imaging*. [2]

magnetoencephalography (MEG)   A method of measuring at the scalp the electrical currents in the brain based on the detection of the magnetic fields produced by those currents. Like EEG, MEG activity is thought to reflect mainly the electrical currents produced in the dendritic trees of the large pyramidal cells in cortex. [2]

magnocellular system   The component of the primary visual processing pathway that is specialized in part for the perception of motion and other aspects of stimulus change; so named because of the relatively large neurons involved. Compare *parvocellular system*. [3]

mammillary bodies   Small prominences on the ventral surface of the diencephalon; functionally, part of the caudal hypothalamus. [Appendix]

McGurk effect   The misperception of speech sounds due to conflicting visual stimuli. [12]

medial geniculate nucleus   The thalamic nucleus in the primary auditory pathway. Compare *lateral geniculate nucleus*. [4]

medulla   The most caudal of the three components of the brainstem, extending from the pons to the spinal cord. Compare *midbrain* and *pons*. [Appendix]

medullary pyramids   Longitudinal bulges on the ventral aspect of the medulla that signify the corticospinal tracts at this level of the nervous system. [5]

MEG   See *magnetoencephalography*.

memory   Processes by which information is encoded (learned), stored, and retrieved. [8]

memory modulation hypothesis   A hypothesis positing that the basolateral amygdala is important for modulating memory processing in other brain regions to enhance the retention of emotional events. [10]

memory search   A process during memory retrieval that explores possible locations of a target memory. [9]

memory trace   See *engram*.

mentalizing   Also called *theory of mind*. The ability to represent the internal mental states of other individuals. [11]

meta-analysis   The approach of combining results from multiple experiments, usually published studies that vary in their research methods, to improve the specificity and generalizability of the inferences that can be drawn. [1]

midbrain   The most rostral of the three components of the brainstem; identified by the superior and inferior colliculi on its dorsal surface, and the cerebral peduncles on its ventral aspect. Compare *medulla* and *pons*. [Appendix]

middle ear   The portion of the ear between the eardrum and the oval window; contains the three small bones that amplify sound stimuli mechanically. [4]

mind   The full spectrum of a person's awareness (one aspect of consciousness) at any point in time, reflecting sensory percepts, as well as thoughts, feelings, goals, desires, and so on. [1]

mirror drawing task   A sensorimotor skill learning task in which the subject is asked to trace the outline of a figure, such as a star, which can be only seen through its reflection on a mirror. Accuracy improves gradually with practice. [8]

mirror neuron   A neuron in the frontal or parietal cortex that shows similar electrophysiological responses to actions executed by oneself or to observation of the same actions being executed by another. [11]

mismatch negativity (MMN)   A negative ERP wave peaking at about 150 to 200 milliseconds following a deviant stimulus in a stream of otherwise identical stimuli (usually sound stimuli). [6]

miss   In recognition memory test, incorrectly classifying an old item as "new." Compare *correct rejection*, *false alarm*, and *hit*. [9]

MMN   See *mismatch negativity*.

modality-specific attention   The focusing attention on the stimulus information specifically within one sensory modality. Compare *supramodal attention*. [6]

monitoring   The process that evaluates the appropriateness of a given behavior for the current context; examples include evaluating the accuracy of answers generated during a memory test or the adequacy of a response rule in an executive function paradigm. [9,13]

monocular   Pertaining to one eye. Compare *binocular*. [3]

mood regulation   The long-term balance between emotional and attentional processing. When these processes become skewed, mood disorders such as depression can occur. [10]

mosaic brain evolution   The proposal that different functional parts of the brain, or modules, evolve at different rates in response to different selective pressures in the environment. [15]

motion   The changing position of an object defined by speed and direction within a frame of reference. [3]

motion aftereffect   The persistence of perceived motion in the opposite direction when a motion stimulus has ceased. [3]

motion parallax   The different degree of movement of near and far objects as a function of moving the head or body while observing a scene. [3]

motor aphasia   See *Broca's aphasia*.

motor cortex   In humans and other mammals, the region of the cerebral cortex anterior to the central sulcus that is concerned with motor behavior; includes the primary motor cortex in the precentral gyrus, and associated premotor cortical areas in the frontal lobe. [Appendix]

motor neuron   A nerve cell that innervates skeletal or smooth muscle. [Appendix]

motor program   The plan to produce a particular motor action, such as writing one's name, that occurs independently of the effectors used to carry out the movement. [5]

motor system   All the components of the central and peripheral nervous systems that support motor behavior. [Appendix]

MRI   See *magnetic resonance imaging*.

MST (middle superior temporal)   In primates, an extrastriate cortical region related to MT that is in part specialized for motion processing. [3]

MT (middle temporal)   In primates, an extrastriate cortical region related to MST that is in part specialized for motion processing. [3]

multiple-trace theory   A theory positing that episodic memories, consolidated or otherwise, always depend on the hippocampus. Compare *standard consolidation theory*. [9]

multisensory integration   The combining of sensory information from different sensory modalities, facilitating the linking of that information together into one perceptual object. [6]

multivoxel pattern analysis (MVPA)   A technique that analyzes patterns of activation across voxels in a particular brain region that consistently correspond to certain stimulus or event types, rather than the overall increase or decrease in activation of the entire region. [2]

MVPA   See *multivoxel pattern analysis*.

myelin   The membranous wrapping of axons by certain classes of glial cells that makes brain regions with axonal pathways look whitish. See *white matter*. [Appendix]

myelination   The process by which glial cells wrap axons to form multiple layers of glial cell membrane that electrically insulate the axon, thereby speeding up the conduction of action potentials. [15]

N2pc wave   A negative-polarity ("N" in N2pc) ERP component elicited by the detection of a pop-out stimulus target in a visual search array, thought to reflect either the shifting and focusing of attention to the location of the pop-out or the filtering of the nearby distracter items. It is elicited over posterior scalp sites ("p"), contralateral ("c") to the side of the target, typically peaking at around 250 ms following the presentation of the stimulus array. [7]

Neanderthals   A subspecies of *Homo sapiens* that lived between 200,000 and 30,000 years ago in the Middle East and Europe. [15]

negative reinforcement   The removal of an aversive outcome following an ation. [14]

nerve cell   See *neuron*.

nervous system   The network of nerve cells throughout the body. [1]

neural circuit   A collection of interconnected neurons mediating a specific function. [Appendix]

neural correlate   A measure of brain function that covaries with the expression of a cognitive function. [1]

neural network   Typically refers to artificial network of interconnected nodes whose connections change in strength as a means of solving problems. Can also be used as a synonym for a neuronal circuit. [12]

neural precursor cell   Also called neural stem cells, these undifferentiated cells are defined by their capacity for self-renewal and ability to generate all the major cell types of the CNS including neurons, astrocytes, oligodendrocytes, and ependymal cells that line the ventricles of the brain. [15]

neural priming   See *repetition suppression*.

neuroeconomics   Also called *decision neuroscience*. An emerging discipline that combines theoretical perspectives from neuroscience and economics, as well as other of the social sciences, in the creation of mechanistic models for behavior. [14]

neuroglial cells   Also called *neuroglia* or *glia*. Any of several types of non-neural cells found in the peripheral and central nervous systems that carry out a variety of functions that do not directly entail signaling. [Appendix]

neuroimaging genomics   Also called *imaging genomics*. A method of relating differences in fMRI activity between people to specific genetic variations. This method can provide accounts of how genetics can influence brain structure and function, and thus in turn cognitive processes. [2]

neuromarketing   The use of measurements of physiology or brain function to shape the branding and advertising of consumer products. [14]

neuron Also called *nerve cell*. A cell specialized for the conduction and transmission of electrical signals in the nervous system. [1,Appendix]

neurorealism The tendency to consider a behavioral or mental phenomenon to be more real based on the presence of neuroscience data. [14]

neurotransmitter A chemical agent released at synapses that mediates signaling between nerve cells. [1,Appendix]

neurotransmitter receptor A molecule embedded in the membrane of a postsynaptic cell that binds a neurotransmitter. [Appendix]

nociceptive system See *pain system*.

nociceptor A cell that responds specifically to potentially harmful stimuli. [4]

noise A sound stimulus that is aperiodic. Compare *tone*. [4]

nondeclarative memory Also called *implicit memory*. Memory expressed through performance; assumed to operate unconsciously. Compare *declarative memory*. [8]

noradrenaline See *norepinephrine*.

norepinephrine Also called *noradrenaline*. A catecholamin-ergic neurotransmitter and hormone released across synapses in postganglionic neurons of the sympathetic nervous system, in the adrenal medulla, and in some parts of the central nervous system. [10]

nucleus (pl. nuclei) An anatomically discrete collection of neurons within the brain; typically serves a particular function. Compare *ganglion*. [Appendix]

nucleus accumbens A subdivision of the *ventral striatum* that contains neurons sensitive to the neurotransmitter dopamine and contributes to learning and reward evaluation. [14]

nucleus of the lateral lemniscus A brainstem nucleus in the primary auditory pathway. [4]

nucleus of the solitary tract A brainstem nucleus that integrates gustatory and other information relevant to the autonomic control of the gut and other autonomic target organs. [4]

occlusion The blocked view of distant objects by nearer objects. [3]

odor The perception elicited by a soluble chemical that interacts with olfactory receptors. [4]

olfactory bulb The olfactory relay station that receives axons from the olfactory cranial nerve and transmits this information via the olfactory tract to higher centers. [4,Appendix]

olfactory epithelium Pseudostratified epithelium that contains olfactory receptor cells, supporting cells, and mucus-secreting glands in the nasal cavity. [4]

olfactory nerve The first cranial nerve; runs from the olfactory mucosa to the olfactory bulb. [Appendix]

olfactory system The sensory system that includes the olfactory epithelium of the nasal cavity, the olfactory tract, and olfactory bulbs; mediates the perception of odors. [4]

olfactory tract The projection from the olfactory bulbs to higher olfactory centers. [4,Appendix]

oligodendrocyte Glial cells with sheetlike processes that form the myelin sheath that insulates nerve axons. [15]

operant conditioning Also called *instrumental learning*. The altered probability of a behavioral response engendered by associating responses with rewards (or punishments). Compare *classical conditioning*. [8]

optic ataxia A neurological condition associated with damage to the dorsal parietal cortex and characterized by deficits in visually guided reaching. [5]

optic chiasm The crossing of optic nerve axons from the nasal portions of the retinas in humans and other mammals such that the temporal visual fields are represented in the contralateral cerebral hemispheres. [Appendix]

optogenetics A method in which genes that code for light-sensitive ion channels or light-sensitive ion transporters are introduced into neurons. Once these genes are expressed, and the channels or transporters are integrated into the cell membrane, the neuron's activity may be controlled by stimulation with light. [2]

orbitofrontal cortex The division of the prefrontal cortex that lies above the orbits in the most rostral and ventral extension of the sagittal fissure; important in emotional processing and decision making. [13]

organelle A subcellular component visible in a light or electron microscope (e.g., nucleus, ribosome, endoplasmic reticulum). [Appendix]

oval window The site where the middle-ear bones transfer vibrational energy to the cochlea. [4]

overt attention The focusing of attention (typically visual) by voluntarily shifting gaze. Compare *covert attention*. [6]

P20–50 attention effect An enhanced positive-polarity ERP wave elicited by an attended auditory stimulus, occurring between 20 and 50 milliseconds after stimulus onset; this effect provided particularly strong support for early-selection models of attention. [6]

P3 See *P300*.

P300 Also called *P3*. A large positive ERP wave elicited by stimuli that are surprising, are of an infrequent event type, or are task-relevant targets, usually when occurring within a stream of other sensory events; typically peaks between 300 and 500 milliseconds after the stimulus. [6,13]

pain The highly unpleasant percepts generated by stimuli that are potentially damaging. [4]

pain system A system for warning an animal about potentially harmful stimuli. While largely responsive to mechanical stimuli, it is also closely related to responses to temperature and noxious chemicals. [4]

parahippocampal gyrus A cortical gyrus in the medial temporal lobe adjacent to the hippocampus; plays a role in declarative memory, emotion, and responses to olfactory stimuli. [Appendix]

parasympathetic division Sometimes referred to as the "rest and digest" system. The component of the autonomic motor system that mediates restorative metabolic functions. Compare *sympathetic division*. [Appendix]

parieto-occipital sulcus Sulcus between the occipital and parietal lobes of the cerebral hemispheres. [Appendix]

Parkinson's disease A neurodegenerative process affecting the substantia nigra that results in a characteristic tremor at rest and a general paucity of movement. [5]

parvocellular system The component of the primary visual processing pathway that is specialized in part for the detection of detail and color; so named because of the relatively small size of the neurons involved. Compare *magnocellular system*. [3]

pediatric amnesia See *childhood amnesia*.

perceptual load The level of processing difficulty or complexity of a task being performed by an individual; usually measured by the time it takes for perceptual analyses of the stimuli. [6]

perceptual priming A form of direct priming in which the test cue and the target are perceptually related. Compare *conceptual priming*. [8]

peripheral nervous system All the nerves and neurons that lie outside the brain and spinal cord. Compare *central nervous system*. [Appendix]

peristimulus time histogram (PSTH) A graph that plots neuronal activity, typically firing rate or number of spikes, as a function of the time of stimulus presentation. [2]

perseveration The repetition of a response despite changing stimuli or rules that make a different response more appropriate. [13]

persistent vegetative state A state that results from profound damage to the brain, perhaps by injury or disease, that is characterized by a lack of awareness. A patient with persistant vegetative state typically can still react to stimuli and exhibit degrees of wakefulness and quiescence. [7]

perspective taking The ability to adopt the viewpoint of another individual. [11]

PET See *positron emission tomography*.

PFC See *prefrontal cortex*.

pheromone A chemical signal produced by an animal such as a rodent, typically from glands, that mediates aspects of social communication. [4]

phone One of about 200 different sound stimuli the human vocal apparatus can produce. A subset of these is used in any given spoken language (approximately 40 in English). [12]

phoneme The basic perceptual unit that distinguishes one utterance from another in a given language. [12]

phrenology Originating in the early nineteenth century, the attempt to create maps of brain function based on the pattern of bumps and valleys on the surface of the skull. [1,13]

pituitary gland An endocrine structure comprising an anterior lobe made up of many different types of hormone-secreting cells, and a posterior lobe that secretes neuropeptides produced by neurons in the hypothalamus. [Appendix]

pons One of the three components of the brainstem, lying between the *midbrain* rostrally and the *medulla* caudally. [Appendix]

pop-out stimulus An item in a visual scene or visual array that differs from all of the other items in the scene (*distracters*) in one featural dimension (such as color, orientation, texture, shape, size). Because the time taken to find a pop-out stimulus is mostly independent of the number of distracter items, its detection is thought to be accomplished by the processing of all the items across the visual field in parallel. Compare *conjunction target*. [7]

positron emission tomography (PET) A method of noninvasive, hemodynamically based brain imaging that uses radio-actively labeled molecules injected into the bloodstream that are taken up to a greater degree by active neurons. [2]

postcentral gyrus The gyrus that lies just posterior to the central sulcus; contains the primary somatosensory cortex. Compare *precentral gyrus*. [Appendix]

posterior parietal cortex The region of the parietal cortex surrounding the intraparietal sulcus. [13]

posttraumatic stress disorder (PTSD) A clinical condition that emerges following the experience of one or more traumatic, stressful events. Symptoms include heightened arousal, emotional numbness, avoidance of event reminders, and persistent reexperiencing of the traumatic event(s). [10]

power motivation An enduring preference for having impact on other people or the world at large. [11]

PPI See *psychophysiological interaction*.

precentral gyrus The gyrus that lies just anterior to the central sulcus; contains the primary motor cortex. Compare *postcentral gyrus*. [Appendix]

prefrontal cortex (PFC) Cortical regions in the frontal lobe that are anterior to the primary motor and premotor cortices; thought to be involved in planning complex cognitive behaviors and in the expression of personality and appropriate social behavior. [13]

premotor cortex Part of the prefrontal cortex lying just anterior to the primary motor cortex; involved in planning movement. [5]

premotor cortical areas Cortical areas, including the premotor cortex, supplementary motor cortex, and parts of the parietal cortex, that provide motor programming signals to the *primary motor cortex*. [5]

premotor theory of attention A cognitive theory proposing that shifts of attention and preparation of goal-directed action are closely linked because they are controlled by shared sensory-motor mechanisms. [7]

primary auditory cortex (A1) The cortical target of the neurons in the medial geniculate nucleus; the terminus of the primary auditory pathway. Compare *secondary auditory cortex*. [4]

primary auditory pathway The pathway from the inner ear to the primary auditory cortex in the temporal lobe. [4]

primary motor cortex A major source of descending projections to motor neurons in the spinal cord and cranial nerve nuclei; located in the precentral gyrus (area 4) and essential for the voluntary control of movement. Compare *premotor cortical areas*. [5]

primary motor neuron See *lower motor neuron*.

primary reinforcer Also called *unconditioned reinforcer*. A stimulus whose rewarding properties come from its salutary effects on homeostatic processes; food, water, warmth, and sex are examples. Compare *secondary reinforcer*. [14]

primary somatosensory cortex (S1) The cortex of the postcentral gyrus of the parietal lobe that receives mechanosensory input from the thalamus. Compare *secondary somatosensory cortex*. [4]

primary visual cortex Also called *striate cortex* or *V1*. The cortex in the calcarine fissure of the parietal lobe that receives visual input from the thalamus. Compare *extrastriate visual cortical areas*. [3]

primary visual pathway The pathway from the retina via the lateral geniculate nucleus of the thalamus to the primary visual cortex; carries the information that allows conscious visual perception. [3]

priming Facilitated processing of a particular stimulus based on previous encounters with the same or a related stimulus. Compare *conditioning* and *skill learning*. [8]

probability weighting   A core assumption of prospect theory, such that the subjective probability of an outcome can differ systematically from the objective probability. [14]

processing negativity   A slow, long-lasting negative-polarity ERP wave that is elicited during auditory selective attention, the amplitude of which reflects how well each stimulus matches an attentional "template." Compare *selection negativity*. [6]

production aphasia   See *Broca's aphasia*.

propranolol   An antagonist of the beta-adrenergic system. [10]

prosodic   Pertaining to the inflection in speech, often associated with emotion. [12]

prosody   The fluctuating pitch of speech; gives emotional and other information to speech. [10]

prosopagnosia   The inability to recognize faces; usually associated with lesions of the right inferior temporal cortex. [3]

prospect theory   A quantitative decision-making model proposing that people make decisions in terms of the anticipated gains and losses from their current state, and that probabilities are subjective. [14]

PSTH   See *peristimulus time histogram*.

psychological construct   A theoretical concept, often generated by converging results across experiments, that cannot be directly observed but serves to explain and unify a body of research. [1]

psychophysiological interaction (PPI) analysis   An fMRI analysis technique that uses the time courses of activity in different brain areas to analyze how interactions between them differ as a function of the cognitive task being performed. For example, it analyzes whether the correlation in activity between two areas, rather than activity itself, differs in one task versus another. [2]

PTSD   See *posttraumatic stress disorder*.

pulvinar   A nucleus of the thalamus that mediates interactions among several sensory association areas of the cortex. [Appendix]

punishment   The delivery of an aversive stimulus. [14]

putamen   One of the three major nuclei that make up the basal ganglia. [Appendix]

pyriform cortex   A component of the cerebral cortex in the temporal lobe pertinent to olfaction; so named because of its pearlike shape. [4,Appendix]

raphe nuclei   Brainstem nuclei involved in the control of the sleep-wake cycle, among other functions related to arousal. [7]

rational choice model   A framework for explaining choice behavior that assumes that decision makers are consistent in their preferences and procedures for generating choices. [14]

rationality   Consistency in decision making that is based on a conscious evaluation of the circumstances. [14]

readiness potential   An electrical potential, recorded from the motor and premotor cortices with EEG electrodes, that signals the intention to initiate a voluntary movement well in advance of actual production of the movement. [5]

recall test   Memory test that requires generating the target information. [9]

receptive aphasia   See *Wernicke's aphasia*.

receptive field   The region of the receptor surface of a sensory neuron that, when stimulated, elicits a response in the neuron being examined. [3]

receptor potential   A membrane potential change that arises at a sensory receptor in the periphery due to a stimulus from the environment. [Appendix]

recollection   Remembering a past event, as well as specific associations and contextual details. Compare *familiarity*. [9]

recovery   During memory retrieval, the process of accessing stored memory traces. [9]

recurrent   See *reentrant*.

reentrant   Also called *recurrent*. Following a stimulus or event, describing a process in which neural activity is fed back to the same brain region, typically a sensory area, that was activated earlier in the processing sequence. [7]

reentrant process   Following a stimulus or event, a process in which neural activity is fed back to the same brain region activated earlier in the processing sequence. [6]

reference dependence   A core assumption of prospect theory, such that outcomes are evaluated in terms of their relative change (positive or negative) from the current state. [14]

reflectance   The percentage of incident light reflected from a surface (often expressed as the *reflectance efficiency function*, in which the reflectance of a surface is measured at different wavelengths). [3]

reflexive attention   See *exogenous attention*.

relational memory theory   A theory positing that the hippocampus is involved primarily in encoding and retrieving associations between items, including spatial associations but also other types of associations. Compare *cognitive map theory* and *episodic memory theory*. [9]

repetition enhancement   The creation of new representations and the increase in activity that result from the repetition of stimuli during priming; associated with priming for novel stimuli. Compare *repetition suppression*. [8]

repetition priming   See *direct priming*.

repetition suppression   Also called *neural priming*. A phenomenon observed in functional neuroimaging studies in which previously encountered stimuli evoke smaller hemodynamic responses than do novel stimuli. Compare *repetition enhancement*. [2,8]

repetitive TMS (rTMS)   A method in which the brain is stimulated with a repeated sequence of magnetic field pulses, ranging from less than 1 per second up to 30 Hz or more. [2]

resonance   The tendency of any physical object to vibrate maximally at a certain frequency. [4]

resting-state connectivity   The patterns of functional connectivity of the brain while a person is awake but not engaged in any specific task or activity. [2]

reticular activating system   A region in the brainstem containing a set of subregions (brainstem "nuclei") that mediate overall arousal and level of awareness. [7]

retinal disparity   The geometrical difference between the same points in the images projected on the two retinas, measured in degrees with respect to the fovea. [3]

retrieval   The recovery or accessing of stored memory traces. Compare *encoding*. [8]

retrieval cue   Any information that leads to the retrieval of memories, such as the hits provided by memory tests. [9]

retrieval mode The mental state of episodic retrieval (the retrieval of episodic memories), which is assumed to be qualitatively different from the mental states of other cognitive abilities. [9]

retrograde amnesia The inability to recall memories for events that happened before the lesion or brain disorder that caused the memory loss. Compare *anterograde amnesia*. [8]

reversal learning The capacities for recognizing that the rules mapping environmental events to behavior have changed and for adjusting behavior accordingly. [13]

reward prediction error (RPE) A quantity given by the difference between the reward that was expected and what actually occurs; the activity of some dopaminergic neurons seems to convey this quantity. [14]

reward value The likelihood that a particular movement will yield a reward, multiplied by the amount of reward expected. [5]

right frontal effect In ERP studies of recognition memory, the phenomenon, occurring at 600 to 1200 milliseconds after the stimulus, whereby old items elicit greater positivity over right frontal regions than do new items. Compare *left parietal effect*. [9]

right-hemisphere hypothesis A hypothesis positing that the right hemisphere is specialized for emotional functions. Compare *valence hypothesis*. [10]

risk aversion The tendency to prefer lower-risk options when making decisions, even in some situations when those options have reduced expected value. [14]

RPE See *reward prediction error*.

rTMS See *repetitive TMS*.

S1 See *primary somatosensory cortex*.

S2 See *secondary somatosensory cortex*.

saccade A ballistic eye movement that changes the point of binocular visual fixation; normally occur at a rate of about three to four per second. [3,5]

saliency map A theoretical construct of visual attention in which the importance of different stimuli in the visual field is set by a combination of top-down processes based on behavioral goals and bottom-up processes resulting from how distinctive the different elements of a stimulus are compared to the background. [7]

satisficing An approach to decision making in which a decision maker does not seek the best possible option, but instead chooses the first option that meets some threshold for acceptability. [14]

savant syndrome A rare clinical condition characterized by extraordinary talent in a particular ability, such as art or math, often in the face of general physical or mental disability. [10]

schizophrenia A heterogeneous psychiatric condition characterized by disordered thought, withdrawal symptoms, and inaccurate beliefs about reality. [13]

SCR See *skin conductance response*.

secondary auditory cortex (A2) Also called *belt areas*. The cortical region surrounding the primary auditory cortex. Compare *primary auditory cortex*. [4]

secondary reinforcer A stimulus that has no direct effects on homeostatic processes but is nevertheless rewarding; money is a paradigmatic example. Compare *primary reinforcer*. [14]

secondary somatosensory cortex (S2) A higher-order somatosensory map in the parietal lobe adjacent to S1. Compare *primary somatosensory cortex*. [4]

selection negativity A slow, sustained, negative-polarity ERP wave, typically starting about 150 milliseconds after an attended visual stimulus, resulting from attention to a nonspatial visual feature of the stimulus. Compare *processing negativity*. [6]

self The subjective sense of existing as an individual. [11]

self-awareness An awareness of oneself as a separate actor in the world. Compare *awareness*. [7]

self-reflexive thought The ability to consider one's own being as an object of thought. [11]

semantic dementia A memory deficit that impairs semantic memory rather than episodic memory and is associated with left-lateralized atrophy of the anterior temporal cortex. [9]

semantic memory Declarative memory that refers to general knowledge about the world, including knowledge of language, facts, and the properties of objects. Compare *episodic memory*. [9]

semantic priming A form of indirect priming in which the prime and the target are semantically related. Compare *conceptual priming*. [8]

sensitization The process by which a behavioral response to an otherwise benign stimulus increases in intensity, frequency, or duration when that stimulus is paired with an aversive stimulus. Compare *habituation*. [8]

sensory adaptation The adjustment of sensory receptors or other elements in a sensory system to different levels of stimulus intensity; allows sensory systems to operate over a wide range of stimulus intensities. [3]

sensory aphasia See *Wernicke's aphasia*.

sensory/functional theory Theory which postulates that semantic memory is organized by sensory and functional properties of real objects. Compare *domain-specific theory*. [9]

sensory ganglia Collections of neurons in the peripheral nervous system that comprise the cell bodies of afferent sensory neurons. [Appendix]

sensory neuron A nerve cell that is involved in sensory processing. [Appendix]

sensory system All the components of the central and peripheral nervous systems concerned with processing information arising from a particular stimulus category (e.g., light, sound stimuli). [Appendix]

septal forebrain nuclei See *basal forebrain nuclei*.

sham rage An emotional reaction elicited in cats by electrical stimulation of the hypothalamus, characterized by hissing, growling, and attack behaviors directed randomly toward innocuous targets. [10]

sharpening theory Priming theory which proposes that when a stimulus is repeated neurons that are not essential fire less, leading to a more efficient "sharpened" representation and a reduction in neural activity. [8]

simultaneous lightness/brightness contrast The ability of contextual information to alter the perception of a visual target, especially in regard to its luminance (i.e., lightness or brightness; *simultaneous brightness contrast*) or its color (*simultaneous color contrast*). [3]

single-unit recording A method of studying the activity of single neurons using a microelectrode. [3]

situation selection   A form of emotion regulation in which individuals select situations that minimize the likelihood of experiencing negative emotions. [10]

skill learning   Gradual improvement in the performance of a motor or cognitive task as a result of extensive experience and repeated practice. Compare *conditioning* and *priming*. [8]

skin conductance response (SCR)   A stimulus-induced increase in the electrical conductance of the skin due to increased hydration. [10]

Skinner box   A device, used in operant conditioning, in which animals such as pigeons or rats learn to press a lever to receive a food pellet. [8]

SMA   See *supplementary motor cortex*.

SME   See *subsequent memory effect*.

SNr   See *substantia nigra pars reticulata*.

social neuroscience   The study of the neural basis of interpersonal and intergroup processes. [10]

social referencing   The use of emotions expressed by another individual to guide one's own behavior. [11]

soma   See *cell body*.

somatic marker hypothesis   A theory, first advocated by Antonio Damasio and his colleagues, that motivated behavior is influenced by neural representations of body states (the "somatic markers"), whose reexperiencing can shape behavior positively or negatively; the hypothesis that evaluation of one's own body states makes important contributions to decision making. [13]

somatic motor system   The components of the motor system that support skeletal movements mediated by the contraction of skeletal muscles. [Appendix]

somatic sensory cortex   Also called *somatosensory cortex*. Region of the parietal lobe that receives information about touch, pressure and vibration at the body surface. [Appendix]

somatotopic   refers to a representation of the body mapped on to the cortex of the brain in a topgraphically preserved way, meaning that adjacent locations on the surface of the body have adjacent representations in the cortex, even if perhaps stretched or distorted. The primary motor cortex and the somatosensory area of the brain are two somatotopically organized areas. [2]

somatotopic map   The corresponding anatomical arrangement of the sensory periphery and its central representation. [4]

sound spectrum   The analysis of a sound stimulus showing the distribution of power as a function of frequency. [4]

sound wave   The periodic compression and rarefaction of air molecules underlying a sound stimulus. [4]

source memory test   Also called *context memory test*. An explicit test of memory that asks participants to remember not merely what events happened in the past but where, when, or how they happened. [9]

source-filter model   A generally accepted model for the production of speech sound stimuli that entails the vocal-fold vibrations as a source and the rest of the vocal tract as a dynamic filter. [12]

specificity   In long-term potentiation, only the synapses activated during stimulation show enhancement; other synapses, even on the same neuron, are not affected. [8]

spinal cord   The portion of the central nervous system that extends from the lower end of the brainstem (the medulla) to the cauda equina. It sits within a protective tube, or column, created by the vertebrae of the spine. [Appendix]

spinal reflex arc   Circuit that includes the afferent to efferent components of a response at the level of the spinal cord. [Appendix]

split-brain patient   An individual whose corpus callosum has been surgically interrupted as a treatment for epilepsy, functionally separating the left and right hemispheres. [12]

spreading activation   Hypothetical mechanism whereby the activation of a node in the semantic network spreads to associated nodes. [8]

standard consolidation theory   A theory positing that the hippocampus rapidly encodes an integrated representation of an event or concept, which is then slowly transferred to the cortex and eventually becomes independent of the hippocampus. Compare *multiple-trace theory*. [9]

startle response   A behavioral reaction to a sudden, intense auditory or visual stimulus that is mediated by a subcortical reflex circuit. [10]

stereopsis   The special sensation of depth that results from fusion of the two eyes' views of relatively nearby objects. [3]

storage   The retention of information over time. [8]

stress hormone   Any of several hormones, including cortisol, epinephrine, and norepinephrine, that are secreted by the adrenal gland when stimulated by its sympathetic innervation. [10]

striate cortex   See *primary visual cortex*.

striatum   The input nuclei of the basal ganglia, consisting of the caudate and the putamen. So called because of the striped appearance of these structures in brain sections. [5,Appendix]

stroke   The clinical and neuropathological result of interruption of the blood supply to one or another region of the brain. [Appendix]

structural equation modeling   A mathematical method of analyzing fMRI data by which two or more models of functional connectivity may be tested against brain data. The method aims at determining the relative likelihood of one model over another given the observed data. [2]

subcortical   Pertaining to brain structures other than the cerebral cortex. [Appendix]

subsequent memory effect (SME)   In functional neuroimaging studies, greater study-phase activity for items that are remembered rather than forgotten in a later memory test. [9]

substantia nigra   A nucleus at the base of the midbrain that receives input from a number of cortical and subcortical structures. The dopaminergic cells of the substantia nigra send their output to the caudate or putamen. [Appendix]

substantia nigra pars reticulata (SNr)   A component of the midbrain substantia nigra nucleus that plays a key role in the suppression and initiation of saccadic eye movements. [5]

sulcus (pl. sulci)   Any of the valleys that arise from the folding of the cerebral hemisphere between *gyri*. See also *fissure*. [Appendix]

superior colliculi (sing. superior colliculus)   Paired structures that form part of the roof of the midbrain; important in orienting movements of the head and eyes. Compare *inferior colliculi*. [5,Appendix]

superior olivary complex   A complex of brainstem nuclei in the primary auditory pathway. [4]

supplementary motor area (SMA)   See *supplementary motor cortex.*

supplementary motor cortex   Also called *supplementary motor area* or *area 6.* A premotor area, lying anterior to the primary motor cortex on the medial surface of the cerebral hemisphere, that plays an important role in movement planning. [5]

supramodal attention   The focusing of attention on stimulus information across multiple modalities at the same time. Compare *modality-specific attention.* [6,7]

Sylvian fissure   See *lateral fissure.*

sympathetic division   Sometimes referred to as the "fight or flight" system. The component of the autonomic motor system that contributes to the mobilization of energy to prepare the body for action. Compare *parasympathetic division.* [Appendix]

sympathy   Having feelings of pity or concern for another individual's plight without experiencing the same feelings expressed by that individual. Compare *empathy.* [11]

synapse   A specialized point of contact between the axon of a neuron (the presynaptic cell) and a target (postsynaptic) cell. Information is transferred between the presynaptic and postsynaptic cells by the release and receipt of biochemical neurotransmitters. [1,Appendix]

synaptic cleft   The small space between a presynaptic and postsynaptic element across which neurotransmitters must diffuse when released. [Appendix]

synaptic consolidation   Memory consolidation involving changes in synapses that presumably allow the persistence of some forms of memory traces at the cellular level. Compare *system consolidation.* [9]

synaptic potential   A membrane potential change (or a conductance change) generated by the action of a chemical transmitter agent. Synaptic potentials allow the transmission of information from one neuron to another. Compare *receptor potential.* [Appendix]

synaptic vesicle   The organelle at a synaptic ending that contains neurotransmitter agents. [Appendix]

synaptogenesis   The elaboration of synapses during neural development. [15]

syntax   The way in which words are combined to form sentences or phrases. [12]

system consolidation   Memory consolidation involving a reorganization of the brain regions that support the memory in question. In the case of declarative memory, refers to a decrease in the role of the hippocampus and an increase in the role of the cortex over time. Compare *synaptic consolidation.* [9]

taste   The sensory modality comprising the perception of substances placed in the mouth. [4]

taste bud   An onion-shaped structure in the mouth or pharynx that contains taste cells. [4]

taste system   See *gustatory system.*

tegmentum   The central gray matter of the brainstem. [Appendix]

temperament   A disposition to react to emotional situations either positively or negatively. [10]

temporal difference learning   A form of learning that modulates behavior according to the difference between an obtained reward and an estimate, compiled over the recent past, of an expected reward. [14]

temporal discounting   Also called *delay discounting.* The reduction in the desirability of an outcome based on the delay in time until it will be delivered. [14]

temporoparietal junction   A region of the neocortex that includes the posterior portion of the superior temporal gyrus and the angular gyrus of the parietal lobe. [11]

thalamus   A collection of nuclei that forms the major component of the diencephalon. Has many functions; a primary role is to relay sensory information from the periphery to the cerebral cortex. [4,10,Appendix]

theory of mind   See *mentalizing.*

third ventricle   Compare *fourth ventricle* and *lateral ventricles.* The midline component of the ventricular system at the level of the diencephalon. [Appendix]

threshold potential   The membrane potential at which a nerve cell fires an action potential. [Appendix]

timbre   The quality of sound by which stimuli that elicit the same pitch and loudness are distinguished; often taken to arise from the distribution of power in the waveform, as opposed to its periodicity. [4]

TMS   *See transcranial magnetic stimu*lation.

tonal   Pertaining to a sound stimulus that, by virtue of its periodic repetition, produces the perception of a tone. [12]

tone   The sound heard in response to a particular frequency of vibration or combination of vibrations that are strongly periodic. Compare *noise.* [4]

tonotopic organization   The central arrangement of tone analysis in the auditory system that roughly corresponds to the peripheral responsiveness of the basilar membrane. [4]

topographical mapping   The specification of spatial relationships in the retina and in other stations of the primary visual pathway. [3]

topography   In vision, the study of spatial relationships at different levels of the primary visual pathway. [3]

trace conditioning   A form of classical conditioning in which there is a brief time interval between the end of the conditioned stimulus and the start of the unconditioned stimulus. Compare *delay conditioning.* [8]

tract   A major white matter (axonal) pathway in the brain. [Appendix]

transcranial magnetic stimulation (TMS)   A method in which a rapidly changing, strong magnetic field is generated next to the skull, thereby delivering transient electrical stimulation to the underlying cortex; the electrical stimulation typically disrupts the local cortical activity, thereby enabling inferences concerning the cognitive function(s) in which that brain area is involved. [2]

transfer-appropriate processing   The hypothesis that memory performance depends on a match between the conditions surrounding the encoding and retrieval of a stimulus. [9]

transmittance   The percentage of light energy that reaches a detector when passed through a filter. [3]

trial   A single occurrence of an experimental event in a study. [2]

trichromat   A person or other animal whose color vision depends on three retinal cone types that absorb long, medium, and short wavelengths of light, respectively. Compare *dichromat.* [3]

trigeminal chemosensory system   The chemosensory system that responds to irritating chemicals that enter the nose or mouth. [4]

tuning curve   The function obtained when a neuron's receptive field is tested with stimuli at different orientations; its peak defines the maximum sensitivity of the neuron in question. [2,3]

tympanic membrane   The eardrum. [4]

unconditioned reinforcer   See *primary reinforcer*. [14]

unconditioned response (UR)   In classical conditioning, the innate reflex that is naturally triggered by a particular stimulus. Compare *conditioned response*. [8]

unconditioned stimulus (US)   In classical conditioning, the stimulus that naturally triggers the innate reflex. Compare *conditioned stimulus*. [8]

uncus   Part of the cerebral cortex near the hippocampus and associated with hippocampal function. [Appendix]

upper motor neuron   A neuron that gives rise to a descending projection that controls the activity of *lower motor neurons* in the brainstem and spinal cord. [5]

UR   See *unconditioned response*.

Urbach-Wiethe syndrome   A rare, congenital dermatological disease that occasionally produces calcifications in temporal lobe structures. [10]

US   See *unconditioned stimulus*.

utility   The personal worth associated with a good; may deviate from the stated value of that good depending on an individual's preferences, biases, or current state. [14]

V1   See *primary visual cortex*.

V4   An area of extrastriate visual cortex that is probably important in color vision, although it processes other information as well. [3]

valence   The degree of pleasantness of a stimulus. [10]

valence hypothesis   A hypothesis postulating that positive emotions are preferentially processed in the left hemisphere and negative emotions are preferentially processed in the right hemisphere. Compare *right-hemisphere hypothesis*. [10]

vector model   A way to graphically represent the relationships among emotions by ordering them along two orthogonal axes of positive and negative valence. Compare *circumplex model*. [10]

ventral horn   The ventral portion of the spinal cord gray matter, which contains the primary motor neurons. Compare *dorsal horn* and *lateral horn*. [Appendix]

ventral posterior nuclear complex   A group of thalamic nuclei that receives the somatosensory projections from the dorsal column nuclei and the trigeminal nuclear complex. [4]

ventral stream   A partially segregated visual processing pathway passing from the primary visual cortex toward the temporal lobe that is especially pertinent to object recognition. Compare *dorsal stream*. [3]

ventral striatum   The portion of the ventral caudate and putamen that encompasses the *nucleus accumbens*. [14]

ventral tegmental area (VTA)   A part of the midbrain that contains many dopaminergic neurons and is important for reward and learning. [14,Appendix]

ventrolateral prefrontal cortex   A functional division of the prefrontal cortex roughly corresponding to the inferior frontal gyrus and surrounding sulci, as located anterior to motor cortex. Compare *dorsolateral prefrontal cortex*. [13]

ventromedial prefrontal cortex   The ventral portion of the prefrontal cortex surrounding the hemispheric midline; plays a key role in the control of emotions and social behavior. Compare *dorsomedial prefrontal cortex*. [13]

vertical integration model   A model of emotion that integrates cortical, subcortical, and visceral processes. [10]

visceral motor system   See *autonomic motor system*.

visual search   The searching in a visual scene with multiple stimulus items for a particular type of item possessing one or more specific feature attributes. [6,7]

visual spatial attention   Attention directed to a location in visual space. [6]

voiced   Pertaining to a speech sound stimulus characterized by laryngeal harmonics—typically a vowel sound. [12]

volatility   The degree to which the rules governing environmental events (e.g., the delivery of rewards) are changing or stable over time. [13]

vowel   Typically a voiced (tonal) element of speech that forms the nucleus of syllables. [12]

VTA   See *ventral tegmental area*.

wakefulness   The state in which one is not asleep. [7]

Weber-Fechner law   The principle that the just-noticeable difference in a stimulus increment is a constant fraction (the *Weber fraction*) of the stimulus; named after two Germans: physiologist-anatomist Ernst Weber, and physicist-philosopher Gustav Fechner. [15]

Wernicke's aphasia   Also called *receptive aphasia* or *sensory aphasia*. A language deficit arising from damage to Wernicke's area in the posterior temporal lobe and characterized by an inability to link objects or ideas and the words that signify them and to subjectively comprehend this relationship. Compare *Broca's aphasia*. [12]

Wernicke's area   An area of cortex in the superior and posterior region of the left temporal lobe that helps mediate language comprehension; named after the nineteenth-century neurologist and psychiatrist Carl Wernicke. Compare *Broca's area*. [12]

white matter   The large axon tracts in the brain and spinal cord; these tracts have a whitish cast when viewed in freshly cut material. Compare *gray matter*. [Appendix]

Wisconsin Card Sorting Test   A cognitive test that involves classifying a set of cards, each showing one or more images of a simple shape, into categories based on rules that periodically change throughout the session. [13]

working memory   Memory held briefly in the mind that enables completion of a particular task (e.g., efficiently searching a room for a lost object). [8,13]

Illustration Credits

Chapter 1: Cognitive Neuroscience: Definitions, Themes, and Approaches

Opener Courtesy of the Duke Institute for Brain Sciences. **1.1** © Everett Collection Inc/Alamy. **1.5** PENFIELD, W. AND T. RASMUSSEN (1950) *The Cerebral Cortex of Man: A Clinical Study of Localization of Function.* New York: Macmillan; Corsi, P., ed. (1991) *The Enchanted Loom: Chapters in the History of Neuroscience.* New York: Oxford University Press.

Chapter 2: The Methods of Cognitive Neuroscience

Opener Courtesy of Marty Woldorff. **2.4B** YIHAR, O, L. I. FENNO, T. J. DAVIDSON, M. MOGRI AND K. DEISSEROTH (2009) Optogenetics in neural systems. *Neuron* 71: 9–34. **2.4C** © Carnett/ Getty Images. **2.5B** COLBY, C. L., J. R. DUHAMEL AND M. E. GOLDBERG (1996) Visual, presaccadic, and cognitive activation of single neurons in monkey lateral intraparietal area. *J. Neurophysiol.* 76: 2841–2852. **2.10D** WOLDORFF, M. G., M. MATZKE, F. ZAMARRIPA AND P. T. FOX (1999) Procedure to extract a weekly pattern of performance of human reaction time. *Hum. Brain Mapp.* 8: 121–127. **2.12B** HUETTEL, S. A., A. W. SONG AND G. MCCARTHY (2009) *Functional Magnetic Resonance Imaging.* Sunderland, MA: Sinauer. **2.14** BUROCK, M. A., R. L. BUCKNER, M. G. WOLDORFF, B. R. ROSEN AND A. M. DALE (1998) Randomized event-related experimental designs allow for extremely rapid presentation rates using functional MRI. *NeuroReport* 9: 3735–3739. **2.15** KOURTZI, Z. AND K. GRILL-SPECTOR (2005) fMRI adaptation: A tool for studying visual representations in the primate brain. In *Fitting the Mind into the World: Adaptation and After-Effects in High Level Vision*, G. Rhodes and C. Clifford (eds.). Oxford: Oxford University Press; photos © Elnur/

Fotolia.com (teacup) and © Eric Isselée/ Fotolia.com (dog).

Chapter 3: Sensory Systems and Perception: Vision

Opener © Terry Smith Images/ Alamy. **3.3** SAKMANN, B. AND O. D. CREUTZFELDT (1969) Scotopic and mesopic light adaptation in the cat's retina. *Plügers Arch.* 313: 168–185. **3.6A** ANDREWS, T. J., S. D. HALPERN AND D. PURVES (1997) Correlated size variations in human visual cortex, lateral geniculate nucleus, and optic tract. *J. Neurosci.* 17: 2859–2868. **3.6B** WATANABE, M. AND R. W. RODIECK (1989) Parasol and midget ganglion cells of the primate retina. *J. Comp. Neurol.* 289: 434–454. **3.7** SERENO, M. I. AND 7 OTHERS (1995) Borders of multiple visual areas in humans revealed by functional magnetic resonance imaging. *Science* 268: 889–893. **3.11A–C** PURVES, D., D. RIDDLE AND A.-S. LaMANTIA (1992) Iterated patterns of brain circuitry (or how the cortex got its spots). *Trends Neurosci.* 15: 362–369. **3.13B** PURVES, D. AND R. B. LOTTO (2003) *Why We See What We Do.* Sunderland, MA: Sinauer. **3.14** WHITE, M. (1979) A new effect of pattern on perceived lightness. *Perception* 8: 413–416. **3.17** PURVES, D. AND R. B. LOTTO (2011) *Why We See What We Do Redux: A Wholly Empirical Theory of Vision.* Sunderland, MA: Sinauer. **3.18** BOUVIER, S. E. AND S. A. ENGEL (2006) Behavioral deficits and cortical damage in cerebral achromatopsia. *Cereb. Cortex* 16: 183–191. **3.19** PURVES, D. AND R. B. LOTTO (2003) *Why We See What We Do.* Sunderland, MA: Sinauer. **3.20** MURRAY, S. O., H. BOYACI AND D. KERSTEN (2006) The representation of perceived angular size in primary visual cortex. *Nat.*

Neurosci. 9: 429–434. **3.23B,C** BLAKE, R. AND N. K. LOGOTHETIS (2002) Visual competition. *Nat. Rev. Neurosci.* 3: 1–11. **3.24** SUGRUE, L. P., G. S. CORRADO AND W. T. NEWSOME (2005) Choosing the greater of two goods: Neural currencies for valuation and decision making. *Nat. Rev. Neurosci.* 6: 363–375. **3.26** TOOTELL, R. B. AND 6 OTHERS (1995) Visual motion aftereffect in human cortical area MT revealed by functional magnetic resonance imaging. *Nature* 375: 139–141. **3.27** DESIMONE, R., T. D. ALBRIGHT, C. G. GROSS AND C. BRUCE (1984) Stimulus-selective properties of ingerior temporal neurons in the macaque. *J. Neurosci.* 4:2051–2062. **3.28** Yarbus, A. L. (1967) *Eye Movements and Vision.* (Translated by B. Haigh; edited by L. A. Riggs.) New York: Plenum. **3.29** ISHAI, A., L. G. UNGERLEIDER AND J. V. HAXBY (2000) Distributed neural systems for the generation of visual images. *Neuron* 28: 979–990.

Chapter 4: Sensory Systems and Perception: Auditory, Mechanical, and Chemical Senses

Opener © Paris Louvre/Alamy. **4.2** Micrograph from KESSEL, R. G. AND R. H. KARDON (1979) *Tissue and Organs: A Text-Atlas of Scanning Electron Microscopy.* San Francisco: W. H. Freeman. **4.7** BENDOR, D. AND X. WANG (2006) Cortical representations of pitch in monkeys and humans. *Curr. Opin. Neurobiol.* 16: 391–399. **4.13** PETROVIC, P., E. KALSO, K. M. PETERSSON AND M. INGVAR (2002) Placebo and opiod analgesia: Imaging a shared neural network. *Science* 295: 1737–1740. **4.15** ROSS, M. H., L. J. ROMMELL AND G. I. KAYE (1995) *Histology, A Text and Atlas.* Baltimore: Williams and Wilkins. **4.16** JENKINS, W. M., M. M. MERZENICH, M. T. OCHS, T. ALLARD AND E. GUICROBLES (1990)

Functional reorganization of primary somatosensory cortex in adult owl monkeys after behaviorally controlled tactile stimulation. *J. Neurophysiol.* 63: 82–104.

Chapter 5: Motor Systems: The Organization of Action

Opener © sampics/Corbis. Introductory Box © Heyday Films/ Zuma Press. **5.1** BERNSTEIN, N. A. (1947) *On the Formation of Movement.* English translation of Russian original. Hillsdale, NJ: Lawrence Erlbaum, p. 83. **5.3** FUCHS, A. F. (1967) Saccadic and smooth pursuit movements in the monkey. *J. Physiol.* (Lond.) 191: 609–630. **5.6** LOTZE, M., M. ERB, H. FLOR, E. HUELSMANN, B. GODDE AND W. GRODD (2000) fMRI evaluation of somatotopic representation in human primary motor cortex. *Neuroimage* 11: 473–481. **5.7** BREEDLOVE, S. M., M. R. ROSENZWEIG AND N. V. WATSON (2007) *Biological Psychology: An Introduction to Behavioral, Cognitive, and Clinical Neuroscience*, 5th Ed. Sunderland, MA: Sinauer. **5.8** GRAZIANO, M. S. A. (2006) The organization of behavioral repertoire in motor cortex. *Ann. Rev. Neurosci.* 29: 105–134. **5.9A** EVARTS, E. V. (1981) Functional studies of the motor cortex. In *The Organization of the Cerebral Cortex*, F. O. Schmitt, F. G. Worden, G. Adelman and S. G. Dennis (eds.). Cambridge, MA: MIT Press, pp. 199–236. **5.9B** PORTER, R. AND R. LEMON (1993) *Corticospinal Function and Voluntary Movement.* Oxford: Oxford University Press. **5.10** LEE, D. L., W. H. ROHRER AND D. L. SPARKS (1988) Population coding of saccadic eye movements by neurons in the superior colliculus. *Nature* 332: 357–360. **5.11** GEORGOPOLOUS, A. P., A. B. SCHWARTZ AND R. E. KETTNER (1986) Neuronal population coding of movement direction. *Science* 233: 1416–1418. **5.13** EAGLEMAN, D. M. (2004) The where and when of intention. *Science* 303: 1144–1146. **5.14** ROITMAN, J. D. AND M. N. SHADLEN (2002) Response of neurons in the lateral intraparietal area during a combined visual discrimination reaction time task. *J. Neurosci.* 22: 9475–9489. **5.15** GOLD, J. I. AND M. N. SHADLEN (2000) Representation of a perceptual decision in developing oculomotor commands. *Nature* 404: 299–308. **5.16** PLATT, M. L. AND P. W. GLIMCHER (1999) Neural correlates of decision variables in parietal cortex. *Nature* 400: 390–394. **5.17** WUNDERLICH, K., A. RANGEL AND J. P. O'DOHERTY (2009) Neural computations underlying action-based decision making in the human brain. *PNAS* 106:

17199–17204. **5.18** TANJI, J. AND K. SHIMA (1994) Role for supplementary motor area cells in planning several move-ments ahead. *Nature* 371: 413–416. **5.19** DEIBER, M. P., M. HONDA, V. IBAÑEZ, N. SADATO AND M. HALLETT (1999) Mesial motor areas in self-initiated versus externally triggered movements examined with fMRI: Effect of movement type and rate. *J. Neurophysiol.* 81: 3065–3077. **5.20B** MILNER, A. D. AND M. A. GOODALE (1995) *The Visual Brain in Action.* Oxford: Oxford University Press. **5.22** HIKOSAKA, O. AND R. H. WURTZ (1989) The basal ganglia. In *The Neurobiology of Saccadic Eye Movements*, R. H. Wurtz and M. E. Goldberg (eds.). New York: Elsevier, pp. 257–281. **5.23** YIN, H. H. AND B. J. KNOWLTON (2006) The role of the basal ganglia in habit formation. *Nat. Rev. Neurosci.* 7: 565–576. **5.24** GRAYDON, F. X., K. J. FRISTON, C. G. THOMAS, V. B. BROOKS AND R. S. MENON (2005) Learning-related fMRI activation associated with a rotational visuomotor transformation. Brain Res. Cogn. Brain Res. 22: 373–383. **5.27** BLUMENFELD, H. (2010) *Neuroanatomy through Clinical Cases*, 2nd Ed. Sunderland, MA: Sinauer. **5.28** IMAMIZU, H. AND 7 OTHERS (2000) Human cerebellar activity reflecting an acquired internal model of a novel tool. *Nature* 403: 192–195. **5.29** RAMNANI, N. (2006) The primate corticocerebellar system: Anatomy and function. *Nat. Rev. Neurosci.* 7: 511–522.

Chapter 6: Attention and Its Effects on Stimulus Processing

Opener © Erin Ryan/Corbis. **6.2A** BROADBENT, D. E. (1958) *Perception and Communication.* London: Pergamon. **6.2B** TREISMAN, A. (1960) Contextual cues in selective listening. *Q. J. Exp. Psychol.* 12: 242–248. **6.3** POSNER, M. I., C. R. R. SNYDER AND B. J. DAVIDSON (1980) Attention and the detection of signals. *J. Exp. Psychol. Gen.* 109: 160–174. **6.4** KLEIN, R. M. (2000) Inhibition of return. *Trends Cogn. Sci.* 4: 138–147; Posner, M. I. and Y. Cohen (1984) Components of visual orienting. In *Attention and Performance, Vol 10: Control of Language Processes*, H. Bouma and D. Bouwhuis (eds.). London: Erlbaum, pp. 531–556. **6.6** PICTON, T. P., S. A. HILLYARD, H. I. KRANSZ AND R. GALAMBOS (1974) Human auditory-evoked potentials. I. Evaluation of components. *Electroenceph. Clin. Neurophysiol.* 36: 179–190. **6.7B,C** HILLYARD, S. A., R. F. HINK, V. L. SCHWENT AND T. W. PICTON (1973) Electrical signs of selective attention in the human brain. *Science*

182: 177–180. **6.8A,B** WOLDORFF, M., J. C. HANSEN AND S. A. HILLYARD (1987) Evidence for effects of selective attention in the mid-latency range of the human auditory event-related potential. In *Current Trends in Event-Related Potential Research*, R. Johnson Jr., R. Parasuraman, and J. W. Rohrbaugh (eds.). Amsterdam: Elsevier, pp. 146–154. **6.8C** WOLDORFF, M. G. AND 6 OTHERS (1993) Modulation of early sensory processing in human auditory cortex during auditory selective attention. *Proc. Natl. Acad. Sci. USA* 90: 8722–8726. **6.9** PETKOV, C. I., X. KANG, K. ALHO, O. BERTRAND, E. W. YUND AND D. L. WOODS (2004) Attentional modulation of human auditory cortex. *Nat. Neurosci.* 7: 658–663. **6.10** WOLDORFF, M. G., S. A. HACKLEY AND S. A. HILLYARD (1991) The effects of channel-selective attention on the mismatch negativity wave elicited by deviant tones. *Psychophysiology* 28: 30–42. **6.13** HEINZE, H. J. AND 11 OTHERS (1994) Combined spatial and temporal imaging of brain activity during visual selective attention in humans. *Nature* 372: 543–546. **6.14** NOESSELT, T. AND 8 OTHERS (2002) Delayed striate cortical activation during spatial attention. *Neuron* 35: 575–587. **6.15** MORAN, J. AND R. DESIMONE (1985) Selective attention gates visual processing in the extrastriate cortex. *Science* 229: 782–784. **6.16** MCADAMS, C. J. AND J. H. R. MAUNSELL (1999) Effects of attention on reliability of individual neurons in monkey visual cortex. *Neuron* 23: 765–773. **6.17** REYNOLDS, J. H., T. PASTERNAK AND R. DESIMONE (2000) Attention increases sensitivity of V4 neurons. *Neuron* 26: 703–714. **6.18** REES, G., C. D. FRITH AND N. LAVIE (1997) Modulating irrelevant motion perception by varying attentional load in an unrelated task. *Science* 278: 1616–1618. **6.19** ZATORRE, R. J., A. C. EVANS, E. MEYER AND A. GJEDDE (1992) Lateralization of phonetic and pitch discrimination in speech processing. *Science* 256: 846–849. **6.20** O'CRAVEN, K. M., B. R. ROSEN, K. K. KWONG, A. TREISMAN AND R. L. SAVOY (1997) Voluntary attention modulates fMRI activity in human MT-MST. *Neuron* 18: 591–598. **6.21** TREUE, S. AND J. C. MARTINEZ-TRUJILLO (1999) Feature-based attention influences motion processing gain in macaque visual cortex. *Nature* 399: 575–579. **6.22** GAZZALEY, A., J. W. COONEY, K. MCKEVOY, R. T. KNIGHT AND M. D'ESPOSITO (2005) Top-down enhancement and suppression of the magnitude and speed of neural activity. *J. Cogn. Neurosci.* 17: 507–517.

Chapter 7: The Control of Attention

Opener © Skip O'Donnell/istockphoto. com. **7.1** FRIEDMAN-HILL, S. R., L. C. ROBERTSON AND A. TREISMAN (1995) Parietal contributions to visual feature binding: Evidence from a patient with bilateral lesions. *Science* 269: 853–855. **7.2A** HUMPHREYS, G. W. AND M. J. RIDDOCH (1993) Interactions between object and space systems revealed through neuropsychology. In *Attention and Performance*, Vol. 14: Synergies in Experimental Psychology, Artificial Intelligence, and Cognitive Neuroscience, D. E. Meyer and S. Kornblum (eds). Cambridge, MA: MIT Press, pp. 183–218. **7.2B** COOPER, A. A. AND G. W. HUMPHREYS (2000) Coding space within but not between objects: Evidence from Balint's syndrome. *Neuropsychologia* 38: 723–733. **7.3** HOPFINGER, J. B., M. H. BUONOCORE AND G. R. MANGUN (2000) The neural mechanisms of top-down attentional control. *Nat. Neurosci.* 3: 284–291. **7.4A** LIU, T., S. D. SLOTNICK, J. T. SERENCES AND S. YANTIS (2003) Cortical mechanisms of feature-based attentional control. *Cereb. Cortex* 13: 1334–1343. **7.4B** SERENCES, J. T., J. SCHWARTBACH, S. M. COURTNEY, X. COLAY AND S. YANTIS (2004) Control of object-based attention in human cortex. *Cereb. Cortex* 14: 1346–1357. **7.5** WOLDORFF, M. G., C. J. HAZLETT, H. M. FICHT-ENHOLTZ, D. H. WEISSMAN, A. M. DALE AND A. W. SONG (2004) Functional parcellation of attentional control regions of the brain. *J. Cogn. Neurosci.* 16: 149–165; GRENT-'T-JONG, T. AND M. G. WOLDORFF (2007) Timing and sequence of brain activity in top-down control of visual-spatial attention. *PLoS Biol.* 5: 114–126. **7.6** COLBY, C. L., J. R. DUHAMEL AND M. E. GOLDBERG (1996) Visual, presaccadic, and cognitive activation of single neurons in monkey lateral intraparietal area. *J. Neurophysiol.* 76: 2841–2852. **7.7** THOMPSON, K. G., K. L. BISCOE AND T. R. SATO (2005) Neuronal basis of covert spatial attention in the frontal eye field. *J. Neurosci.* 25: 9479–9487. **7.8** BUSCHMAN, T. J. AND E. K. MILLER (2007) Top-down versus bottom-up control of attention in the prefrontal and posterior parietal cortices. *Science* 315: 1860–1862. **7.9A** HOPFINGER, J. B., M. H. BUONOCORE AND G. R. MANGUN (2000) The neural mechanisms of top-down attentional control. *Nat. Neurosci.* 3: 284–291. **7.9B** LUCK, S. J., L. CHELAZZI, S. A. HILLYARD AND R. DESIMONE (1997) Neural mechanisms of spatial selective attention in areas V1, V2, and V4 of macaque visual cortex. *J. Neurophysiol.*

77: 24–42. **7.9C** GRENT-'T-JONG, T. AND M. G. WOLDORFF (2007) Timing and sequence of brain activity in top-down control of visual-spatial attention. *PLoS Biol.* 5: 114–126. **7.10** CORBETTA, M., J. M. KINCADE, J. M. OLLINGER, M. P. MCAVOY AND G. L. SHULMAN (2000) Voluntary orienting is dissociated from target detection in human posterior parietal cortex. *Nat. Neurosci.* 3: 292–297. **7.11** TREISMAN, A. AND G. GELADE (1980) A feature integration theory of attention. *Cogn. Psychol.* 12: 97–136. **7.12** LUCK, S. J. AND S. A. HILLYARD (1994) Spatial filtering during visual search: Evidence from human electrophysiology. *J. Exp. Psychol. Hum. Percept. Perform.* 20: 1000–1014. **7.13** CORBETTA, M. AND G. L. SHULMAN (2002) Control of goal-directed and stimulus-driven attention in the brain. *Nat. Rev. Neurosci.* 3: 201–215. **7.14** MOORE, T., K. M. ARMSTRONG AND M. FALLAH (2003) Visuomotor origins of covert spatial attention. *Neuron* 40: 671–683. **7.15** CORBETTA, M., AND 10 OTHERS (1998) A common network of functional areas for attention and eye movements. *Neuron* 21: 761–773. **7.18** TONG, F., K. NAKAYAMA, J. T. VAUGHAN AND N. KANWISHER (1998) Binocular rivalry and visual awareness in human extrastriate cortex. *Neuron* 21: 753–759. **7.19** OWEN, A. M., M. R. COLEMAN, M. BOLY, M. H. DAVIS, S. LAUREYS AND J. D. PICKARD (2006) Detecting awareness in the vegetative state. *Science* 313: 1402.

Chapter 8: Memory: Varieties and Mechanisms

Opener © Jeff Greenberg/Alamy. **8.2A** WARRINGTON, E. K. AND T. SHALLICE (1969) The selective impairment of auditory-verbal short-term memory. *Brain* 92: 885–896. **8.2B** DRACHMAN, D. A. AND J. ARBIT (1966) Memory and the hippocampal complex. II. Is memory a multiple process? *Arch. Neurol.* 15: 52–61. **8.3** GABRIELI, J. D. E., D. A. FLEISHMAN, M. M. KEANE, S. L. REMINGER AND F. MORRELL (1995) Double dissociation between memory systems underlying explicit and implicit memory in the human brain. *Psychol. Sci.* 6: 76–82. **8.5A** WELDON, M. S. AND H. L. ROEDIGER (1987) Altering retrieval demands reverses the picture superiority effect. *Mem. Cogn.* 15: 269–280. **8.5B** GRAF, P. AND G. MANDLER (1984) Activation makes words more accessible, but not necessarily more retrievable. *J. Verb. Learn. Verb. Behav.* 23: 553–568. **8.6** KOUTSTAAL, W., A. D. WAGNER, M. ROTTE, A. MARIL, R. L. BUCKNER AND D. L. SCHACTER (2001) Perceptual

specificity in visual object priming: Functional magnetic resonance imaging evidence for a laterality difference in fusiform cortex. *Neuropsychologia* 39: 184–199. **8.7** HENSON, R. N. A. AND M. D. RUGG (2003) Neural response suppression, haemodynamic repetition effects, and behavioural priming. *Neuropsychologia* 41: 263–270. **8.8** WAGNER, A. D., W. KOUTSTAAL, A. MARIL, D. L. SCHACTER AND R. L. BUCKNER (2000) Task-specific repetition priming in left inferior prefrontal cortex. *Cereb. Cortex* 10: 1176–1184. **8.10** ROSSELL, S. L., C. J. PRICE AND A. C. NOBRE (2003) The anatomy and time course of semantic priming investigated by fMRI and ERPs. *Neuropsychologia* 41: 550–564. **8.11** HENSON, R., T. SHALLICE AND R. DOLAN (2000) Neuroimaging evidence for dissociable forms of repetition priming. *Science* 287: 1269–1272. **8.13** STEELE, C. J. AND V. B. PENHUME (2010) Specific increases within global decreases: A functional magnetic resonance imaging investigation of five days of motor sequence learning. *J. Neurosci.* 30: 8332–8341. **8.14** DELLA-MAGGIORE, V., N. MALFAIT, D. J. OSTRY AND T. PAUS (2004) Stimulation of the posterior parietal cortex interferes with arm trajectory adjustments during the learning of new dynamics. *J. Neurosci.* 24: 9971–9976. **8.15B** GAUTHIER, I., M. J. TARR, A. W. ANDERSON, P. SKUDLARSKI AND J. C. GORE (1999) Activation of the middle fusiform "face area" increases with expertise in recognizing novel objects. *Nat. Neurosci.* 2: 568–573. **8.15C** GAUTHIER, I., P. SKUDLARSKI, J. C. GORE AND A. W. ANDERSON (2000) Expertise for cars and birds recruits brain areas involved in face recognition. *Nat. Neurosci.* 3: 191–197. **8.16** POLLMANN, S. AND M. MAERTENS (2005) Shift of activity from attention to motor-related brain areas during visual learning. *Nat. Neurosci.* 8: 1494–1496. **8.17** KNOWLTON, B. J., J. A. MANGELS AND L. R. SQUIRE (1996) A neostriatal habit learning system in humans. *Science* 262: 1747–1749. **8.18** POLDRACK, R. A. AND 7 OTHERS (2001) Interactive memory systems in the human brain. *Nature* 414: 546–550. **8.20** DAUM, I., M. M. SCHUGENS, H. ACKERMANN, W. LUTZENBERGER, J. DICHGAN AND N. BIRBAUMER (1993) Classical conditioning after cerebellar lesions in humans. *Behav. Neurosci.* 107: 748–756. **8.21** CLARK, R. E. AND L. R. SQUIRE (1998) Classical conditioning and brain systems: The role of awareness. *Science* 280: 77–81. **8.22** YIN, H. H. AND B. J.

KNOWLTON (2006) The role of the basal ganglia in habit formation. *Nat. Rev. Neurosci.* 7: 464–476.   **8.23** SQUIRE, L. R. AND E. R. KANDEL (1999) *Memory: From Mind to Molecules.* New York: Scientific American Library.   **8.24** MALINOW, R., H. SCHULMAN AND R. W. TSIEN (1989) Inhibition of postsynaptic PKC or CaMKII blocks induction but not expression of LTP. *Science* 245: 862–866.   **8.25** TSIEN, J. Z., P. T. HUERTA AND S. TONEGAWA (1996) The essential role of hippocampal CA1 NMDA receptor-dependent synaptic plasticity in spatial memory. *Cell* 87: 1327–1338.   **8.26A–C** LAMPRECHT, R. AND J. LEDOUX (2004) Structural plasticity and memory. *Nat. Rev. Neurosci.* 5: 45–54.   **8.26D** ENGERT, F. AND T. BONHOEFFER (1999) Dendritic spine changes associated with hippocampal long-term synaptic plasticity. *Nature* 399: 66–70.

Chapter 9: Declarative Memory

Opener © Steve Skjold/Alamy.
9.3B EKSTROM, A. AND 6 OTHERS (2003) Cellular networks underlying human spatial navigation. *Nature* 425: 184–187.   **9.4** DUSEK, J. AND H. EICHENBAUM (1997) The hippocampus and memory for orderly stimulus relations. *Proc. Natl. Acad. Sci. USA* 94: 7109–7114.   **9.5A** TULVING, E. (2002) Episodic memory: From mind to brain. *Annu. Rev. Psychol.* 53: 1–25.   **9.5B** ROSENBAUM, R. S. AND 6 OTHERS (2000) Remote spatial memory in amnesic person with extensive bilateral hippocampal lesions. *Nat. Neurosci.* 3: 1044–1048.   **9.6A** HODGES, J. R. AND K. S. GRAHAM (2001) Episodic memory: Insights from semantic dementia. *Phil. Trans. R. Soc. Lond. B* 356: 1423–1434.   **9.7A** ELDRIDGE, L. L., B. J. KNOWLTON, C. S. FURMANSKI, S. Y. BOOKHEIMER AND S. A. ENGLE (2000) Remembering episodes: A selective role for the hippocampus during retrieval. *Nat. Neurosci.* 3: 1149–1152.   **9.7B** FORTIN, N. J., S. P. WRIGHT AND H. EICHENBAUM (2004) Recollection-like memory retrieval in rats is dependent on the hippocampus. *Nature* 431: 188–191.   **9.8A** XIANG, J.-Z. AND M. W. BROWN (1998) Differential neuronal encoding of novelty, familiarity, and recency in regions of the anterior temporal lobe. *Neuropharmacology* 37: 657–676.   **9.8B** DASELAAR, S. M., M. S. FLECK AND R. CABEZA (2006) Triple dissociation within the medial temporal lobes: Recollection, familiarity, and novelty. *J. Neurophysiol.* 96: 1902–1911.   **9.9** DAVACHI, L. (2006) Item, context and relational episodic encoding in humans. *Curr. Opin. Neurobiol.* 16: 693–700; photo (bananas) © DNY59/istock.   **9.10A** BINDER, J. R. AND R. H. DESAI (2011) The neurobiology of semantic memory. *Trends Cogn. Sci.* 15: 527–536.   **9.10B** HAUK, O., I. JOHNSRUDE AND F. PULVERMÜLLER (2004) Somatotopic representation of action words in human motor and premotor cortex. *Neuron* 41: 301–307.   **9.10C** MAHON, B. Z. AND A. CARAMAZZA (2011) What drives the organization of object recognition in the brain? *Trends Cogn. Sci.* 15: 97–103.   **9.11A–C** PATTERSON, K., P. J. NESTOR AND T. T. ROGERS (2007) Where do you know what you know? The representation of semantic knowledge in the human brain. *Nat. Rev. Neurosci.* 8: 976–987.   **9.11D** SIMMONS, W. K., M. REDDISH, P. S. F. BELLGOWAN AND A. MARTIN (2010) The selectivity and functional connectivity of the anterior temporal lobes. *Cereb. Cortex* 20: 813–825.   **9.12** SAKAI, K. AND Y. MIYASHITA (1991) Neural organization for the long-term memory of paired associates. *Nature* 354: 152–155.   **9.13A** DANKER, J. F. AND J. R. ANDERSON (2010) The ghosts of brain states past: Remembering reactivates the brain regions engaged during encoding. *Psychol. Bull.* 136: 87–102; brain images from WHEELER, M. E., S. E. PETERSEN AND R. L. BUCKNER (2000) Memory's echo: Vivid remembering reactivates sensory-specific cortex. *Proc. Natl. Acad. Sci USA* 97: 11125–11129; photo (banjo) © Rasmus Rasmussen/istock.   **9.13B** JOHNSON, J. D. AND M. D. RUGG (2007) Recollection and the reinstatement of encoding-related cortical activity. *Cereb. Cortex* 17: 2507–2515.   **9.13C** POLYN, S. M., V. S. NATU, J. D. COHEN AND K. A. NORMAN (2006) Category-specific cortical activity precedes retrieval during memory search. *Science* 310: 1963–1966.   **9.14A** PALLER, K. A. AND A. D. WAGNER (2002) Observing the transformation of experience into memory. *Trends Cogn. Sci.* 6: 92–102.   **9.14B** MCDERMOTT, K. B., S. E. PETERSEN, J. M. WATSON AND J. G. OJEMANN (2003) A procedure for identifying regions preferentially activated by attention to semantic and phonological relations using fMRI. *Neuropsychologia* 41: 293–304.   **9.15** BLUMENFELD, R. S. AND C. RANGANATH (2006) Dorsolateral prefrontal cortex promotes long-term memory formation through its role in working memory organization. *J. Neurosci.* 26: 916–925.   **9.16A** SPANIOL, J., P. S. R. DAVIDSON, A. S. N. KIM, H. HAN, M. MOSCOVITCH AND C. L. GRADY (2009) Event-related fMRI studies of episodic encoding and retrieval: Meta-analyses using activation likelihood estimation. *Neuropsychologia* 47: 1765–1779.   **9.16B** FLECK, M. S., S. M. DASELAAR, I. G. DOBBINS AND R. CABEZA (2006) Role of prefrontal and anterior cingulate regions in decision-making processes shared by memory and nonmemory tasks. *Cereb. Cortex* 16: 1623–1630.   **9.16C** VELANOVA, K., L. L. JACOBY, M. E. WHEELER, M. P. MCAVOY, S. E. PETERSEN AND R. L. BUCKNER (2003) Functional-anatomic correlates of sustained and transient processing components engaged during controlled retrieval. *J. Neurosci.* 23: 8460–8470.   **9.17A** JANOWSKY, J. S., A. P. SHIMAMURA, M. KRITCHEVSKY AND L. R. SQUIRE (1989) Cognitive impairment following frontal lobe damage and its relevance to human amnesia. *Behav. Neurosci.* 103: 548–560.   **9.17B** SCHACTER, D. L., N. M. ALPERT, C. R. SAVAGE, S. L. RAUCH AND M. S. ALBERT (1996) Conscious recollection and the human hippocampal formation: Evidence from positron emission tomography. *Proc. Natl. Acad. Sci. USA* 93: 321–325.   **9.17C** GILBOA, A., C. ALAIN, D. T. STUSS, B. MELO, S. MILLER AND M. MOSCOVITCH (2006) Mechanisms of spontaneous confabulations: A strategic account. *Brain* 129: 1399–1414.   **9.19A** CABEZA, R., E. CIARAMELLI, I. R. OLSON AND M. MOSCOVITCH (2008) The parietal cortex and episodic memory: An attentional account. *Nat. Rev. Neurosci.* 9: 613–625.   **9.19B** UNCAPHER, M. R. AND A. D. WAGNER (2009) Posterior parietal cortex and episodic encoding: Insights from fMRI subsequent memory effects and dual-attention theory. *Neurobiol. Learn. Mem.* 91: 139–154.   **9.19C** DASELAAR, S. M., S. E. PRINCE, N. A., DENNIS, S. M. HAYES, H. KIM AND R. CABEZA (2009) Posterior midline and ventral parietal activity is associated with retrieval success and encoding failure. *Front. Hum. Neurosci.* 3: 13.   **9.20** DUDAI, Y. (2004) The neurobiology of consolidations, or, how stable is the engram? *Annu. Rev. Psychol.* 55: 51–86; AGRANOFF, B., R. DAVIS AND J. BRINK (1966) Chemical studies on memory formation in goldfish. *Brain Res.* 1: 303–309; KIM, J. J. AND M. S. FANSELOW (1992) Modality-specific retrograde amnesia of fear following hippocampal lesions. *Science* 256: 675–677.   **9.21** FRANKLAND, P. W. AND B. BONTEMPI (2005) The organization of recent and remote memories. *Nat. Rev. Neurosci.* 6: 119–130.   **9.22A** JI, D. Y. AND M. A. WILSON (2007) Coordinated memory replay in the visual cortex and hippocampus during sleep. *Nat.*

Neurosci. 10: 100–107.   **9.22B** RUDOY, J. D., J. L. VOSS, C. E. WESTERBERG AND K. A. PALLER (2009) Strengthening individual memories by reactivating them during sleep. *Science* 326: 1079; photos © Georgiy Pashin/istock (cat) and © caimacanul/istock (teakettle).   **9.22C** TAMBINI, A., N. KETZ AND L. DAVACHI (2010) Enhanced brain correlations during rest are related to memory for recent experiences. *Neuron* 65: 280–290.

Chapter 10: Emotion

Opener © Irina Behr/istock.   **10.3A** LANG, P. J., M. K. GREENWALD, M. M. BRADLEY AND A. O. HAMM (1993) Looking at pictures: Affective, facial, visceral, and behavioral reactions. *Psychophysiology* 30: 261–273.   **10.3B** RUSSELL, J. A. (1980) A circumplex model of affect. *J. Pers. Soc. Psychol.* 39: 1161–1178.   **10.8A** MACLEAN, P. D. (1949) Psychosomatic disease and the "visceral brain": Recent developments bearing on the Papez theory of emotion. *Psychosom. Med.* 11: 338–353.   **10.9** ROSS, E. D. (1997) The aprosodias. In *Behavioral Neurology and Neuropsychology*, T. E. Feinberg and M. J. Farah (eds.). New York: McGraw-Hill, pp. 699–710.   **10.11A** SHACKMAN, A. J., B. W. MCMENAMIN, J. S. MAXWELL, L. L. GREISCHAR AND R. J. DAVIDSON (2010) Right dorsolateral prefrontal cortical activity and behavioral inhibition. *Psychol. Sci.* 20: 1500–1506.   **10.11B** KALIN, N. H., C. LARSON, S. E. SHELTON AND R. J. DAVIDSON (1998) Asymmetric frontal brain activity, cortisol, and behavior associated with fearful temperament in rhesus monkeys. *Behav. Neurosci.* 112: 286–292.   **10.13A** BECHARA, A., D. TRANEL, H. DAMASIO, R. ADOLPHS, C. ROCKLAND AND A. R. DAMASIO (1995) Double dissociation of conditioning and declarative knowledge relative to the amygdala and hippocampus in humans. *Science* 269: 1115–1118.   **10.13B** PHILLIPS, R. G. AND J. E. LEDOUX (1992) Differential contribution of amygdala and hippocampus to cued and contextual fear conditioning. *Behav. Neurosci.* 106: 274–285.   **10.14A** ANDERSON, S. W., A. BECHARA, H. DAMASIO, D. TRANEL AND A. R. DAMASIO (1999) Impairment of social and moral behavior related to early damage in the human prefrontal cortex. *Nat. Neurosci.* 2: 1032–1037.   **10.14B,C** BECHARA, A., A. R. DAMASIO, H. DAMASIO AND S. W. ANDERSON (1994) Insensitivity to future consequences following damage to the human prefrontal cortex.

Cognition 50: 7–15.   **10.15A** CRAIG, A. D. (2007) Interoception and emotion: A neuroanatomical perspective. In *Handbook of Emotions*, 3rd Ed., M. Lewis, J. M. Haviland-Jones and L. F. Barrett (eds.). New York: Guilford, pp. 395–408.   **10.15B** CRITCHLEY, H. D., S. WIENS, P. ROTSHTEIN, A. ÖHMAN AND R. J. DOLAN (2004) Neural systems supporting interoceptive awareness. *Nat. Neurosci.* 7: 189–195.   **10.16A** CALDER, A. J., J. KEANE, F. MANES, N. ANTOUN AND A. W. YOUNG (2000) Impaired recognition and experience of disgust following brain injury. *Nat. Neurosci.* 3: 1077–1078.   **10.16B** ADOLPHS, R. AND 8 OTHERS (1999) Recognition of facial emotion in nine individuals with bilateral amygdala damage. *Neuropsychologia* 37: 1111–1117.   **10.17A** WHALEN, P. J. AND 10 OTHERS (2004) Human amygdala responsivity to masked fearful eye whites. *Science* 306: 2061.   **10.17B** WILLIAMS, M. A., A. P. MORRIS, F. MCGLONE, D. F. ABBOTT AND J. B. MATTINGLEY (2004) Amygdala responses to fearful and happy facial expressions under conditions of binocular suppression. *J. Neurosci.* 24: 2898–2904.   **10.18** ANDERSON, A. K. AND E. A. PHELPS (2001) Lesions of the human amygdala impair enhanced perception of emotionally salient events. *Nature* 411: 305–309.   **10.20** VUILLEUMIER, P. AND J. DRIVER (2007) Modulation of visual processing by attention and emotion: Windows on causal interactions between human brain regions. *Phil. Trans. R. Soc. B: Biol. Sci.* 362: 837–855.   **10.21** FICHTENHOLTZ, H. M. AND K. S. LABAR (2012) Emotional influences on visuospatial attention. In *Neuroscience of Attention: Attentional Control and Selection*, G. R. Mangun (ed.). New York: Oxford University Press, pp. 250–266.   **10.22** MCGAUGH, J. L. (2000) Memory: A century of consolidation. *Science* 287: 248–251.   **10.23** LABAR, K. S. AND R. CABEZA (2006) Cognitive neuroscience of emotional memory. *Nat. Rev Neurosci.* 7: 54–64.   **10.24A** MURTY, V. P., M. RITCHEY, R. A. ADCOCK AND K. S. LABAR (2010) fMRI studies of emotional memory encoding: A quantitative meta-analysis. *Neuropsychologia* 49: 695–705.   **10.24B** DOLCOS, F., K. S. LABAR AND R. CABEZA (2004) Interaction between the amygdala and the medial temporal lobe memory system predicts better memory for emotional events. *Neuron* 42: 855–863.   **10.25** OCHSNER, K. N. AND 6 OTHERS (2004) For better or for worse: Neural systems supporting the cognitive down- and up-regulation of negative emotion. *Neuroimage* 23: 483–499.

Chapter 11: Social Cognition

Opener © Jonathan Larsen/Diadem Images/Alamy.   **11.1A** HEATHERTON, T. F., C. L. WYLAND, C. N. MACRAE, K. E. DEMOS, B. T. DENNY AND W. M. KELLEY (2006) Medial pre-frontal activity differentiates self from close others. *Soc. Cogn. Affect. Neurosci.* 1: 18–24.   **11.1B** CABEZA, R. AND 7 OTHERS (2004) Brain activity during episodic retrieval of autobiographical and laboratory events: An fMRI study using a novel photo paradigm. *J. Cogn. Neurosci.* 16: 1583–1594.   **11.2A** ARZY, S., G. THUT, C. MOHR, C. M. MICHEL AND O. BLANKE (2006) Neural basis of embodiment: Distinct contributions of temporoparietal junction and extrastriate body area. *J. Neurosci.* 26: 8074–8081.   **11.2B** BLANKE, O. AND 7 OTHERS (2005) Linking out-of-body experience and self processing to mental own-body imagery at the temporoparietal junction. *J. Neurosci.* 25: 550–557.   **11.3A** HAXBY, J. V., E. A. HOFFMAN AND I. GOBBINI (2000) The distributed human neural system for face perception. *Trends Cogn. Sci.* 4: 223–233.   **11.3B** HASSELMO, M. E., E. T. ROLLS AND G. C. BAYLIS (1989) The role of expression and identity in the face-selective responses of neurons in the temporal visual cortex of the monkey. *Behav. Brain Res.* 32: 203–218.   **11.3C** LABAR, K. S., M. J. CRUPAIN, J. B. VOYVODIC AND G. MCCARTHY (2003) Dynamic perception of facial affect and identity in the human brain. *Cereb. Cortex* 13: 1023–1033.   **11.4** ADAMS, R. B., JR., H. L. GORDON, A. A. BAIRD, N. AMBADY AND R. E. KLECK (2003) Effects of gaze on amygdala sensitivity to anger and fear faces. *Science* 300: 1536.   **11.5** ALLISON, T., A. PUCE AND G. MCCARTHY (2000) Social perception from visual cues: Role of the STS region. *Trends Cogn. Sci.* 4: 267–278.   **11.6A** PELPHREY, K. A., J. D. SINGERMAN, T. ALLISON AND G. MCCARTHY (2003) Brain activation evoked by perception of gaze shifts: The influence of context. *Neuropsychologia* 41: 156–170.   **11.6B** ZUCKER, N. L. AND 6 OTHERS (2011) Neural signaling of mixed messages during a social exchange. *Neuroreport* 22: 413–418.   **11.7** SCHULLER, A. M. AND B. ROSSION (2001) Spatial attention triggered by eye gaze increases and speeds up early visual activity. *Neuroreport* 12: 2381–2386.   **11.8** PHELPS, E. A. AND 6 OTHERS (2000) Performance on indirect measures of race evaluation predicts amygdala activation. *J. Cogn. Neurosci.* 12: 729–738.   **11.9A,B** AMODIO, D. M. (2008) The social neuroscience of intergroup relations. *Eur. J. Soc. Psychol.* 19: 1–54.   **11.9C** AMODIO, D. M., P. G. DEVINE AND E. HARMON-JONES

(2008) Individual differences in the regulation of intergroup bias: The role of conflict monitoring and neural signals for control. *J. Pers. Soc. Psychol.* 94: 60–74. **11.10** RICHESON, J. A. AND 6 OTHERS (2003) An fMRI investigation of the impact of interracial contact on executive function. *Nat. Neurosci.* 6: 1323–1328. **11.11A** SAID, C. P., S. G. BARON AND A. TODOROV (2008) Nonlinear amygdala response to face trustworthiness: Contributions of high and low spatial frequency information. *J. Cogn. Neurosci.* 21: 519–528. **11.11B** ADOLPHS, R., D. TRANEL AND A. R. DAMASIO (1998) The human amygdala in social judgment. *Nature* 393: 470–474. **11.12** RIZZOLATTI, G., L. FADIGA, V. GALLESE AND L. FOGASSI (1996) Premotor cortex and the recognition of motor actions. *Cogn. Brain Res.* 3: 131–141. **11.13A** RIZZOLATTI, G. AND C. SINIGAGLIA (2010) The functional role of the parieto-frontal mirror circuit: Interpretations and misinterpretations. *Nat. Rev. Neurosci.* 11: 264–274. **11.13B** KEYSERS, C., J. H. KAAS AND V. GAZZOLA (2010) Somatosensation in social perception. *Nat. Rev. Neurosci.* 11: 417–428. **11.14** FRITH, U. AND C. D. FRITH (2003) Development and neurophysiology of mentalizing. *Philos. Trans. R. Soc. Lond. B* 358: 459–473. **11.15** HARE, B., J. CALL AND M. TOMASELLO (2001) Do chimpanzees know what conspecifics know? *Anim. Behav.* 61: 139–151. **11.17** HEIN, G. AND T. SINGER (2008) I feel how you feel but not always: The empathic brain and its modulation. *Curr. Opin. Neurobiol.* 18: 153–158. **11.18** GESQUIERE, L. R., N. H. LEARN, C. M. SIMAO, P. O. ONYANGO, S. C. ALBERTS AND J. ALTMANN (2011) Life at the top: Rank and stress in wild male baboons. *Science* 333: 357–360.

Chapter 12: Language
Opener © Jim West/Alamy. **12.1B** MILLER, G. A. (1991) *The Science of Words.* New York: Scientific American Library. **12.2** SCHWARTZ, D. A., C. Q. HOWE AND D. PURVES (2003) The statistical structure of human speech sounds predicts musical universals. *J. Neurosci.* 23: 7160–7168. **12.4A** JOHNSON, J. S. AND E. L. NEWPORT (1989) Critical period effects in second language learning: The influence of maturational state on the acquisition of English as a second language. *Cogn. Psychol.* 21: 60–99. **12.4B** BROWN, T. T., H. M. LUGAR, R. S. COALSON, F. M. MIEZIN, S. E. PETERESEN AND B. L. SCHLAGGER (2005) Developmental changes in human cerebral functional

organization for word generation. *Cereb. Cortex* 15: 275–290. **12.5** KUHL, P. K., K. A. WILLIAMS, F. LACERDA, K. N. STEVENS AND B. LINDBLOM (1992) Linguistic experience alters phonetic perception in infants 6 months of age. *Science* 255: 606–608. **12.10A** PENFIELD, W. AND L. ROBERTS (1959) *Speech and Brain Mechanisms.* Princeton, NJ: Princeton University Press, 1959. **12.10B** OJEMANN, G. A., I. FRIED AND E. LETTICH (1989) Electrocorticographic (EcoG) correlates of language. *Electroencephalogr. Clin. Neurophysiol.* 73: 453–463. **12.11** KUTAS, M. AND S. A. HILLYARD (1980) Reading senseless sentences: Brain potentials reflect semantic incongruity. *Science* 207: 203–205. **12.12A** POSNER, M. I. AND M. E. RAICHLE (1994) *Images of Mind.* New York: Scientific American Library. **12.12B** BINDER, J. R., H. RUTVIK, W. DESAL, W. GRAVES AND L. CONANT (2009) Where is the semantic system? A critical review and meta-analysis of 120 functional neuroimaging studies. *Cereb. Cortex* 19: 2767–2796. **12.13** CHAO, L. L., J. V. HAXBY AND A. MARTIN (1999) Attribute-based neural substrates in temporal cortex for perceiving and knowing about objects. *Nat. Neurosci.* 2: 913–919. **12.14** BELLUGI, U., H. POIZNER AND E. S. KLIMA (1989) Language, modality, and the brain. *Trends Neurosci.* 12: 380–388. **12.15** GHAZANFAR, A. A. AND N. LOGOTHETIS (2003) Facial expressions linked to monkey calls. *Nature* 423: 937. **12.16** SAVAGE-RUMBAUGH, S., S. G. SHANKER AND T. J. TAYLOR (1998) *Apes, Language, and the Human Mind.* New York: Oxford University Press. **Box 12D** Photograph by David McIntyre.

Chapter 13: Executive Functions
Opener © epa european pressphoto agency b.v./Alamy. **13.4A** DAMASIO, H., T. GRABOWSKI, R. FRANK, A. M. GALABURDA AND A. R. DAMASIO (1994) The return of Phineas Gage: Clues about the brain from the skull of a famous patient. *Science* 264: 1102–1105. **13.4B** WILGUS, J. AND B. WILGUS (2009) Face to face with Phineas Gage. *J. Hist. Neurosci.* 18: 340–345. **13.5** MILLER, E. K. AND J. D. COHEN (2001) An integrative theory of prefrontal cortex function. *Annu. Rev. Neurosci.* 24: 167–202. **13.6** WALLIS, J. D., K. C. ANDERSON AND E. K. MILLER (2001) Single neurons in prefrontal cortex encode abstract rules. *Nature* 411: 953–956. **13.8** COOLS, R., L. CLARK AND T. W. ROBBINS (2004) Differential responses in human striatum and

prefrontal cortex to changes in object and rule relevance. *J. Neurosci.* 24: 1129–1135. **13.9A** HUETTEL, S. A., A. W. SONG AND G. MCCARTHY (2004) *Functional Magnetic Resonance Imaging.* Sunderland, MA: Sinauer. **13.9B** POLICH, J. (2007) Updating P300: An integrative theory of P3a and P3b. *Clin. Neurophysiol.* 118: 2128–2148. **13.9C** HUETTEL, S. A. AND G. MCCARTHY (2004) What is the oddball task? Prefrontal cortex is activated by dynamic changes in response strategy. *Neuropsychologia* 42: 379–386. **13.11** SMITH, R., K. KERAMATIAN AND K. CHRISTOFF (2007) Localizing the rostrolateral prefrontal cortex at the individual level. *Neuroimage* 36: 1387–1396. **13.12** SHALLICE, T. (1982) Specific impairments of planning. *Philos. Trans. R. Soc. Lond. B Biol. Sci.* 298: 199–209. **13.13** BADRE, D. AND M. D'ESPOSITO (2009) Is the rostro-caudal axis of the frontal lobe hierarchical? *Nat. Rev. Neurosci.* 10: 659–669. **13.14B** BUSH, G., P. J. WHALEN, B. R. ROSEN, M. A. JENIKE, S. C. MCINERNEY AND S. L. RAUCH (1998) The counting Stroop: An interference task specialized for functional neuroimaging—Validation study with functional MRI. *Hum. Brain Mapp.* 6: 270–282. **13.14C** KERNS, J. G., J. D. COHEN, A. W. MACDONALD III, R. Y. CHO, V. A. STENGER AND C. S. CARTER (2004) Anterior cingulate conflict monitoring and adjustments in control. *Science* 303: 1023–1026. **13.15** BUSH, G., P. LUU AND M. I. POSNER (2000) Cognitive and emotional influences in anterior cingulate cortex. *Trends Cogn. Sci.* 4: 215–222. **13.16** FELLOWS, L. K. AND M. J. FARAH (2005) Is anterior cingulate cortex necessary for cognitive control? *Brain* 128: 788–796. **13.17** BEHRENS, T. E., M. W. WOOLRICH, M. E. WALTON AND M. F. RUSHWORTH (2007) Learning the value of information in an uncertain world. *Nat. Neurosci.* 10: 1214–1221. **13.18** VENKATRAMAN, V., A. G. ROSATI, A. A. TAREN AND S. A. HUETTEL (2009) Resolving response, decision, and strategic control: Evidence for a functional topography in dorsomedial prefrontal cortex. *J. Neurosci.* 29: 13158–13164. **13.19** TAREN, A. A., V. VENKATRAMAN AND S. A. HUETTEL (2011) A parallel functional topography between medial and lateral prefrontal cortex: Evidence and implications for cognitive control. *J. Neurosci.* 31: 5026–5031. **13.20** BADDELEY, A. (2003) Working memory: Looking back and looking forward. *Nat. Rev. Neurosci.* 4: 829–839. **13.21** COWAN, N. (1998) Visual and auditory working memory capacity. *Trends Cogn. Sci.*

2: 77–78. **13.22** FUNAHASHI, S., C. J. BRUCE AND P. S. GOLDMAN-RAKIC (1989) Mnemonic coding of visual space in the monkey's dorsolateral prefrontal cortex. *J. Neurophysiol.* 61: 331. **13.23** D'ESPOSITO M., B. R. POSTLE AND B. RYPMA (2000) Prefrontal cortical contributions to working memory: Evidence from event–related fMRI studies. *Exp. Brain Res.* 133: 3–11. **13.24** HARRISON, S. A. AND F. TONG (2009) Decoding reveals the contents of visual working memory in early visual areas. *Nature* 458: 632–635. **Box 13B Figure B** © The Behavioural Ecology Research Group, University of Oxford.

Chapter 14: Decision Making

Opener © Ed Eckstein/Corbis. **14.2** TVERSKY, A. AND D. KAHNEMAN (1992) Advances in prospect theory: Cumulative representation of uncertainty. *J. Risk Uncertain.* 5: 297–323. **14.4** BERRIDGE, K. C. AND T. E. ROBINSON (1998) What is the role of dopamine in reward: Hedonic impact, reward learning, or incentive salience? *Brain Res. Rev.* 28: 309–369. **14.5** MURAYAMA, K., M. MATSUMOTO, K. IZUMA AND K. MATSUMOTO (2010) Neural basis of the undermining effect of monetary reward on intrinsic motivation. *Proc. Natl. Acad. Sci. USA* 107: 20911–20916. **14.6, 14.7** SCHULTZ, W., P. DAYAN AND P. R. MONTAGUE (1997) A neural substrate of prediction and reward. *Science* 275: 1593–1599. **14.8** GEHRING, W. J. AND A. R. WILLOUGHBY (2002) The medial frontal cortex and the rapid processing of monetary gains and losses. *Science* 295: 2279–2282. **14.9** VICKERY, T. J., M. M. CHUN AND D. LEE (2011) Ubiquity and specificity of reinforcement signals throughout the human brain. *Neuron* 72: 166–177. **14.10** MATSUMOTO, M. AND O. HIKOSAKA (2009) Two types of dopamine neuron distinctly convey positive and negative motivational signals. *Nature* 459: 837–841. **14.11** MOHR, P. N., G. BIELE AND H. R. HEEKEREN (2010) Neural processing of risk. *J. Neurosci.* 30: 6613–6619. **14.12A** HSU, M., M. BHATT, R. ADOLPHS, D. TRANEL AND C. F. CAMERER (2005) Neural systems responding to degrees of uncertainty in human decision-making. *Science* 310: 1680–1683. **14.12B** HUETTEL, S. A., C. J. STOWE, E. M. GORDON, B. T. WARNER AND M. L. PLATT (2006) Neural signatures of economic preferences for risk and ambiguity. *Neuron* 49: 765–775. **14.13B** MCCLURE, S. M., D. I. LAIBSON, G. LOEWENSTEIN AND J. D. COHEN (2004) Separate neural

systems value immediate and delayed monetary rewards. *Science* 306: 503–507. **14.13C** KABLE, J. W. AND P. W. GLIMCHER (2007) The neural correlates of subjective value during intertemporal choice. *Nat. Neurosci.* 10: 1625–1633. **14.14** DEANER, R. O., A. V. KHERA AND M. L. PLATT (2005) Monkeys pay per view: Adaptive valuation of social images by rhesus macaques. *Curr. Biol.* 15: 543–548. **14.15A** HARBAUGH, W. T., U. MAYR AND D. R. BURGHART (2007) Neural responses to taxation and voluntary giving reveal motives for charitable donations. *Science* 316: 1622–1625. **14.15B** TANKERSLEY, D., C. J. STOWE AND S. A. HUETTEL (2007) Altruism is associated with an increased neural response to agency. *Nat. Neurosci.* 10: 150–151. **14.15C** WAYTZ, A., J. ZAKI AND J. P. MITCHELL (2012) Response of dorsomedial prefrontal cortex predicts altruistic behavior. *J. Neurosci.* 32: 7646–7650. **14.17B–D** KING-CASAS, B., D. TOMLIN, C. ANEN, C. F. CAMERER, S. R. QUARTZ AND P. R. MONTAGUE (2005) Getting to know you: Reputation and trust in a two-person economic exchange. *Science* 308: 78–83. **14.18** KNOCH, D., A. PASCUAL-LEONE, K. MEYER, V. TREYER AND E. FEHR (2006) Diminishing reciprocal fairness by disrupting the right prefrontal cortex. *Science* 314: 829–832. **14.19** HEEKEREN, H. R., S. MARRETT, P. A. BANDETTINI AND L. G. UNDERLEIDER (2004) A general mechanism for perceptual decision-making in the human brain. *Nature* 431: 856–862. **14.20A** BECHARA, A., H. DAMASIO AND A. R. DAMASIO (2000) Emotion, decision making and the orbitofrontal cortex. *Cereb. Cortex* 10: 295–307. **14.20B** SHIV, B., G. LOEWENSTEIN, A. BECHARA, H. DAMASIO AND A. R. DAMASIO (2005) Investment behavior and the negative side of emotion. *Psychol. Sci.* 16: 435–439. **14.21** PADOA-SCHIOPPA, C. AND J. A. ASSAD (2006) Neurons in the orbitofrontal cortex encode economic value. *Nature* 441: 223–226. **14.22A** PLASSMANN, H., J. O'DOHERTY AND A. RANGEL (2007) Orbitofrontal cortex encodes willingness to pay in everyday economic transactions. *J. Neurosci.* 27: 9984–9988. **14.22B** SMITH, D. V., B. Y. HAYDEN, T.-K. TRUONG, A. W. SONG, M. L. PLATT AND S. A. HUETTEL (2010) Distinct value signals in anterior and posterior ventromedial prefrontal cortex. *J. Neurosci.* 30: 2490–2495. **14.24** DE MARTINO, B. D. KUMARAN, B. SEYMOUR AND R. J. DOLAN (2006) Frames, biases,

and rational decision-making in the human brain. *Science* 313: 684–687.

Chapter 15: Evolution and Development of Brain and Cognition

Opener Courtesy of Michael Platt. **15.2** COWAN, W. M. (1979) The development of the brain. *Sci. Am.* 241(3): 113–133. **15.3A** CASEY, B. J., N. TOTTENHAM, C. LISTON AND S. DURSTON (2005) Imaging the developing brain: What have we learned about cognitive development? *Trends Cogn. Sci.* 9: 104–110. **15.3B** BOURGEOIS, J. AND P. RAKIC (1993) Changes of synaptic density in the primary visual cortex of the macaque monkey from fetal to adult stage. *J. Neurosci.* 13: 2801–2820. **15.4A** DEKABAN, A. S. AND D. SADOWSKY (1978) Changes in brain weights during the span of human life: Relation of brain weights to body heights and body weights. *Ann. Neurol.* 4: 345–356. **15.4B,C** LENROOT, R. K. AND J. N. GIEDD (2006) Brain development in children and adolescents: Insights from anatomical brain magnetic resonance imaging. *Neurosci. Behav. Rev.* 30: 718–729. **15.5** SHAW, P. AND 8 OTHERS (2006) Intellectual ability and cortical development in children and adolescents. *Nature* 440: 676–679. **15.7A** JERISON, H. J. (1977) The theory of encephalization. *Ann. N.Y. Acad. Sci.* 299: 146–160. **15.7B** STRIEDTER, G. F. (2005) *Principles of Brain Evolution.* Sunderland, MA: Sinauer. **15.8A** University of Wisconsin and Michigan State Comparative Mammalian Brain Collections. **15.8B** STEPHAN, H., H. FRAHM AND G. BARON (1981) New and revised data on volumes of brain structures in insectivores and primates. *Folia Primatol.* 35: 1–29. **15.9** STRIEDTER, G. F. (2005) *Principles of Brain Evolution.* Sunderland, MA: Sinauer. **15.10** GILBERT, S. L., W. B. DOBYNS AND B. T. LAHN (2005) Genetic links between brain development and brain evolution. *Nat. Rev. Genet.* 6: 581. **15.11A** CLANCY, B., R. B. DARLINGTON AND B. L. FINLAY (2001) The course of human events: predicting the timing of primate neural development. *Dev. Sci.* 3: 57–66. **15.11B** FINLAY, B. AND R. DARLINGTON (1995) Linked regularities in the development and evolution of mammalian brains. *Science* 268: 1578–1584. **15.12A** WOOLSEY, T. A. AND H. VAN DER LOOS (1970) The structural organization of layer IV in the somatosensory region (SI) of mouse cerebral cortex. The description of a cortical field composed of discrete cytoarchitectonic units. *Brain Res.* 17:

53–66. **15.12B** PENFIELD, W. AND E. BOULDREY (1937) Somatic motor and sensory representation in the cerebral cortex of man as studied by electrical stimulation. *Brain* 60: 389-443. **15.13** KREBS, J. R., D. F. SHERRY, S. D. HEALY, V. H. PERRY AND A. L. VACCARINO (1989) Hippocampal specialization of food-storing birds. *Proc. Natl. Acad. Sci. USA* 86: 1388–1392; photos courtesy of John and Karen Hollingsworth (Clark's nutcracker) and Lee Carney (scrub jay), U.S. Fish and Wildlife Service. **15.14A** Photos © David Tipling (howler monkey) and Mike Lane (spider monkey) Alamy Photo. **15.14B** STEPHAN, H., H. FRAHM AND G. BARON (1981) New and revised data on volumes of brain structures in insectivores and primates. *Folia Primatol.* 35: 1-29. **15.15** BAUER, P. J., S. A. WIEBE, L. J. CARVER, J. M. WATERS AND C. A. NELSON (2003) Developments in longterm explicit memory late in the first year of life: Behavioral and electrophysiological indices. *Psychol. Sci.* 14: 629–635. **15.16** CANTLON, J. AND E. M. BRANNON (2006) Shared system for ordering small and large numbers in monkeys and humans. *Psychol. Sci.* 17: 401–406. **15.17** LIBERTUS, M. E. AND E. M. BRANNON (2010) Stable individual differences in number discrimination in infancy. *Dev.*

Sci. 13: 900–906. **15.18** CANTLON, J., E. M. BRANNON, E. J. CARTER AND K. PELPHREY (2006) Notation-independent number processing in the intraparietal sulcus in adults and young children. *PLoS Biology* 4: e125, 1–11. **15.19** NIEDER, A. AND E. K. MILLER (2004) A parietofrontal network for visual numerical information in the monkey. *Proc. Natl. Acad. Sci. USA* 101: 7457–7462. **15.20A** BYRNE, R. W. AND N. CORP (2004) Neocortex size predicts deception rate in primates. *Proc. R. Soc. Lond. B* 271: 1693–1699. **15.20B** KUDO, H. AND R. I. M. DUNBAR (2001) Neocortex size and social network size in primates. *Anim. Behav.* 62: 711–722; photo © Andrey Novikov/istockphoto. com. **15.20C** READER, S. M. AND K. N. LALAND (2002) Social intelligence, innovation, and enhanced brain size in primates. *Proc. Natl. Acad. Sci. USA* 99: 4436–4441. **15.21A** TSAO, D. T., W. A. FREIWALD, R. B. H. TOOTELL AND M. S. LIVINGSTONE (2006) A cortical region consisting entirely of face-selective cells. *Science* 311: 670–674. **15.21B** KENDRICK, K. M., A. P. DA COSTA, A. E. LEIGH, M. R. HINTON AND J. W. PEIRCE (2001) Sheep don't forget a face. *Nature* 414: 165–166. **15.22** SALLET, J. AND 9 OTHERS (2011) Social network size affects neural circuits in macaques. *Science* 334(6056): 697–700. **15.23** PASCALIS,

O., M. DEHAAN AND C. A. NELSON (2002) Is face processing species specific during the first year of life? *Science* 296: 1321–1323. **15.24A** PREUSS, T. M. AND P. S. GOLDMAN-RAKIC (1991) Myelo- and cytoarchitecture of the granular frontal cortex and surrounding regions in the strepsirhine primate *Galago* and the anthropoid primate *Macaca*. *J. Comp. Neurol.* 310: 429–474. **15.24B** PETRIDES, M., G. CADORET AND S. MACKEY (2005) Orofacial somatomotor responses in the macaque monkey homologue of Broca's area. *Nature* 435: 1235–1238. **15.25** GIL-DA-COSTA, R., A. MARTIN, M. A. LOPES, M. MUÑOZ, J. FRITZ AND A. R. BRAUN (2006) Species-specific calls activate homologs of Broca's and Wernicke's areas in the macaque. *Nat. Neurosci.* 9: 1064–1070. **Box 15C** Cave painting photo © Robert Harding Picture Library Ltd/Alamy.

Appendix: The Human Nervous System

The art in the Appendix, along with much of the anatomical art in the rest of the book, is adapted from the Fifth Edition of *Neuroscience* (2012) by D. Purves, G. J. Augustine, D. Fitzpatrick, W. C. Hall, A.-S. LaMantia and L. E. White. Sunderland, MA: Sinauer Associates, Inc., Publishers.

Index